American Medical Association

Physicians dedicated to the health of America

Current Procedural Terminology

cpt®
2003

Michael Beebe, MS	Grace M. Kotowicz, RN, BS	Desiree Rozell, MPA
Joyce A. Dalton	Elizabeth Lumakovska, RHIT, BS	Lianne Stancik, RHIT
Catherine Duffy, RHIT, BS	Marie L. Mindeman, BA, RHIT	Ada Walker, AS
Desiree Evans, AS	Karen E. O'Hara, BS, CCS-P	Arletrice A. Watkins, RHIA
Rejina L. Glenn	Mary R. O'Heron, RHIA, CCS-P	Joan Zacharias, RHIT
DeHandro Hayden, BS	Dan Reyes, BA	

AMA press

Standard ISBN: 1-57947-302-4
ISSN: 0276-8283

1st Edition printed 1966
2nd Edition printed 1970
3rd Edition printed 1973
4th Edition printed 1977
Revised: 1978, 1979, 1980, 1981, 1982, 1984, 1985,
1986, 1987, 1988, 1989, 1990, 1991, 1992, 1993, 1994,
1995, 1996, 1997, 1998, 1999, 2000, 2001, 2002

For questions regarding the use of CPT codes, please contact the American Medical Association CPT
Information and Education Services at 800 634-6922.

To purchase additional CPT products, contact the American Medical Association Customer Service
at 800 621-8335.

To request a license for distribution of products containing or reprinting CPT, please see our Web site
at *www.ama-assn.org/cpt* or contact the American Medical Association CPT Intellectual Property
Services, 515 N. State Street, Chicago, Illinois 60610, 312 464-5022.

AC25:02-P-001:10/02

Foreword

Current Procedural Terminology, Fourth Edition (*CPT*®) is a listing of descriptive terms and identifying codes for reporting medical services and procedures performed by physicians. The purpose of the terminology is to provide a uniform language that will accurately describe medical, surgical, and diagnostic services, and will thereby provide an effective means for reliable nationwide communication among physicians, patients, and third parties. *CPT 2003* is the most recent revision of a work that first appeared in 1966.

CPT descriptive terms and identifying codes currently serve a wide variety of important functions in the field of medical nomenclature. The *CPT* book is useful for administrative management purposes such as claims processing and for the development of guidelines for medical care review. The uniform language is also applicable to medical education and outcomes, health services and quality research by providing a useful basis for local, regional, and national utilization comparisons. The *CPT* book is the most widely accepted nomenclature for the reporting of physician procedures and services under government and private health insurance programs. In 2000 the CPT Code Set was designated by the Department of Health and Human Services as the national coding standard for physician and other health care professional services and procedures under the Health Insurance Portability and Accountability Act (HIPAA). This means that for all financial and administrative health care transactions sent electronically, the CPT Code Set will need to be used.

The changes that appear in this revision have been prepared by the CPT Editorial Panel with the assistance of physicians representing all specialties of medicine, and with important contributions from many third party payors and governmental agencies.

The American Medical Association trusts that this revision will continue the usefulness of its predecessors in identifying, describing, and coding medical, surgical, and diagnostic services.

Michael D. Maves, MD, MBA
Executive Vice President, CEO

Acknowledgments

Publication of the annual *CPT* book represents many challenges and opportunities. From reconciling the many differences of opinion about the best way to describe a procedure, to the last details on placement of a semicolon, many individuals and organizations devote their energies and expertise to the preparation of this revision.

The editorial staff wishes to express sincere thanks to the many national medical specialty societies, health insurance organizations and agencies, and to the many individual physicians and other health professionals who have made contributions.

Thanks are due to Robert A. Musacchio, PhD, Sr VP, American Medical Association; Claudia Bonnell, Blue Cross and Blue Shield Association; Nelly Leon-Chisen, American Hospital Association; Thomas Musco, Health Insurance Association of America; and Sue Prophet, RHIA, American Health Information Management Association, for their invaluable assistance in enhancing CPT.

And finally, our gratitude to AMA Press of the American Medical Association for their assistance in producing the books, diskettes, and CD-ROMs that contain CPT: Anthony J. Frankos, Vice President, Business Products, Mary Lou White, Executive Director, Editorial, Elise Schumacher, Senior Acquisition Editor, J. D. Kinney, Director of Marketing, Jean Roberts, Director, Production and Manufacturing, Erin Kalitowski, Marketing Manager, Pat Lee, Technical Developmental Editor, Rosalyn Carlton, Senior Production Coordinator, Boon Ai Tan, Senior Production Coordinator, Ronnie Summers, Senior Print Coordinator, and Todd Feinstein, Application Developer.

AMA CPT Editorial Panel

Chair
Tracy R. Gordy, MD*
Vice-Chair
Karen R. Borman, MD*
James S. Adamson, Jr, MD
Simon Philip Cohn, MD
Lee D. Eisenberg, MD*
Helene M. Fearon, PT
Laurie Feinberg, MD
Blair C. Filler, MD
Diller B. Groff, MD
Samuel Hassenbusch, MD
Lee Harold Hilborne, MD
Glenn D. Littenberg, MD
Gerald E. Silverstein, MD*
Stanley W. Stead, MD
William T. Thorwarth, MD*
James M. Tucker, MD**
James A. Zalla, MD

Secretary
Michael Beebe, MS
*Member of the CPT Executive Committee
**New Panel Member August 2002

AMA CPT Advisory Committee

American Academy of Allergy, Asthma and Immunology
Donald W. Aaronson, MD
American Academy of Child & Adolescent Psychiatry
David I. Berland, MD
American Academy of Dermatology
Allen S. Wirtzer, MD
American Academy of Facial Plastic and Reconstructive Surgery
Mark V. Connelly, MD
American Academy of Family Physicians
A. Clinton MacKinney, MD, MS
American Academy of Insurance Medicine
Nigel K. Roberts, MD (In Memoriam)
American Academy of Neurology
Marc Nuwer, MD, PhD
American Academy of Ophthalmology
Michael X. Repka, MD
American Academy of Orthopaedic Surgeons
Richard L. Wixson, MD
American Academy of Otolaryngic Allergy
Harold R. Wright, MD
American Academy of Otolaryngology Head and Neck Surgery
Richard Waguespack, MD
American Academy of Pediatrics
Joel F. Bradley, Jr, MD
American Academy of Physical Medicine and Rehabilitation
Frank J.E. Falco, MD
American Academy of Physician Assistants
Patrick J. Cafferty, PA-C
American Academy of Sleep Medicine
David P. Franco, MD
American Association for Thoracic Surgery
James M. Levett, MD
American Association for Vascular Surgery
Anton N. Sidawy, MD
American Association of Clinical Endocrinologists
Satti Sethu-Kumar Reddy, MD

American Association of Electrodiagnostic Medicine
Neil A. Busis, MD
Kyle W. Ruffling, MD*
American Association of Gynecologic Laparoscopists
Andrew I. Brill, MD
Jodi Kaigh, MD*
American Association of Neurological Surgeons
Jeffrey Cozzens, MD
American Association of Public Health Physicians
Arvind K. Goyal, MD, MPH
American Chiropractic Association
Craig S. Little, DC
American Clinical Neurophysiology Society
Marc Nuwer, MD, PhD
American College of Allergy, Asthma and Immunology
Gary N. Gross, MD
American College of Cardiology
Douglas L. Wood, MD
American College of Chest Physicians
Walter J. O'Donohue, Jr, MD
American College of Emergency Physicians
Peter L. Sawchuk, MD
American College of Medical Genetics
David B. Flannery, MD
American College of Medical Quality
William N. Werner, MD, MPH
American College of Obstetricians and Gynecologists
Philip N. Eskew, Jr, MD
American College of Occupational and Environmental Medicine
Elizabeth Genovese, MD
American College of Physicians-American Society of Internal Medicine
H. Christopher Alexander III, MD
American College of Preventive Medicine
Fred T. Nobrega, MD
American College of Radiation Oncology
Thomas J. Weatherall, Jr, MD
American College of Radiology
Gordon S. Perlmutter, MD
American College of Rheumatology
David A. Cooley, MD
American College of Surgeons
John T. Preskitt, MD
American Dental Association
Jeffery B. Carter, MD, DMD
American Dietetic Association
Jane White, PhD
American Gastroenterological Association
Joel V. Brill, MD
American Geriatric Society
Peter A. Hollmann, MD
American Institute of Ultrasound in Medicine
Harvey L. Nisenbaum, MD
American Medical Directors Association
Dennis L. Stone, MD
American Medical Group Association
Susan K. Turney, MD
American Nurses Association
Ann M. Thrailkill, RM
American Occupational Therapy Association
Linda Botten, OTR, CHT, ATP

American Optometric Association
Mike Todd, DO
American Orthopaedic Association
Robert H. Haralson III, MD
American Orthopaedic Foot and Ankle Society
Walter J. Pedowitz, MD
American Osteopathic Association
Boyd R. Buser, DO
American Pediatric Surgical Association
John P. Crow, MD
American Physical Therapy Association
Rhea Cohn, PT
American Podiatric Medical Association
Robert D. Sowell, DPM
American Psychiatric Association
Chester W. Schmidt, Jr, MD
American Psychological Association
Antonio Puente, PhD
American Roentgen Ray Society
Geraldine B. McGinty
American Society for Aesthetic Plastic Surgery
Paul R. Weiss, MD
American Society for Dermatologic Surgery
Pamela K. Phillips, MD
American Society for Gastrointestinal Endoscopy
Maurits J. Wiersema, MD
American Society for Reproductive Medicine
John T. Queenan, Jr, MD
American Society for Surgery of the Hand
Daniel J. Nagle, MD
American Society for Therapeutic Radiology, and Oncology
Paul E. Wallner, DO
American Society of Abdominal Surgeons
Louis F. Alfano, Jr, MD
American Society of Anesthesiologists
H. J. Przybylo, MD
American Society of Cataract and Refractive Surgery
Stephen S. Lane, MD
American Society of Clinical Oncology
Dean Gesme, MD
American Society of Clinical Pathologists
Mark S. Synovec, MD
American Society of Colon and Rectal Surgeons
David A. Margolin, MD
American Society of Cytopathology
David C. Hoak, MD
American Society of General Surgeons
Charles Drueck, MD
American Society of Hematology
Sameul M. Silver, MD
American Society of Neuroradiology
Robert A. Murray, MD
American Society of Ophthalmic Plastic and Reconstructive Surgery
David M. Reifler, MD
American Society of Plastic Surgeons
Raymond V. Janevicius, MD
American Speech-Language Hearing Association
R. Wayne Holland, EdD
American Thoracic Society
Scott Manaker, MD
American Urological Association
Jeffrey A. Dann, MD
Association of University Radiologists
Bob W. Gayler, MD

College of American Pathologists
Stephen N. Bauer, MD
Congress of Neurological Surgeons
R. Patrick Jacob, MD
Contact Lens Association of Ophthalmologists
Charles B. Slonim, MD, FACS
National Association of Social Workers
Nelda Spyres, ACSW, LCSW
North American Spine Society
Francis P. Lagattuta, MD
Radiologic Society of North American
Richard E. Fulton, MD
Renal Physicians Association
Richard J. Hamburger, MD
Society for Investigative Dermatology
Stephen P. Stone, MD
Society for Radiologists in Ultrasound
Robert L. Bree, MD
Society of American Gastrointestinal Endoscopic Surgeons
Eric G. Weiss, MD
Society of Critical Care Medicine
George A. Sample, MD
Society of Interventional Radiology
Gary S. Dorfman, MD
Society of Nuclear Medicine
Kenneth A. McKusick, MD
Society of Thoracic Surgeons
Keith S. Naunheim, MD
United States and Canadian Academy of Pathology
Beverly P. Nelson, MD
*New Advisors April 2002

AMA Health Care Professionals Advisory Committee (HCPAC)

Tracy R. Gordy, MD, Co-Chair
AMA CPT Editorial Panel
Helene Fearon, PT, Co-Chair
Linda Botten, OTR, CHT
American Occupational Therapy Association
Patrick J. Cafferty, PA-C
American Academy of Physician Assistants
Rhea Cohn, PT
American Physical Therapy Association
R. Wayne Holland, EdD
American Speech-Language Hearing Association
Stephen S. Lane, MD
American Society of Cataract and Refractive Surgery
Craig S. Little, DC
American Chiropractic Association
Antonio Puente, PhD
American Psychological Association
Robert D. Sowell, DPM
American Podiatric Medical Association
Nelda Spyres, ACSW, LCSW
National Association of Social Workers
Ann M. Thrailkill, RN
American Nurses Association
Mike Todd, DO
American Optometric Association
Jane V. White, PhD, RD, FADA
American Dietetic Association

CPT 2003 Book Enhancements

Each year we look for ways to improve or enhance features to the *CPT* book that respond to the needs of the users. The *CPT 2003* book contains several improvements that are designed to make the book more user-friendly.

This year's enhancements to the Standard edition include the following:

Summary of Additions, Deletions, and Revisions Included in Appendix B

In past additions of the *CPT* book, Appendix B contained code numbers and indicated whether a code was added, revised, or deleted. This year we updated Appendix B to show the changes that occurred in the code descriptors. Deleted language appears with a ~~strikethrough~~, while new text appears underlined. This enhancement will give users a quick reference to the changes, without having to refer to the previous edition for the original code language.

Black "Bleed" Tabs for Sections

For 2003, "bleed" tabs have been added to give users a visual reference to the sections of the CPT book.

Note: Appendix C (Update to Short Descriptors) has been deleted in *CPT 2003*. Because of this deletion, Appendices D, E, and F, now become C, D, and E, respectively.

The following enhancements appear only in *CPT 2003* Professional Edition:

Place-of-Service Codes

For the first time, the *CPT* book contains the list of Place-of-Service codes. The list contains the code, name, and description. These codes are used on professional claims to specify the entity where service(s) are rendered. Users are required to check with their individual payers to determine whether a particular code will be recognized for payment purposes.

Color to Indicate Changed Text

This year we added green to indicate changed text. We continue to use the ▶◀ to indicate specific words or sections that contain changes, but by using color, the changed text will now be easier to notice.

Color "Bleeds" for Sections

We also added vertical color bleeds to each page of the book. This feature will make it even easier to navigate through the book, giving users a visual guide. While we added the color bars we also kept the thumb notches, for those who prefer the tactile approach.

Category III Codes Thumb Notch

As the number of Category III codes continue to increase, in *CPT 2003*, we added a separate "thumb notch" so users can quickly locate the section. Last year this section was added to the end of the Medicine section.

Legend for References

Since 1998, the *CPT* book has contained the "➋" symbol located under many of the codes throughout the body of the book. This year we have added a legend that directs users to page xv, where the publications are explained and users are instructed as to how to obtain the referenced publications.

Contents

Contents

Introduction

Current Procedural Terminology, Fourth Edition (*CPT*®) is a systematic listing and coding of procedures and services performed by physicians. Each procedure or service is identified with a five-digit code. The use of CPT codes simplifies the reporting of services. With this code set, the procedure or service rendered by the physician is accurately identified.

Inclusion of a descriptor and its associated specific five-digit identifying code number in the *CPT* book is generally based upon the procedure being consistent with contemporary medical practice and being performed by many physicians in clinical practice in multiple locations. Inclusion in the *CPT* book does not represent endorsement by the American Medical Association of any particular diagnostic or therapeutic procedure. Inclusion or exclusion of a procedure does not imply any health insurance coverage or reimbursement policy.

The main body of the material is listed in six sections. Within each section are subsections with anatomic, procedural, condition, or descriptor subheadings. The procedures and services with their identifying codes are presented in numeric order with one exception—the entire **Evaluation and Management** section (99201-99499) has been placed at the beginning of the listed procedures. These items are used by most physicians in reporting a significant portion of their services. The **Medicine** (procedures) section now follows **Pathology and Laboratory.**

Section Numbers and Their Sequences

Evaluation and Management ....99201 to 99499

Anesthesiology ....00100 to 01999, 99100 to 99140

Surgery ....10021 to 69990

Radiology (Including Nuclear Medicine and Diagnostic
    Ultrasound) ....70010 to 79999

Pathology and Laboratory ....80048 to 89399

Medicine
(except Anesthesiology) ...90281 to 99199, 99500-99600

The first and last code numbers and the subsection name of the items appear at the top of each page (eg, "11000-11313 Surgery/Integumentary System"). The continuous pagination of the *CPT* book is found on the lower, outer margin of each page along with the section name.

Instructions for Use of the *CPT* Book

Select the name of the procedure or service that accurately identifies the service performed. Do not select a CPT code that merely approximates the service provided. If no such procedure or service exists, then report the service using the appropriate unlisted procedure or service code. In surgery, it may be an operation; in medicine, a diagnostic or therapeutic procedure; in radiology, a radiograph. Other additional procedures performed or pertinent special services are also listed. When necessary, any modifying or extenuating circumstances are added. Any service or procedure should be adequately documented in the medical record.

It is important to recognize that the listing of a service or procedure and its code number in a specific section of this book does not restrict its use to a specific specialty group. Any procedure or service in any section of this book may be used to designate the services rendered by any qualified physician or other qualified health care professional.

Format of the Terminology

CPT procedure terminology has been developed as stand-alone descriptions of medical procedures. However, some of the procedures in the *CPT* book are not printed in their entirety but refer back to a common portion of the procedure listed in a preceding entry. This is evident when an entry is followed by one or more indentations. This is done in an effort to conserve space.

Example

25100   Arthrotomy, wrist joint; with biopsy

25105   with synovectomy

Note that the common part of code 25100 (that part before the semicolon) should be considered part of code 25105. Therefore, the full procedure represented by code 25105 should read:

25105   Arthrotomy, wrist joint; for synovectomy

Requests to Update the CPT Nomenclature

The effectiveness of the *Current Procedural Terminology* (*CPT*®) nomenclature is dependent upon constant updating to reflect changes in medical practice. This can only be accomplished through the interest and timely suggestions of practicing physicians, medical specialty societies, state medical associations, and other organizations and agencies. Accordingly, the American Medical Association welcomes correspondence, inquiries, and suggestions concerning old and new procedures, as well as other matters such as codes and indices.

For suggestions concerning the introduction of new procedures, or the coding, deleting, or revising of procedures contained in *CPT 2003*, correspondence requesting an application for coding change should be directed to:

CPT Editorial Research & Development
American Medical Association
515 North State Street
Chicago, Illinois 60610

Coding change request forms to introduce new procedures or to delete or revise procedures already in the CPT nomenclature are also available at the AMA/CPT website http://www.ama-assn.org/ama/pub/article/3866-3846.html.

All proposed additions to, or modifications of, *CPT 2003* will be by decision of the CPT Editorial Panel after consultation with appropriate medical specialty societies.

Guidelines

Specific "Guidelines" are presented at the beginning of each of the six sections. These guidelines define items that are necessary to appropriately interpret and report the procedures and services contained in that section. For example, in the **Medicine** section, specific instructions are provided for handling unlisted services or procedures, special reports, and supplies and materials provided. Guidelines also provide explanations regarding terms that apply only to a particular section. For instance, **Surgery Guidelines** provides an explanation of the use of the star, while in **Radiology**, the unique term, "radiological supervision and interpretation" is defined.

Starred Procedures

The star "∗" is used to identify certain surgical procedures. A description of this reporting mechanism will be found in the **Surgery Guidelines**.

Add-on Codes

Some of the listed procedures are commonly carried out in addition to the primary procedure performed. These additional or supplemental procedures are designated as "add-on" codes with a "✚" symbol, and are listed in Appendix D of the *CPT* book (formerly Appendix E). Add-on codes in *CPT 2003* can be readily identified by specific descriptor nomenclature which includes phrases such as "each additional" or "(List separately in addition to primary procedure)".

The "add-on" code concept in *CPT 2003* applies only to add-on procedures/services performed by the same physician. Add-on codes describe additional intra-service work associated with the primary procedure (eg, additional digit(s), lesion(s), neurorrhaphy(s), vertebral segment(s), tendon(s), joint(s)).

Add-on codes are always performed in addition to the primary service/procedure, and must never be reported as a stand-alone code. All add-on codes found in the *CPT* book are exempt from the multiple procedure concept (see modifier '-51' definition of **Surgery Guidelines**).

Modifiers

A modifier provides the means by which the reporting physician can indicate that a service or procedure that has been performed has been altered by some specific circumstance but not changed in its definition or code. The judicious application of modifiers obviates the necessity for separate procedure listings that may describe the modifying circumstance. Modifiers may be used to indicate to the recipient of a report that:

- A service or procedure has both a professional and technical component.
- A service or procedure was performed by more than one physician and/or in more than one location.
- A service or procedure has been increased or reduced.
- Only part of a service was performed.
- An adjunctive service was performed.
- A bilateral procedure was performed.
- A service or procedure was provided more than once.
- Unusual events occurred.

Example

A physician providing diagnostic or therapeutic radiology services, ultrasound or nuclear medicine services in a hospital would modifier '-26' to report the professional component.

73090-26 = Professional component only for an x-ray of the forearm

Example

Two surgeons may be required to manage a specific surgical problem. When two surgeons work together as primary surgeons performing distinct part(s) of a procedure, each surgeon should report his/her distinct operative work by adding the modifier '-62' to the procedure code and any associated code(s) for that procedure as long as both surgeons continue to work together as primary surgeons. Each surgeon should report the co-surgery once using the same procedure code. The modifier '-62' would be applicable. For instance, a neurological surgeon and an otolaryngologist are working as co-surgeons in performing transphenoidal excision of a pituitary neoplasm.

61548-62 = Hypophysectomy or excision of pituitary tumor, transnasal or transseptal approach, nonstereotactic + two surgeons modifier

AND the second surgeon would report:

61548-62 = Hypophysectomy or excision of pituitary tumor, transnasal or transseptal approach, nonstereotactic + two surgeons modifier

If additional procedure(s) (including add-on procedure(s)) are performed during the same surgical session, separate code(s) may also be reported with the modifier '-62' added. **Note:** If a co-surgeon acts as an assistant in the performance of additional procedure(s) during the same surgical session, those services may be reported using separate procedure code(s) with the modifier '-80' or modifier '-82' added, as appropriate. A complete listing of modifiers is found in Appendix A.

Unlisted Procedure or Service

It is recognized that there may be services or procedures performed by physicians that are not found in the *CPT* book. Therefore, a number of specific code numbers have been designated for reporting unlisted procedures. When an unlisted procedure number is used, the service or procedure should be described. Each of these unlisted procedural code numbers (with the appropriate accompanying topical entry) relates to a specific section of the book and is presented in the Guidelines of that section.

Special Report

A service that is rarely provided, unusual, variable, or new may require a special report in determining medical appropriateness of the service. Pertinent information should include an adequate definition or description of the nature, extent, and need for the procedure; and the time, effort, and equipment necessary to provide the service. Additional items which may be included are: complexity of symptoms, final diagnosis, pertinent physical findings, diagnostic and therapeutic procedures, concurrent problems, and follow-up care.

Code Changes

A summary listing of additions, deletions, and revisions applicable to *CPT 2003* is found in **Appendix B**. New procedure numbers added to the *CPT* book are identified throughout the text with the symbol "●" placed before the code number. In instances where a code revision has resulted in a substantially altered procedure descriptor, the symbol "▲" is placed before the code number. The symbols "► ◄" are used to indicate new and revised text other than the procedure descriptors. CPT add-on codes are annotated by a "✚" symbol and are listed in **Appendix D** (formerly Appendix E). The "⊘" symbol is used to identify codes that are exempt from the use of modifier '-51', but have not been designated as CPT add-on procedures/services. A list of codes exempt from modifier '-51' usage is included in **Appendix E** (formerly Appendix F).

Alphabetical Reference Index

A new, expanded alphabetical index is found in the back of the book. It includes listings by procedure and anatomic site. Procedures and services commonly known by their eponyms or other designations are also included.

CPT in Electronic Formats

CPT 2003 procedure codes and descriptors are also available on diskettes and CD-ROM in various formats. For more information call 800 621-8335.

Visit CPT on the AMA Website
http://www.ama-assn.org/cpt

Notes

Evaluation and Management (E/M) Services Guidelines

In addition to the information presented in the **Introduction,** several other items unique to this section are defined or identified here.

Classification of Evaluation and Management (E/M) Services

The E/M section is divided into broad categories such as office visits, hospital visits, and consultations. Most of the categories are further divided into two or more subcategories of E/M services. For example, there are two subcategories of office visits (new patient and established patient) and there are two subcategories of hospital visits (initial and subsequent). The subcategories of E/M services are further classified into levels of E/M services that are identified by specific codes. This classification is important because the nature of physician work varies by type of service, place of service, and the patient's status.

The basic format of the levels of E/M services is the same for most categories. First, a unique code number is listed. Second, the place and/or type of service is specified, eg, office consultation. Third, the content of the service is defined, eg, comprehensive history and comprehensive examination. (See "Levels of E/M Services," page 2, for details on the content of E/M services.) Fourth, the nature of the presenting problem(s) usually associated with a given level is described. Fifth, the time typically required to provide the service is specified. (A detailed discussion of time is provided on page 3.)

Definitions of Commonly Used Terms

Certain key words and phrases are used throughout the E/M section. The following definitions are intended to reduce the potential for differing interpretations and to increase the consistency of reporting by physicians in differing specialties.

New and Established Patient

Solely for the purposes of distinguishing between new and established patients, **professional services** are those face-to-face services rendered by a physician and reported by a specific CPT code(s). A new patient is one who has not received any professional services from the physician or another physician of the same specialty who belongs to the same group practice, within the past three years.

An established patient is one who has received professional services from the physician or another physician of the same specialty who belongs to the same group practice, within the past three years.

In the instance where a physician is on call for or covering for another physician, the patient's encounter will be classified as it would have been by the physician who is not available.

No distinction is made between new and established patients in the emergency department. E/M services in the emergency department category may be reported for any new or established patient who presents for treatment in the emergency department.

Chief Complaint

A concise statement describing the symptom, problem, condition, diagnosis or other factor that is the reason for the encounter, usually stated in the patient's words.

Concurrent Care

Concurrent care is the provision of similar services, eg, hospital visits, to the same patient by more than one physician on the same day. When concurrent care is provided, no special reporting is required. Modifier '-75' has been deleted.

Counseling

Counseling is a discussion with a patient and/or family concerning one or more of the following areas:

■ diagnostic results, impressions, and/or recommended diagnostic studies;

■ prognosis;

■ risks and benefits of management (treatment) options;

■ instructions for management (treatment) and/or follow-up;

Evaluation and Management Guidelines

- importance of compliance with chosen management (treatment) options;
- risk factor reduction; and
- patient and family education.

(For psychotherapy, see 90804-90857)

Family History

A review of medical events in the patient's family that includes significant information about:

- the health status or cause of death of parents, siblings, and children;
- specific diseases related to problems identified in the Chief Complaint or History of the Present Illness, and/or System Review;
- diseases of family members which may be hereditary or place the patient at risk.

History of Present Illness

A chronological description of the development of the patient's present illness from the first sign and/or symptom to the present. This includes a description of location, quality, severity, timing, context, modifying factors and associated signs and symptoms significantly related to the presenting problem(s).

Levels of E/M Services

Within each category or subcategory of E/M service, there are three to five levels of E/M services available for reporting purposes. Levels of E/M services are **not** interchangeable among the different categories or subcategories of service. For example, the first level of E/M services in the subcategory of office visit, new patient, does not have the same definition as the first level of E/M services in the subcategory of office visit, established patient.

The levels of E/M services include examinations, evaluations, treatments, conferences with or concerning patients, preventive pediatric and adult health supervision, and similar medical services, such as the determination of the need and/or location for appropriate care. Medical screening includes the history, examination, and medical decision-making required to determine the need and/or location for appropriate care and treatment of the patient (eg, office and other outpatient setting, emergency department, nursing facility, etc.). The levels of E/M services encompass the wide variations in skill, effort, time, responsibility and medical knowledge required for the prevention or diagnosis and treatment of illness or injury and the promotion of optimal health. Each level of E/M services may be used by all physicians.

The descriptors for the levels of E/M services recognize seven components, six of which are used in defining the levels of E/M services. These components are:

- history;
- examination;

- medical decision making;
- counseling;
- coordination of care;
- nature of presenting problem; and
- time.

The first three of these components (history, examination, and medical decision making) are considered the **key** components in selecting a level of E/M services. (See "Determine the Extent of History Obtained," page 5.)

The next three components (counseling, coordination of care, and the nature of the presenting problem) are considered **contributory** factors in the majority of encounters. Although the first two of these contributory factors are important E/M services, it is not required that these services be provided at every patient encounter.

Coordination of care with other providers or agencies without a patient encounter on that day is reported using the case management codes.

The final component, time, is discussed in detail (see page 3).

Any specifically identifiable procedure (ie, identified with a specific CPT code) performed on or subsequent to the date of initial or subsequent "E/M Services" should be reported separately.

The actual performance and/or interpretation of diagnostic tests/studies ordered during a patient encounter are not included in the levels of E/M services. Physician performance of diagnostic tests/studies for which specific CPT codes are available may be reported separately, in addition to the appropriate E/M code. The physician's interpretation of the results of diagnostic tests/studies (ie, professional component) with preparation of a separate distinctly identifiable signed written report may also be reported separately, using the appropriate CPT code with the modifier '-26' appended.

The physician may need to indicate that on the day a procedure or service identified by a CPT code was performed, the patient's condition required a significant separately identifiable E/M service above and beyond other services provided or beyond the usual preservice and postservice care associated with the procedure that was performed. The E/M service may be caused or prompted by the symptoms or condition for which the procedure and/or service was provided. This circumstance may be reported by adding the modifier '-25' to the appropriate level of E/M service. As such, different diagnoses are not required for reporting of the procedure and the E/M services on the same date.

Nature of Presenting Problem

A presenting problem is a disease, condition, illness, injury, symptom, sign, finding, complaint, or other reason for encounter, with or without a diagnosis being established at the time of the encounter. The E/M codes recognize five types of presenting problems that are defined as follows:

Minimal: A problem that may not require the presence of the physician, but service is provided under the physician's supervision.

Self-limited or minor: A problem that runs a definite and prescribed course, is transient in nature, and is not likely to permanently alter health status OR has a good prognosis with management/compliance.

Low severity: A problem where the risk of morbidity without treatment is low; there is little to no risk of mortality without treatment; full recovery without functional impairment is expected.

Moderate severity: A problem where the risk of morbidity without treatment is moderate; there is moderate risk of mortality without treatment; uncertain prognosis OR increased probability of prolonged functional impairment.

High severity: A problem where the risk of morbidity without treatment is high to extreme; there is a moderate to high risk of mortality without treatment OR high probability of severe, prolonged functional impairment.

Past History

A review of the patient's past experiences with illnesses, injuries, and treatments that includes significant information about:

- prior major illnesses and injuries;
- prior operations;
- prior hospitalizations;
- current medications;
- allergies (eg, drug, food);
- age appropriate immunization status;
- age appropriate feeding/dietary status.

Social History

An age appropriate review of past and current activities that includes significant information about:

- marital status and/or living arrangements;
- current employment;
- occupational history;
- use of drugs, alcohol, and tobacco;
- level of education;
- sexual history;
- other relevant social factors.

System Review (Review of Systems)

An inventory of body systems obtained through a series of questions seeking to identify signs and/or symptoms which the patient may be experiencing or has experienced. For the purposes of CPT the following elements of a system review have been identified:

- Constitutional symptoms (fever, weight loss, etc.)
- Eyes
- Ears, Nose, Mouth, Throat
- Cardiovascular
- Respiratory
- Gastrointestinal
- Genitourinary
- Musculoskeletal
- Integumentary (skin and/or breast)
- Neurological
- Psychiatric
- Endocrine
- Hematologic/Lymphatic
- Allergic/Immunologic

The review of systems helps define the problem, clarify the differential diagnosis, identify needed testing, or serves as baseline data on other systems that might be affected by any possible management options.

Time

The inclusion of time in the definitions of levels of E/M services has been implicit in prior editions of *CPT*. The inclusion of time as an explicit factor beginning in *CPT 1992* is done to assist physicians in selecting the most appropriate level of E/M services. It should be recognized that the specific times expressed in the visit code descriptors are averages, and therefore represent a range of times which may be higher or lower depending on actual clinical circumstances.

Time is **not** a descriptive component for the emergency department levels of E/M services because emergency department services are typically provided on a variable intensity basis, often involving multiple encounters with several patients over an extended period of time. Therefore, it is often difficult for physicians to provide accurate estimates of the time spent face-to-face with the patient.

Studies to establish levels of E/M services employed surveys of practicing physicians to obtain data on the amount of time and work associated with typical E/M services. Since "work" is not easily quantifiable, the codes must rely on other objective, verifiable measures that correlate with physicians' estimates of their "work". It has been demonstrated that physicians' estimations of **intraservice time** (as explained on the next page), both within and across specialties, is a variable that is predictive of the "work" of E/M services. This same research has shown there is a strong relationship between intra-service time and total time for E/M services. Intra-service time, rather than total time, was chosen for inclusion with the codes because of its relative ease of measurement and because of its direct correlation with measurements of the total amount of time and work associated with typical E/M services.

Intra-service times are defined as **face-to-face** time for office and other outpatient visits and as **unit/floor** time for hospital and other inpatient visits. This distinction is necessary because most of the work of typical office visits takes place during the face-to-face time with the patient, while most of the work of typical hospital visits takes place during the time spent on the patient's floor or unit.

Face-to-face time (office and other outpatient visits and office consultations): For coding purposes, face-to-face time for these services is defined as only that time that the physician spends face-to-face with the patient and/or family. This includes the time in which the physician performs such tasks as obtaining a history, performing an examination, and counseling the patient.

Physicians also spend time doing work before or after the face-to-face time with the patient, performing such tasks as reviewing records and tests, arranging for further services, and communicating further with other professionals and the patient through written reports and telephone contact.

This **non-face-to-face** time for office services—also called pre- and post-encounter time—is not included in the time component described in the E/M codes. However, the pre- and post-face-to-face work associated with an encounter was included in calculating the total work of typical services in physician surveys.

Thus, the face-to-face time associated with the services described by any E/M code is a valid proxy for the total work done before, during, and after the visit.

Unit/floor time (hospital observation services, inpatient hospital care, initial and follow-up hospital consultations, nursing facility): For reporting purposes, intra-service time for these services is defined as unit/floor time, which includes the time that the physician is present on the patient's hospital unit and at the bedside rendering services for that patient. This includes the time in which the physician establishes and/or reviews the patient's chart, examines the patient, writes notes and communicates with other professionals and the patient's family.

In the hospital, pre- and post-time includes time spent off the patient's floor performing such tasks as reviewing pathology and radiology findings in another part of the hospital.

This pre- and post-visit time is not included in the time component described in these codes. However, the pre- and post-work performed during the time spent off the floor or unit was included in calculating the total work of typical services in physician surveys.

Thus, the unit/floor time associated with the services described by any code is a valid proxy for the total work done before, during, and after the visit.

Unlisted Service

An E/M service may be provided that is not listed in this section of *CPT*. When reporting such a service, the appropriate "Unlisted" code may be used to indicate the service, identifying it by "Special Report", as discussed in the following paragraph. The "Unlisted Services" and accompanying codes for the E/M section are as follows:

99429	Unlisted preventive medicine service
99499	Unlisted evaluation and management service
▶**99600**◀	Unlisted home visit service or procedure

Special Report

An unlisted service or one that is unusual, variable, or new may require a special report demonstrating the medical appropriateness of the service. Pertinent information should include an adequate definition or description of the nature, extent, and need for the procedure; and the time, effort, and equipment necessary to provide the service. Additional items which may be included are complexity of symptoms, final diagnosis, pertinent physical findings, diagnostic and therapeutic procedures, concurrent problems, and follow-up care.

Clinical Examples

Clinical examples of the codes for E/M services are provided to assist physicians in understanding the meaning of the descriptors and selecting the correct code. The clinical examples are listed in Appendix C. Each example was developed by physicians in the specialties shown.

The same problem, when seen by physicians in different specialties, may involve different amounts of work. Therefore, the appropriate level of encounter should be reported using the descriptors rather than the examples.

The examples have been tested for validity and approved by the CPT Editorial Panel. Physicians were given the examples and asked to assign a code or assess the amount of time and work involved. Only those examples that were rated consistently have been included in Appendix C.

Table 1
Categories and Subcategories of Service

Category/Subcategory	Code Numbers	Category/Subcategory	Code Numbers
Office or Other Outpatient Services		Subsequent Nursing Facility Care	99311-99313
New Patient	99201-99205	Nursing Facility Discharge Services	99315-99316
Established Patient	99211-99215	Domiciliary, Rest Home or	
Hospital Observation Discharge Services	99217	Custodial Care Services	
Hospital Observation Services	99218-99220	New Patient	99321-99323
Hospital Observation or Inpatient Care		Established Patient	99331-99333
Services (Including Admission and		Home Services	
Discharge Services)	99234-99236	New Patient	99341-99345
Hospital Inpatient Services		Established Patient	99347-99350
Initial Hospital Care	99221-99223	Prolonged Services	
Subsequent Hospital Care	99231-99233	With Direct Patient Contact	99354-99357
Hospital Discharge Services	99238-99239	Without Direct Patient Contact	99358-99359
Consultations		Standby Services	99360
Office Consultations	99241-99245	Case Management Services	
Initial Inpatient Consultations	99251-99255	Team Conferences	99361-99362
Follow-up Inpatient Consultations	99261-99263	Telephone Calls	99371-99373
Confirmatory Consultations	99271-99275	Care Plan Oversight Services	99374-99380
Emergency Department Services	99281-99288	Preventive Medicine Services	
▶Pediatric◀ Patient Transport	99289-99290	New Patient	99381-99387
Critical Care Services		Established Patient	99391-99397
▶Adult (over 24 months of age)	99291-99292◀	Individual Counseling	99401-99404
▶Pediatric◀	99293-99294	Group Counseling	99411-99412
▶Neonatal◀	99295-99296	Other	99420-99429
▶Intensive Care (Low Birth Weight)	99298-99299◀	Newborn Care	99431-99440
Nursing Facility Services		Special E/M Services	99450-99456
Comprehensive Nursing Facility		Other E/M Services	99499
Assessments	99301-99303		

Instructions for Selecting a Level of E/M Service

Identify the Category and Subcategory of Service

The categories and subcategories of codes available for reporting E/M services are shown in Table 1 above.

Review the Reporting Instructions for the Selected Category or Subcategory

Most of the categories and many of the subcategories of service have special guidelines or instructions unique to that category or subcategory. Where these are indicated, eg, "Inpatient Hospital Care," special instructions will be presented preceding the levels of E/M services.

Review the Level of E/M Service Descriptors and Examples in the Selected Category or Subcategory

The descriptors for the levels of E/M services recognize seven components, six of which are used in defining the levels of E/M services. These components are:

- history;
- examination;
- medical decision making;
- counseling;
- coordination of care;
- nature of presenting problem; and
- time.

The first three of these components (ie, history, examination, and medical decision making) should be considered the **key** components in selecting the level of E/M services. An exception to this rule is in the case of visits which consist predominantly of counseling or coordination of care (See numbered paragraph 3, page 7.)

The nature of the presenting problem and time are provided in some levels to assist the physician in determining the appropriate level of E/M service.

Determine the Extent of History Obtained

The extent of the history is dependent upon clinical judgment and on the nature of the presenting problems(s). The levels of E/M services recognize four types of history that are defined as follows:

Problem focused: chief complaint; brief history of present illness or problem.

Expanded problem focused: chief complaint; brief history of present illness; problem pertinent system review.

Detailed: chief complaint; extended history of present illness; problem pertinent system review extended to include a review of a limited number of additional systems; **pertinent** past, family, and/or social history **directly related to the patient's problems.**

Comprehensive: chief complaint; extended history of present illness; review of systems which is directly related to the problem(s) identified in the history of the present illness plus a review of all additional body systems; **complete** past, family, and social history.

The comprehensive history obtained as part of the preventive medicine evaluation and management service is not problem-oriented and does not involve a chief complaint or present illness. It does, however, include a comprehensive system review and comprehensive or interval past, family, and social history as well as a comprehensive assessment/history of pertinent risk factors.

Determine the Extent of Examination Performed

The extent of the examination performed is dependent on clinical judgment and on the nature of the presenting problem(s). The levels of E/M services recognize four types of examination that are defined as follows:

Problem focused: a limited examination of the affected body area or organ system.

Expanded problem focused: a limited examination of the affected body area or organ system and other symptomatic or related organ system(s).

Detailed: an extended examination of the affected body area(s) and other symptomatic or related organ system(s).

Comprehensive: a general multi-system examination or a complete examination of a single organ system. **Note:** The comprehensive examination performed as part of the preventive medicine evaluation and management service is multisystem, but its extent is based on age and risk factors identified.

For the purposes of these CPT definitions, the following body areas are recognized:

- Head, including the face
- Neck
- Chest, including breasts and axilla
- Abdomen
- Genitalia, groin, buttocks
- Back
- Each extremity

For the purposes of these CPT definitions, the following organ systems are recognized:

- Eyes
- Ears, Nose, Mouth, and Throat
- Cardiovascular
- Respiratory
- Gastrointestinal
- Genitourinary
- Musculoskeletal
- Skin
- Neurologic
- Psychiatric
- Hematologic/Lymphatic/Immunologic

Determine the Complexity of Medical Decision Making

Medical decision making refers to the complexity of establishing a diagnosis and/or selecting a management option as measured by:

- the number of possible diagnoses and/or the number of management options that must be considered;
- the amount and/or complexity of medical records, diagnostic tests, and/or other information that must be obtained, reviewed, and analyzed; and
- the risk of significant complications, morbidity, and/or mortality, as well as comorbidities, associated with the patient's presenting problems(s), the diagnostic procedure(s) and/or the possible management options.

Four types of medical decision making are recognized: straightforward; low complexity; moderate complexity; and high complexity. To qualify for a given type of decision making, two of the three elements in Table 2 on the following page must be met or exceeded.

Comorbidities/underlying diseases, in and of themselves, are not considered in selecting a level of E/M services *unless* their presence significantly increases the complexity of the medical decision making.

Select the Appropriate Level of E/M Services Based on the Following

1. For the following categories/subcategories, **all of the key components,** ie, history, examination, and medical decision making, must meet or exceed the stated requirements to qualify for a particular level of E/M service: office, new patient; hospital observation services; initial hospital care; office consultations; initial inpatient consultations; confirmatory consultations; emergency department services; comprehensive nursing facility assessments; domiciliary care, new patient; and home, new patient.

Evaluation and Management Guidelines

Table 2
Complexity of Medical Decision Making

Number of Diagnoses or Management Options	Amount and/or Complexity of Data to be Reviewed	Risk of Complications and/or Morbidity or Mortality	Type of Decision Making
minimal	minimal or none	minimal	**straightforward**
limited	limited	low	**low complexity**
multiple	moderate	moderate	**moderate complexity**
extensive	extensive	high	**high complexity**

2. For the following categories/subcategories, **two of the three key components** (ie, history, examination, and medical decision making) must meet or exceed the stated requirements to qualify for a particular level of E/M services: office, established patient; subsequent hospital care; follow-up inpatient consultations; subsequent nursing facility care; domiciliary care, established patient; and home, established patient.

3. When counseling and/or coordination of care dominates (more than 50%) the physician/patient and/or family encounter (face-to-face time in the office or other outpatient setting or floor/unit time in the hospital or nursing facility), then **time** may be considered the key or controlling factor to qualify for a particular level of E/M services. This includes time spent with parties who have assumed responsibility for the care of the patient or decision making whether or not they are family members (eg, foster parents, person acting in locum parentis, legal guardian). The extent of counseling and/or coordination of care must be documented in the medical record.

Evaluation and Management Guidelines

Notes

⊘=Modifier '-51' Exempt   ▶◀ or ▶ ◀=New or Revised Text   ✚=Add-on Code

Evaluation and Management

Office or Other Outpatient Services

The following codes are used to report evaluation and management services provided in the physician's office or in an outpatient or other ambulatory facility. A patient is considered an outpatient until inpatient admission to a health care facility occurs.

To report services provided to a patient who is admitted to a hospital or nursing facility in the course of an encounter in the office or other ambulatory facility, see the notes for initial hospital inpatient care (page 11) or comprehensive nursing facility assessments (page 22).

For services provided by physicians in the emergency department, see 99281-99285.

For observation care, see 99217-99220.

For observation or inpatient care services (including admission and discharge services), see 99234-99236.

New Patient

99201 **Office or other outpatient visit** for the evaluation and management of a new patient, which requires these three key components:

■ **a problem focused history;**

■ **a problem focused examination; and**

■ **straightforward medical decision making.**

Counseling and/or coordination of care with other providers or agencies are provided consistent with the nature of the problem(s) and the patient's and/or family's needs.

Usually, the presenting problems are self limited or minor. Physicians typically spend 10 minutes face-to-face with the patient and/or family.

99202 **Office or other outpatient visit** for the evaluation and management of a new patient, which requires these three key components:

■ **an expanded problem focused history;**

■ **an expanded problem focused examination; and**

■ **straightforward medical decision making.**

Counseling and/or coordination of care with other providers or agencies are provided consistent with the nature of the problem(s) and the patient's and/or family's needs.

Usually, the presenting problem(s) are of low to moderate severity. Physicians typically spend 20 minutes face-to-face with the patient and/or family.

99203 **Office or other outpatient visit** for the evaluation and management of a new patient, which requires these three key components:

■ **a detailed history;**

■ **a detailed examination; and**

■ **medical decision making of low complexity.**

Counseling and/or coordination of care with other providers or agencies are provided consistent with the nature of the problem(s) and the patient's and/or family's needs.

Usually, the presenting problem(s) are of moderate severity. Physicians typically spend 30 minutes face-to-face with the patient and/or family.

99204 **Office or other outpatient visit** for the evaluation and management of a new patient, which requires these three key components:

■ **a comprehensive history;**

■ **a comprehensive examination; and**

■ **medical decision making of moderate complexity.**

Counseling and/or coordination of care with other providers or agencies are provided consistent with the nature of the problem(s) and the patient's and/or family's needs.

Usually, the presenting problem(s) are of moderate to high severity. Physicians typically spend 45 minutes face-to-face with the patient and/or family.

99205 **Office or other outpatient visit** for the evaluation and management of a new patient, which requires these three key components:

■ **a comprehensive history;**

■ **a comprehensive examination; and**

■ **medical decision making of high complexity.**

Counseling and/or coordination of care with other providers or agencies are provided consistent with the nature of the problem(s) and the patient's and/or family's needs.

Usually, the presenting problem(s) are of moderate to high severity. Physicians typically spend 60 minutes face-to-face with the patient and/or family.

Established Patient

99211 **Office or other outpatient visit** for the evaluation and management of an established patient, that may not require the presence of a physician. Usually, the presenting problem(s) are minimal. Typically, 5 minutes are spent performing or supervising these services.

Evaluation and Management

99212 **Office or other outpatient visit** for the evaluation and management of an established patient, which requires at least two of these three key components:

- **a problem focused history;**
- **a problem focused examination;**
- **straightforward medical decision making.**

Counseling and/or coordination of care with other providers or agencies are provided consistent with the nature of the problem(s) and the patient's and/or family's needs.

Usually, the presenting problem(s) are self limited or minor. Physicians typically spend 10 minutes face-to-face with the patient and/or family.

99213 **Office or other outpatient visit** for the evaluation and management of an established patient, which requires at least two of these three key components:

- **an expanded problem focused history;**
- **an expanded problem focused examination;**
- **medical decision making of low complexity.**

Counseling and coordination of care with other providers or agencies are provided consistent with the nature of the problem(s) and the patient's and/or family's needs.

Usually, the presenting problem(s) are of low to moderate severity. Physicians typically spend 15 minutes face-to-face with the patient and/or family.

99214 **Office or other outpatient visit** for the evaluation and management of an established patient, which requires at least two of these three key components:

- **a detailed history;**
- **a detailed examination;**
- **medical decision making of moderate complexity.**

Counseling and/or coordination of care with other providers or agencies are provided consistent with the nature of the problem(s) and the patient's and/or family's needs.

Usually, the presenting problem(s) are of moderate to high severity. Physicians typically spend 25 minutes face-to-face with the patient and/or family.

99215 **Office or other outpatient visit** for the evaluation and management of an established patient, which requires at least two of these three key components:

- **a comprehensive history;**
- **a comprehensive examination;**
- **medical decision making of high complexity.**

Counseling and/or coordination of care with other providers or agencies are provided consistent with the nature of the problem(s) and the patient's and/or family's needs.

Usually, the presenting problem(s) are of moderate to high severity. Physicians typically spend 40 minutes face-to-face with the patient and/or family.

Hospital Observation Services

The following codes are used to report evaluation and management services provided to patients designated/admitted as "observation status" in a hospital. It is not necessary that the patient be located in an observation area designated by the hospital.

If such an area does exist in a hospital (as a separate unit in the hospital, in the emergency department, etc.), these codes are to be utilized if the patient is placed in such an area.

For definitions of key components and commonly used terms, please see **Evaluation and Management Services Guidelines.**

Typical times have not yet been established for this category of services.

Observation Care Discharge Services

Observation care discharge of a patient from "observation status" includes final examination of the patient, discussion of the hospital stay, instructions for continuing care, and preparation of discharge records. For observation or inpatient hospital care including the admission and discharge of the patient on the same date, see codes 99234-99236 as appropriate.

99217 **Observation care discharge** day management (This code is to be utilized by the physician to report all services provided to a patient on discharge from "observation status" if the discharge is on other than the initial date of "observation status." To report services to a patient designated as "observation status" or "inpatient status" and discharged on the same date, use the codes for Observation or Inpatient Care Services [including Admission and Discharge Services, 99234-99236 as appropriate.])

Initial Observation Care

New or Established Patient

The following codes are used to report the encounter(s) by the supervising physician with the patient when designated as "observation status." This refers to the initiation of observation status, supervision of the care plan for observation and performance of periodic reassessments. For observation encounters by other physicians, see Office or Other Outpatient Consultation codes (99241-99245).

To report services provided to a patient who is admitted to the hospital after receiving hospital observation care services on the same date, see the notes for initial hospital inpatient care (page 12). For a patient admitted to the hospital on a date subsequent to the date of observation status, the hospital admission would be reported with the appropriate Initial Hospital Care codes (99221-99223). For a patient admitted and discharged from observation or inpatient status on the same date, the services should be reported with codes 99234-99236 as appropriate. Do not report observation discharge (99217) in conjunction with a hospital admission.

When "observation status" is initiated in the course of an encounter in another site of service (eg, hospital emergency department, physician's office, nursing facility) all evaluation and management services provided by the supervising physician in conjunction with initiating "observation status" are considered part of the initial observation care when performed on the same date. The observation care level of service reported by the supervising physician should include the services related to initiating "observation status" provided in the other sites of service as well as in the observation setting.

Evaluation and management services on the same date provided in sites that are related to initiating "observation status" should NOT be reported separately.

These codes may not be utilized for post-operative recovery if the procedure is considered part of the surgical "package." These codes apply to all evaluation and management services that are provided on the same date of initiating "observation status."

99218   **Initial observation care,** per day, for the evaluation and management of a patient which requires these three key components:

- a detailed or comprehensive history;
- a detailed or comprehensive examination; and
- medical decision making that is straightforward or of low complexity.

Counseling and/or coordination of care with other providers or agencies are provided consistent with the nature of the problem(s) and the patient's and/or family's needs.

Usually, the problem(s) requiring admission to "observation status" are of low severity.

99219   **Initial observation care,** per day, for the evaluation and management of a patient, which requires these three key components:

- a comprehensive history;
- a comprehensive examination; and
- medical decision making of moderate complexity.

Counseling and/or coordination of care with other providers or agencies are provided consistent with the nature of the problem(s) and the patient's and/or family's needs.

Usually, the problem(s) requiring admission to "observation status" are of moderate severity.

99220   **Initial observation care,** per day, for the evaluation and management of a patient, which requires these three key components:

- a comprehensive history;
- a comprehensive examination; and
- medical decision making of high complexity.

Counseling and/or coordination of care with other providers or agencies are provided consistent with the nature of the problem(s) and the patient's and/or family's needs.

Usually, the problem(s) requiring admission to "observation status" are of high severity.

Hospital Inpatient Services

The following codes are used to report evaluation and management services provided to hospital inpatients. Hospital inpatient services include those services provided to patients in a "partial hospital" setting. These codes are to be used to report these partial hospitalization services. See also psychiatry notes in the full text of *CPT.*

For definitions of key components and commonly used terms, please see **Evaluation and Management Services Guidelines.** For Hospital Observation Services, see 99218-99220. For a patient admitted and discharged from observation or inpatient status on the same date, the services should be reported with codes 99234-99236 as appropriate.

Initial Hospital Care

New or Established Patient

The following codes are used to report the first hospital inpatient encounter with the patient by the admitting physician.

For initial inpatient encounters by physicians other than the admitting physician, see initial inpatient consultation codes (99251-99255) or subsequent hospital care codes (99231-99233) as appropriate.

When the patient is admitted to the hospital as an inpatient in the course of an encounter in another site of service (eg, hospital emergency department, observation status in a hospital, physician's office, nursing facility) all evaluation and management services provided by that physician in conjunction with that admission are considered part of the initial hospital care when performed on the same date as the admission. The inpatient care level of service reported by the admitting physician should include the services related to the admission he/she provided in the other sites of service as well as in the inpatient setting.

Evaluation and Management

Evaluation and management services on the same date provided in sites that are related to the admission "observation status" should NOT be reported separately. For a patient admitted and discharged from observation or inpatient status on the same date, the services should be reported with codes 99234-99236 as appropriate.

99221   **Initial hospital care,** per day, for the evaluation and management of a patient which requires these three key components:

- **a detailed or comprehensive history;**
- **a detailed or comprehensive examination; and**
- **medical decision making that is straightforward or of low complexity.**

Counseling and/or coordination of care with other providers or agencies are provided consistent with the nature of the problem(s) and the patient's and/or family's needs.

Usually, the problem(s) requiring admission are of low severity. Physicians typically spend 30 minutes at the bedside and on the patient's hospital floor or unit.

99222   **Initial hospital care,** per day, for the evaluation and management of a patient, which requires these three key components:

- **a comprehensive history;**
- **a comprehensive examination; and**
- **medical decision making of moderate complexity.**

Counseling and/or coordination of care with other providers or agencies are provided consistent with the nature of the problem(s) and the patient's and/or family's needs.

Usually, the problem(s) requiring admission are of moderate severity. Physicians typically spend 50 minutes at the bedside and on the patient's hospital floor or unit.

99223   **Initial hospital care,** per day, for the evaluation and management of a patient, which requires these three key components:

- **a comprehensive history;**
- **a comprehensive examination; and**
- **medical decision making of high complexity.**

Counseling and/or coordination of care with other providers or agencies are provided consistent with the nature of the problem(s) and the patient's and/or family's needs.

Usually, the problem(s) requiring admission are of high severity. Physicians typically spend 70 minutes at the bedside and on the patient's hospital floor or unit.

Subsequent Hospital Care

All levels of subsequent hospital care include reviewing the medical record and reviewing the results of diagnostic studies and changes in the patient's status, (ie, changes in history, physical condition and response to management) since the last assessment by the physician.

99231   **Subsequent hospital care,** per day, for the evaluation and management of a patient, which requires at least two of these three key components:

- **a problem focused interval history;**
- **a problem focused examination;**
- **medical decision making that is straightforward or of low complexity.**

Counseling and/or coordination of care with other providers or agencies are provided consistent with the nature of the problem(s) and the patient's and/or family's needs.

Usually, the patient is stable, recovering or improving. Physicians typically spend 15 minutes at the bedside and on the patient's hospital floor or unit.

99232   **Subsequent hospital care,** per day, for the evaluation and management of a patient, which requires at least two of these three key components:

- **an expanded problem focused interval history;**
- **an expanded problem focused examination;**
- **medical decision making of moderate complexity.**

Counseling and/or coordination of care with other providers or agencies are provided consistent with the nature of the problem(s) and the patient's and/or family's needs.

Usually, the patient is responding inadequately to therapy or has developed a minor complication. Physicians typically spend 25 minutes at the bedside and on the patient's hospital floor or unit.

99233   **Subsequent hospital care,** per day, for the evaluation and management of a patient, which requires at least two of these three key components:

- **a detailed interval history;**
- **a detailed examination;**
- **medical decision making of high complexity.**

Counseling and/or coordination of care with other providers or agencies are provided consistent with the nature of the problem(s) and the patient's and/or family's needs.

Usually, the patient is unstable or has developed a significant complication or a significant new problem. Physicians typically spend 35 minutes at the bedside and on the patient's hospital floor or unit.

Observation or Inpatient Care Services (Including Admission and Discharge Services)

The following codes are used to report observation or inpatient hospital care services provided to patients admitted and discharged on the same date of service. When a patient is admitted to the hospital from observation status on the same date, the physician should report only the initial hospital care code. The initial hospital care code reported by the admitting physician should include the services related to the observation status services he/she provided on the same date of inpatient admission.

When "observation status" is initiated in the course of an encounter in another site of service (eg, hospital emergency department, physician's office, nursing facility) all evaluation and management services provided by the supervising physician in conjunction with initiating "observation status" are considered part of the initial observation care when performed on the same date. The observation care level of service should include the services related to initiating "observation status" provided in the other sites of service as well as in the observation setting when provided by the same physician.

For patients admitted to observation or inpatient care and discharged on a different date, see codes 99218-99220 and 99217, or 99221-99223 and 99238-99239.

99234   **Observation or inpatient hospital care,** for the evaluation and management of a patient including admission and discharge on the same date which requires these three key components:

- **a detailed or comprehensive history;**
- **a detailed or comprehensive examination; and**
- **medical decision making that is straightforward or of low complexity.**

Counseling and/or coordination of care with other providers or agencies are provided consistent with the nature of the problem(s) and the patient's and/or family's needs.

Usually the presenting problem(s) requiring admission are of low severity.

99235   **Observation or inpatient hospital care,** for the evaluation and management of a patient including admission and discharge on the same date which requires these three key components:

- **a comprehensive history;**
- **a comprehensive examination; and**
- **medical decision making of moderate complexity.**

Counseling and/or coordination of care with other providers or agencies are provided consistent with the nature of the problem(s) and the patient's and/or family's needs.

Usually the presenting problem(s) requiring admission are of moderate severity.

99236   **Observation or inpatient hospital care,** for the evaluation and management of a patient including admission and discharge on the same date which requires these three key components:

- **a comprehensive history;**
- **a comprehensive examination; and**
- **medical decision making of high complexity.**

Counseling and/or coordination of care with other providers or agencies are provided consistent with the nature of the problem(s) and the patient's and/or family's needs.

Usually the presenting problem(s) requiring admission are of high severity.

Hospital Discharge Services

The hospital discharge day management codes are to be used to report the total duration of time spent by a physician for final hospital discharge of a patient. The codes include, as appropriate, final examination of the patient, discussion of the hospital stay, even if the time spent by the physician on that date is not continuous, instructions for continuing care to all relevant caregivers, and preparation of discharge records, prescriptions and referral forms. For a patient admitted and discharged from observation or inpatient status on the same date, the services should be reported with codes 99234-99236 as appropriate.

99238   **Hospital discharge day management;** 30 minutes or less

99239   more than 30 minutes

(These codes are to be utilized by the physician to report all services provided to a patient on the date of discharge, if other than the initial date of inpatient status. To report services to a patient who is admitted as an inpatient, and discharged on the same date, see codes 99234-99236 for observation or inpatient hospital care including the admission and discharge of the patient on the same date. To report concurrent care services provided by a physician(s) other than the attending physician, use subsequent hospital care codes (99231-99233) on the day of discharge.)

(For Observation Care Discharge, use 99217)

(For observation or inpatient hospital care including the admission and discharge of the patient on the same date, see 99234-99236)

(For Nursing Facility Care Discharge, see 99315, 99316)

(For discharge services provided to newborns admitted and discharged on the same date, use 99435)

Consultations

A consultation is a type of service provided by a physician whose opinion or advice regarding evaluation and/or management of a specific problem is requested by another physician or other appropriate source.

A physician consultant may initiate diagnostic and/or therapeutic services at the same or subsequent visit.

The written or verbal request for a consult may be made by a physician or other appropriate source and documented in the patient's medical record.

The consultant's opinion and any services that were ordered or performed must also be documented in the patient's medical record and communicated by written report to the requesting physician or other appropriate source.

A "consultation" initiated by a patient and/or family, and not requested by a physician, is not reported using the initial consultation codes but may be reported using the codes for confirmatory consultation or office visits, as appropriate.

If a confirmatory consultation is required, eg, by a third party payor, the modifier '-32', mandated services, should also be reported.

Any specifically identifiable procedure (ie, identified with a specific CPT code) performed on or subsequent to the date of the initial consultation should be reported separately.

If subsequent to the completion of a consultation, the consultant assumes responsibility for management of a portion or all of the patient's condition(s), the follow-up consultation codes should not be used. In the hospital setting, the consulting physician should use the appropriate inpatient hospital consultation code for the initial encounter and then subsequent hospital care codes (not follow-up consultation codes). In the office setting, the appropriate established patient code should be used.

There are four subcategories of consultations: office, initial inpatient, follow-up inpatient, and confirmatory. See each subcategory for specific reporting instructions.

For definitions of key components and commonly used terms, please see **Evaluation and Management Services Guidelines**.

Office or Other Outpatient Consultations

New or Established Patient

The following codes are used to report consultations provided in the physician's office or in an outpatient or other ambulatory facility, including hospital observation services, home services, domiciliary, rest home, custodial care, or emergency department (see consultation definition, above). Follow-up visits in the consultant's office or other outpatient facility that are initiated by the physician consultant are reported using office visit codes for established patients (99211-99215). If an additional request for an opinion or advice regarding the same or a new problem is received from the attending physician and documented in the medical record, the office consultation codes may be used again.

99241 **Office consultation** for a new or established patient, which requires these three key components:

- **a problem focused history;**
- **a problem focused examination; and**
- **straightforward medical decision making.**

Counseling and/or coordination of care with other providers or agencies are provided consistent with the nature of the problem(s) and the patient's and/or family's needs.

Usually, the presenting problem(s) are self limited or minor. Physicians typically spend 15 minutes face-to-face with the patient and/or family.

99242 **Office consultation** for a new or established patient, which requires these three key components:

- **an expanded problem focused history;**
- **an expanded problem focused examination; and**
- **straightforward medical decision making.**

Counseling and/or coordination of care with other providers or agencies are provided consistent with the nature of the problem(s) and the patient's and/or family's needs.

Usually, the presenting problem(s) are of low severity. Physicians typically spend 30 minutes face-to-face with the patient and/or family.

99243 **Office consultation** for a new or established patient, which requires these three key components:

- **a detailed history;**
- **a detailed examination; and**
- **medical decision making of low complexity.**

Counseling and/or coordination of care with other providers or agencies are provided consistent with the nature of the problem(s) and the patient's and/or family's needs.

Usually, the presenting problem(s) are of moderate severity. Physicians typically spend 40 minutes face-to-face with the patient and/or family.

99244 **Office consultation** for a new or established patient, which requires these three key components:

- **a comprehensive history;**
- **a comprehensive examination; and**
- **medical decision making of moderate complexity.**

Counseling and/or coordination of care with other providers or agencies are provided consistent with the nature of the problem(s) and the patient's and/or family's needs.

Usually, the presenting problem(s) are of moderate to high severity. Physicians typically spend 60 minutes face-to-face with the patient and/or family.

99245 Office consultation for a new or established patient, which requires these three key components:

- **a comprehensive history;**
- **a comprehensive examination; and**
- **medical decision making of high complexity.**

Counseling and/or coordination of care with other providers or agencies are provided consistent with the nature of the problem(s) and the patient's and/or family's needs.

Usually, the presenting problem(s) are of moderate to high severity. Physicians typically spend 80 minutes face-to-face with the patient and/or family.

Initial Inpatient Consultations

New or Established Patient

The following codes are used to report physician consultations provided to hospital inpatients, residents of nursing facilities, or patients in a partial hospital setting. Only one initial consultation should be reported by a consultant per admission.

99251   **Initial inpatient consultation** for a new or established patient, which requires these three key components:

- **a problem focused history;**
- **a problem focused examination; and**
- **straightforward medical decision making.**

Counseling and/or coordination of care with other providers or agencies are provided consistent with the nature of the problem(s) and the patient's and/or family's needs.

Usually, the presenting problem(s) are self limited or minor. Physicians typically spend 20 minutes at the bedside and on the patient's hospital floor or unit.

99252   **Initial inpatient consultation** for a new or established patient, which requires these three key components:

- **an expanded problem focused history;**
- **an expanded problem focused examination; and**
- **straightforward medical decision making.**

Counseling and/or coordination of care with other providers or agencies are provided consistent with the nature of the problem(s) and the patient's and/or family's needs.

Usually, the presenting problem(s) are of low severity. Physicians typically spend 40 minutes at the bedside and on the patient's hospital floor or unit.

99253   **Initial inpatient consultation** for a new or established patient, which requires these three key components:

- **a detailed history;**
- **a detailed examination; and**
- **medical decision making of low complexity.**

Counseling and/or coordination of care with other providers or agencies are provided consistent with the nature of the problem(s) and the patient's and/or family's needs.

Usually, the presenting problem(s) are of moderate severity. Physicians typically spend 55 minutes at the bedside and on the patient's hospital floor or unit.

99254   **Initial inpatient consultation** for a new or established patient, which requires three key components:

- **a comprehensive history;**
- **a comprehensive examination; and**
- **medical decision making of moderate complexity.**

Counseling and/or coordination of care with other providers or agencies are provided consistent with the nature of the problem(s) and the patient's and/or family's needs.

Usually, the presenting problem(s) are of moderate to high severity. Physicians typically spend 80 minutes at the bedside and on the patient's hospital floor or unit.

99255   **Initial inpatient consultation** for a new or established patient, which requires these three key components:

- **a comprehensive history;**
- **a comprehensive examination; and**
- **medical decision making of high complexity.**

Counseling and/or coordination of care with other providers or agencies are provided consistent with the nature of the problem(s) and the patient's and/or family's needs.

Usually, the presenting problem(s) are of moderate to high severity. Physicians typically spend 110 minutes at the bedside and on the patient's hospital floor or unit.

Follow-Up Inpatient Consultations

Established Patient

Follow-up consultations are visits to complete the initial consultation OR subsequent consultative visits requested by the attending physician.

A follow-up consultation includes monitoring progress, recommending management modifications or advising on a new plan of care in response to changes in the patient's status.

If the physician consultant has initiated treatment at the initial consultation, and participates thereafter in the patient's management, the codes for subsequent hospital care should be used (99231-99233).

The following codes are used to report follow-up consultations provided to hospital inpatients or nursing facility residents only. For consultative services provided in other settings, the codes for office or other outpatient consultations should be reported (99241-99245).

99261   **Follow-up inpatient consultation** for an established patient, which requires at least two of these three key components:

- **a problem focused interval history;**
- **a problem focused examination;**
- **medical decision making that is straightforward or of low complexity.**

Counseling and/or coordination of care with other providers or agencies are provided consistent with nature of the problem(s) and the patient's and/or family's needs.

Usually, the patient is stable, recovering or improving. Physicians typically spend 10 minutes at the bedside and on the patient's hospital floor or unit.

99262 **Follow-up inpatient consultation** for an established patient which requires at least two of these three key components:

- **an expanded problem focused interval history;**
- **an expanded problem focused examination;**
- **medical decision making of moderate complexity.**

Counseling and/or coordination of care with other providers or agencies are provided consistent with the nature of the problem(s) and the patient's and/or family's needs.

Usually, the patient is responding inadequately to therapy or has developed a minor complication. Physicians typically spend 20 minutes at the bedside and on the patient's hospital floor or unit.

99263 **Follow-up inpatient consultation** for an established patient which requires at least two of these three key components:

- **a detailed interval history;**
- **a detailed examination;**
- **medical decision making of high complexity.**

Counseling and/or coordination of care with other providers or agencies are provided consistent with the nature of the problem(s) and the patient's and/or family's needs.

Usually, the patient is unstable or has developed a significant complication or a significant new problem. Physicians typically spend 30 minutes at the bedside and on the patient's hospital floor or unit.

Confirmatory Consultations

New or Established Patient

The following codes are used to report the evaluation and management services provided to patients when the consulting physician is aware of the confirmatory nature of the opinion sought (eg, when a second/third opinion is requested or required on the necessity or appropriateness of a previously recommended medical treatment or surgical procedure).

Confirmatory consultations may be provided in any setting.

A physician consultant providing a confirmatory consultation is expected to provide an opinion and/or advice only. Any services subsequent to the opinion are coded at the appropriate level of office visit, established patient, or subsequent hospital care. If a confirmatory

consultation is required, eg, by a third party payor, the modifier '-32', mandated services, should also be reported. (See also Consultation notes, page 13.) Typical times have not yet been established for this subcategory of services.

99271 **Confirmatory consultation** for a new or established patient, which requires these three key components:

- **a problem focused history;**
- **a problem focused examination; and**
- **straightforward medical decision making.**

Counseling and/or coordination of care with other providers or agencies are provided consistent with the nature of the problem(s) and the patient's and/or family's needs.

Usually, the presenting problem(s) are self limited or minor.

99272 **Confirmatory consultation** for a new or established patient, which requires these three key components:

- **an expanded problem focused history;**
- **an expanded problem focused examination; and**
- **straightforward medical decision making.**

Counseling and/or coordination of care with other providers or agencies are provided consistent with the nature of the problem(s) and the patient's and/or family's needs.

Usually, the presenting problem(s) are of low severity.

99273 **Confirmatory consultation** for a new or established patient, which requires these three key components:

- **a detailed history;**
- **a detailed examination; and**
- **medical decision making of low complexity.**

Counseling and/or coordination of care with other providers or agencies are provided consistent with the nature of the problem(s) and the patient's and/or family's needs.

Usually, the presenting problem(s) are of moderate severity.

99274 **Confirmatory consultation** for a new or established patient, which requires these three key components:

- **a comprehensive history;**
- **a comprehensive examination; and**
- **medical decision making of moderate complexity.**

Counseling and/or coordination of care with other providers or agencies are provided consistent with the nature of the problem(s) and the patient's and/or family's needs.

Usually, the presenting problem(s) are of moderate to high severity.

99275   **Confirmatory consultation** for a new or established patient, which requires these three key components:

- **a comprehensive history;**
- **a comprehensive examination; and**
- **medical decision making of high complexity.**

Counseling and/or coordination of care with other providers or agencies are provided consistent with the nature of the problem(s) and the patient's and/or family's needs.

Usually, the presenting problem(s) are of moderate to high severity.

Emergency Department Services

New or Established Patient

The following codes are used to report evaluation and management services provided in the emergency department. No distinction is made between new and established patients in the emergency department.

An emergency department is defined as an organized hospital-based facility for the provision of unscheduled episodic services to patients who present for immediate medical attention. The facility must be available 24 hours a day.

For critical care services provided in the emergency department, see Critical Care notes and 99291, 99292.

For evaluation and management services provided to a patient in an observation area of a hospital, see 99217-99220.

For observation or inpatient care services (including admission and discharge services), see 99234-99236.

99281   **Emergency department visit** for the evaluation and management of a patient, which requires these three key components:

- **a problem focused history;**
- **a problem focused examination; and**
- **straightforward medical decision making.**

Counseling and/or coordination of care with other providers or agencies are provided consistent with the nature of the problem(s) and the patient's and/or family's needs.

Usually, the presenting problem(s) are self limited or minor.

99282   **Emergency department visit** for the evaluation and management of a patient, which requires these three key components:

- **an expanded problem focused history;**
- **an expanded problem focused examination; and**
- **medical decision making of low complexity.**

Counseling and/or coordination of care with other providers or agencies are provided consistent with the nature of the problem(s) and the patient's and/or family's needs.

Usually, the presenting problem(s) are of low to moderate severity.

99283   **Emergency department visit** for the evaluation and management of a patient, which requires these three key components:

- **an expanded problem focused history;**
- **an expanded problem focused examination; and**
- **medical decision making of moderate complexity.**

Counseling and/or coordination of care with other providers or agencies are provided consistent with the nature of the problem(s) and the patient's and/or family's needs.

Usually, the presenting problem(s) are of moderate severity.

99284   **Emergency department visit** for the evaluation and management of a patient, which requires these three key components:

- **a detailed history;**
- **a detailed examination; and**
- **medical decision making of moderate complexity.**

Counseling and/or coordination of care with other providers or agencies are provided consistent with the nature of the problem(s) and the patient's and/or family's needs.

Usually, the presenting problem(s) are of high severity, and require urgent evaluation by the physician but do not pose an immediate significant threat to life or physiologic function.

99285   **Emergency department visit** for the evaluation and management of a patient, which requires these three key components within the constraints imposed by the urgency of the patient's clinical condition and/or mental status:

- **a comprehensive history;**
- **a comprehensive examination; and**
- **medical decision making of high complexity.**

Counseling and/or coordination of care with other providers or agencies are provided consistent with the nature of the problem(s) and the patient's and/or family's needs.

Usually, the presenting problem(s) are of high severity and pose an immediate significant threat to life or physiologic function.

Other Emergency Services

In physician directed emergency care, advanced life support, the physician is located in a hospital emergency or critical care department, and is in two-way voice communication with ambulance or rescue personnel outside the hospital. The physician directs the performance of necessary medical procedures, including but not limited to: telemetry of cardiac rhythm; cardiac and/or pulmonary resuscitation; endotracheal or esophageal obturator airway intubation; administration of intravenous fluids and/or administration of intramuscular, intratracheal or subcutaneous drugs; and/or electrical conversion of arrhythmia.

99288 **Physician direction of** emergency medical systems (EMS) emergency care, advanced life support

►Pediatric Critical Care◄ Patient Transport

The following codes 99289 and 99290 are used to report the physical attendance and direct face-to-face care by a physician during the interfacility transport of a critically ill or ►critically◄ injured ►pediatric◄ patient. For the purpose of reporting codes 99289 and 99290, face-to-face care begins when the physician assumes primary responsibility of the ►pediatric◄ patient at the referring hospital/facility, and ends when the receiving hospital/facility accepts responsibility for the ►pediatric◄ patient's care. Only the time the physician spends in direct face-to-face contact with the patient during the transport should be reported. ►Pediatric◄ patient transport services involving less than 30 minutes of face-to-face physician care should not be reported using codes 99289, 99290. Procedure(s) or service(s) performed by other members of the transporting team may not be reported by the supervising physician.

►The following services are included when performed during the pediatric patient transport by the physician providing critical care and may not be reported separately: routine monitoring evaluations (eg, heart rate, respiratory rate, blood pressure, and pulse oximetry), the interpretation of cardiac output measurements (93561, 93562), chest x-rays (71010, 71015, 71020), pulse oximetry (94760, 94761, 94762), blood gases and information data stored in computers (eg, ECGs, blood pressures, hematologic data) (99090), gastric intubation (43752, 91105), temporary transcutaneous pacing (92953), ventilatory management (94656, 94660, 94662) and vascular access procedures (36000, 36400, 36405, 36406, 36410, 36415, 36540, 36600). Any services performed which are not listed above should be reported separately.

Critical care is the direct delivery by a physician(s) of medical care for a critically ill or critically injured patient. A critical illness or injury acutely impairs one or more

vital organ systems such that there is a high probability of imminent or life threatening deterioration in the patient's condition. Critical care involves high complexity decision making to assess, manipulate, and support vital system function(s) to treat single or multiple vital organ system failure and/or to prevent further life threatening deterioration of the patient's condition. Examples of vital organ system failure include, but are not limited to: central nervous system failure, circulatory failure, shock, renal, hepatic, metabolic, and/or respiratory failure.

Providing medical care to a critically ill, injured, or post-operative patient qualifies as a critical care service only if both the illness or injury and the treatment being provided meet the above requirements.◄

The direction of emergency care to transporting staff by a physician located in a hospital or other facility by two-way communication is not considered direct face-to-face care and should not be reported with codes 99289, 99290. Physician directed emergency care through outside voice communication to transporting staff personnel is reported with code 99288.

The emergency department services codes (99281-99285), initial hospital care codes (99221-99223), hourly critical care codes (99291, 99292), or initial date neonatal intensive care code (99295) are only reported after the patient has been admitted to the emergency department, the inpatient floor or the critical care unit of the receiving facility.

Code 99289 is used to report the first 30-74 minutes of direct face-to-face time with the transport ►pediatric◄ patient and should be reported only once on a given date. Code 99290 is used to report each additional 30 minutes provided on a given date. Face-to-face services less than 30 minutes should not be reported with these codes.

▲ **99289** Critical care services delivered by a physician, face-to-face, during an interfacility transport of critically ill or critically injured pediatric patient, 24 months of age or less; first 30-74 minutes of hands on care during transport

✛ **99290** each additional 30 minutes (List separately in addition to code for primary service)

(Use 99290 in conjunction with 99289)

►(Critical care of less than 30 minutes total duration should be reported with the appropriate E/M code)◄

Critical Care Services

Critical care is the direct delivery by a physician(s) of medical care for a critically ill or critically injured patient. A critical illness or injury acutely impairs one or more vital organ systems such that there is a high probability of imminent or life threatening deterioration in the patient's condition. Critical care involves high complexity decision making to assess, manipulate, and support vital system function(s) to treat single or multiple vital organ system failure and/or to prevent further life threatening deterioration of the patient's condition. Examples of vital organ system failure include, but are not limited to: central nervous system failure, circulatory failure, shock, renal, hepatic, metabolic, and/or respiratory failure. Although critical care typically requires interpretation of multiple physiologic parameters and/or application of advanced technology(s), critical care may be provided in life threatening situations when these elements are not present. Critical care may be provided on multiple days, even if no changes are made in the treatment rendered to the patient, provided that the patient's condition continues to require the level of physician attention described above.

Providing medical care to a critically ill, injured, or post-operative patient qualifies as a critical care service only if both the illness or injury and the treatment being provided meet the above requirements. Critical care is usually, but not always, given in a critical care area, such as the coronary care unit, intensive care unit, pediatric intensive care unit, respiratory care unit, or the emergency care facility.

Critical care services provided to infants ▶31 days up through 24 months of age◀ are reported with ▶pediatric critical care codes 99293 and 99294. The pediatric critical care codes are reported as long as the infant/young child qualifies for critical care services during the hospital stay.◀ Critical care services provided to neonates (30 days of age or less) are reported with the neonatal critical care codes 99295 ▶and◀ 99296. The neonatal critical care codes are reported as long as the neonate qualifies for critical care services ▶through the 30th postnatal day.◀ The reporting of ▶the pediatric and◀ neonatal critical care services is not based on time ▶or◀ the type of unit (eg, pediatric or neonatal critical care unit) ▶and it is not dependent upon◀ the type of provider delivering the care. For additional instructions on reporting these services, see the Neonatal ▶and Pediatric Critical Care◀ section and codes ▶99293-99296.◀

Services for a patient who is not critically ill but happens to be in a critical care unit are reported using other appropriate E/M codes.

Critical care and other E/M services may be provided to the same patient on the same date by the same physician.

The following services are included in reporting critical care when performed during the critical period by the physician(s) providing critical care: the interpretation of cardiac output measurements (93561, 93562), chest x-rays (71010, 71015, 71020), pulse oximetry (94760, 94761, 94762), blood gases, and information data stored in computers (eg, ECGs, blood pressures, hematologic data (99090)); gastric intubation (43752, 91105); temporary transcutaneous pacing (92953); ventilatory management (94656, 94657, 94660, 94662); and

vascular access procedures (36000, 36410, 36415, 36540, 36600). Any services performed which are not listed above should be reported separately.

Codes 99291-99292 should be reported for the physician's attendance during the transport of critically ill or ▶critically◀ injured patients ▶over 24 months of age◀ to or from a facility or hospital. ▶For◀ physician transport services of critically ill or ▶critically◀ injured ▶pediatric◀ patients ▶24 months of age or less◀ see 99289, 99290.

The critical care codes 99291 and 99292 are used to report the total duration of time spent by a physician providing critical care services to a critically ill or critically injured patient, even if the time spent by the physician on that date is not continuous. For any given period of time spent providing critical care services, the physician must devote his or her full attention to the patient and, therefore, cannot provide services to any other patient during the same period of time.

Time spent with the individual patient should be recorded in the patient's record. The time that can be reported as critical care is the time spent engaged in work directly related to the individual patient's care whether that time was spent at the immediate bedside or elsewhere on the floor or unit. For example, time spent on the unit or at the nursing station on the floor reviewing test results or imaging studies, discussing the critically ill patient's care with other medical staff or documenting critical care services in the medical record would be reported as critical care, even though it does not occur at the bedside. Also, when the patient is unable or clinically incompetent to participate in discussions, time spent on the floor or unit with family members or surrogate decision makers obtaining a medical history, reviewing the patient's condition or prognosis, or discussing treatment or limitation(s) of treatment may be reported as critical care, provided that the conversation bears directly on the management of the patient.

Time spent in activities that occur outside of the unit or off the floor (eg, telephone calls, whether taken at home, in the office, or elsewhere in the hospital) may not be reported as critical care since the physician is not immediately available to the patient. Time spent in activities that do not directly contribute to the treatment of the patient may not be reported as critical care, even if they are performed in the critical care unit (eg, participation in administrative meetings or telephone calls to discuss other patients). Time spent performing separately reportable procedures or services should not be included in the time reported as critical care time.

Code 99291 is used to report the first 30-74 minutes of critical care on a given date. It should be used only once per date even if the time spent by the physician is not continuous on that date. Critical care of less than 30 minutes total duration on a given date should be reported with the appropriate E/M code.

Evaluation and Management

Code 99292 is used to report additional block(s) of time, of up to 30 minutes each beyond the first 74 minutes. (See table below.)

The following examples illustrate the correct reporting of critical care services:

Total Duration of Critical Care	Codes
less than 30 minutes (less than 1/2 hour)	appropriate E/M codes
30-74 minutes (1/2 hr. - 1 hr. 14 min.)	99291 X 1
75-104 minutes (1 hr. 15 min. - 1 hr. 44 min.)	99291 X 1 AND 99292 X 1
105-134 minutes (1 hr. 45 min. - 2 hr. 14 min.)	99291 X 1 AND 99292 X 2
135 - 164 minutes (2 hr. 15 min. - 2 hr. 44 min.)	99291 X 1 AND 99292 X 3
165 - 194 minutes (2 hr. 45 min. - 3 hr. 14 min.)	99291 X 1 AND 99292 X 4
194 minutes or longer (3 hr. 14 min. - etc.)	99291 and 99292 as appropriate (see illustrated reporting examples above)

99291   **Critical care, evaluation and management** of the critically ill or critically injured patient; first 30-74 minutes

+ 99292   each additional 30 minutes (List separately in addition to code for primary service)

(Use 99292 in conjunction with 99291)

Neonatal and Pediatric Critical Care Services

The following codes ▶(99293-99296)◀ are used to report services provided by a physician directing the care of a critically ill ▶neonate/infant. The same definitions for critical care services apply for the adult, child, and neonate.◀

▶The initial day◀ neonatal critical care code ▶(99295) can◀ be used in addition to codes 99360, 99436 or 99440 as appropriate, when the physician is present for the delivery and newborn resuscitation is required. ▶Other procedures performed as a necessary part of the resuscitation (eg, endotracheal intubation) are also reported separately.◀

▶Codes 99295, 99296 are used to report services provided by a physician directing the care of a critically ill neonate through the first 30 days of life. They represent care starting with the date of admission (99295) and subsequent day(s) (99296) and may be reported only once per day, per patient. Once the neonate is no longer considered to be critically ill, the Intensive Low Birth Weight Services codes for those with present body weight of less than 2500 grams (99298, 99299) or the codes for Subsequent Hospital Care (99231-99233) for those with present body weight over 2500 grams should be utilized.◀

▶Codes 99293, 99294 are used to report services provided by a physician directing the care of a critically ill infant or young child from 31 days of postnatal age up through 24 months of age. They represent care starting with the date of admission (99293) and subsequent day(s) (99294) and may be reported by a single physician only once per day, per patient in a given setting. The critically ill or critically injured child older than two years when admitted to an intensive care unit would be reported with hourly critical care service codes (99291, 99292). Once an infant is no longer considered to be critically ill but continues to require intensive care, the Intensive Low Birth Weight Services codes (99298, 99299) should be used to report services for infants with present body weight of less than 2500 grams. When the present body weight of those infants exceeds 2500 grams, the Subsequent Hospital Care (99231-99233) codes should be utilized.◀

Care rendered ▶under 99293-99296◀ includes management, monitoring, and treatment of the patient including ▶respiratory, pharmacologic control of the circulatory system,◀ enteral and parenteral nutrition, metabolic and hematologic maintenance, parent/ ▶family◀ counseling, case management services, and personal direct supervision of the health care team in the performance of cognitive and procedural activities.

▶The pediatric and neonatal critical care codes include those procedures◀ listed above for ▶the◀ hourly ▶critical care◀ codes ▶(99291, 99292). In addition,◀ the following procedures are also included in the bundled (global) ▶pediatric and◀ neonatal ▶critical care service◀ codes ▶(99293-99296):◀ umbilical venous (36510) and umbilical arterial ▶(36660)◀ catheters, central (36488, 36490) or peripheral vessel catheterization (36000), other arterial catheters (36140, 36620), oral or nasogastric tube placement ▶(43752),◀ endotracheal intubation (31500), lumbar puncture (62270), suprapubic bladder aspiration (51000), bladder catheterization (53670), initiation and management of mechanical ventilation (94656, 94657) or continuous positive airway pressure (CPAP) (94660), surfactant administration, intravascular fluid administration ▶(90780, 90781)◀, transfusion of blood components (36430, 36440), vascular punctures (36420, 36600), invasive or non-invasive electronic monitoring of vital signs, bedside pulmonary function testing ►(94375)◄, and/or monitoring or interpretation of blood gases or oxygen saturation (94760-94762). Any services performed which are not listed above should be reported separately.

For additional instructions, see descriptions listed for 99293-►99296◄

►Pediatric Critical Care◄

● **99293**   **Initial pediatric critical care,** 31 days up through 24 months of age, per day, for the evaluation and management of a critically ill infant or young child

● **99294**   **Subsequent pediatric critical care,** 31 days up through 24 months of age, per day, for the evaluation and management of a critically ill infant or young child

►Neonatal Critical Care◄

▲ **99295**   **Initial neonatal critical care,** per day, for the evaluation and management of a critically ill neonate, 30 days of age or less

This code is reserved for the date of admission for neonates who are critically ill. Critically ill neonates require cardiac and/or respiratory support (including ventilator or nasal CPAP when indicated), continuous or frequent vital sign monitoring, laboratory and blood gas interpretations, follow-up physician reevaluations, and constant observation by the health care team under direct physician supervision. Immediate preoperative evaluation and stabilization of neonates with life threatening surgical or cardiac conditions are included under this code. ►Neonates with life threatening surgical or cardiac conditions are included under this code.◄

►Care for neonates who require an intensive care setting but who are not critically ill is reported using the initial hospital care codes (99221-99223).◄

▲ **99296**   **Subsequent neonatal critical care,** per day, for the evaluation and management of a critically ill neonate, 30 days of age or less

A critically ill neonate will require cardiac and/or respiratory support (including ventilator or nasal CPAP when indicated), continuous or frequent vital sign monitoring, laboratory and blood gas interpretations, follow-up physician re-evaluations throughout a 24-hour period, and constant observation by the health care team under direct physician supervision.

►(99297 has been deleted. To report, use 99296)◄

►Intensive (Non-Critical) Low Birth Weight Services◄

►Codes 99298-99299 are used to report services subsequent to the day of admission provided by a physician directing the continuing intensive care of the low birth weight (LBW) or very low birth weight (VLBW) infant who no longer meets the definition of critically ill. They represent subsequent day(s) of care and may be reported only once per day, per patient. Low birth weight services are reported for those neonates less than 2500 grams who do not meet the definition of critical care but continue to require intensive observation and frequent services and interventions only available in an intensive care setting. The level and frequency of services required for the LBW and the VLBW infant exceed those available in less intensive hospital areas or medical floors. Codes 99298-99299 are global 24-hour codes with the same services bundled as outlined under codes 99293-99296.◄

►For additional instructions, see descriptions listed for 99298-99299.◄

▲ **99298**   **Subsequent intensive care,** per day, for the evaluation and management of the recovering very low birth weight infant (present body weight less than 1500 grams)

►Infants with present body weight less than 1500 grams◄ who are no longer critically ill continue to require intensive cardiac and respiratory monitoring, continuous and/or frequent vital sign monitoring, heat maintenance, enteral and/or parenteral nutritional adjustments, laboratory and oxygen monitoring and constant observation by the health care team under direct physician supervision.

● **99299**   **Subsequent intensive care,** per day, for the evaluation and management of the recovering low birth weight infant (present body weight of 1500-2500 grams)

Infants with present body weight of 1500-2500 grams who are no longer critically ill continue to require intensive cardiac and respiratory monitoring, continuous and/or frequent vital sign monitoring, heat maintenance, enteral and/or parenteral nutritional adjustments, laboratory and oxygen monitoring, and constant observation by the health care team under direct physician supervision.

Nursing Facility Services

The following codes are used to report evaluation and management services to patients in Nursing Facilities (formerly called Skilled Nursing Facilities (SNFs), Intermediate Care Facilities (ICFs) or Long Term Care Facilities (LTCFs)).

These codes should also be used to report evaluation and management services provided to a patient in a psychiatric residential treatment center (a facility or a distinct part of a facility for psychiatric care, which provides a 24-hour therapeutically planned and professionally staffed group living and learning environment). If procedures such as medical psychotherapy are provided in addition to evaluation and management services, these should be reported in addition to the evaluation and management services provided.

Nursing facilities that provide convalescent, rehabilitative, or long term care are required to conduct comprehensive, accurate, standardized, and reproducible assessments of each resident's functional capacity using a Resident Assessment Instrument (RAI). All RAIs include the Minimum Data Set (MDS), Resident Assessment Protocols (RAPs) and utilization guidelines. The MDS is the primary screening and assessment tool; the RAPs trigger the identification of potential problems and provide guidelines for follow-up assessments.

Physicians have a central role in assuring that all residents receive thorough assessments and that medical plans of care are instituted or revised to enhance or maintain the residents' physical and psychosocial functioning.

Two subcategories of nursing facility services are recognized: Comprehensive Nursing Facility Assessments and Subsequent Nursing Facility Care. Both subcategories apply to new or established patients. Comprehensive Assessments may be performed at one or more sites in the assessment process: the hospital, observation unit, office, nursing facility, domiciliary/non-nursing facility or patient's home.

For definitions of key components and commonly used terms, please see **Evaluation and Management Services Guidelines.**

Comprehensive Nursing Facility Assessments

New or Established Patient

When the patient is admitted to the nursing facility in the course of an encounter in another site of service (eg, hospital emergency department, physician's office), all evaluation and management services provided by that physician in conjunction with that admission are considered part of the initial nursing facility care when performed on the same date as the admission or readmission. The nursing facility care level of service reported by the admitting physician should include the services related to the admission he/she provided in the other sites of service as well as in the nursing facility setting.

Hospital discharge or observation discharge services performed on the same date of nursing facility admission or readmission may be reported separately. For a patient discharged from inpatient status on the same date of nursing facility admission or readmission, the hospital discharge services should be reported with codes 99238-99239 as appropriate. For a patient discharged from observation status on the same date of nursing facility admission or readmission, the observation care discharge services should be reported with code 99217. For a patient admitted and discharged from observation or inpatient status on the same date, see codes 99234-99236.

(For nursing facility care discharge, see 99315, 99316)

More than one comprehensive assessment may be necessary during an inpatient confinement.

99301   **Evaluation and management** of a new or established patient involving an annual nursing facility assessment which requires these three key components:

- **a detailed interval history;**
- **a comprehensive examination; and**
- **medical decision making that is straightforward or of low complexity.**

Counseling and/or coordination of care with other providers or agencies are provided consistent with the nature of the problem(s) and the patient's and/or family's needs.

Usually, the patient is stable, recovering or improving. The review and affirmation of the medical plan of care is required. Physicians typically spend 30 minutes at the bedside and on the patient's facility floor or unit.

99302   **Evaluation and management** of a new or established patient involving a nursing facility assessment which requires these three key components:

- **a detailed interval history;**
- **a comprehensive examination; and**
- **medical decision making of moderate to high complexity.**

Counseling and/or coordination of care with other providers or agencies are provided consistent with the nature of the problem(s) and the patient's and/or family's needs.

Usually, the patient has developed a significant complication or a significant new problem and has had a major permanent change in status.

The creation of a new medical plan of care is required. Physicians typically spend 40 minutes at the bedside and on the patient's facility floor or unit.

99303 **Evaluation and management** of a new or established patient involving a nursing facility assessment at the time of initial admission or readmission to the facility, which requires these three key components:

- **a comprehensive history;**
- **a comprehensive examination; and**
- **medical decision making of moderate to high complexity.**

Counseling and/or coordination of care with other providers or agencies are provided consistent with the nature of the problem(s) and the patient's and/or family's needs.

The creation of a medical plan of care is required. Physicians typically spend 50 minutes at the bedside and on the patient's facility floor or unit.

Subsequent Nursing Facility Care

New or Established Patient

The following codes are used to report the services provided to residents of nursing facilities who do not require a comprehensive assessment, and/or who have not had a major, permanent change of status.

All levels include reviewing the medical record, noting changes in the resident's status since the last visit, and reviewing and signing orders.

99311 **Subsequent nursing facility care,** per day, for the evaluation and management of a new or established patient, which requires at least two of these three key components:

- **a problem focused interval history;**
- **a problem focused examination;**
- **medical decision making that is straightforward or of low complexity.**

Counseling and/or coordination of care with other providers or agencies are provided consistent with the nature of the problem(s) and the patient's and/or family's needs.

Usually, the patient is stable, recovering or improving. Physicians typically spend 15 minutes at the bedside and on the patient's facility floor or unit.

99312 **Subsequent nursing facility care,** per day, for the evaluation and management of a new or established patient, which requires at least two of these three key components:

- **an expanded problem focused interval history;**
- **an expanded problem focused examination;**
- **medical decision making of moderate complexity.**

Counseling and/or coordination of care with other providers or agencies are provided consistent with the nature of the problem(s) and the patient's and/or family's needs.

Usually, the patient is responding inadequately to therapy or has developed a minor complication. Physicians typically spend 25 minutes at the bedside and on the patient's facility floor or unit.

99313 **Subsequent nursing facility care,** per day, for the evaluation and management of a new or established patient, which requires at least two of these three key components:

- **a detailed interval history;**
- **a detailed examination;**
- **medical decision making of moderate to high complexity.**

Counseling and/or coordination of care with other providers or agencies are provided consistent with the nature of the problem(s) and the patient's and/or family's needs.

Usually, the patient has developed a significant complication or a significant new problem. Physicians typically spend 35 minutes at the bedside and on the patient's facility floor or unit.

Nursing Facility Discharge Services

The nursing facility discharge day management codes are to be used to report the total duration of time spent by a physician for the final nursing facility discharge of a patient. The codes include, as appropriate, final examination of the patient, discussion of the nursing facility stay, even if the time spent by the physician on that date is not continuous. Instructions are given for continuing care to all relevant caregivers, and preparation of discharge records, prescriptions and referral forms.

99315 Nursing facility discharge day management; 30 minutes or less

99316 more than 30 minutes

Domiciliary, Rest Home (eg, Boarding Home), or Custodial Care Services

The following codes are used to report evaluation and management services in a facility which provides room, board and other personal assistance services, generally on a long-term basis. The facility's services do not include a medical component.

For definitions of key components and commonly used terms, please see **Evaluation and Management Services Guidelines.**

Typical times have not yet been established for this category of services.

Evaluation and Management

New Patient

99321 **Domiciliary or rest home visit** for the evaluation and management of a new patient which requires these three key components:

- **a problem focused history;**
- **a problem focused examination; and**
- **medical decision making that is straightforward or of low complexity.**

Counseling and/or coordination of care with other providers or agencies are provided consistent with the nature of the problem(s) and the patient's and/or family's needs.

Usually, the presenting problem(s) are of low severity.

99322 **Domiciliary or rest home visit** for the evaluation and management of a new patient, which requires these three key components:

- **an expanded problem focused history;**
- **an expanded problem focused examination; and**
- **medical decision making of moderate complexity.**

Counseling and/or coordination of care with other providers or agencies are provided consistent with the nature of the problem(s) and the patient's and/or family's needs.

Usually, the presenting problem(s) are of moderate severity.

99323 **Domiciliary or rest home visit** for the evaluation and management of a new patient, which requires these three key components:

- **a detailed history;**
- **a detailed examination; and**
- **medical decision making of high complexity.**

Counseling and/or coordination of care with other providers or agencies are provided consistent with the nature of the problem(s) and the patient's and/or family's needs.

Usually, the presenting problem(s) are of high complexity.

Established Patient

99331 **Domiciliary or rest home visit** for the evaluation and management of an established patient, which requires at least two of these three key components:

- **a problem focused interval history;**
- **a problem focused examination;**
- **medical decision making that is straightforward or of low complexity.**

Counseling and/or coordination of care with other providers or agencies are provided consistent with the nature of the problem(s) and the patient's and/or family's needs.

Usually, the patient is stable, recovering or improving.

99332 **Domiciliary or rest home visit** for the evaluation and management of an established patient, which requires at least two of these three key components:

- **an expanded problem focused interval history;**
- **an expanded problem focused examination;**
- **medical decision making of moderate complexity.**

Counseling and/or coordination of care with other providers or agencies are provided consistent with the nature of the problem(s) and the patient's and/or family's needs.

Usually, the patient is responding inadequately to therapy or has developed a minor complication.

99333 **Domiciliary or rest home visit** for the evaluation and management of an established patient, which requires at least two of these three key components:

- **a detailed interval history;**
- **a detailed examination;**
- **medical decision making of high complexity.**

Counseling and/or coordination of care with other providers or agencies are provided consistent with the nature of the problem(s) and the patient's and/or family's needs.

Usually, the patient is unstable or has developed a significant complication or a significant new problem.

Home Services

The following codes are used to report evaluation and management services provided in a private residence.

For definitions of key components and commonly used terms, please see **Evaluation and Management Services Guidelines.**

New Patient

99341 **Home visit** for the evaluation and management of a new patient, which requires these three key components:

- **a problem focused history;**
- **a problem focused examination; and**
- **straightforward medical decision making.**

Counseling and/or coordination of care with other providers or agencies are provided consistent with the nature of the problem(s) and the patient's and/or family's needs.

Usually, the presenting problem(s) are of low severity. Physicians typically spend 20 minutes face-to-face with the patient and/or family.

99342   **Home visit** for the evaluation and management of a new patient, which requires these three key components:

- **an expanded problem focused history;**
- **an expanded problem focused examination; and**
- **medical decision making of low complexity.**

Counseling and/or coordination of care with other providers or agencies are provided consistent with the nature of the problem(s) and the patient's and/or family's needs.

Usually, the presenting problem(s) are of moderate severity. Physicians typically spend 30 minutes face-to-face with the patient and/or family.

99343   **Home visit** for the evaluation and management of a new patient, which requires these three key components:

- **a detailed history;**
- **a detailed examination; and**
- **medical decision making of moderate complexity.**

Counseling and/or coordination of care with other providers or agencies are provided consistent with the nature of the problem(s) and the patient's and/or family's needs.

Usually, the presenting problem(s) are of moderate to high severity. Physicians typically spend 45 minutes face-to-face with the patient and/or family.

99344   **Home visit** for the evaluation and management of a new patient, which requires these three components:

- **a comprehensive history;**
- **a comprehensive examination; and**
- **medical decision making of moderate complexity.**

Counseling and/or coordination of care with other providers or agencies are provided consistent with the nature of the problem(s) and the patient's and/or family's needs.

Usually, the presenting problem(s) are of high severity. Physicians typically spend 60 minutes face-to-face with the patient and/or family.

99345   **Home visit** for the evaluation and management of a new patient, which requires these three key components:

- **a comprehensive history;**
- **a comprehensive examination; and**
- **medical decision making of high complexity.**

Counseling and/or coordination of care with other providers or agencies are provided consistent with the nature of the problem(s) and the patient's and/or family's needs.

Usually, the patient is unstable or has developed a significant new problem requiring immediate physician attention. Physicians typically spend 75 minutes face-to-face with the patient and/or family.

Established Patient

99347   **Home visit** for the evaluation and management of an established patient, which requires at least two of these three key components:

- **a problem focused interval history;**
- **a problem focused examination;**
- **straightforward medical decision making.**

Counseling and/or coordination of care with other providers or agencies are provided consistent with the nature of the problem(s) and the patient's and/or family's needs.

Usually, the presenting problem(s) are self limited or minor. Physicians typically spend 15 minutes face-to-face with the patient and/or family.

99348   **Home visit** for the evaluation and management of an established patient, which requires at least two of these three key components:

- **an expanded problem focused interval history;**
- **an expanded problem focused examination;**
- **medical decision making of low complexity.**

Counseling and/or coordination of care with other providers or agencies are provided consistent with the nature of the problem(s) and the patient's and/or family's needs.

Usually, the presenting problem(s) are of low to moderate severity. Physicians typically spend 25 minutes face-to-face with the patient and/or family.

99349   **Home visit** for the evaluation and management of an established patient, which requires at least two of these three key components:

- **a detailed interval history;**
- **a detailed examination;**
- **medical decision making of moderate complexity.**

Counseling and/or coordination of care with other providers or agencies are provided consistent with the nature of the problem(s) and the patient's and/or family's needs.

Usually, the presenting problem(s) are moderate to high severity. Physicians typically spend 40 minutes face-to-face with the patient and/or family.

99350   **Home visit** for the evaluation and management of an established patient, which requires at least two of these three key components:

- **a comprehensive interval history;**
- **a comprehensive examination;**
- **medical decision making of moderate to high complexity.**

Counseling and/or coordination of care with other providers or agencies are provided consistent with the nature of the problem(s) and the patient's and/or family's needs.

Evaluation and Management

Usually, the presenting problem(s) are of moderate to high severity. The patient may be unstable or may have developed a significant new problem requiring immediate physician attention. Physicians typically spend 60 minutes face-to-face with the patient and/or family.

(99351 has been deleted. To report, use 99347)

(99352 has been deleted. To report, use 99348)

(99353 has been deleted. To report, use 99349)

Prolonged Services

Prolonged Physician Service With Direct (Face-To-Face) Patient Contact

Codes 99354-99357 are used when a physician provides prolonged service involving direct (face-to-face) patient contact that is beyond the usual service in either the inpatient or outpatient setting. This service is reported in addition to other physician services, including evaluation and management services at any level. Appropriate codes should be selected for supplies provided or procedures performed in the care of the patient during this period.

Codes 99354-99357 are used to report the total duration of face-to-face time spent by a physician on a given date providing prolonged service, even if the time spent by the physician on that date is not continuous.

Code 99354 or 99356 is used to report the first hour of prolonged service on a given date, depending on the place of service.

Either code also may be used to report a total duration of prolonged service of 30-60 minutes on a given date. Either code should be used only once per date, even if the time spent by the physician is not continuous on that date. Prolonged service of less than 30 minutes total duration on a given date is not separately reported because the work involved is included in the total work of the evaluation and management codes.

Code 99355 or 99357 is used to report each additional 30 minutes beyond the first hour, depending on the place of service. Either code may also be used to report the final 15-30 minutes of prolonged service on a given date. Prolonged service of less than 15 minutes beyond the first hour or less than 15 minutes beyond the final 30 minutes is not reported separately.

The following examples illustrate the correct reporting of prolonged physician service with direct patient contact in the office setting:

Total Duration of Prolonged Services	Code(s)
less than 30 minutes (less than 1/2 hour)	Not reported separately
30-74 minutes (1/2 hr. - 1 hr. 14 min.)	99354 X 1
75-104 minutes (1 hr. 15 min. - 1 hr. 44 min.)	99354 X 1 AND 99355 X 1
105-134 minutes (1 hr. 45 min. - 2 hr. 14 min.)	99354 X 1 AND 99355 X 2
135-164 minutes (2 hr. 15 min. - 2 hr. 44 min.)	99354 X 1 AND 99355 X 3
165-194 minutes (2 hr. 45 min. - 3 hr. 14 min.)	99354 X 1 AND 99355 X 4

+ **99354** Prolonged physician service in the office or other outpatient setting requiring direct (face-to-face) patient contact beyond the usual service (eg, prolonged care and treatment of an acute asthmatic patient in an outpatient setting); first hour (List separately in addition to code for office or other outpatient Evaluation and Management service)

(Use 99354 in conjunction with codes 99201-99215, 99241-99245, 99301-99350)

+ **99355** each additional 30 minutes (List separately in addition to code for prolonged physician service)

(Use 99355 in conjunction with codes 99354)

+ **99356** Prolonged physician service in the inpatient setting, requiring direct (face-to-face) patient contact beyond the usual service (eg, maternal fetal monitoring for high risk delivery or other physiological monitoring, prolonged care of an acutely ill inpatient); first hour (List separately in addition to code for inpatient Evaluation and Management service)

(Use 99356 in conjunction with codes 99221-99233, 99251-99255, 99261-99263)

+ **99357** each additional 30 minutes (List separately in addition to code for prolonged physician service)

(Use 99357 in conjunction with code 99356)

Prolonged Physician Service Without Direct (Face-To-Face) Patient Contact

Codes 99358 and 99359 are used when a physician provides prolonged service not involving direct (face-to-face) care that is beyond the usual service in either the inpatient or outpatient setting.

This service is to be reported in addition to other physician service, including evaluation and management services at any level.

Codes 99358 and 99359 are used to report the total duration of non-face-to-face time spent by a physician on a given date providing prolonged service, even if the time spent by the physician on that date is not continuous. Code 99358 is used to report the first hour of prolonged service on a given date regardless of the place of service.

It may also be used to report a total duration of prolonged service of 30-60 minutes on a given date. It should be used only once per date even if the time spent by the physician is not continuous on that date.

Prolonged service of less than 30 minutes total duration on a given date is not separately reported.

Code 99359 is used to report each additional 30 minutes beyond the first hour regardless of the place of service. It may also be used to report the final 15-30 minutes of prolonged service on a given date.

Prolonged service of less than 15 minutes beyond the first hour or less than 15 minutes beyond the final 30 minutes is not reported separately.

+ **99358**   **Prolonged evaluation and management service** before and/or after direct (face-to-face) patient care (eg, review of extensive records and tests, communication with other professionals and/or the patient/family); first hour (List separately in addition to code(s) for other physician service(s) and/or inpatient or outpatient Evaluation and Management service)

+ **99359**   each additional 30 minutes (List separately in addition to code for prolonged physician service)

(Use 99359 in conjunction with code 99358)

(To report telephone calls, see 99371-99373)

Physician Standby Services

Code 99360 is used to report physician standby service that is requested by another physician and that involves prolonged physician attendance without direct (face-to-face) patient contact. The physician may not be providing care or services to other patients during this period. This code is not used to report time spent proctoring another physician. It is also not used if the period of standby ends with the performance of a procedure subject to a "surgical" package by the physician who was on standby.

Code 99360 is used to report the total duration of time spent by a physician on a given date on standby. Standby service of less than 30 minutes total duration on a given date is not reported separately.

Second and subsequent periods of standby beyond the first 30 minutes may be reported only if a full 30 minutes of standby was provided for each unit of service reported.

99360   **Physician standby service,** requiring prolonged physician attendance, each 30 minutes (eg, operative standby, standby for frozen section, for cesarean/high risk delivery, for monitoring EEG)

▶(For hospital mandated on call services, see 99026, 99027)◀

(99360 may be reported in addition to 99431, 99440 as appropriate)

(99360 may not be reported in addition to 99436)

Case Management Services

Physician case management is a process in which a physician is responsible for direct care of a patient, and for coordinating and controlling access to or initiating and/or supervising other health care services needed by the patient.

Team Conferences

99361   **Medical conference** by a physician with interdisciplinary team of health professionals or representatives of community agencies to coordinate activities of patient care (patient not present); approximately 30 minutes

99362   approximately 60 minutes

Telephone Calls

99371   **Telephone call** by a physician to patient or for consultation or medical management or for coordinating medical management with other health care professionals (eg, nurses, therapists, social workers, nutritionists, physicians, pharmacists); simple or brief (eg, to report on tests and/or laboratory results, to clarify or alter previous instructions, to integrate new information from other health professionals into the medical treatment plan, or to adjust therapy)

99372   intermediate (eg, to provide advice to an established patient on a new problem, to initiate therapy that can be handled by telephone, to discuss test results in detail, to coordinate medical management of a new problem in an established patient, to discuss and evaluate new information and details, or to initiate new plan of care)

99373   complex or lengthy (eg, lengthy counseling session with anxious or distraught patient, detailed or prolonged discussion with family members regarding seriously ill patient, lengthy communication necessary to coordinate complex services of several different health professionals working on different aspects of the total patient care plan)

Care Plan Oversight Services

Care Plan Oversight Services are reported separately from codes for office/outpatient, hospital, home, nursing facility or domiciliary services. The complexity and approximate physician time of the care plan oversight services provided within a 30-day period determine code selection. Only one physician may report services for a given period of time, to reflect that physician's sole or predominant supervisory role with a particular patient. These codes should not be reported for supervision of patients in nursing facilities or under the care of home health agencies unless they require recurrent supervision of therapy.

The work involved in providing very low intensity or infrequent supervision services is included in the pre- and post-encounter work for home, office/outpatient and nursing facility or domiciliary visit codes.

99374 **Physician supervision** of a patient under care of home health agency (patient not present) in home, domiciliary or equivalent environment (eg, Alzheimer's facility) requiring complex and multidisciplinary care modalities involving regular physician development and/or revision of care plans, review of subsequent reports of patient status, review of related laboratory and other studies, communication (including telephone calls) for purposes of assessment or care decisions with health care professional(s), family member(s), surrogate decision maker(s) (eg, legal guardian) and/or key caregiver(s) involved in patient's care, integration of new information into the medical treatment plan and/or adjustment of medical therapy, within a calendar month; 15-29 minutes

99375 30 minutes or more

(99376 has been deleted. To report, see 99375, 99378, 99380)

99377 **Physician supervision** of a hospice patient (patient not present) requiring complex and multidisciplinary care modalities involving regular physician development and/or revision of care plans, review of subsequent reports of patient status, review of related laboratory and other studies, communication (including telephone calls) for purposes of assessment or care decisions with health care professional(s), family member(s), surrogate decision maker(s) (eg, legal guardian) and/or key caregiver(s) involved in patient's care, integration of new information into the medical treatment plan and/or adjustment of medical therapy, within a calendar month; 15-29 minutes

99378 30 minutes or more

99379 **Physician supervision** of a nursing facility patient (patient not present) requiring complex and multidisciplinary care modalities involving regular physician development and/or revision of care plans, review of subsequent reports of patient status, review of related laboratory and other studies, communication (including telephone calls) for purposes of assessment or care decisions with health care professional(s), family member(s), surrogate decision maker(s) (eg, legal guardian) and/or key caregiver(s) involved in patient's care, integration of new information into the medical treatment plan and/or adjustment of medical therapy, within a calendar month; 15-29 minutes

99380 30 minutes or more

Preventive Medicine Services

The following codes are used to report the preventive medicine evaluation and management of infants, children, adolescents and adults.

The extent and focus of the services will largely depend on the age of the patient.

If an abnormality/ies is encountered or a preexisting problem is addressed in the process of performing this preventive medicine evaluation and management service, and if the problem/abnormality is significant enough to require additional work to perform the key components of a problem-oriented E/M service, then the appropriate Office/Outpatient code 99201-99215 should also be reported. Modifier '-25' should be added to the Office/Outpatient code to indicate that a significant, separately identifiable Evaluation and Management service was provided by the same physician on the same day as the preventive medicine service. The appropriate preventive medicine service is additionally reported.

An insignificant or trivial problem/abnormality that is encountered in the process of performing the preventive medicine evaluation and management service and which does not require additional work and the performance of the key components of a problem-oriented E/M service should not be reported.

The "comprehensive" nature of the Preventive Medicine Services codes 99381-99397 reflects an age and gender appropriate history/exam and is NOT synonymous with the "comprehensive" examination required in Evaluation and Management codes 99201-99350.

Codes 99381-99397 include counseling/anticipatory guidance/risk factor reduction interventions which are provided at the time of the initial or periodic comprehensive preventive medicine examination. (Refer to codes 99401-99412 for reporting those counseling/anticipatory guidance/risk factor reduction interventions that are provided at an encounter separate from the preventive medicine examination.)

Immunizations and ancillary studies involving laboratory, radiology, other procedures, or screening tests identified with a specific CPT code are reported separately. For immunizations, see 90471-90474 and 90476-90749.

New Patient

99381 **Initial comprehensive preventive medicine** evaluation and management of an individual including an age and gender appropriate history, examination, counseling/anticipatory guidance/risk factor reduction interventions, and the ordering of appropriate immunization(s), laboratory/diagnostic procedures, new patient; infant (age under 1 year)

99382 early childhood (age 1 through 4 years)

99383	late childhood (age 5 through 11 years)
99384	adolescent (age 12 through 17 years)
99385	18-39 years
99386	40-64 years
99387	65 years and over

Established Patient

99391   **Periodic comprehensive preventive medicine** reevaluation and management of an individual including an age and gender appropriate history, examination, counseling/anticipatory guidance/risk factor reduction interventions, and the ordering of appropriate immunization(s), laboratory/diagnostic procedures, established patient; infant (age under 1 year)

99392	early childhood (age 1 through 4 years)
99393	late childhood (age 5 through 11 years)
99394	adolescent (age 12 through 17 years)
99395	18-39 years
99396	40-64 years
99397	65 years and over

Counseling and/or Risk Factor Reduction Intervention

New or Established Patient

These codes are used to report services provided to individuals at a separate encounter for the purpose of promoting health and preventing illness or injury.

Preventive medicine counseling and risk factor reduction interventions provided as a separate encounter will vary with age and should address such issues as family problems, diet and exercise, substance abuse, sexual practices, injury prevention, dental health, and diagnostic and laboratory test results available at the time of the encounter.

These codes are not to be used to report counseling and risk factor reduction interventions provided to patients with symptoms or established illness. For counseling individual patients with symptoms or established illness, use the appropriate office, hospital or consultation or other evaluation and management codes. For counseling groups of patients with symptoms or established illness, use 99078.

Preventive Medicine, Individual Counseling

99401   **Preventive medicine counseling** and/or risk factor reduction intervention(s) provided to an individual (separate procedure); approximately 15 minutes

99402	approximately 30 minutes
99403	approximately 45 minutes
99404	approximately 60 minutes

Preventive Medicine, Group Counseling

99411   **Preventive medicine counseling** and/or risk factor reduction intervention(s) provided to individuals in a group setting (separate procedure); approximately 30 minutes

| 99412 | approximately 60 minutes |

Other Preventive Medicine Services

99420   **Administration and interpretation** of health risk assessment instrument (eg, health hazard appraisal)

99429   **Unlisted preventive** medicine service

Newborn Care

The following codes are used to report the services provided to newborns in several different settings.

For newborn hospital discharge services provided on a date subsequent to the admission date of the newborn, use 99238.

For discharge services provided to newborns admitted and discharged on the same date, use 99435.

99431   **History and examination** of the normal newborn infant, initiation of diagnostic and treatment programs and preparation of hospital records. (This code should also be used for birthing room deliveries.)

99432   **Normal newborn care** in other than hospital or birthing room setting, including physical examination of baby and conference(s) with parent(s)

99433   **Subsequent hospital care,** for the evaluation and management of a normal newborn, per day

99435   **History and examination** of the normal newborn infant, including the preparation of medical records. (This code should only be used for newborns assessed and discharged from the hospital or birthing room on the same date.)

99436   **Attendance** at delivery (when requested by delivering physician) and initial stabilization of newborn

(99436 may be reported in addition to 99431)

(99436 may not be reported in addition to 99440)

(99438 has been deleted)

99440   **Newborn resuscitation:** provision of positive pressure ventilation and/or chest compressions in the presence of acute inadequate ventilation and/or cardiac output

Evaluation and Management

Evaluation and Management

Special Evaluation and Management Services

The following codes are used to report evaluations performed to establish baseline information prior to life or disability insurance certificates being issued. This service is performed in the office or other setting, and applies to both new and established patients. When using these codes, no active management of the problem(s) is undertaken during the encounter.

If other evaluation and management services and/or procedures are performed on the same date, the appropriate E/M or procedure code(s) should be reported in addition to these codes.

Basic Life and/or Disability Evaluation Services

99450   **Basic life** and/or disability examination that includes:

- measurement of height, weight and blood pressure;
- completion of a medical history following a life insurance pro forma;
- collection of blood sample and/or urinalysis complying with "chain of custody" protocols; and
- completion of necessary documentation/certificates.

Work Related or Medical Disability Evaluation Services

99455   **Work related** or medical disability examination by the treating physician that includes:

- completion of a medical history commensurate with the patient's condition;
- performance of an examination commensurate with the patient's condition;
- formulation of a diagnosis, assessment of capabilities and stability, and calculation of impairment;
- development of future medical treatment plan; and
- completion of necessary documentation/certificates and report.

99456   **Work related** or medical disability examination by other than the treating physician that includes:

- completion of a medical history commensurate with the patient's condition;
- performance of an examination commensurate with the patient's condition;
- formulation of a diagnosis, assessment of capabilities and stability, and calculation of impairment;
- development of future medical treatment plan; and
- completion of necessary documentation/certificates and report.

Other Evaluation and Management Services

99499   **Unlisted evaluation and management** service

Anesthesia Guidelines

Services involving administration of anesthesia are reported by the use of the anesthesia five digit procedure code (00100-01999) plus modifier codes (defined under "Anesthesia Modifiers" later in these Guidelines).

The reporting of anesthesia services is appropriate by or under the responsible supervision of a physician. These services may include but are not limited to general, regional, supplementation of local anesthesia, or other supportive services in order to afford the patient the anesthesia care deemed optimal by the anesthesiologist during any procedure. These services include the usual preoperative and postoperative visits, the anesthesia care during the procedure, the administration of fluids and/or blood and the usual monitoring services (eg, ECG, temperature, blood pressure, oximetry, capnography, and mass spectrometry). Unusual forms of monitoring (eg, intra-arterial, central venous, and Swan-Ganz) are not included.

Items used by all physicians in reporting their services are presented in the **Introduction.** Some of the commonalities are repeated here for the convenience of those physicians referring to this section on **Anesthesia.** Other definitions and items unique to anesthesia are also listed.

To report sedation with or without analgesia (conscious sedation) provided by a physician also performing the service for which conscious sedation is being provided, see codes 99141, 99142.

To report regional or general anesthesia provided by a physician also performing the services for which the anesthesia is being provided, see modifier '-47,' Anesthesia by Surgeon, in Appendix A.

Time Reporting

Time for anesthesia procedures may be reported as is customary in the local area. Anesthesia time begins when the anesthesiologist begins to prepare the patient for the induction of anesthesia in the operating room or in an equivalent area and ends when the anesthesiologist is no longer in personal attendance, that is, when the patient may be safely placed under postoperative supervision.

Physician's Services

Physician's services rendered in the office, home, or hospital, consultation, and other medical services are listed in the section entitled **Evaluation and Management Services** (99200 series) found in the front of the book, beginning on page 1. "Special Services and Reporting" (99000 series) are presented in the **Medicine** section.

Materials Supplied by Physician

Supplies and materials provided by the physician (eg, sterile trays, drugs) over and above those usually included with the office visit or other services rendered may be listed separately. List drugs, tray supplies, and materials provided. Identify as 99070.

Separate or Multiple Procedures

It is appropriate to designate multiple procedures that are rendered on the same date by separate entries. This can be reported by using the multiple procedure modifier '-51'. See "Anesthesia Modifiers" for modifier definitions.

Special Report

A service that is rarely provided, unusual, variable, or new may require a special report in determining medical appropriateness of the service. Pertinent information should include an adequate definition or description of the nature, extent, and need for the procedure; and the time, effort, and equipment necessary to provide the service. Additional items which may be included are:

- complexity of symptoms;
- final diagnosis;
- pertinent physical findings;
- diagnostic and therapeutic procedures;
- concurrent problems;
- follow-up care.

Anesthesia Modifiers

All anesthesia services are reported by use of the anesthesia five digit procedure code (00100-01999) plus the addition of a physical status modifier. The use of other optional modifiers may be appropriate.

Physical Status Modifiers

Physical Status modifiers are represented by the initial letter 'P' followed by a single digit from 1 to 6 defined below.

P1-A normal healthy patient.

P2-A patient with mild systemic disease.

P3-A patient with severe systemic disease.

P4-A patient with severe systemic disease that is a constant threat to life.

P5-A moribund patient who is not expected to survive without the operation.

P6-A declared brain-dead patient whose organs are being removed for donor purposes.

The above six levels are consistent with the American Society of Anesthesiologists (ASA) ranking of patient physical status. Physical status is included in CPT to distinguish among various levels of complexity of the anesthesia service provided.

Example: 00100-P1

Qualifying Circumstances

More than one may be selected.

Many anesthesia services are provided under particularly difficult circumstances, depending on factors such as extraordinary condition of patient, notable operative conditions, and/or unusual risk factors. This section includes a list of important qualifying circumstances that significantly impact on the character of the anesthesia service provided. These procedures would not be reported alone but would be reported as additional procedure numbers qualifying an anesthesia procedure or service.

+ **99100**   Anesthesia for patient of extreme age, under 1 year and over 70 (List separately in addition to code for primary anesthesia procedure)

►(For procedure performed on infants less than 1 year of age at time of surgery, see 00833, 00834)◄

+ **99116**   Anesthesia complicated by utilization of total body hypothermia (List separately in addition to code for primary anesthesia procedure)

+ **99135**   Anesthesia complicated by utilization of controlled hypotension (List separately in addition to code for primary anesthesia procedure)

+ **99140**   Anesthesia complicated by emergency conditions (specify) (List separately in addition to code for primary anesthesia procedure)

(An emergency is defined as existing when delay in treatment of the patient would lead to a significant increase in the threat to life or body part.)

Anesthesia

Head

00100	Anesthesia for procedures on salivary glands, including biopsy
00102	Anesthesia for procedures on plastic repair of cleft lip
00103	Anesthesia for reconstructive procedures of eyelid (eg, blepharoplasty, ptosis surgery)
00104	Anesthesia for electroconvulsive therapy
00120	Anesthesia for procedures on external, middle, and inner ear including biopsy; not otherwise specified

(00122 has been deleted. To report, use 00120)

00124	otoscopy
00126	tympanotomy
00140	Anesthesia for procedures on eye; not otherwise specified
00142	lens surgery
00144	corneal transplant
00145	vitreoretinal surgery

(00146 has been deleted. To report, use 00140)

00147	iridectomy
00148	ophthalmoscopy
00160	Anesthesia for procedures on nose and accessory sinuses; not otherwise specified
00162	radical surgery
00164	biopsy, soft tissue
00170	Anesthesia for intraoral procedures, including biopsy; not otherwise specified
00172	repair of cleft palate
00174	excision of retropharyngeal tumor
00176	radical surgery
00190	Anesthesia for procedures on facial bones or skull; not otherwise specified
00192	radical surgery (including prognathism)
00210	Anesthesia for intracranial procedures; not otherwise specified
00212	subdural taps
00214	burr holes, including ventriculography
00215	cranioplasty or elevation of depressed skull fracture, extradural (simple or compound)
00216	vascular procedures
00218	procedures in sitting position
00220	cerebrospinal fluid shunting procedures
00222	electrocoagulation of intracranial nerve

Neck

00300	Anesthesia for all procedures on the integumentary system, muscles and nerves of head, neck, and posterior trunk, not otherwise specified
▲ 00320	Anesthesia for all procedures on esophagus, thyroid, larynx, trachea and lymphatic system of neck; not otherwise specified, age 1 year or older
00322	needle biopsy of thyroid

(For procedures on cervical spine and cord, see 00600, 00604, 00670)

● 00326	Anesthesia for all procedures on the larynx and trachea in children less than 1 year of age

▶(Do not report 00326 in conjunction with code 99100)◀

00350	Anesthesia for procedures on major vessels of neck; not otherwise specified
00352	simple ligation

(For arteriography, use 01916)

Thorax (Chest Wall and Shoulder Girdle)

00400	Anesthesia for procedures on the integumentary system on the extremities, anterior trunk and perineum; not otherwise specified
00402	reconstructive procedures on breast (eg, reduction or augmentation mammoplasty, muscle flaps)
00404	radical or modified radical procedures on breast
00406	radical or modified radical procedures on breast with internal mammary node dissection
00410	electrical conversion of arrhythmias

(00420 has been deleted. To report, use 00300)

00450	Anesthesia for procedures on clavicle and scapula; not otherwise specified
00452	radical surgery
00454	biopsy of clavicle

Anesthesia

00470   Anesthesia for partial rib resection; not otherwise specified

00472   thoracoplasty (any type)

00474   radical procedures (eg, pectus excavatum)

       (00476 has been deleted. To report, use 00470)

Intrathoracic

00500   Anesthesia for all procedures on esophagus

00520   Anesthesia for closed chest procedures; (including bronchoscopy) not otherwise specified

00522   needle biopsy of pleura

00524   pneumocentesis

       (00526 has been deleted. To report, use 00520)

00528   mediastinoscopy and diagnostic thoracoscopy

       ▶(For tracheobronchial reconstruction, use 00539)◀

00530   Anesthesia for permanent transvenous pacemaker insertion

00532   Anesthesia for access to central venous circulation

00534   Anesthesia for transvenous insertion or replacement of pacing cardioverter-defibrillator

       (For transthoracic approach, use 00560)

00537   Anesthesia for cardiac electrophysiologic procedures including radiofrequency ablation

● 00539   Anesthesia for tracheobronchial reconstruction

00540   Anesthesia for thoracotomy procedures involving lungs, pleura, diaphragm, and mediastinum (including surgical thoracoscopy); not otherwise specified

● 00541   utilizing one lung ventilation

00542   decortication

00544   pleurectomy

00546   pulmonary resection with thoracoplasty

00548   intrathoracic procedures on the trachea and bronchi

00550   Anesthesia for sternal debridement

00560   Anesthesia for procedures on heart, pericardial sac, and great vessels of chest; without pump oxygenator

00562   with pump oxygenator

00563   with pump oxygenator with hypothermic circulatory arrest

00566   Anesthesia for direct coronary artery bypass grafting without pump oxygenator

00580   Anesthesia for heart transplant or heart/lung transplant

Spine and Spinal Cord

00600   Anesthesia for procedures on cervical spine and cord; not otherwise specified

       (For myelography and diskography, see radiological procedures 01905)

00604   procedures with patient in the sitting position

00620   Anesthesia for procedures on thoracic spine and cord; not otherwise specified

00622   thoracolumbar sympathectomy

00630   Anesthesia for procedures in lumbar region; not otherwise specified

00632   lumbar sympathectomy

00634   chemonucleolysis

       (00650 has been deleted. To report, use 00220)

00635   diagnostic or therapeutic lumbar puncture

● 00640   Anesthesia for manipulation of the spine or for closed procedures on the cervical, thoracic or lumbar spine

00670   Anesthesia for extensive spine and spinal cord procedures (eg, spinal instrumentation or vascular procedures)

Upper Abdomen

00700   Anesthesia for procedures on upper anterior abdominal wall; not otherwise specified

00702   percutaneous liver biopsy

00730   Anesthesia for procedures on upper posterior abdominal wall

00740   Anesthesia for upper gastrointestinal endoscopic procedures, endoscope introduced proximal to duodenum

00750   Anesthesia for hernia repairs in upper abdomen; not otherwise specified

00752   lumbar and ventral (incisional) hernias and/or wound dehiscence

00754   omphalocele

00756   transabdominal repair of diaphragmatic hernia

00770   Anesthesia for all procedures on major abdominal blood vessels

00790   Anesthesia for intraperitoneal procedures in upper abdomen including laparoscopy; not otherwise specified

00792   partial hepatectomy or management of liver hemorrhage (excluding liver biopsy)

00794   pancreatectomy, partial or total (eg, Whipple procedure)

00796   liver transplant (recipient)

(For harvesting of liver, use 01990)

00797   gastric restrictive procedure for morbid obesity

Lower Abdomen

00800   Anesthesia for procedures on lower anterior abdominal wall; not otherwise specified

00802   panniculectomy

(00806 has been deleted. To report, see 00790, 00840)

00810   Anesthesia for lower intestinal endoscopic procedures, endoscope introduced distal to duodenum

00820   Anesthesia for procedures on lower posterior abdominal wall

00830   Anesthesia for hernia repairs in lower abdomen; not otherwise specified

00832   ventral and incisional hernias

▶(For hernia repairs in the infant 1 year of age or younger, see 00834, 00836)◀

● **00834**   Anesthesia for hernia repairs in the lower abdomen not otherwise specified, under 1 year of age

▶(Do not report 00834 in conjunction with code 99100)◀

● **00836**   Anesthesia for hernia repairs in the lower abdomen not otherwise specified, infants less than 37 weeks gestational age at birth and less than 50 weeks gestational age at time of surgery

▶(Do not report 00836 in conjunction with code 99100)◀

00840   Anesthesia for intraperitoneal procedures in lower abdomen including laparoscopy; not otherwise specified

00842   amniocentesis

00844   abdominoperineal resection

00846   radical hysterectomy

00848   pelvic exenteration

(00850 has been deleted. To report, use 01961)

00851   tubal ligation/transection

(00855 has been deleted. To report, use 01963)

(00857 has been deleted. To report, use 01968, 01969)

00860   Anesthesia for extraperitoneal procedures in lower abdomen, including urinary tract; not otherwise specified

00862   renal procedures, including upper 1/3 of ureter, or donor nephrectomy

00864   total cystectomy

00865   radical prostatectomy (suprapubic, retropubic)

00866   adrenalectomy

00868   renal transplant (recipient)

(For donor nephrectomy, use 00862)

(For harvesting kidney from brain-dead patient, use 01990)

▶(00869 has been deleted. To report, use 00921)◀

00870   cystolithotomy

00872   Anesthesia for lithotripsy, extracorporeal shock wave; with water bath

00873   without water bath

00880   Anesthesia for procedures on major lower abdominal vessels; not otherwise specified

00882   inferior vena cava ligation

(00884 has been deleted. To report, use 01930)

Perineum

(00900 has been deleted. To report, see 00300, 00400)

00902   Anesthesia for; anorectal procedure

00904   radical perineal procedure

00906   vulvectomy

00908   perineal prostatectomy

00910   Anesthesia for transurethral procedures (including urethrocystoscopy); not otherwise specified

00912   transurethral resection of bladder tumor(s)

00914   transurethral resection of prostate

00916   post-transurethral resection bleeding

00918   with fragmentation, manipulation and/or removal of ureteral calculus

00920   Anesthesia for procedures on male genitalia (including open urethral procedures); not otherwise specified

● **00921**   vasectomy, unilateral/bilateral

00922   seminal vesicles

00924   undescended testis, unilateral or bilateral

00926   radical orchiectomy, inguinal

00928   radical orchiectomy, abdominal

00930   orchiopexy, unilateral or bilateral

00932   complete amputation of penis

00934   radical amputation of penis with bilateral inguinal lymphadenectomy

00936   radical amputation of penis with bilateral inguinal and iliac lymphadenectomy

00938   insertion of penile prosthesis (perineal approach)

00940 Anesthesia for vaginal procedures (including biopsy of labia, vagina, cervix or endometrium); not otherwise specified

00942 colpotomy, vaginectomy, colporrhaphy, and open urethral procedures

00944 vaginal hysterectomy

(00946 has been deleted. To report, use 01960)

00948 cervical cerclage

00950 culdoscopy

00952 hysteroscopy and/or hysterosalpingography

(00955 has been deleted. To report, use 01967)

Pelvis (Except Hip)

(01000 has been deleted. To report, use 00400)

(01110 has been deleted. To report, use 00300)

01112 Anesthesia for bone marrow aspiration and/or biopsy, anterior or posterior iliac crest

01120 Anesthesia for procedures on bony pelvis

(01122 has been deleted. To report, use 01120)

01130 Anesthesia for body cast application or revision

01140 Anesthesia for interpelviabdominal (hindquarter) amputation

01150 Anesthesia for radical procedures for tumor of pelvis, except hindquarter amputation

01160 Anesthesia for closed procedures involving symphysis pubis or sacroiliac joint

01170 Anesthesia for open procedures involving symphysis pubis or sacroiliac joint

01180 Anesthesia for obturator neurectomy; extrapelvic

01190 intrapelvic

Upper Leg (Except Knee)

01200 Anesthesia for all closed procedures involving hip joint

01202 Anesthesia for arthroscopic procedures of hip joint

01210 Anesthesia for open procedures involving hip joint; not otherwise specified

01212 hip disarticulation

01214 total hip arthroplasty

01215 revision of total hip arthroplasty

01220 Anesthesia for all closed procedures involving upper 2/3 of femur

01230 Anesthesia for open procedures involving upper 2/3 of femur; not otherwise specified

01232 amputation

01234 radical resection

(01240 has been deleted. To report, use 00400)

01250 Anesthesia for all procedures on nerves, muscles, tendons, fascia, and bursae of upper leg

01260 Anesthesia for all procedures involving veins of upper leg, including exploration

01270 Anesthesia for procedures involving arteries of upper leg, including bypass graft; not otherwise specified

01272 femoral artery ligation

01274 femoral artery embolectomy

(01276 has been deleted. To report, use 00880)

Knee and Popliteal Area

►Surgical endoscopy/arthroscopy always includes a diagnostic endoscopy/arthroscopy.◄

(01300 has been deleted. To report, use 00400)

01320 Anesthesia for all procedures on nerves, muscles, tendons, fascia, and bursae of knee and/or popliteal area

01340 Anesthesia for all closed procedures on lower 1/3 of femur

01360 Anesthesia for all open procedures on lower 1/3 of femur

01380 Anesthesia for all closed procedures on knee joint

▲**01382** Anesthesia for diagnostic arthroscopic procedures of knee joint

01390 Anesthesia for all closed procedures on upper ends of tibia, fibula, and/or patella

01392 Anesthesia for all open procedures on upper ends of tibia, fibula, and/or patella

▲**01400** Anesthesia for open or surgical arthroscopic procedures on knee joint; not otherwise specified

01402 total knee arthroplasty

01404 disarticulation at knee

01420 Anesthesia for all cast applications, removal, or repair involving knee joint

01430 Anesthesia for procedures on veins of knee and popliteal area; not otherwise specified

01432 arteriovenous fistula

01440 Anesthesia for procedures on arteries of knee and popliteal area; not otherwise specified

01442 popliteal thromboendarterectomy, with or without patch graft

01444 popliteal excision and graft or repair for occlusion or aneurysm

Lower Leg (Below Knee, Includes Ankle and Foot)

▶Surgical endoscopy/arthroscopy always includes a diagnostic endoscopy/arthroscopy.◀

(01460 has been deleted. To report, use 00400)

01462   Anesthesia for all closed procedures on lower leg, ankle, and foot

▲ **01464**   Anesthesia for arthroscopic procedures of ankle and/or foot

01470   Anesthesia for procedures on nerves, muscles, tendons, and fascia of lower leg, ankle, and foot; not otherwise specified

01472   repair of ruptured Achilles tendon, with or without graft

01474   gastrocnemius recession (eg, Strayer procedure)

01480   Anesthesia for open procedures on bones of lower leg, ankle, and foot; not otherwise specified

01482   radical resection (including below knee amputation)

01484   osteotomy or osteoplasty of tibia and/or fibula

01486   total ankle replacement

01490   Anesthesia for lower leg cast application, removal, or repair

01500   Anesthesia for procedures on arteries of lower leg, including bypass graft; not otherwise specified

01502   embolectomy, direct or with catheter

01520   Anesthesia for procedures on veins of lower leg; not otherwise specified

01522   venous thrombectomy, direct or with catheter

Shoulder and Axilla

▶Surgical endoscopy/arthroscopy always includes a diagnostic endoscopy/arthroscopy.◀

Includes humeral head and neck, sternoclavicular joint, acromioclavicular joint, and shoulder joint.

(01600 has been deleted. To report, use 00400)

01610   Anesthesia for all procedures on nerves, muscles, tendons, fascia, and bursae of shoulder and axilla

01620   Anesthesia for all closed procedures on humeral head and neck, sternoclavicular joint, acromioclavicular joint, and shoulder joint

▲ **01622**   Anesthesia for diagnostic arthroscopic procedures of shoulder joint

▲ **01630**   Anesthesia for open or surgical arthroscopic procedures on humeral head and neck, sternoclavicular joint, acromioclavicular joint, and shoulder joint; not otherwise specified

01632   radical resection

01634   shoulder disarticulation

01636   interthoracoscapular (forequarter) amputation

01638   total shoulder replacement

01650   Anesthesia for procedures on arteries of shoulder and axilla; not otherwise specified

01652   axillary-brachial aneurysm

01654   bypass graft

01656   axillary-femoral bypass graft

01670   Anesthesia for all procedures on veins of shoulder and axilla

01680   Anesthesia for shoulder cast application, removal or repair; not otherwise specified

01682   shoulder spica

Upper Arm and Elbow

▶Surgical endoscopy/arthroscopy always includes a diagnostic endoscopy/arthroscopy.◀

(01700 has been deleted. To report, use 00400)

01710   Anesthesia for procedures on nerves, muscles, tendons, fascia, and bursae of upper arm and elbow; not otherwise specified

01712   tenotomy, elbow to shoulder, open

01714   tenoplasty, elbow to shoulder

01716   tenodesis, rupture of long tendon of biceps

01730   Anesthesia for all closed procedures on humerus and elbow

▲ **01732**   Anesthesia for diagnostic arthroscopic procedures of elbow joint

▲ **01740**   Anesthesia for open or surgical arthroscopic procedures of the elbow; not otherwise specified

01742   osteotomy of humerus

01744   repair of nonunion or malunion of humerus

01756   radical procedures

01758   excision of cyst or tumor of humerus

01760   total elbow replacement

01770   Anesthesia for procedures on arteries of upper arm and elbow; not otherwise specified

01772   embolectomy

Anesthesia

Anesthesia

01780   Anesthesia for procedures on veins of upper arm and elbow; not otherwise specified

01782   phleborrhaphy

(01784 has been deleted. To report, see 01770, 01780)

Forearm, Wrist, and Hand

(01800 has been deleted. To report, use 00400)

01810   Anesthesia for all procedures on nerves, muscles, tendons, fascia, and bursae of forearm, wrist, and hand

01820   Anesthesia for all closed procedures on radius, ulna, wrist, or hand bones

● **01829**   Anesthesia for diagnostic arthroscopic procedures on the wrist

▲ **01830**   Anesthesia for open or surgical arthroscopic/endoscopic procedures on distal radius, distal ulna, wrist, or hand joints; not otherwise specified

01832   total wrist replacement

01840   Anesthesia for procedures on arteries of forearm, wrist, and hand; not otherwise specified

01842   embolectomy

01844   Anesthesia for vascular shunt, or shunt revision, any type (eg, dialysis)

01850   Anesthesia for procedures on veins of forearm, wrist, and hand; not otherwise specified

01852   phleborrhaphy

01860   Anesthesia for forearm, wrist, or hand cast application, removal, or repair

Radiological Procedures

(01900 has been deleted. To report, use 00952)

(01902 has been deleted. To report, use 00214)

(01904 has been deleted. To report, use 01905)

01905   Anesthesia for myelography, diskography, vertebroplasty

(01906 has been deleted. To report, use 01905)

(01908 has been deleted. To report, use 01905)

(01910 has been deleted. To report, use 01905)

(01912 has been deleted. To report, use 01905)

(01914 has been deleted. To report, use 01905)

01916   Anesthesia for diagnostic arteriography/venography

(Do not report 01916 in conjunction with therapeutic codes 01924-01926, 01930-01933)

(01918 has been deleted. To report, use 01916)

01920   Anesthesia for cardiac catheterization including coronary angiography and ventriculography (not to include Swan-Ganz catheter)

(01921 has been deleted. To report, see 01924-01926)

01922   Anesthesia for non-invasive imaging or radiation therapy

01924   Anesthesia for therapeutic interventional radiologic procedures involving the arterial system; not otherwise specified

01925   carotid or coronary

01926   intracranial, intracardiac, or aortic

01930   Anesthesia for therapeutic interventional radiologic procedures involving the venous/lymphatic system (not to include access to the central circulation); not otherwise specified

01931   intrahepatic or portal circulation (eg, transcutaneous porto-caval shunt (TIPS))

01932   intrathoracic or jugular

01933   intracranial

Burn Excisions or Debridement

01951   Anesthesia for second and third degree burn excision or debridement with or without skin grafting, any site, for total body surface area (TBSA) treated during anesthesia and surgery; less than four percent total body surface area

01952   between four and nine percent of total body surface area

+ **01953**   each additional nine percent total body surface area or part thereof (List separately in addition to code for primary procedure)

(Use 01953 in conjunction with code 01952)

Obstetric

01960   Anesthesia for vaginal delivery only

▲ **01961**   Anesthesia for cesarean delivery only

▲ **01962**   Anesthesia for urgent hysterectomy following delivery

▲ **01963**   Anesthesia for cesarean hysterectomy without any labor analgesia/anesthesia care

▲ **01964**   Anesthesia for abortion procedures

01967   Neuraxial labor analgesia/anesthesia for planned vaginal delivery (this includes any repeat subarachnoid needle placement and drug injection and/or any necessary replacement of an epidural catheter during labor)

+ ▲ 01968   Anesthesia for cesarean delivery following neuraxial labor analgesia/anesthesia (List separately in addition to code for primary procedure performed)

(Use 01968 in conjunction with code 01967)

+ ▲ 01969   Anesthesia for cesarean hysterectomy following neuraxial labor analgesia/anesthesia (List separately in addition to code for primary procedure performed)

(Use 01969 in conjunction with code 01967)

Other Procedures

01990   Physiological support for harvesting of organ(s) from brain-dead patient

● 01991   Anesthesia for diagnostic or therapeutic nerve blocks and injections (when block or injection is performed by a different provider); other than the prone position

● 01992   prone position

▶(Do not report code 01991or 01992 in conjunction with 99141)◀

01995   Regional intravenous administration of local anesthetic agent or other medication (upper or lower extremity)

(For intra-arterial or intravenous therapy for pain management, see 90783, 90784)

▲ 01996   Daily hospital management of epidural or subarachnoid continuous drug administration

▶(Report code 01996 for daily hospital management of continuous epidural or subarachnoid drug administration performed after insertion of an epidural or subarachnoid catheter placed primarily for anesthesia administration during an operative session, but retained for post-operative pain management)◀

01999   Unlisted anesthesia procedure(s)

Notes

⊘ =Modifier '-51' Exempt   ▶◀ or ▶ ◀=New or Revised Text   ✦=Add-on Code

Surgery Guidelines

Items used by all physicians in reporting their services are presented in the **Introduction.** Some of the commonalities are repeated here for the convenience of those physicians referring to this section on **Surgery.** Other definitions and items unique to Surgery are also listed.

Physicians' Services

Physicians' services rendered in the office, home, or hospital, consultations, and other medical services are listed in the section entitled **Evaluation and Management Services** (99200 series) found in the front of the book, beginning on page 9. "Special Services and Reports" (99000 series) is presented in the **Medicine** section.

CPT Surgical Package Definition

The services provided by the physician to any patient by their very nature are variable. The CPT codes that represent a readily identifiable surgical procedure thereby include, on a procedure-by-procedure basis, a variety of services. In defining the specific services "included" in a given CPT surgical code, the following services are always included in addition to the operation per se:

- local infiltration, metacarpal/metatarsal/digital block or topical anesthesia;
- subsequent to the decision for surgery, one related E/M encounter on the date immediately prior to or on the date of procedure (including history and physical);
- immediate postoperative care, including dictating operative notes, talking with the family and other physicians;
- writing orders;
- evaluating the patient in the postanesthesia recovery area;
- typical postoperative follow-up care.

Follow-Up Care for Diagnostic Procedures

Follow-up care for diagnostic procedures (eg, endoscopy, arthroscopy, injection procedures for radiography) includes only that care related to recovery from the diagnostic procedure itself. Care of the condition for which the diagnostic procedure was performed or of other concomitant conditions is not included and may be listed separately.

Follow-Up Care for Therapeutic Surgical Procedures

Follow-up care for therapeutic surgical procedures includes only that care which is usually a part of the surgical service. Complications, exacerbations, recurrence, or the presence of other diseases or injuries requiring additional services should be separately reported.

Materials Supplied by Physician

Supplies and materials provided by the physician (eg, sterile trays/drugs), over and above those usually included with the procedure(s) rendered are reported separately. List drugs, trays, supplies, and materials provided. Identify as 99070 or specific supply code.

Reporting More Than One Procedure/Service

When a physician performs more than one procedure/service on the same date, same session or during a post-operative period (subject to the "surgical package" concept), several CPT modifiers may apply. (See Appendix A for definition.)

-27 Multiple Outpatient Hospital E/M Encounters on the Same Date

For hospital outpatient reporting purposes, utilization of hospital resources related to separate and distinct E/M encounters performed in multiple outpatient hospital settings on the same date may be reported by adding the modifier '-27' to each appropriate level outpatient and/or emergency department E/M code(s). This modifier provides a means of reporting circumstances involving evaluation and management services provided by physician(s) in more than one (multiple) outpatient hospital setting(s) (eg, hospital emergency department, clinic). **Note:** This modifier is not to be used for physician reporting of multiple E/M services performed by the same physician on the same date. For physician reporting of all outpatient evaluation and management services provided by the same physician on the same date and performed in multiple outpatient setting(s) (eg, hospital emergency department, clinic), see **Evaluation and Management, Emergency Department,** or **Preventive Medicine Services** codes.

-51 Multiple Procedures

When multiple procedures/services (other than evaluation and management) are performed at the same session, report the most significant procedure first, with all other procedures listed with the '-51' modifier appended. For a list of procedures exempt from the use of the '-51' modifier, see Appendices D and E.

-58 Staged or Related Procedure or Service by the Same Physician During the Postoperative Period

When a procedure(s) is prospectively planned as a staged procedure, or when the secondary and subsequent procedure(s) is more extensive, or to indicate therapy following a diagnostic surgical procedure, use the '-58' modifier with the staged procedure(s).

-59 Distinct Procedural Service

For procedure(s)/service(s) not ordinarily performed or encountered on the same day by the same physician, but appropriate under certain circumstances (eg, different site or organ system, separate excision or lesion), use the '-59' modifier.

-76 Repeat Procedure by Same Physician

When a procedure or service is repeated by the same physician subsequent to the original service, use the '-76' modifier.

-77 Repeat Procedure by Another Physician

When a procedure is repeated by another physician subsequent to the original service, use the '-77' modifier.

-78 Return to the Operating Room for a Related Procedure During the Postoperative Period

When a procedure, related to the initial procedure, requires a return to the operating room during the postoperative period of that initial procedure, use the '-78' modifier.

-79 Unrelated Procedure or Service by the Same Physician During the Postoperative Period

When a procedure, unrelated to the initial procedure, is performed by the same physician during the postoperative period of the initial procedure, use the '-79' modifier.

-91 Repeat Clinical Diagnostic Laboratory Test

In the course of treatment of the patient, it may be necessary to repeat the same laboratory test on the same day to obtain subsequent (multiple) test results. Under these circumstances, the laboratory test performed can be identified by its usual procedure number and the addition of the modifier '-91'. **Note:** This modifier may not be used when tests are rerun to confirm initial results; due to testing problems with specimens or equipment; or for any other reason when a normal, one-time, reportable result is all that is required. This modifier may not be used when other code(s) describe a series of test results (eg, glucose tolerance tests, evocative/suppression testing). This modifier may only be used for laboratory test(s) performed more than once on the same day on the same patient.

Separate Procedure

Some of the procedures or services listed in *CPT* that are commonly carried out as an integral component of a total service or procedure have been identified by the inclusion of the term "separate procedure." The codes designated as "separate procedure" should not be reported in addition to the code for the total procedure or service of which it is considered an integral component.

However, when a procedure or service that is designated as a "separate procedure" is carried out independently or considered to be unrelated or distinct from other procedures/services provided at that time, it may be reported by itself, or in addition to other procedures/ services by appending the modifier '-59' to the specific "separate procedure" code to indicate that the procedure is not considered to be a component of another procedure, but is a distinct, independent procedure. This may represent a different session or patient encounter, different procedure or surgery, different site or organ system, separate incision/excision, separate lesion, or separate injury (or area of injury in extensive injuries).

Subsection Information

Several of the subheadings or subsections have special needs or instructions unique to that section. Where these are indicated (eg, "Maternity Care and Delivery"), special **"Notes"** will be presented preceding those procedural terminology listings, referring to that subsection specifically. If there is an "Unlisted Procedure" code number (see below) for the individual subsection, it will also be shown. Those subsections within the **Surgery** section that have **"Notes"** are as follows:

Removal of Skin Tags	11200-11201
Shaving of Lesions	11300-11313
Excision—Benign Lesions	11400-11471
Excision—Malignant Lesions	11600-11646
Repair (Closure)	12001-13160
Adjacent Tissue Transfer or Rearrangement	14000-14350
Free Skin Grafts	15000-15400
Flaps (Skin and/or Deep Tissue)	15570-15999
Burns, Local Treatment	16000-16042
Destruction, Benign Lesions	17000-17250
Destruction, Malignant Lesions	17260-17286
Mohs Micrographic Surgery	17304-17310
Musculoskeletal	20000-29909
Wound Exploration—Trauma	20100-20103
Grafts (or Implants)	20900-20999
Spine: Excision	22100-22116
Spine: Osteotomy	22210-22226
Spine: Fracture/Dislocation	22305-22328
Spine: Arthrodesis	22548-22812
Spinal Instrumentation	22840-22855
Casting and Strapping	29000-29750
Cardiovascular System	33010-37799
Pacing Cardioverter-Pacemaker or Defibrillator	33200-33249
Venous—CABG	33510-33516
Arterial—Venous—CABG	33517-33530
Arterial—CABG	33533-33545
Endovascular Repair of Abdominal Aortic Aneurysm	34800-34826
Transluminal Angioplasty	35450-35476
Transluminal Atherectomy	35480-35495
Composite Grafts	35681-35683
Arteries and Veins	34001-35907
Vascular Injection Procedures:	
Intravenous	36000-36015
Intra-Arterial/Intra-Aortic	36100-36299
Endoscopy	31505-31579, 32601-32665, 43200-43272, 44360-44397, 45300-45387, 46600-46615, 47550-47556
Herniotomy	49491-49611
Urodynamics	51725-51797
Endoscopy	
Urinary	50945-50980, 51990-52400
Testis	54690-54699
Female Genital	58550-58579, 58660-58679
Endocrine	60650-60659
Ureter and Pelvis	52320-52339
Maternity Care and Delivery	59000-59899
Surgery of Skull Base	61580-61619
Neurostimulators (Intracranial)	61850-61888
Neurostimulators (Spinal)	63650-63688
Neurostimulators (Peripheral Nerve)	64553-64595
Secondary Implants(s)	65125-65175
Removal Cataract	66830-66999
Prophylaxis	67141-67145
Operating Microscope	69990

Unlisted Service or Procedure

A service or procedure may be provided that is not listed in this edition of *CPT*. When reporting such a service, the appropriate "Unlisted Procedure" code may be used to indicate the service, identifying it by "Special Report" as discussed in the section below. The "Unlisted Procedures" and accompanying codes for **Surgery** are as follows:

15999 Unlisted procedure, excision pressure ulcer

17999 Unlisted procedure, skin, mucous membrane and subcutaneous tissue

19499 Unlisted procedure, breast

20999 Unlisted procedure, musculoskeletal system, general

21089 Unlisted maxillofacial prosthetic procedure

21299 Unlisted craniofacial and maxillofacial procedure

21499 Unlisted musculoskeletal procedure, head

21899 Unlisted procedure, neck or thorax

22899 Unlisted procedure, spine

22999 Unlisted procedure, abdomen, musculoskeletal system

23929 Unlisted procedure, shoulder

24999 Unlisted procedure, humerus or elbow

25999 Unlisted procedure, forearm or wrist

26989 Unlisted procedure, hands or fingers

27299 Unlisted procedure, pelvis or hip joint

27599 Unlisted procedure, femur or knee

27899 Unlisted procedure, leg or ankle

28899 Unlisted procedure, foot or toes

29799 Unlisted procedure, casting or strapping

29999 Unlisted procedure, arthroscopy

30999 Unlisted procedure, nose

31299 Unlisted procedure, accessory sinuses

31599 Unlisted procedure, larynx

31899 Unlisted procedure, trachea, bronchi

32999 Unlisted procedure, lungs and pleura

Surgery Guidelines

Code	Description
33999	Unlisted procedure, cardiac surgery
36299	Unlisted procedure, vascular injection
▶ 37501	Unlisted vascular endoscopy procedure◀
37799	Unlisted procedure, vascular surgery
38129	Unlisted laparoscopy procedure, spleen
38589	Unlisted laparoscopy procedure, lymphatic system
38999	Unlisted procedure, hemic or lymphatic system
39499	Unlisted procedure, mediastinum
39599	Unlisted procedure, diaphragm
40799	Unlisted procedure, lips
40899	Unlisted procedure, vestibule of mouth
41599	Unlisted procedure, tongue, floor of mouth
41899	Unlisted procedure, dentoalveolar structures
42299	Unlisted procedure, palate, uvula
42699	Unlisted procedure, salivary glands or ducts
42999	Unlisted procedure, pharynx, adenoids, or tonsils
43289	Unlisted laparoscopy procedure, esophagus
43499	Unlisted procedure, esophagus
43659	Unlisted laparoscopy procedure, stomach
43999	Unlisted procedure, stomach
▶ 44238	Unlisted laparoscopy procedure, intestine (except rectum)◀
▶ 44239	Unlisted laparoscopy procedure, rectum◀
44899	Unlisted procedure, Meckels diverticulum and the mesentery
44979	Unlisted laparoscopy procedure, appendix
45999	Unlisted procedure, rectum
46999	Unlisted procedure, anus
47379	Unlisted laparoscopic procedure, liver
47399	Unlisted procedure, liver
47579	Unlisted laparoscopy procedure, biliary tract
47999	Unlisted procedure, biliary tract
48999	Unlisted procedure, pancreas
49329	Unlisted laparoscopy procedure, abdomen, peritoneum and omentum
49659	Unlisted laparoscopy procedure, hernioplasty, herniorrhaphy, herniotomy
49999	Unlisted procedure, abdomen, peritoneum and omentum
50549	Unlisted laparoscopy procedure, renal
50949	Unlisted laparoscopy procedure, ureter
53899	Unlisted procedure, urinary system
54699	Unlisted laparoscopy procedure, testis
55559	Unlisted laparoscopy procedure, spermatic cord
55899	Unlisted procedure, male genital system
58578	Unlisted laparoscopy procedure, uterus
58579	Unlisted hysteroscopy procedure, uterus
58679	Unlisted laparoscopy procedure, oviduct, ovary
58999	Unlisted procedure, female genital system (nonobstetrical)
59898	Unlisted laparoscopy procedure, maternity care and delivery
59899	Unlisted procedure, maternity care and delivery
60659	Unlisted laparoscopy procedure, endocrine system
60699	Unlisted procedure, endocrine system
64999	Unlisted procedure, nervous system
66999	Unlisted procedure, anterior segment of eye
67299	Unlisted procedure, posterior segment
67399	Unlisted procedure, ocular muscle
67599	Unlisted procedure, orbit
67999	Unlisted procedure, eyelids
68399	Unlisted procedure, conjunctiva
68899	Unlisted procedure, lacrimal system
69399	Unlisted procedure, external ear
69799	Unlisted procedure, middle ear
69949	Unlisted procedure, inner ear
69979	Unlisted procedure, temporal bone, middle fossa approach

Special Report

A service that is rarely provided, unusual, variable, or new may require a special report in determining medical appropriateness of the service. Pertinent information should include an adequate definition or description of the nature, extent, and need for the procedure, and the time, effort, and equipment necessary to provide the service. Additional items which may be included are:

- complexity of symptoms;
- final diagnosis;
- pertinent physical findings (such as size, locations, and number of lesion(s), if appropriate);
- diagnostic and therapeutic procedures (including major and supplementary surgical procedures, if appropriate);
- concurrent problems;
- follow-up care.

Starred (∗) Procedures or Items

Certain relatively small surgical services involve a readily identifiable surgical procedure but include variable preoperative and postoperative services (eg, incision and drainage of an abscess, injection of a tendon sheath, manipulation of a joint under anesthesia, dilation of the urethra). Because of the indefinite pre- and postoperative services the usual "package" concept for surgical services (see above) cannot be applied. Such procedures are identified by a star (∗) following the procedure code number.

When a star (*****) follows a surgical procedure code number, the following rules apply:

1. *The service as listed includes the surgical procedure only.* Associated pre- and postoperative services are not included in the service as listed.

2. *Preoperative services are considered as one of the following:*

■ When the starred (*****) procedure is carried out at the time of an initial visit (new patient) and this procedure constitutes the major service at that visit, procedure number 99025 is listed in lieu of the usual initial visit as an additional service.

■ When the starred (*****) procedure is carried out at the time of an initial or established patient visit involving significant identifiable services, the appropriate visit is listed with the modifier '-25' appended in addition to the starred (*****) procedure and its follow-up care.

■ When the starred (*****) procedure requires hospitalization, an appropriate hospital visit is listed in addition to the starred (*****) procedure and its follow-up care.

3. *All postoperative care is added on a service-by-service basis (eg, office or hospital visit, cast change).*

4. *Complications are added on a service-by-service basis (as with all surgical procedures).*

Surgical Destruction

Surgical destruction is a part of a surgical procedure and different methods of destruction are not ordinarily listed separately unless the technique substantially alters the standard management of a problem or condition. Exceptions under special circumstances are provided for by separate code numbers.

Notes

Surgery

General

(10000-10020 have been deleted. To report see 10060, 10061)

10021 Fine needle aspiration; without imaging guidance

10022   with imaging guidance

(For radiological supervision and interpretation, see 76003, 76360, ▶76393,◀ 76942)

(For percutaneous needle biopsy ▶other than fine needle aspiration,◀ see ▶20206 for muscle, 32400 for pleura,◀ 32405 for lung ▶or mediastinum, 42400 for salivary gland,◀ 47000, 47001 for liver, 48102 for pancreas, 49180 for abdominal or retroperitoneal mass, ▶60100 for thyroid, 62269 for spinal cord)◀

(For evaluation of fine needle aspirate, see 88172, 88173)

Integumentary System

Skin, Subcutaneous and Accessory Structures

Incision and Drainage

(For excision, see 11400, et seq)

10040* Acne surgery (eg, marsupialization, opening or removal of multiple milia, comedones, cysts, pustules)

10060* Incision and drainage of abscess (eg, carbuncle, suppurative hidradenitis, cutaneous or subcutaneous abscess, cyst, furuncle, or paronychia); simple or single

10061   complicated or multiple

10080* Incision and drainage of pilonidal cyst; simple

10081   complicated

(For excision of pilonidal cyst, see 11770-11772)

(10100, 10101 have been deleted. To report, see 10060, 10061)

10120* Incision and removal of foreign body, subcutaneous tissues; simple

10121   complicated

(To report wound exploration due to penetrating trauma without laparotomy or thoracotomy, see 20100-20103, as appropriate)

(To report debridement associated with open fracture(s) and/or dislocation(s), use 11010-11012, as appropriate)

10140* Incision and drainage of hematoma, seroma or fluid collection

(If imaging guidance is performed, see 76360, 76393, 76942)

(10141 has been deleted. To report, use 10140)

10160* Puncture aspiration of abscess, hematoma, bulla, or cyst

(If imaging guidance is performed, see 76360, 76393, 76942)

10180 Incision and drainage, complex, postoperative wound infection

(For secondary closure of surgical wound, see 12020, 12021, 13160)

Excision—Debridement

(For dermabrasions, see 15780-15783)

(For nail debridement, see 11720-11721)

(For burn(s), see 16000-16035)

11000* Debridement of extensive eczematous or infected skin; up to 10% of body surface

+ 11001   each additional 10% of the body surface (List separately in addition to code for primary procedure)

(Use 11001 in conjunction with code 11000)

11010 Debridement including removal of foreign material associated with open fracture(s) and/or dislocation(s); skin and subcutaneous tissues

11011   skin, subcutaneous tissue, muscle fascia, and muscle

11012   skin, subcutaneous tissue, muscle fascia, muscle, and bone

11040 Debridement; skin, partial thickness

11041   skin, full thickness

11042   skin, and subcutaneous tissue

11043   skin, subcutaneous tissue, and muscle

11044   skin, subcutaneous tissue, muscle, and bone

(Do not report 11040-11044 in addition to 97601, 97602)

Paring or Cutting

(11050-11052 have been deleted. To report paring, see 11055-11057, or to report destruction, see 17000-17004)

11055 Paring or cutting of benign hyperkeratotic lesion (eg, corn or callus); single lesion

11056   two to four lesions

11057   more than four lesions

(11060-11062 have been deleted. To report, see 11300-11313)

Surgery: Integumentary System

Biopsy

11100   Biopsy of skin, subcutaneous tissue and/or mucous membrane (including simple closure), unless otherwise listed (separate procedure); single lesion

+ 11101   each separate/additional lesion (List separately in addition to code for primary procedure)

(Use 11101 in conjunction with code 11100)

(For biopsy of conjunctiva, use 68100; eyelid, use 67810)

Removal of Skin Tags

Removal by scissoring or any sharp method, ligature strangulation, electrosurgical destruction or combination of treatment modalities including chemical or electrocauterization of wound, with or without local anesthesia.

11200*   Removal of skin tags, multiple fibrocutaneous tags, any area; up to and including 15 lesions

+ 11201   each additional ten lesions (List separately in addition to code for primary procedure)

(Use 11201 in conjunction with code 11200)

Shaving of Epidermal or Dermal Lesions

Shaving is the sharp removal by transverse incision or horizontal slicing to remove epidermal and dermal lesions without a full-thickness dermal excision. This includes local anesthesia, chemical or electrocauterization of the wound. The wound does not require suture closure.

11300*   Shaving of epidermal or dermal lesion, single lesion, trunk, arms or legs; lesion diameter 0.5 cm or less

11301   lesion diameter 0.6 to 1.0 cm

11302   lesion diameter 1.1 to 2.0 cm

11303   lesion diameter over 2.0 cm

11305*   Shaving of epidermal or dermal lesion, single lesion, scalp, neck, hands, feet, genitalia; lesion diameter 0.5 cm or less

11306   lesion diameter 0.6 to 1.0 cm

11307   lesion diameter 1.1 to 2.0 cm

11308   lesion diameter over 2.0 cm

11310*   Shaving of epidermal or dermal lesion, single lesion, face, ears, eyelids, nose, lips, mucous membrane; lesion diameter 0.5 cm or less

11311   lesion diameter 0.6 to 1.0 cm

11312   lesion diameter 1.1 to 2.0 cm

11313   lesion diameter over 2.0 cm

Excision—Benign Lesions

Excision (including simple closure) of benign lesions of skin ►(eg, neoplasm,◄ cicatricial, fibrous, inflammatory, congenital, cystic lesions), ►includes◄ local anesthesia. See appropriate size and area below. ►For shave removal, see 11300 et seq., and for electrosurgical and other methods see 17000 et seq.◄

Excision is defined as full-thickness (through the dermis) removal of ►a lesion, including margins,◄ and includes simple (non-layered) closure ►when performed. Report separately each benign lesion excised. Code selection is determined by measuring the greatest clinical diameter of the apparent lesion plus that margin required for complete excision (lesion diameter plus the most narrow margins required equals the excised diameter). The margins refer to the most narrow margin required to adequately excise the lesion, based on the physician's judgment. The measurement of lesion plus margin is made prior to excision. The excised diameter is the same whether the surgical defect is repaired in a linear fashion, or reconstructed (eg with a skin graft).◄

The closure of defects created by incision, excision, or trauma may require intermediate or complex closure. Repair by intermediate or complex closure should be reported separately. ►For excision of benign lesions requiring more than simple closure, ie, requiring intermediate or complex closure, report 11400-11466 in addition to appropriate intermediate (12031-12057) or complex closure (13100-13153) codes. For reconstructive closure, see 11400-14300, 15000-15261, 15570-15770.◄ See page 50 for definition of intermediate or complex closure.

▲ 11400   Excision, benign lesion including margins, except skin tag (unless listed elsewhere), trunk, arms or legs; excised diameter 0.5 cm or less

▲ 11401   excised diameter 0.6 to 1.0 cm

▲ 11402   excised diameter 1.1 to 2.0 cm

▲ 11403   excised diameter 2.1 to 3.0 cm

▲ 11404   excised diameter 3.1 to 4.0 cm

▲ 11406   excised diameter over 4.0 cm

(For unusual or complicated excision, add modifier '-22')

▲ 11420   Excision, benign lesion including margins, except skin tag (unless listed elsewhere), scalp, neck, hands, feet, genitalia; excised diameter 0.5 cm or less

▲ 11421   excised diameter 0.6 to 1.0 cm

▲ 11422   excised diameter 1.1 to 2.0 cm

▲ 11423   excised diameter 2.1 to 3.0 cm

▲ 11424   excised diameter 3.1 to 4.0 cm

▲ 11426   excised diameter over 4.0 cm

(For unusual or complicated excision, add modifier '-22')

▲**11440**   Excision, other benign lesion including margins (unless listed elsewhere), face, ears, eyelids, nose, lips, mucous membrane; excised diameter 0.5 cm or less

▲**11441**   excised diameter 0.6 to 1.0 cm

▲**11442**   excised diameter 1.1 to 2.0 cm

▲**11443**   excised diameter 2.1 to 3.0 cm

▲**11444**   excised diameter 3.1 to 4.0 cm

▲**11446**   excised diameter over 4.0 cm

(For unusual or complicated excision, add modifier '-22')

(For eyelids involving more than skin, see also 67800 et seq)

11450   Excision of skin and subcutaneous tissue for hidradenitis, axillary; with simple or intermediate repair

11451   with complex repair

11462   Excision of skin and subcutaneous tissue for hidradenitis, inguinal; with simple or intermediate repair

11463   with complex repair

11470   Excision of skin and subcutaneous tissue for hidradenitis, perianal, perineal, or umbilical; with simple or intermediate repair

11471   with complex repair

(When skin graft or flap is used for closure, use appropriate procedure code in addition)

(For bilateral procedure, add modifier '-50')

Excision—Malignant Lesions

Excision (including simple closure) of malignant ►lesions◄ of skin ►(eg, basal cell carcinoma, squamous cell carcinoma, melanoma) includes◄ local anesthesia. ►(See appropriate size and body area below.)◄ For ►destruction◄ of malignant lesions of skin, see destruction codes ►17260-17286.◄

Excision is defined as full-thickness (through the dermis) removal of ►a lesion including margins, and includes simple (non-layered) closure when performed. Report separately each malignant lesion excised. Code selection is determined by measuring the greatest clinical diameter of the apparent lesion plus that margin required for complete excision (lesion diameter plus the most narrow margins required equals the excised diameter). The margins refer to the most narrow margin required to adequately excise the lesion, based on the physician's judgment. The measurement of lesion plus margin is made prior to excision. The excised diameter is the same whether the surgical defect is repaired in a linear fashion, or reconstructed (eg with a skin graft).◄

The closure of defects created by incision, excision, or trauma may require intermediate or complex closure. Repair by intermediate or complex closure should be reported separately. ►For excision of malignant lesions requiring more than simple closure, ie, requiring intermediate or complex closure, report 11600-11646 in addition to appropriate intermediate (12031-12057) or complex closure (13100-13153) codes. For reconstructive closure, see 14000-14300, 15000-15261, 15570-15770.◄ See page 50 for definition of intermediate or complex closure.

►When frozen section pathology shows the margins of excision were not adequate, an additional excision may be necessary for complete tumor removal. Use only one code to report the additional excision and re-excision(s) based on the final widest excised diameter required for complete tumor removal at the same operative session. To report a re-excision procedure performed to widen margins at a subsequent operative session, see codes 11600-11646, as appropriate. Append the modifier '-58' if the re-excision procedure is performed during the postoperative period of the primary excision procedure.◄

▲**11600**   Excision, malignant lesion including margins, trunk, arms, or legs; excised diameter 0.5 cm or less

▲**11601**   excised diameter 0.6 to 1.0 cm

▲**11602**   excised diameter 1.1 to 2.0 cm

▲**11603**   excised diameter 2.1 to 3.0 cm

▲**11604**   excised diameter 3.1 to 4.0 cm

▲**11606**   excised diameter over 4.0 cm

▲**11620**   Excision, malignant lesion including margins, scalp, neck, hands, feet, genitalia; excised diameter 0.5 cm or less

▲**11621**   excised diameter 0.6 to 1.0 cm

▲**11622**   excised diameter 1.1 to 2.0 cm

▲**11623**   excised diameter 2.1 to 3.0 cm

▲**11624**   excised diameter 3.1 to 4.0 cm

▲**11626**   excised diameter over 4.0 cm

▲**11640**   Excision, malignant lesion including margins, face, ears, eyelids, nose, lips; excised diameter 0.5 cm or less

▲**11641**   excised diameter 0.6 to 1.0 cm

▲**11642**   excised diameter 1.1 to 2.0 cm

▲**11643**   excised diameter 2.1 to 3.0 cm

▲**11644**   excised diameter 3.1 to 4.0 cm

▲**11646**   excised diameter over 4.0 cm

(For eyelids involving more than skin, see also 67800 et seq)

Surgery: Integumentary System

Nails

(For drainage of paronychia or onychia, see 10060, 10061)

(11700, 11701 have been deleted. To report, use 11720, 11721)

(11710, 11711 have been deleted. To report, use 11720, 11721)

11719 Trimming of nondystrophic nails, any number

11720 Debridement of nail(s) by any method(s); one to five

11721   six or more

11730* Avulsion of nail plate, partial or complete, simple; single

(11731 has been deleted. To report, use 11732)

+ 11732   each additional nail plate (List separately in addition to code for primary procedure)

(Use 11732 in conjunction with code 11730)

11740 Evacuation of subungual hematoma

11750 Excision of nail and nail matrix, partial or complete, (eg, ingrown or deformed nail) for permanent removal;

11752   with amputation of tuft of distal phalanx

(For skin graft, if used, use 15050)

11755 Biopsy of nail unit (eg, plate, bed, matrix, hyponychium, proximal and lateral nail folds) (separate procedure)

11760 Repair of nail bed

11762 Reconstruction of nail bed with graft

11765 Wedge excision of skin of nail fold (eg, for ingrown toenail)

(For incision of pilonidal cyst, see 10080, 10081)

11770 Excision of pilonidal cyst or sinus; simple

11771   extensive

11772   complicated

Introduction

11900* Injection, intralesional; up to and including seven lesions

11901*   more than seven lesions

(11900, 11901 are not to be used for preoperative local anesthetic injection)

(For veins, see 36470, 36471)

(For intralesional chemotherapy administration, see 96405, 96406)

11920 Tattooing, intradermal introduction of insoluble opaque pigments to correct color defects of skin, including micropigmentation; 6.0 sq cm or less

11921   6.1 to 20.0 sq cm

+ 11922   each additional 20.0 sq cm (List separately in addition to code for primary procedure)

(Use 11922 in conjunction with code 11921)

11950 Subcutaneous injection of filling material (eg, collagen); 1 cc or less

11951   1.1 to 5.0 cc

11952   5.1 to 10.0 cc

11954   over 10.0 cc

11960 Insertion of tissue expander(s) for other than breast, including subsequent expansion

(For breast reconstruction with tissue expander(s), use 19357)

11970 Replacement of tissue expander with permanent prosthesis

11971 Removal of tissue expander(s) without insertion of prosthesis

11975 Insertion, implantable contraceptive capsules

11976 Removal, implantable contraceptive capsules

11977 Removal with reinsertion, implantable contraceptive capsules

11980 Subcutaneous hormone pellet implantation (implantation of estradiol and/or testosterone pellets beneath the skin)

11981 Insertion, non-biodegradable drug delivery implant

11982 Removal, non-biodegradable drug delivery implant

11983 Removal with reinsertion, non-biodegradable drug delivery implant

Repair (Closure)

Use the codes in this section to designate wound closure utilizing sutures, staples, or tissue adhesives (eg, 2-cyanoacrylate), either singly or in combination with each other, or in combination with adhesive strips. Wound closure utilizing adhesive strips as the sole repair material should be coded using the appropriate E/M code.

Definitions

The repair of wounds may be classified as Simple, Intermediate, or Complex.

Simple repair is used when the wound is superficial; eg, involving primarily epidermis or dermis, or subcutaneous tissues without significant involvement of deeper structures, and requires simple one layer closure. This includes local anesthesia and chemical or electrocauterization of wounds not closed.

Intermediate repair includes the repair of wounds that, in addition to the above, require layered closure of one or more of the deeper layers of subcutaneous tissue and superficial (non-muscle) fascia, in addition to the skin (epidermal and dermal) closure. Single-layer closure of heavily contaminated wounds that have required extensive cleaning or removal of particulate matter also constitutes intermediate repair.

Complex repair includes the repair of wounds requiring more than layered closure, viz., scar revision, debridement, (eg, traumatic lacerations or avulsions), extensive undermining, stents or retention sutures. Necessary preparation includes creation of a defect for repairs (eg, excision of a scar requiring a complex repair) or the debridement of complicated lacerations or avulsions. Complex repair does not include excision of benign (11400-11446) or malignant (11600-11646) lesions.

Instructions for listing services at time of wound repair:

1. The repaired wound(s) should be measured and recorded in centimeters, whether curved, angular, or stellate.

2. When multiple wounds are repaired, add together the lengths of those in the same classification (see above) and from all anatomic sites that are grouped together into the same code descriptor. For example, add together the lengths of intermediate repairs to the trunk and extremities. Do not add lengths of repairs from different groupings of anatomic sites (eg, face and extremities). Also, do not add together lengths of different classifications (eg, intermediate and complex repairs).

When more than one classification of wounds is repaired, list the more complicated as the primary procedure and the less complicated as the secondary procedure, using modifier '-51'.

3. Decontamination and/or debridement: Debridement is considered a separate procedure only when gross contamination requires prolonged cleansing, when appreciable amounts of devitalized or contaminated tissue are removed, or when debridement is carried out separately without immediate primary closure. (For extensive debridement of soft tissue and/or bone, see 11040-11044.)

(For extensive debridement of soft tissue and/or bone, not associated with open fracture(s) and/or dislocation(s) resulting from penetrating and/or blunt trauma, see 11040-11044.)

(For extensive debridement of subcutaneous tissue, muscle fascia, muscle, and/or bone associated with open fracture(s) and/or dislocation(s), see 11010-11012.)

4. Involvement of nerves, blood vessels and tendons: Report under appropriate system (Nervous, Cardiovascular, Musculoskeletal) for repair of these structures. The repair of these associated wounds is included in the primary procedure unless it qualifies as a complex wound, in which case modifier '-51' applies.

Simple ligation of vessels in an open wound is considered as part of any wound closure.

Simple "exploration" of nerves, blood vessels or tendons exposed in an open wound is also considered part of the essential treatment of the wound and is not a separate procedure unless appreciable dissection is required. If the wound requires enlargement, extension of dissection (to determine penetration), debridement, removal of foreign body(s), ligation or coagulation of minor subcutaneous and/or muscular blood vessel(s) of the subcutaneous tissue, muscle fascia, and/or muscle, not requiring thoracotomy or laparotomy, use codes 20100-20103, as appropriate.

Repair—Simple

Sum of lengths of repairs for each group of anatomic sites.

12001*	Simple repair of superficial wounds of scalp, neck, axillae, external genitalia, trunk and/or extremities (including hands and feet); 2.5 cm or less
12002*	2.6 cm to 7.5 cm
12004*	7.6 cm to 12.5 cm
12005	12.6 cm to 20.0 cm
12006	20.1 cm to 30.0 cm
12007	over 30.0 cm
12011*	Simple repair of superficial wounds of face, ears, eyelids, nose, lips and/or mucous membranes; 2.5 cm or less
12013*	2.6 cm to 5.0 cm
12014	5.1 cm to 7.5 cm
12015	7.6 cm to 12.5 cm
12016	12.6 cm to 20.0 cm
12017	20.1 cm to 30.0 cm
12018	over 30.0 cm
12020	Treatment of superficial wound dehiscence; simple closure
12021	with packing

(For extensive or complicated secondary wound closure, use 13160)

Repair—Intermediate

Sum of lengths of repairs for each group of anatomic sites.

12031*	Layer closure of wounds of scalp, axillae, trunk and/or extremities (excluding hands and feet); 2.5 cm or less
12032*	2.6 cm to 7.5 cm
12034	7.6 cm to 12.5 cm
12035	12.6 cm to 20.0 cm
12036	20.1 cm to 30.0 cm
12037	over 30.0 cm

12041*   Layer closure of wounds of neck, hands, feet and/or external genitalia; 2.5 cm or less

12042   2.6 cm to 7.5 cm

12044   7.6 cm to 12.5 cm

12045   12.6 cm to 20.0 cm

12046   20.1 cm to 30.0 cm

12047   over 30.0 cm

12051*   Layer closure of wounds of face, ears, eyelids, nose, lips and/or mucous membranes; 2.5 cm or less

12052   2.6 cm to 5.0 cm

12053   5.1 cm to 7.5 cm

12054   7.6 cm to 12.5 cm

12055   12.6 cm to 20.0 cm

12056   20.1 cm to 30.0 cm

12057   over 30.0 cm

Repair—Complex

Reconstructive procedures, complicated wound closure.

Sum of lengths of repairs for each group of anatomic sites.

(For full thickness repair of lip or eyelid, see respective anatomical subsections)

13100   Repair, complex, trunk; 1.1 cm to 2.5 cm

(For 1.0 cm or less, see simple or intermediate repairs)

13101   2.6 cm to 7.5 cm

+ 13102   each additional 5 cm or less (List separately in addition to code for primary procedure)

(Use 13102 in conjunction with code 13101)

13120   Repair, complex, scalp, arms, and/or legs; 1.1 cm to 2.5 cm

(For 1.0 cm or less, see simple or intermediate repairs)

13121   2.6 cm to 7.5 cm

+ 13122   each additional 5 cm or less (List separately in addition to code for primary procedure)

(Use 13122 in conjunction with code 13121)

13131   Repair, complex, forehead, cheeks, chin, mouth, neck, axillae, genitalia, hands and/or feet; 1.1 cm to 2.5 cm

(For 1.0 cm or less, see simple or intermediate repairs)

13132   2.6 cm to 7.5 cm

+ 13133   each additional 5 cm or less (List separately in addition to code for primary procedure)

(Use 13133 in conjunction with code 13132)

13150   Repair, complex, eyelids, nose, ears and/or lips; 1.0 cm or less

(See also 40650-40654, 67961-67975)

13151   1.1 cm to 2.5 cm

13152   2.6 cm to 7.5 cm

+ 13153   each additional 5 cm or less (List separately in addition to code for primary procedure)

(Use 13153 in conjunction with code 13152)

13160   Secondary closure of surgical wound or dehiscence, extensive or complicated

(For packing or simple secondary wound closure, see 12020, 12021)

(13300 has been deleted. To report, see 13102, 13122, 13133 and 13153)

Adjacent Tissue Transfer or Rearrangement

For full thickness repair of lip or eyelid, see respective anatomical subsections.

Excision (including lesion) and/or repair by adjacent tissue transfer or rearrangement (eg, Z-plasty, W-plasty, V-Y plasty, rotation flap, advancement flap, double pedicle flap). When applied in repairing lacerations, the procedures listed must be developed by the surgeon to accomplish the repair. They do not apply when direct closure or rearrangement of traumatic wounds incidentally result in these configurations.

Skin graft necessary to close secondary defect is considered an additional procedure.

14000   Adjacent tissue transfer or rearrangement, trunk; defect 10 sq cm or less

14001   defect 10.1 sq cm to 30.0 sq cm

14020   Adjacent tissue transfer or rearrangement, scalp, arms and/or legs; defect 10 sq cm or less

14021   defect 10.1 sq cm to 30.0 sq cm

14040   Adjacent tissue transfer or rearrangement, forehead, cheeks, chin, mouth, neck, axillae, genitalia, hands and/or feet; defect 10 sq cm or less

14041   defect 10.1 sq cm to 30.0 sq cm

14060   Adjacent tissue transfer or rearrangement, eyelids, nose, ears and/or lips; defect 10 sq cm or less

14061   defect 10.1 sq cm to 30.0 sq cm

(For eyelid, full thickness, see 67961 et seq)

14300   Adjacent tissue transfer or rearrangement, more than 30 sq cm, unusual or complicated, any area

14350   Filleted finger or toe flap, including preparation of recipient site

Free Skin Grafts

Identify by size and location of the defect (recipient area) and the type of graft; includes simple debridement of granulations or recent avulsion.

When a primary procedure such as orbitectomy, radical mastectomy, or deep tumor removal requires skin graft for definitive closure, see appropriate anatomical subsection for primary procedure and this section for skin graft.

Use 15000 for initial wound preparation.

Use 15100-15261 for autogenous skin grafts. For autogenous tissue-cultured skin grafts, use 15100-15121. These codes include harvesting of keratinocytes and their subsequent application. Procedures are coded by recipient site. Use codes 15342 and 15343 for application of skin substitute/neodermis. Use modifier '-58' for staged application procedure(s).

Repair of donor site requiring skin graft or local flaps is to be added as an additional procedure.

Codes 15000, 15001, 15350, 15351, 15400, 15401 describe burn and wound preparation and management procedures. The following definition should be applied to codes 15000, 15001, 15100, 15101, 15120, 15121 when determining the involvement of body size. The measurement of 100 sq cm is applicable to adults and children age 10 and over, percentages apply to infants and children under the age of 10.

(For microvascular flaps, see 15756-15758)

15000   Surgical preparation or creation of recipient site by excision of open wounds, burn eschar, or scar (including subcutaneous tissues); first 100 sq cm or one percent of body area of infants and children

(For appropriate skin grafts, see 15050-15261; list the free graft separately by its procedure number when the graft, immediate or delayed, is applied)

+ 15001   each additional 100 sq cm or each additional one percent of body area of infants and children (List separately in addition to code for primary procedure)

(Use code 15001 in conjunction with code 15000)

(For excision of benign lesions, see 11400-11471)

(For excision of malignant lesions, see 11600-11646)

(For excision with alloplastic dressing, use 15000 only)

(For excision with immediate skin grafting use 15050-15261 in addition to 15000)

(For excision with immediate allograft placement use 15350 in addition to 15000)

(For excision with immediate xenograft placement use 15400 in addition to 15000)

15050   Pinch graft, single or multiple, to cover small ulcer, tip of digit, or other minimal open area (except on face), up to defect size 2 cm diameter

15100   Split graft, trunk, arms, legs; first 100 sq cm or less, or one percent of body area of infants and children (except 15050)

+ 15101   each additional 100 sq cm, or each additional one percent of body area of infants and children, or part thereof (List separately in addition to code for primary procedure)

(Use 15101 in conjunction with code 15100)

15120   Split graft, face, scalp, eyelids, mouth, neck, ears, orbits, genitalia, hands, feet and/or multiple digits; first 100 sq cm or less, or one percent of body area of infants and children (except 15050)

+ 15121   each additional 100 sq cm, or each additional one percent of body area of infants and children, or part thereof (List separately in addition to code for primary procedure)

(Use 15121 in conjunction with code 15120)

(For eyelids, see also 67961 et seq)

15200   Full thickness graft, free, including direct closure of donor site, trunk; 20 sq cm or less

+ 15201   each additional 20 sq cm (List separately in addition to code for primary procedure)

(Use 15201 in conjunction with code 15200)

15220   Full thickness graft, free, including direct closure of donor site, scalp, arms, and/or legs; 20 sq cm or less

+ 15221   each additional 20 sq cm (List separately in addition to code for primary procedure)

(Use 15221 in conjunction with code 15220)

15240   Full thickness graft, free, including direct closure of donor site, forehead, cheeks, chin, mouth, neck, axillae, genitalia, hands, and/or feet; 20 sq cm or less

(For finger tip graft, use 15050)

(For repair of syndactyly, fingers, see 26560-26562)

+ 15241   each additional 20 sq cm (List separately in addition to code for primary procedure)

(Use 15241 in conjunction with code 15240)

15260   Full thickness graft, free, including direct closure of donor site, nose, ears, eyelids, and/or lips; 20 sq cm or less

+ 15261   each additional 20 sq cm (List separately in addition to code for primary procedure)

(Use 15261 in conjunction with code 15260)

(For eyelids, see also 67961 et seq)

(Repair of donor site requiring skin graft or local flaps, to be added as additional separate procedure)

15342   Application of bilaminate skin substitute/neodermis; 25 sq cm

+ 15343   each additional 25 sq cm (List separately in addition to code for primary procedure)

(Use 15343 in conjunction with code 15342)

Surgery: Integumentary System

15350 Application of allograft, skin; 100 sq cm or less

(For staged tissue graft implantation, use modifier '-58')

+ 15351 each additional 100 sq cm (List separately in addition to code for primary procedure)

(Use 15351 in conjunction with code 15350)

15400 Application of xenograft, skin; 100 sq cm or less

+ 15401 each additional 100 sq cm (List separately in addition to code for primary procedure)

(Use 15401 in conjunction with code 15400)

(15410-15416 have been deleted. To report, see 15756-15758)

Flaps (Skin and/or Deep Tissues)

Regions listed refer to recipient area (not donor site) when flap is being attached in transfer or to final site.

Regions listed refer to donor site when tube is formed for later or when "delay" of flap is prior to transfer.

Procedures 15570-15738 do not include extensive immobilization (eg, large plaster casts and other immobilizing devices are considered additional separate procedures).

Repair of donor site requiring skin graft or local flaps is considered an additional separate procedure.

(For microvascular flaps, see 15756-15758)

(15500-15515 have been deleted. To report, use 15000)

(15540-15555 have been deleted. To report, see 15570-15576)

15570 Formation of direct or tubed pedicle, with or without transfer; trunk

15572 scalp, arms, or legs

15574 forehead, cheeks, chin, mouth, neck, axillae, genitalia, hands or feet

15576 eyelids, nose, ears, lips, or intraoral

(15580 has been deleted. To report, use 15574)

15600 Delay of flap or sectioning of flap (division and inset); at trunk

15610 at scalp, arms, or legs

15620 at forehead, cheeks, chin, neck, axillae, genitalia, hands, or feet

(15625 has been deleted. To report, use 15620)

15630 at eyelids, nose, ears, or lips

15650 Transfer, intermediate, of any pedicle flap (eg, abdomen to wrist, Walking tube), any location

(15700-15730 have been deleted. To report, see 15570-15576)

(For eyelids, nose, ears, or lips, see also anatomical area)

(For revision, defatting or rearranging of transferred pedicle flap or skin graft, see 13100-14300)

(Procedures 15732-15738 are described by donor site of the muscle, myocutaneous, or fasciocutaneous flap)

15732 Muscle, myocutaneous, or fasciocutaneous flap; head and neck (eg, temporalis, masseter muscle, sternocleidomastoid, levator scapulae)

15734 trunk

15736 upper extremity

15738 lower extremity

Other Flaps and Grafts

Repair of donor site requiring skin graft or local flaps should be reported as an additional procedure.

15740 Flap; island pedicle

(15745 has been deleted. To report, see 15732-15738)

15750 neurovascular pedicle

(15755 has been deleted. To report, see 15756-15758)

▲ 15756 Free muscle or myocutaneous flap with microvascular anastomosis

(Do not report code 69990 in addition to code 15756)

15757 Free skin flap with microvascular anastomosis

(Do not report code 69990 in addition to code 15757)

15758 Free fascial flap with microvascular anastomosis

(Do not report code 69990 in addition to code 15758)

15760 Graft; composite (eg, full thickness of external ear or nasal ala), including primary closure, donor area

15770 derma-fat-fascia

15775 Punch graft for hair transplant; 1 to 15 punch grafts

15776 more than 15 punch grafts

(For strip transplant, use 15220)

Other Procedures

15780 Dermabrasion; total face (eg, for acne scarring, fine wrinkling, rhytids, general keratosis)

15781 segmental, face

15782 regional, other than face

15783 superficial, any site, (eg, tattoo removal)

(15785 has been deleted. To report, see 15781, 15782)

15786* Abrasion; single lesion (eg, keratosis, scar)

+ 15787 each additional four lesions or less (List separately in addition to code for primary procedure)

(Use 15787 in conjunction with code 15786)

15788   Chemical peel, facial; epidermal

15789   dermal

         (15790, 15791 have been deleted. To report, see 15788-
         15793)

15792   Chemical peel, nonfacial; epidermal

15793   dermal

         (15800 has been deleted)

15810   Salabrasion; 20 sq cm or less

15811   over 20 sq cm

15819   Cervicoplasty

15820   Blepharoplasty, lower eyelid;

15821   with extensive herniated fat pad

15822   Blepharoplasty, upper eyelid;

15823   with excessive skin weighting down lid

         (For bilateral blepharoplasty, add modifier '-50')

         (See also 67916, 67917, 67923, 67924)

15824   Rhytidectomy; forehead

         (For repair of brow ptosis, use 67900)

15825   neck with platysmal tightening (platysmal flap, P-flap)

15826   glabellar frown lines

         (15827 has been deleted. To report, use 15838)

15828   cheek, chin, and neck

15829   superficial musculoaponeurotic system (SMAS) flap

         (For bilateral rhytidectomy, add modifier '-50')

15831   Excision, excessive skin and subcutaneous tissue
         (including lipectomy); abdomen (abdominoplasty)

15832   thigh

15833   leg

15834   hip

15835   buttock

15836   arm

15837   forearm or hand

15838   submental fat pad

15839   other area

         (For bilateral procedure, add modifier '-50')

15840   Graft for facial nerve paralysis; free fascia graft
         (including obtaining fascia)

         (For bilateral procedure, add modifier '-50')

15841   free muscle graft (including obtaining graft)

15842   free muscle flap by microsurgical technique

         (Do not report code 69990 in addition to code 15842)

15845   regional muscle transfer

         (For intravenous fluorescein examination of blood flow in
         graft or flap, use 15860)

         (For nerve transfers, decompression, or repair, see 64831-
         64876, 64905, 64907, 69720, 69725, 69740, 69745,
         69955)

15850   Removal of sutures under anesthesia (other than local),
         same surgeon

15851   Removal of sutures under anesthesia (other than local),
         other surgeon

15852   Dressing change (for other than burns) under anesthesia
         (other than local)

15860   Intravenous injection of agent (eg, fluorescein) to test
         vascular flow in flap or graft

         (15875 has been deleted. To report, see 15876-15879)

15876   Suction assisted lipectomy; head and neck

15877   trunk

15878   upper extremity

15879   lower extremity

Pressure Ulcers (Decubitus Ulcers)

15920   Excision, coccygeal pressure ulcer, with coccygectomy;
         with primary suture

15922   with flap closure

         (15930 has been deleted. To report, use 15934)

15931   Excision, sacral pressure ulcer, with primary suture;

         (15932 has been deleted)

15933   with ostectomy

15934   Excision, sacral pressure ulcer, with skin flap closure;

15935   with ostectomy

15936   Excision, sacral pressure ulcer, in preparation for muscle
         or myocutaneous flap or skin graft closure;

15937   with ostectomy

         (For repair of defect using muscle or myocutaneous flap,
         use code(s) 15734 and/or 15738 in addition to 15936,
         15937. For repair of defect using split skin graft, use
         codes 15100 and/or 15101 in addition to 15936, 15937)

15940   Excision, ischial pressure ulcer, with primary suture;

15941   with ostectomy (ischiectomy)

         (15942, 15943 have been deleted. To report, see 15944-
         15946)

15944   Excision, ischial pressure ulcer, with skin flap closure;

15945   with ostectomy

15946   Excision, ischial pressure ulcer, with ostectomy, in preparation for muscle or myocutaneous flap or skin graft closure

(For repair of defect using muscle or myocutaneous flap, use code(s) 15734 and/or 15738 in addition to 15946. For repair of defect using split skin graft, use codes 15100 and/or 15101 in addition to 15946)

15950   Excision, trochanteric pressure ulcer, with primary suture;

15951   with ostectomy

15952   Excision, trochanteric pressure ulcer, with skin flap closure;

15953   with ostectomy

(15954 and 15955 have been deleted. To report, use appropriate debridement, closure or flap codes)

15956   Excision, trochanteric pressure ulcer, in preparation for muscle or myocutaneous flap or skin graft closure;

15958   with ostectomy

(For repair of defect using muscle or myocutaneous flap, use code(s) 15734 and/or 15738 in addition to 15956, 15958. For repair of defect using split skin graft, use codes 15100 and/or 15101 in addition to 15956, 15958)

(15960-15983 have been deleted. To report, use appropriate debridement, closure or flap codes)

15999   Unlisted procedure, excision pressure ulcer

(For free skin graft to close ulcer or donor site, see 15000 et seq)

Burns, Local Treatment

Procedures 16000-16036 refer to local treatment of burned surface only.

List percentage of body surface involved and depth of burn.

For necessary related medical services (eg, hospital visits, detention) in management of burned patients, see appropriate services in **Evaluation and Management** and **Medicine** sections.

(For skin graft, see 15100-15650)

16000   Initial treatment, first degree burn, when no more than local treatment is required

16010   Dressings and/or debridement, initial or subsequent; under anesthesia, small

16015   under anesthesia, medium or large, or with major debridement

16020*   without anesthesia, office or hospital, small

16025*   without anesthesia, medium (eg, whole face or whole extremity)

16030   without anesthesia, large (eg, more than one extremity)

16035   Escharotomy; initial incision

16036   each additional incision (List separately in addition to code for primary procedure)

(Use 16036 in conjunction with code 16035)

(For debridement, curettement of burn wound, see 16010-16030)

(16040-16042 have been deleted. To report, use 15000)

Destruction

Destruction means the ablation of benign, premalignant or malignant tissues by any method, with or without curettement, including local anesthesia, and not usually requiring closure.

Any method includes electrosurgery, cryosurgery, laser and chemical treatment. Lesions include condylomata, papillomata, molluscum contagiosum, herpetic lesions, warts (ie, common, plantar, flat), milia, or other benign, premalignant (eg, actinic keratoses), or malignant lesions.

(For destruction of lesion(s) in specific anatomic sites, see 40820, 46900-46917, 46924, 54050-54057, 54065, 56501, 56515, 57061, 57065, 67850, 68135)

(For paring or cutting of benign hyperkeratotic lesions (eg, corns or calluses), see 11055-11057)

(For sharp removal or electrosurgical destruction of skin tags and fibrocutaneous tags, see 11200, 11201)

(For cryotherapy of acne, use 17340)

(For initiation or follow-up care of topical chemotherapy (eg, 5-FU or similar agents), see appropriate office visits)

(For shaving of epidermal or dermal lesions, see 11300-11313)

Destruction, Benign or Premalignant Lesions

17000*   Destruction (eg, laser surgery, electrosurgery, cryosurgery, chemosurgery, surgical curettement), all benign or premalignant lesions (eg, actinic keratoses) other than skin tags or cutaneous vascular proliferative lesions; first lesion

(17001, 17002 have been deleted. To report, see 17003, 17004)

+ 17003   second through 14 lesions, each (List separately in addition to code for first lesion)

(Use 17003 in conjunction with code 17000)

⊘ **17004**   Destruction (eg, laser surgery, electrosurgery, cryosurgery, chemosurgery, surgical curettement), all benign or premalignant lesions (eg, actinic keratoses) other than skin tags or cutaneous vascular proliferative lesions; 15 or more lesions

(Do not report 17004 in conjunction with codes 17000-17003)

(17010 has been deleted. To report, see specific anatomic site code)

(17100-17105 have been deleted. To report, see 17000, 17003, 17004)

17106   Destruction of cutaneous vascular proliferative lesions (eg, laser technique); less than 10 sq cm

17107   10.0 to 50.0 sq cm

17108   over 50.0 sq cm

17110*   Destruction (eg, laser surgery, electrosurgery, cryosurgery, chemosurgery, surgical curettement), of flat warts, molluscum contagiosum, or milia; up to 14 lesions

17111   15 or more lesions

(For destruction of common or plantar warts, see 17000, 17003, 17004)

(17200, 17201 have been deleted. To report, see 11200, 11201)

17250*   Chemical cauterization of granulation tissue (proud flesh, sinus or fistula)

(17250 is not to be used with removal or excision codes for the same lesion)

Destruction, Malignant Lesions, Any Method

17260*   Destruction, malignant lesion (eg, laser surgery, electrosurgery, cryosurgery, chemosurgery, surgical curettement), trunk, arms or legs; lesion diameter 0.5 cm or less

17261   lesion diameter 0.6 to 1.0 cm

17262   lesion diameter 1.1 to 2.0 cm

17263   lesion diameter 2.1 to 3.0 cm

17264   lesion diameter 3.1 to 4.0 cm

17266   lesion diameter over 4.0 cm

17270*   Destruction, malignant lesion (eg, laser surgery, electrosurgery, cryosurgery, chemosurgery, surgical curettement), scalp, neck, hands, feet, genitalia; lesion diameter 0.5 cm or less

17271   lesion diameter 0.6 to 1.0 cm

17272   lesion diameter 1.1 to 2.0 cm

17273   lesion diameter 2.1 to 3.0 cm

17274   lesion diameter 3.1 to 4.0 cm

17276   lesion diameter over 4.0 cm

17280*   Destruction, malignant lesion (eg, laser surgery, electrosurgery, cryosurgery, chemosurgery, surgical curettement), face, ears, eyelids, nose, lips, mucous membrane; lesion diameter 0.5 cm or less

17281   lesion diameter 0.6 to 1.0 cm

17282   lesion diameter 1.1 to 2.0 cm

17283   lesion diameter 2.1 to 3.0 cm

17284   lesion diameter 3.1 to 4.0 cm

17286   lesion diameter over 4.0 cm

Mohs Micrographic Surgery

Mohs micrographic surgery, for the removal of complex or ill-defined skin cancer, requires a single physician to act in two integrated, but separate and distinct capacities: surgeon and pathologist. If either of these responsibilities are delegated to another physician who reports his services separately, these codes are not appropriate. If repair is performed, use separate repair, flap, or graft codes. ►If a biopsy of a suspected skin cancer is performed on the same day as Mohs surgery because there was no prior pathology confirmation of a diagnosis, then report diagnostic skin biopsy (11100, 11101) and frozen section pathology (88331) with modifier '-59' to distinguish from the subsequent definitive surgical procedure of Mohs surgery.◄

(17300-17302 have been deleted. To report, use 17304-17310)

(17303 has been deleted)

⊘ ▲ **17304**   Chemosurgery (Mohs micrographic technique), including removal of all gross tumor, surgical excision of tissue specimens, mapping, color coding of specimens, microscopic examination of specimens by the surgeon, and complete histopathologic preparation including the first routine stain (eg, hematoxylin and eosin, toluidine blue); first stage, fresh tissue technique, up to 5 specimens

►(If additional special pathology procedures, stains or immunostains are required, use 88311-88314, 88342)◄

⊘ **17305**   second stage, fixed or fresh tissue, up to 5 specimens

⊘ **17306**   third stage, fixed or fresh tissue, up to 5 specimens

⊘ **17307**   additional stage(s), up to 5 specimens, each stage

+ ▲ **17310**   each additional specimen, after the first 5 specimens, fixed or fresh tissue, any stage (List separately in addition to code for primary procedure)

►(Use 17310 in conjunction with codes 17304-17307)◄

Other Procedures

17340*   Cryotherapy (CO_2 slush, liquid N_2) for acne

17360*   Chemical exfoliation for acne (eg, acne paste, acid)

17380*   Electrolysis epilation, each 1/2 hour

(For actinotherapy, use 96900)

17999   Unlisted procedure, skin, mucous membrane and subcutaneous tissue

Breast

Incision

19000* Puncture aspiration of cyst of breast;

+ 19001 each additional cyst (List separately in addition to code for primary procedure)

(Use 19001 in conjunction with code 19000)

(If imaging guidance is performed, see 76095, 76096, 76393, 76942)

19020 Mastotomy with exploration or drainage of abscess, deep

19030 Injection procedure only for mammary ductogram or galactogram

(For radiological supervision and interpretation, see 76086, 76088)

Excision

(All codes for bilateral procedures have been deleted. To report, add modifier '-50')

19100* Biopsy of breast; percutaneous, needle core, not using imaging guidance (separate procedure)

(For fine needle aspiration, use 10021)

(For image guided breast biopsy, see 19102, 19103, 10022)

19101 open, incisional

19102 percutaneous, needle core, using imaging guidance

(For placement of percutaneous localization clip, use 19295)

19103 percutaneous, automated vacuum assisted or rotating biopsy device, using imaging guidance

(For imaging guidance performed in conjunction with 19102, 19103, see 76095, 76096, 76360, 76393, 76942)

(For placement of percutaneous localization clip, use 19295)

19110 Nipple exploration, with or without excision of a solitary lactiferous duct or a papilloma lactiferous duct

19112 Excision of lactiferous duct fistula

19120 Excision of cyst, fibroadenoma, or other benign or malignant tumor, aberrant breast tissue, duct lesion, nipple or areolar lesion (except 19140), open, male or female, one or more lesions

19125 Excision of breast lesion identified by preoperative placement of radiological marker, open; single lesion

+ 19126 each additional lesion separately identified by a preoperative radiological marker (List separately in addition to code for primary procedure)

(Use 19126 in conjunction with code 19125)

19140 Mastectomy for gynecomastia

19160 Mastectomy, partial;

19162 with axillary lymphadenectomy

19180 Mastectomy, simple, complete

(For immediate or delayed insertion of implant, use 19340 or 19342)

(For gynecomastia, use 19140)

19182 Mastectomy, subcutaneous

(19184-19187 have been deleted. To report, use 19182 with 19340 or 19342)

19200 Mastectomy, radical, including pectoral muscles, axillary lymph nodes

(19211-19216 have been deleted. To report, use 19200 with 19340 or 19342)

19220 Mastectomy, radical, including pectoral muscles, axillary and internal mammary lymph nodes (Urban type operation)

(19224-19229 have been deleted. To report, use 19220 with 19340 or 19342)

19240 Mastectomy, modified radical, including axillary lymph nodes, with or without pectoralis minor muscle, but excluding pectoralis major muscle

(19250-19255 have been deleted. To report, use 19240 with 19340 or 19342)

19260 Excision of chest wall tumor including ribs

19271 Excision of chest wall tumor involving ribs, with plastic reconstruction; without mediastinal lymphadenectomy

19272 with mediastinal lymphadenectomy

Introduction

19290 Preoperative placement of needle localization wire, breast;

+ 19291 each additional lesion (List separately in addition to code for primary procedure)

(Use 19291 in conjunction with code 19290)

(For radiological supervision and interpretation, see 76095, 76096, 76942)

+ 19295 Image guided placement, metallic localization clip, percutaneous, during breast biopsy (List separately in addition to code for primary procedure)

(Use 19295 in conjunction with codes 19102, 19103)

Repair and/or Reconstruction

(19300-19304 have been deleted. To report, see 19316, 19318)

(19310, 19311 have been deleted. To report, use 19325)

(All codes for bilateral procedures have been deleted. To report, add modifier '-50')

19316   Mastopexy

19318   Reduction mammaplasty

19324   Mammaplasty, augmentation; without prosthetic implant

19325   with prosthetic implant

(For flap or graft, use also appropriate number)

19328   Removal of intact mammary implant

19330   Removal of mammary implant material

19340   Immediate insertion of breast prosthesis following mastopexy, mastectomy or in reconstruction

19342   Delayed insertion of breast prosthesis following mastopexy, mastectomy or in reconstruction

(For supply of implant, use 99070)

(For preparation of custom breast implant, use 19396)

19350   Nipple/areola reconstruction

19355   Correction of inverted nipples

19357   Breast reconstruction, immediate or delayed, with tissue expander, including subsequent expansion

(19360 has been deleted)

19361   Breast reconstruction with latissimus dorsi flap, with or without prosthetic implant

(19362 has been deleted. To report, see 19367-19369)

19364   Breast reconstruction with free flap

(Do not report code 69990 in addition to code 19364)

(19364 includes harvesting of the flap, microvascular transfer, closure of the donor site, and inset shaping the flap into a breast)

19366   Breast reconstruction with other technique

(For operating microscope, use 69990)

(For insertion of prosthesis, use also 19340 or 19342)

19367   Breast reconstruction with transverse rectus abdominis myocutaneous flap (TRAM), single pedicle, including closure of donor site;

19368   with microvascular anastomosis (supercharging)

(Do not report code 69990 in addition to code 19368)

19369   Breast reconstruction with transverse rectus abdominis myocutaneous flap (TRAM), double pedicle, including closure of donor site

19370   Open periprosthetic capsulotomy, breast

19371   Periprosthetic capsulectomy, breast

19380   Revision of reconstructed breast

19396   Preparation of moulage for custom breast implant

Other Procedures

19499   Unlisted procedure, breast

Notes

Musculoskeletal System

Cast and strapping procedures appear at the end of this section.

The services listed below include the application and removal of the first cast or traction device only. Subsequent replacement of cast and/or traction device may require an additional listing.

Definitions

The terms "closed treatment," "open treatment," and "percutaneous skeletal fixation" have been carefully chosen to accurately reflect current orthopaedic procedural treatments. ▶Treatment is used when a fracture is stabilized by an intramedullary implant, as this procedure may be performed either "open" or "closed". In "closed" intramedullary nailing, the fracture fragments are not visualized, but an intramedullary nail is inserted across the fracture site, with the aid of x-ray imaging. As such, a closed nailing procedure is neither open (where the fracture site is visualized and reduced under direct vision) nor is it strictly closed (because the fracture hematoma can communicate with the outside environment).◀

Closed treatment specifically means that the fracture site is not surgically opened (exposed to the external environment and directly visualized). This terminology is used to describe procedures that treat fractures by three methods: 1) without manipulation 2) with manipulation 3) with or without traction.

Open treatment is used when the ▶fractured bone is either (1)◀ surgically opened (exposed to the external environment) ▶and◀ the fracture (bone ends) visualized and internal fixation may be used ▶or (2) the fractured bone is opened remote from the fracture site in order to insert an intramedullary nail across the fracture site (the fracture site is not opened and visualized).◀

Percutaneous skeletal fixation describes fracture treatment which is neither open nor closed. In this procedure, the fracture fragments are not visualized, but fixation (eg, pins) is placed across the fracture site, usually under x-ray imaging.

The type of fracture (eg, open, compound, closed) does not have any coding correlation with the type of treatment (eg, closed, open, or percutaneous) provided.

The codes for treatment of fractures and joint injuries (dislocations) are categorized by the type of manipulation (reduction) and stabilization (fixation or immobilization). These codes can apply to either open (compound) or closed fractures or joint injuries.

Skeletal traction is the application of a force (distracting or traction force) to a limb segment through a wire, pin, screw, or clamp that is attached (eg, penetrates) to bone.

Skin traction is the application of a force (longitudinal) to a limb using felt or strapping applied directly to skin only.

External fixation is the usage of skeletal pins plus an attaching mechanism/device used for temporary or definitive treatment of acute or chronic bony deformity.

Codes for obtaining autogenous bone grafts, cartilage, tendon, fascia lata grafts or other tissues through separate incisions are to be used only when the graft is not already listed as part of the basic procedure.

Re-reduction of a fracture and/or dislocation performed by the primary physician may be identified by the addition of the modifier '-76' to the usual procedure number to indicate "Repeat Procedure by Same Physician." (See guidelines.)

Codes for external fixation are to be used only when external fixation is not already listed as part of the basic procedure.

All codes for suction irrigation have been deleted. To report, list only the primary surgical procedure performed (eg, sequestrectomy, deep incision).

Manipulation is used throughout the musculoskeletal fracture and dislocation subsections to specifically mean the attempted reduction or restoration of a fracture or joint dislocation to its normal anatomic alignment by the application of manually applied forces.

General

Incision

20000*   Incision of soft tissue abscess (eg, secondary to osteomyelitis); superficial

20005   deep or complicated

        (20010 has been deleted)

Wound Exploration—Trauma (eg, Penetrating Gunshot, Stab Wound)

20100-20103 relate to wound(s) resulting from penetrating trauma. These codes describe surgical exploration and enlargement of the wound, extension of dissection (to determine penetration), debridement, removal of foreign body(s), ligation or coagulation of minor subcutaneous and/or muscular blood vessel(s), of the subcutaneous tissue, muscle fascia, and/or muscle, not requiring thoracotomy or laparotomy. If a repair is done to major structure(s) or major blood vessel(s) requiring thoracotomy or laparotomy, then those specific code(s) would supersede the use of codes 20100-20103.
To report Simple, Intermediate, or Complex repair of wound(s) that do not require enlargement of the wound, extension of dissection, etc., as stated above, use specific Repair code(s) in the Integumentary System section.

20100 Exploration of penetrating wound (separate procedure); neck

20101 chest

20102 abdomen/flank/back

20103 extremity

Excision

20150 Excision of epiphyseal bar, with or without autogenous soft tissue graft obtained through same fascial incision

(For aspiration of bone marrow, use 38220)

20200 Biopsy, muscle; superficial

20205 deep

20206* Biopsy, muscle, percutaneous needle

(If imaging guidance is performed, see 76360, 76393, 76942)

(For fine needle aspiration, use 10021 or 10022)

(For evaluation of fine needle aspirate, see 88172-88173)

(For excision of muscle tumor, deep, see specific anatomic section)

20220 Biopsy, bone, trocar, or needle; superficial (eg, ilium, sternum, spinous process, ribs)

20225 deep (eg, vertebral body, femur)

(For bone marrow biopsy, use 38221)

(For radiologic supervision and interpretation, see 76003, 76360, 76393)

20240 Biopsy, bone, excisional; superficial (eg, ilium, sternum, spinous process, ribs, trochanter of femur)

20245 deep (eg, humerus, ischium, femur)

20250 Biopsy, vertebral body, open; thoracic

20251 lumbar or cervical

(For sequestrectomy, osteomyelitis or drainage of bone abscess, see anatomical area)

Introduction or Removal

(For injection procedure for arthrography, see anatomical area)

20500* Injection of sinus tract; therapeutic (separate procedure)

20501* diagnostic (sinogram)

(For radiological supervision and interpretation, use 76080)

20520* Removal of foreign body in muscle or tendon sheath; simple

20525* deep or complicated

20526 Injection, therapeutic (eg, local anesthetic, corticosteroid), carpal tunnel

▲**20550*** Injection(s); tendon sheath, ligament

20551 tendon origin/insertion

▲**20552** single or multiple trigger point(s), one or two muscle(s)

▲**20553** single or multiple trigger point(s), three or more muscle(s)

(If imaging guidance is performed, see 76003, 76393, 76942)

▲**20600*** Arthrocentesis, aspiration and/or injection; small joint or bursa (eg, fingers, toes)

▲**20605*** intermediate joint or bursa (eg, temporomandibular, acromioclavicular, wrist, elbow or ankle, olecranon bursa)

20610* major joint or bursa (eg, shoulder, hip, knee joint, subacromial bursa)

(If imaging guidance is performed, see 76003, 76360, 76393, 76942)

●**20612** Aspiration and/or injection of ganglion cyst(s) any location

▶(To report multiple ganglion cyst aspirations/injections, use 20612 and append modifier '-59')◀

20615 Aspiration and injection for treatment of bone cyst

20650* Insertion of wire or pin with application of skeletal traction, including removal (separate procedure)

⊘**20660** Application of cranial tongs, caliper, or stereotactic frame, including removal (separate procedure)

20661 Application of halo, including removal; cranial

20662 pelvic

20663 femoral

20664 Application of halo, including removal, cranial, 6 or more pins placed, for thin skull osteology (eg, pediatric patients, hydrocephalus, osteogenesis imperfecta), requiring general anesthesia

20665* Removal of tongs or halo applied by another physician

20670* Removal of implant; superficial, (eg, buried wire, pin or rod) (separate procedure)

20680 deep (eg, buried wire, pin, screw, metal band, nail, rod or plate)

⊘**20690** Application of a uniplane (pins or wires in one plane), unilateral, external fixation system

(20691 has been deleted. To report, use 20690)

⊘**20692** Application of a multiplane (pins or wires in more than one plane), unilateral, external fixation system (eg, Ilizarov, Monticelli type)

20693 Adjustment or revision of external fixation system requiring anesthesia (eg, new pin(s) or wire(s) and/or new ring(s) or bar(s))

20694 Removal, under anesthesia, of external fixation system

Replantation

20802   Replantation, arm (includes surgical neck of humerus through elbow joint), complete amputation

         (20804 has been deleted. To report, see specific code(s) for repair of bone(s), ligament(s), tendon(s), nerve(s), or blood vessel(s) with modifier '-52')

20805   Replantation, forearm (includes radius and ulna to radial carpal joint), complete amputation

         (20806 has been deleted. To report, see specific code(s) for repair of bone(s), ligament(s), tendon(s), nerve(s), or blood vessel(s) with modifier '-52')

20808   Replantation, hand (includes hand through metacarpophalangeal joints), complete amputation

         (20812 has been deleted. To report, see specific code(s) for repair of bone(s), ligament(s), tendon(s), nerve(s), or blood vessel(s) with modifier '-52')

20816   Replantation, digit, excluding thumb (includes metacarpophalangeal joint to insertion of flexor sublimis tendon), complete amputation

         (20820 has been deleted. To report, see specific code(s) for repair of bone(s), ligament(s), tendon(s), nerve(s), or blood vessel(s) with modifier '-52')

20822   Replantation, digit, excluding thumb (includes distal tip to sublimis tendon insertion), complete amputation

         (20823 has been deleted. To report, see specific code(s) for repair of bone(s), ligament(s), tendon(s), nerve(s), or blood vessel(s) with modifier '-52')

20824   Replantation, thumb (includes carpometacarpal joint to MP joint), complete amputation

         (20826 has been deleted. To report, see specific code(s) for repair of bone(s), ligament(s), tendon(s), nerve(s), or blood vessel(s) with modifier '-52')

20827   Replantation, thumb (includes distal tip to MP joint), complete amputation

         (20828 has been deleted. To report, see specific code(s) for repair of bone(s), ligament(s), tendon(s), nerve(s), or blood vessel(s) with modifier '-52')

         (20832 has been deleted. To report, see specific code(s) for repair of bone(s), ligament(s), tendon(s), nerve(s), or blood vessel(s) with modifier '-52')

         (20834 has been deleted. To report, see specific code(s) for repair of bone(s), ligament(s), tendon(s), nerve(s), or blood vessel(s) with modifier '-52')

20838   Replantation, foot, complete amputation

         (20840 has been deleted. To report, see specific code(s) for repair of bone(s), ligament(s), tendon(s), nerve(s), or blood vessel(s) with modifier '-52')

Grafts (or Implants)

Codes for obtaining autogenous bone, cartilage, tendon, fascia lata grafts, or other tissues through separate incisions are to be used only when graft is not already listed as part of basic procedure.

Do not append modifier '-62' to bone graft codes 20900-20938.

         (For spinal surgery bone graft(s) see codes 20930-20938)

⊘ **20900**   Bone graft, any donor area; minor or small (eg, dowel or button)

⊘ **20902**   major or large

⊘ **20910**   Cartilage graft; costochondral

⊘ **20912**   nasal septum

         (For ear cartilage, use 21235)

⊘ **20920**   Fascia lata graft; by stripper

⊘ **20922**   by incision and area exposure, complex or sheet

⊘ **20924**   Tendon graft, from a distance (eg, palmaris, toe extensor, plantaris)

⊘ **20926**   Tissue grafts, other (eg, paratenon, fat, dermis)

         (Codes 20930-20938 are reported in addition to codes for the definitive procedure(s) without modifier '-51')

⊘ **20930**   Allograft for spine surgery only; morselized

⊘ **20931**   structural

⊘ **20936**   Autograft for spine surgery only (includes harvesting the graft); local (eg, ribs, spinous process, or laminar fragments) obtained from same incision

⊘ **20937**   morselized (through separate skin or fascial incision)

⊘ **20938**   structural, bicortical or tricortical (through separate skin or fascial incision)

         (For needle aspiration of bone marrow for the purpose of bone grafting, use 38220)

Other Procedures

20950   Monitoring of interstitial fluid pressure (includes insertion of device, eg, wick catheter technique, needle manometer technique) in detection of muscle compartment syndrome

20955   Bone graft with microvascular anastomosis; fibula

20956   iliac crest

20957   metatarsal

         (20960 has been deleted. To report, use 20962)

20962   other than fibula, iliac crest, or metatarsal

         (Do not report code 69990 in addition to codes 20955-20962)

Surgery: Musculoskeletal System

20969 Free osteocutaneous flap with microvascular anastomosis; other than iliac crest, metatarsal, or great toe

20970 iliac crest

(20971 has been deleted. To report, use 20969)

20972 metatarsal

20973 great toe with web space

(Do not report code 69990 in addition to codes 20969-20973)

(For great toe, wrap-around procedure, use 26551)

⊘ **20974** Electrical stimulation to aid bone healing; noninvasive (nonoperative)

⊘ **20975** invasive (operative)

(20976 has been deleted)

20979 Low intensity ultrasound stimulation to aid bone healing, noninvasive (nonoperative)

20999 Unlisted procedure, musculoskeletal system, general

Head

Skull, facial bones and temporomandibular joint.

Incision

(For drainage of superficial abscess and hematoma, use 20000)

(For removal of embedded foreign body from dentoalveolar structure, see 41805, 41806)

21010 Arthrotomy, temporomandibular joint

(21011 has been deleted. To report, use 21010 with modifier '-50')

Excision

(For biopsy, see 20220, 20240)

21015 Radical resection of tumor (eg, malignant neoplasm), soft tissue of face or scalp

(21020 has been deleted. To report, use 61501)

21025 Excision of bone (eg, for osteomyelitis or bone abscess); mandible

21026 facial bone(s)

21029 Removal by contouring of benign tumor of facial bone (eg, fibrous dysplasia)

▲**21030** Excision of benign tumor or cyst of maxilla or zygoma by enucleation and curettage

21031 Excision of torus mandibularis

21032 Excision of maxillary torus palatinus

▲**21034** Excision of malignant tumor of maxilla or zygoma

▲ **21040** Excision of benign tumor or cyst of mandible, by enucleation and/or curettage

▶(21041 has been deleted. For enucleation and/or curettage of benign cysts or tumors of mandible not requiring osteotomy, use 21040)◀

▶(For excision of benign tumor or cyst of mandible requiring osteotomy, see 21046-21047)◀

21044 Excision of malignant tumor of mandible;

21045 radical resection

(For bone graft, use 21215)

● **21046** Excision of benign tumor or cyst of mandible; requiring intra-oral osteotomy (eg, locally aggressive or destructive lesion(s))

● **21047** requiring extra-oral osteotomy and partial mandibulectomy (eg, locally aggressive or destructive lesion(s))

● **21048** Excision of benign tumor or cyst of maxilla; requiring intra-oral osteotomy (eg, locally aggressive or destructive lesion(s))

● **21049** requiring extra-oral osteotomy and partial maxillectomy (eg, locally aggressive or destructive lesion(s))

21050 Condylectomy, temporomandibular joint (separate procedure)

(21051 has been deleted. To report, use 21050 with modifier '-50')

21060 Meniscectomy, partial or complete, temporomandibular joint (separate procedure)

(21061 has been deleted. To report, use 21060 with modifier '-50')

21070 Coronoidectomy (separate procedure)

(21071 has been deleted. To report, use 21070 with modifier '-50')

Introduction or Removal

(For application or removal of caliper or tongs, see 20660, 20665.) Codes 21076-21089 describe professional services for the rehabilitation of patients with oral, facial or other anatomical deficiencies by means of prostheses such as an artificial eye, ear, or nose or intraoral obturator to close a cleft. Codes 21076-21089 should only be used when the physician actually designs and prepares the prosthesis (ie, not prepared by an outside laboratory).

21076 Impression and custom preparation; surgical obturator prosthesis

21077 orbital prosthesis

21079 interim obturator prosthesis

21080 definitive obturator prosthesis

21081	mandibular resection prosthesis
21082	palatal augmentation prosthesis
21083	palatal lift prosthesis
21084	speech aid prosthesis
21085	oral surgical splint
21086	auricular prosthesis
21087	nasal prosthesis
21088	facial prosthesis

21089 Unlisted maxillofacial prosthetic procedure

21100* Application of halo type appliance for maxillofacial fixation, includes removal (separate procedure)

21110 Application of interdental fixation device for conditions other than fracture or dislocation, includes removal

(For removal of interdental fixation by another physician, see 20670-20680)

21116 Injection procedure for temporomandibular joint arthrography

(For radiological supervision and interpretation, use 70332. Do not report 76003 in addition to 70332)

Repair, Revision, and/or Reconstruction

(For cranioplasty, see 21179, 21180 and 62116, 62120, 62140-62147)

21120 Genioplasty; augmentation (autograft, allograft, prosthetic material)

21121 sliding osteotomy, single piece

21122 sliding osteotomies, two or more osteotomies (eg, wedge excision or bone wedge reversal for asymmetrical chin)

21123 sliding, augmentation with interpositional bone grafts (includes obtaining autografts)

21125 Augmentation, mandibular body or angle; prosthetic material

21127 with bone graft, onlay or interpositional (includes obtaining autograft)

21137 Reduction forehead; contouring only

21138 contouring and application of prosthetic material or bone graft (includes obtaining autograft)

21139 contouring and setback of anterior frontal sinus wall

21141 Reconstruction midface, LeFort I; single piece, segment movement in any direction (eg, for Long Face Syndrome), without bone graft

21142 two pieces, segment movement in any direction, without bone graft

21143 three or more pieces, segment movement in any direction, without bone graft

(21144 has been deleted. To report, use 21141)

21145 single piece, segment movement in any direction, requiring bone grafts (includes obtaining autografts)

21146 two pieces, segment movement in any direction, requiring bone grafts (includes obtaining autografts) (eg, ungrafted unilateral alveolar cleft)

21147 three or more pieces, segment movement in any direction, requiring bone grafts (includes obtaining autografts) (eg, ungrafted bilateral alveolar cleft or multiple osteotomies)

21150 Reconstruction midface, LeFort II; anterior intrusion (eg, Treacher-Collins Syndrome)

21151 any direction, requiring bone grafts (includes obtaining autografts)

21154 Reconstruction midface, LeFort III (extracranial), any type, requiring bone grafts (includes obtaining autografts); without LeFort I

21155 with LeFort I

21159 Reconstruction midface, LeFort III (extra and intracranial) with forehead advancement (eg, mono bloc), requiring bone grafts (includes obtaining autografts); without LeFort I

21160 with LeFort I

21172 Reconstruction superior-lateral orbital rim and lower forehead, advancement or alteration, with or without grafts (includes obtaining autografts)

(For frontal or parietal craniotomy performed for craniosynostosis, use 61556)

21175 Reconstruction, bifrontal, superior-lateral orbital rims and lower forehead, advancement or alteration (eg, plagiocephaly, trigonocephaly, brachycephaly), with or without grafts (includes obtaining autografts)

(For bifrontal craniotomy performed for craniosynostosis, use 61557)

21179 Reconstruction, entire or majority of forehead and/or supraorbital rims; with grafts (allograft or prosthetic material)

21180 with autograft (includes obtaining grafts)

(For extensive craniectomy for multiple suture craniosynostosis, use only 61558 or 61559)

21181 Reconstruction by contouring of benign tumor of cranial bones (eg, fibrous dysplasia), extracranial

21182 Reconstruction of orbital walls, rims, forehead, nasoethmoid complex following intra- and extracranial excision of benign tumor of cranial bone (eg, fibrous dysplasia), with multiple autografts (includes obtaining grafts); total area of bone grafting less than 40 sq cm

21183 total area of bone grafting greater than 40 sq cm but less than 80 sq cm

21184 total area of bone grafting greater than 80 sq cm

(For excision of benign tumor of cranial bones, see 61563, 61564)

21188   Reconstruction midface, osteotomies (other than LeFort type) and bone grafts (includes obtaining autografts)

21193   Reconstruction of mandibular rami, horizontal, vertical, C, or L osteotomy; without bone graft

21194   with bone graft (includes obtaining graft)

21195   Reconstruction of mandibular rami and/or body, sagittal split; without internal rigid fixation

21196   with internal rigid fixation

21198   Osteotomy, mandible, segmental;

21199   with genioglossus advancement

(21200, 21202, 21203 have been deleted. To report, see 21193-21198)

(21204 has been deleted. To report, see 21141-21160)

21206   Osteotomy, maxilla, segmental (eg, Wassmund or Schuchard)

(21207 has been deleted. To report, use 21209)

21208   Osteoplasty, facial bones; augmentation (autograft, allograft, or prosthetic implant)

21209   reduction

21210   Graft, bone; nasal, maxillary or malar areas (includes obtaining graft)

(For cleft palate repair, see 42200-42225)

21215   mandible (includes obtaining graft)

21230   Graft; rib cartilage, autogenous, to face, chin, nose or ear (includes obtaining graft)

21235   ear cartilage, autogenous, to nose or ear (includes obtaining graft)

(21239 has been deleted. To report, use 21208)

21240   Arthroplasty, temporomandibular joint, with or without autograft (includes obtaining graft)

(21241 has been deleted. To report, use 21240)

21242   Arthroplasty, temporomandibular joint, with allograft

21243   Arthroplasty, temporomandibular joint, with prosthetic joint replacement

21244   Reconstruction of mandible, extraoral, with transosteal bone plate (eg, mandibular staple bone plate)

21245   Reconstruction of mandible or maxilla, subperiosteal implant; partial

21246   complete

21247   Reconstruction of mandibular condyle with bone and cartilage autografts (includes obtaining grafts) (eg, for hemifacial microsomia)

21248   Reconstruction of mandible or maxilla, endosteal implant (eg, blade, cylinder); partial

21249   complete

(21250, 21254 have been deleted. To report, see 21141-21160)

21255   Reconstruction of zygomatic arch and glenoid fossa with bone and cartilage (includes obtaining autografts)

21256   Reconstruction of orbit with osteotomies (extracranial) and with bone grafts (includes obtaining autografts) (eg, micro-ophthalmia)

21260   Periorbital osteotomies for orbital hypertelorism, with bone grafts; extracranial approach

21261   combined intra- and extracranial approach

21263   with forehead advancement

21267   Orbital repositioning, periorbital osteotomies, unilateral, with bone grafts; extracranial approach

21268   combined intra- and extracranial approach

21270   Malar augmentation, prosthetic material

(For malar augmentation with bone graft, use 21210)

21275   Secondary revision of orbitocraniofacial reconstruction

21280   Medial canthopexy (separate procedure)

(For medial canthoplasty, use 67950)

21282   Lateral canthopexy

21295   Reduction of masseter muscle and bone (eg, for treatment of benign masseteric hypertrophy); extraoral approach

21296   intraoral approach

Other Procedures

21299   Unlisted craniofacial and maxillofacial procedure

Fracture and/or Dislocation

21300   Closed treatment of skull fracture without operation

(For operative repair, see 62000-62010)

21310   Closed treatment of nasal bone fracture without manipulation

21315*   Closed treatment of nasal bone fracture; without stabilization

21320   with stabilization

21325   Open treatment of nasal fracture; uncomplicated

21330   complicated, with internal and/or external skeletal fixation

21335   with concomitant open treatment of fractured septum

21336   Open treatment of nasal septal fracture, with or without stabilization

21337   Closed treatment of nasal septal fracture, with or without stabilization

21338   Open treatment of nasoethmoid fracture; without external fixation

21339   with external fixation

21340   Percutaneous treatment of nasoethmoid complex fracture, with splint, wire or headcap fixation, including repair of canthal ligaments and/or the nasolacrimal apparatus

21343   Open treatment of depressed frontal sinus fracture

21344   Open treatment of complicated (eg, comminuted or involving posterior wall) frontal sinus fracture, via coronal or multiple approaches

21345   Closed treatment of nasomaxillary complex fracture (LeFort II type), with interdental wire fixation or fixation of denture or splint

21346   Open treatment of nasomaxillary complex fracture (LeFort II type); with wiring and/or local fixation

21347   requiring multiple open approaches

21348   with bone grafting (includes obtaining graft)

(21350 has been deleted. If necessary to report, use appropriate Evaluation and Management code)

21355*   Percutaneous treatment of fracture of malar area, including zygomatic arch and malar tripod, with manipulation

21356   Open treatment of depressed zygomatic arch fracture (eg, Gillies approach)

21360   Open treatment of depressed malar fracture, including zygomatic arch and malar tripod

21365   Open treatment of complicated (eg, comminuted or involving cranial nerve foramina) fracture(s) of malar area, including zygomatic arch and malar tripod; with internal fixation and multiple surgical approaches

21366   with bone grafting (includes obtaining graft)

(21380 has been deleted. If necessary to report, use appropriate Evaluation and Management code)

21385   Open treatment of orbital floor blowout fracture; transantral approach (Caldwell-Luc type operation)

21386   periorbital approach

21387   combined approach

21390   periorbital approach, with alloplastic or other implant

21395   periorbital approach with bone graft (includes obtaining graft)

21400   Closed treatment of fracture of orbit, except blowout; without manipulation

21401   with manipulation

21406   Open treatment of fracture of orbit, except blowout; without implant

21407   with implant

21408   with bone grafting (includes obtaining graft)

(21420 has been deleted. If necessary to report, use appropriate Evaluation and Management code)

21421   Closed treatment of palatal or maxillary fracture (LeFort I type), with interdental wire fixation or fixation of denture or splint

21422   Open treatment of palatal or maxillary fracture (LeFort I type);

21423   complicated (comminuted or involving cranial nerve foramina), multiple approaches

21431   Closed treatment of craniofacial separation (LeFort III type) using interdental wire fixation of denture or splint

21432   Open treatment of craniofacial separation (LeFort III type); with wiring and/or internal fixation

21433   complicated (eg, comminuted or involving cranial nerve foramina), multiple surgical approaches

21435   complicated, utilizing internal and/or external fixation techniques (eg, head cap, halo device, and/or intermaxillary fixation)

(For removal of internal or external fixation device, use 20670)

21436   complicated, multiple surgical approaches, internal fixation, with bone grafting (includes obtaining graft)

21440   Closed treatment of mandibular or maxillary alveolar ridge fracture (separate procedure)

21445   Open treatment of mandibular or maxillary alveolar ridge fracture (separate procedure)

21450   Closed treatment of mandibular fracture; without manipulation

21451   with manipulation

21452   Percutaneous treatment of mandibular fracture, with external fixation

21453   Closed treatment of mandibular fracture with interdental fixation

21454   Open treatment of mandibular fracture with external fixation

(21455 has been deleted. To report, use 21453)

21461   Open treatment of mandibular fracture; without interdental fixation

21462   with interdental fixation

21465   Open treatment of mandibular condylar fracture

21470   Open treatment of complicated mandibular fracture by multiple surgical approaches including internal fixation, interdental fixation, and/or wiring of dentures or splints

21480   Closed treatment of temporomandibular dislocation; initial or subsequent

21485   complicated (eg, recurrent requiring intermaxillary fixation or splinting), initial or subsequent

21490   Open treatment of temporomandibular dislocation

(For interdental wire fixation, use 21497)

Surgery: Musculoskeletal System

21493   Closed treatment of hyoid fracture; without manipulation

21494   with manipulation

21495   Open treatment of hyoid fracture

(For treatment of fracture of larynx, see 31584-31586)

21497   Interdental wiring, for condition other than fracture

Other Procedures

21499   Unlisted musculoskeletal procedure, head

(For unlisted craniofacial or maxillofacial procedure, use 21299)

Neck (Soft Tissues) and Thorax

(For cervical spine and back, see 21920 et seq)

(For injection of fracture site or trigger point, use 20550)

Incision

(For incision and drainage of abscess or hematoma, superficial, see 10060, 10140)

21501   Incision and drainage, deep abscess or hematoma, soft tissues of neck or thorax;

21502   with partial rib ostectomy

21510   Incision, deep, with opening of bone cortex (eg, for osteomyelitis or bone abscess), thorax

(21511 has been deleted)

Excision

(For bone biopsy, see 20220-20251)

21550   Biopsy, soft tissue of neck or thorax

(For needle biopsy of soft tissue, use 20206)

21555   Excision tumor, soft tissue of neck or thorax; subcutaneous

21556   deep, subfascial, intramuscular

21557   Radical resection of tumor (eg, malignant neoplasm), soft tissue of neck or thorax

21600   Excision of rib, partial

(For radical resection of chest wall and rib cage for tumor, use 19260)

(For radical debridement of chest wall and rib cage for injury, see 11040-11044)

21610   Costotransversectomy (separate procedure)

21615   Excision first and/or cervical rib;

21616   with sympathectomy

21620   Ostectomy of sternum, partial

21627   Sternal debridement

(For debridement and closure, use 21750)

21630   Radical resection of sternum;

21632   with mediastinal lymphadenectomy

(21633 has been deleted. To report, use 21630)

Repair, Revision, and/or Reconstruction

(For superficial wound, see **Integumentary System** section under Repair—Simple)

21700   Division of scalenus anticus; without resection of cervical rib

21705   with resection of cervical rib

21720   Division of sternocleidomastoid for torticollis, open operation; without cast application

(For transection of spinal accessory and cervical nerves, see 63191, 64722)

21725   with cast application

▲ **21740**   Reconstructive repair of pectus excavatum or carinatum; open

(21741 has been deleted. To report, use 21899)

● **21742**   minimally invasive approach (Nuss procedure), without thoracoscopy

● **21743**   minimally invasive approach (Nuss procedure), with thoracoscopy

21750   Closure of median sternotomy separation with or without debridement (separate procedure)

Fracture and/or Dislocation

21800   Closed treatment of rib fracture, uncomplicated, each

21805   Open treatment of rib fracture without fixation, each

21810   Treatment of rib fracture requiring external fixation (flail chest)

21820   Closed treatment of sternum fracture

21825   Open treatment of sternum fracture with or without skeletal fixation

(For sternoclavicular dislocation, see 23520-23532)

Other Procedures

21899   Unlisted procedure, neck or thorax

Back and Flank

Excision

21920   Biopsy, soft tissue of back or flank; superficial

21925   deep

(For needle biopsy of soft tissue, use 20206)

21930   Excision, tumor, soft tissue of back or flank

21935   Radical resection of tumor (eg, malignant neoplasm), soft tissue of back or flank

Spine (Vertebral Column)

Cervical, thoracic, and lumbar spine.

Within the SPINE section, bone grafting procedures are reported separately and in addition to arthrodesis. For bone grafts in other Musculoskeletal sections, see specific code(s) descriptor(s) and/or accompanying guidelines.

To report bone grafts performed after arthrodesis, see codes 20930-20938. Bone graft codes are reported without modifier '-51' (multiple procedure). Do not append modifier '-62' to bone graft codes 20900-20938.

Example:

Posterior arthrodesis of L5-S1 for degenerative disc disease utilizing morselized autogenous iliac bone graft harvested through a separate fascial incision.

Report as 22612 and 20937.

Within the SPINE section, instrumentation is reported separately and in addition to arthrodesis. To report instrumentation procedures performed with definitive vertebral procedure(s), see codes 22840-22855. Instrumentation procedure codes 22840-22848 and 22851 are reported in addition to the definitive procedure(s) without modifier '-51'. The modifier '-62' may not be appended to the definitive or add-on spinal instrumentation procedure code(s) 22840-►22848 and 22850-22852.◄

Example:

Posterior arthrodesis of L4-S1, utilizing morselized autogenous iliac bone graft harvested through separate fascial incision, and pedicle screw fixation.

Report as 22612, 22614, 22842, and 20937.

Vertebral procedures are sometimes followed by arthrodesis and in addition may include bone grafts and instrumentation.

When arthrodesis is performed in addition to another procedure, the arthrodesis should be reported in addition to the original procedure with a modifier '-51' (multiple procedures). Examples are after osteotomy, fracture care, vertebral corpectomy and laminectomy. Since bone grafts and instrumentation are never performed without arthrodesis, modifier '-51' (multiple procedures) is not used.

Arthrodesis, however, may be performed in the absence of other procedures and therefore when it is combined with another definitive procedure, modifier '-51' (multiple procedure) is appropriate.

Example:

Treatment of a burst fracture of L2 by corpectomy followed by arthrodesis of L1-L3, utilizing anterior instrumentation L1-L3 and structural allograft.

Report as 63090, 22558-51, 22585, 22845, and 20931.

When two surgeons work together as primary surgeons performing distinct part(s) of a single reportable procedure, each surgeon should report his/her distinct operative work by appending the modifier '-62' to the single definitive procedure code. If additional procedure(s) (including add-on procedure(s)) are performed during the same surgical session, separate code(s) may be reported by each co-surgeon, without the modifier '-62' appended (see Appendix A).

Example:

A 42-year-old male with a history of posttraumatic degenerative disc disease at L3-4 and L4-5 (internal disc disruption) underwent surgical repair. Surgeon A performed an anterior exposure of the spine with mobilization of the great vessels. Surgeon B performed anterior (minimal) diskectomy and fusion at L3-4 and L4-5 using anterior interbody technique.

Report surgeon A: 22558-62, 22585-62
Report surgeon B: 22558-62, 22585-62, 20931

> (Do not append modifier -62 to bone graft code 20931)
>
> (For injection procedure for myelography, use 62284)
>
> (For injection procedure for diskography, see 62290, 62291)
>
> (For injection procedure, chemonucleolysis, single or multiple levels, use 62292)
>
> (For injection procedure for facet joints, see 64470-64476, 64622-64627)
>
> (For needle or trocar biopsy, see 20220-20225)

Excision

For the following codes, when two surgeons work together as primary surgeons performing distinct part(s) of partial vertebral body excision, each surgeon should report his/her distinct operative work by appending the modifier '-62' to the procedure code. In this situation, the modifier '-62' may be appended to the procedure code(s) 22100-22102, 22110-22114 and, as appropriate, to the associated additional vertebral segment add-on code(s) 22103, 22116 as long as both surgeons continue to work together as primary surgeons.

> (For bone biopsy, see 20220-20251)
>
> (22010 has been deleted. To report, use 21920)
>
> (22011 has been deleted. To report, use 21925)
>
> (22012 has been deleted. To report, use 20206)
>
> (22030-22033 have been deleted. To report, use 21930)

22100	Partial excision of posterior vertebral component (eg, spinous process, lamina or facet) for intrinsic bony lesion, single vertebral segment; cervical
22101	thoracic
22102	lumbar

Surgery: Musculoskeletal System

+ 22103 each additional segment (List separately in addition to code for primary procedure)

(Use 22103 in conjunction with codes 22100, 22101, 22102)

(22105 has been deleted. To report, use 22100)

(22106 has been deleted. To report, use 22101)

(22107 has been deleted. To report, use 22102)

22110 Partial excision of vertebral body, for intrinsic bony lesion, without decompression of spinal cord or nerve root(s), single vertebral segment; cervical

(22111 has been deleted)

22112 thoracic

(22113 has been deleted)

22114 lumbar

(22115 has been deleted)

+ 22116 each additional vertebral segment (List separately in addition to code for primary procedure)

(Use 22116 in conjunction with codes 22110, 22112, 22114)

(22120-22130 have been deleted. For complete or near complete resection of vertebral body, see vertebral corpectomy, 63081-63091)

(22140 has been deleted. To report, use 63081 and 22554 and 20931 or 20938)

(22141 has been deleted. To report, use 63085 or 63087 and 22556 and 20931 or 20938)

(22142 has been deleted. To report, use 63087 or 63090 and 22558 and 20931 or 20938)

(22145 has been deleted. To report, use 63082 or 63086 or 63088 or 63091, and 22585)

(22148 has been deleted. To report, see 20931 or 20938)

(22150 has been deleted. To report, use 63081 and 22554 and 20931 or 20938 and 22851)

(22151 has been deleted. To report, use 63085 or 63087 and 22556 and 20931 or 20938 and 22851)

(22152 has been deleted. To report, use 63087 or 63090 and 22558, and 20931 or 20938 and 22851)

(22200-22207 have been deleted. For osteotomy of spine, see 22210-22226)

Osteotomy

To report arthrodesis, see codes 22590-22632. (Report in addition to code(s) for the definitive procedure with modifier '-51'.)

To report instrumentation procedures, see codes 22840-22855. (Report in addition to code(s) for the definitive procedure(s) without modifier '-51'.) Do not append modifier '-62' to spinal instrumentation codes 22840-▶22848 and 22850-22852.◀

To report bone graft procedures, see codes 20930-20938. (Report in addition to code(s) for the definitive procedure(s) without modifier '-51'.) Do not append modifier '-62' to bone graft codes 20900-20938.

For the following codes, when two surgeons work together as primary surgeons performing distinct part(s) of an anterior spine osteotomy, each surgeon should report his/her distinct operative work by appending the modifier '-62' to the procedure code. In this situation, the modifier '-62' may be appended to the procedure code(s) 22210-22214, 22220-22224 and, as appropriate, to associated additional segment add-on code(s) 22216, 22226 as long as both surgeons continue to work together as primary surgeons.

22210 Osteotomy of spine, posterior or posterolateral approach, one vertebral segment; cervical

22212 thoracic

22214 lumbar

+ 22216 each additional vertebral segment (List separately in addition to primary procedure)

(Use 22216 in conjunction with codes 22210, 22212, 22214)

22220 Osteotomy of spine, including diskectomy, anterior approach, single vertebral segment; cervical

22222 thoracic

22224 lumbar

+ 22226 each additional vertebral segment (List separately in addition to code for primary procedure)

(Use 22226 in conjunction with codes 22220, 22222, 22224)

(22230 has been deleted. To report, use 22216 or 22226)

(22250, 22251 have been deleted. For vertebral corpectomy, see 63081-63091)

Fracture and/or Dislocation

To report arthrodesis, see codes 22590-22632. (Report in addition to code(s) for the definitive procedure with modifier '-51'.)

To report instrumentation procedures, see codes 22840-22855. (Report in addition to code(s) for the definitive procedure(s) without modifier '-51'.) Do not append modifier '-62' to spinal instrumentation codes 22840-▶22848 and 22850-22852.◀

To report bone graft procedures, see codes 20930-20938. (Report in addition to code(s) for the definitive procedure(s) without modifier '-51'.) Do not append modifier '-62' to bone graft codes 20900-20938.

For the following codes, when two surgeons work together as primary surgeons performing distinct part(s) of open fracture and/or dislocation procedure(s), each surgeon should report his/her distinct operative work by appending the modifier '-62' to the procedure code. In this situation, the modifier '-62' may be appended to the procedure code(s) 22318-22327 and, as appropriate, the associated additional fracture vertebrae or dislocated segment add-on code 22328 as long as both surgeons continue to work together as primary surgeons.

22305   Closed treatment of vertebral process fracture(s)

22310   Closed treatment of vertebral body fracture(s), without manipulation, requiring and including casting or bracing

22315   Closed treatment of vertebral fracture(s) and/or dislocation(s) requiring casting or bracing, with and including casting and/or bracing, with or without anesthesia, by manipulation or traction

     (For spinal subluxation, use 97140)

22318   Open treatment and/or reduction of odontoid fracture(s) and or dislocation(s) (including os odontoideum), anterior approach, including placement of internal fixation; without grafting

22319   with grafting

22325   Open treatment and/or reduction of vertebral fracture(s) and/or dislocation(s), posterior approach, one fractured vertebrae or dislocated segment; lumbar

22326   cervical

22327   thoracic

+ 22328   each additional fractured vertebrae or dislocated segment (List separately in addition to code for primary procedure)

     (Use 22328 in conjunction with codes 22325, 22326, 22327)

     (For treatment of vertebral fracture by the anterior approach, see corpectomy 63081-63091, and appropriate arthrodesis, bone graft and instrument codes)

     (22330-22379 have been deleted. For decompression of spine following fracture, see 63001-63091; for arthrodesis of spine following fracture, see 22548-22632)

Manipulation

     (22500 has been deleted. To report, use 97140)

22505   Manipulation of spine requiring anesthesia, any region

Vertebral Body, Embolization or Injection

22520   Percutaneous vertebroplasty, one vertebral body, unilateral or bilateral injection; thoracic

22521   lumbar

22522   each additional thoracic or lumbar vertebral body (List separately in addition to code for primary procedure)

     (Use 22522 in conjunction with codes 22520, 22521 as appropriate)

     (For radiological supervision and interpretation, see 76012, 76013)

Arthrodesis

Arthrodesis may be performed in the absence of other procedures and therefore when it is combined with another definitive procedure (eg, osteotomy, fracture care, vertebral corpectomy or laminectomy), modifier '-51' is appropriate. However, arthrodesis codes 22585, 22614, and 22632 are considered add-on procedure codes and should not be used with modifier '-51'.

To report instrumentation procedures, see codes 22840-22855. (Report in addition to code(s) for the definitive procedure(s) without modifier '-51'.) Do not append modifier '-62' to spinal instrumentation codes 22840-▶22848 and 22850-22852.◀

To report bone graft procedures, see codes 20930-20938. (Report in addition to code(s) for the definitive procedure(s) without modifier '-51'.) Do not append modifier '-62' to bone graft codes 20900-20938.

Anterior or Anterolateral Approach Technique

Procedure codes 22554-22558 are for SINGLE interspace; for additional interspaces, use 22585. A vertebral interspace is the non-bony compartment between two adjacent vertebral bodies, which contains the intervertebral disk, and includes the nucleus pulposus, annulus fibrosus, and two cartilagenous endplates.

For the following codes, when two surgeons work together as primary surgeons performing distinct part(s) of an anterior interbody arthrodesis, each surgeon should report his/her distinct operative work by appending the modifier '-62' to the procedure code. In this situation, the modifier '-62' may be appended to the procedure code(s) 22548-22558 and, as appropriate, to the associated additional interspace add-on code 22585 as long as both surgeons continue to work together as primary surgeons.

22548   Arthrodesis, anterior transoral or extraoral technique, clivus-C1-C2 (atlas-axis), with or without excision of odontoid process

     (22550, 22552, 22555, 22560, 22561, 22565 have been deleted. For intervertebral disk excision by laminotomy or laminectomy, see 63020-63042. For arthrodesis, see 22548-22632)

22554   Arthrodesis, anterior interbody technique, including minimal diskectomy to prepare interspace (other than for decompression); cervical below C2

22556   thoracic

22558   lumbar

+ 22585   each additional interspace (List separately in addition to code for primary procedure)

     (Use 22585 in conjunction with codes 22554, 22556, 22558)

Surgery: Musculoskeletal System

Surgery: Musculoskeletal System

Posterior, Posterolateral or Lateral Transverse Process Technique

To report instrumentation procedures, see codes 22840-22855. (Report in addition to code(s) for the definitive procedure(s) without modifier '-51'.) Do not append modifier '-62' to spinal instrumentation codes 22840-▶22848 and 22850-22852.◀

To report bone graft procedures, see codes 20930-20938. (Report in addition to code(s) for the definitive procedure(s) without modifier '-51'.) Do not append modifier '-62' to bone graft codes 20900-20938.

A vertebral segment describes the basic constituent part into which the spine may be divided. It represents a single complete vertebral bone with its associated articular processes and laminae. A vertebral interspace is the non-bony compartment between two adjacent vertebral bodies which contains the intervertebral disk, and includes the nucleus pulposus, annulus fibrosus, and two cartilagenous endplates.

22590   Arthrodesis, posterior technique, craniocervical (occiput-C2)

22595   Arthrodesis, posterior technique, atlas-axis (C1-C2)

22600   Arthrodesis, posterior or posterolateral technique, single level; cervical below C2 segment

(22605 has been deleted. To report, use 22600)

22610   thoracic (with or without lateral transverse technique)

22612   lumbar (with or without lateral transverse technique)

+ 22614   each additional vertebral segment (List separately in addition to code for primary procedure)

(Use 22614 in conjunction with codes 22600, 22610, 22612)

(22615 has been deleted. To report, use 22554 and 20930-20938)

(22617 has been deleted. To report, use 22548 and 20930-20938)

(22620 has been deleted. To report, use 22590 and 20930-20938)

(22625 has been deleted. To report, use 22612 and 22840-22855, and 20930-20938)

22630   Arthrodesis, posterior interbody technique, including laminectomy and/or diskectomy to prepare interspace (other than for decompression), single interspace; lumbar

+ 22632   each additional interspace (List separately in addition to code for primary procedure)

(Use 22632 in conjunction with code 22630)

(22640-22645 have been deleted. To report, see 22610, 22612, and 20930-20938)

(22650 has been deleted. To report, use 22614)

(22655 has been deleted. To report, see 22630, 22632 and 20930-20938)

(22670 has been deleted. To report, see 22610 or 22612 and 22840-22855, and 20930-20938)

(22680 has been deleted. To report, see 22556-22585 and 20930-20938)

(22700 has been deleted. To report, see 22558 and 20930-20938)

(22720 has been deleted. To report, see 22612 and 20930-20938)

(22730 has been deleted. To report, see 22585, 22614)

(22735 has been deleted. To report, see 22585, 22614)

Spine Deformity (eg, Scoliosis, Kyphosis)

To report instrumentation procedures, see codes 22840-22855. (Report in addition to code(s) for the definitive procedure(s) without modifier '-51'.) Do not append modifier '-62' to spinal instrumentation codes 22840-▶22848 and 22850-22852.◀

To report bone graft procedures, see codes 20930-20938. (Report in addition to code(s) for the definitive procedure(s) without modifier '-51'.) Do not append modifier '-62' to bone graft codes 20900-20938.

A vertebral segment describes the basic constituent part into which the spine may be divided. It represents a single complete vertebral bone with its associated articular processes and laminae.

For the following codes, when two surgeons work together as primary surgeons performing distinct part(s) of an arthrodesis for spinal deformity, each surgeon should report his/her distinct operative work by appending the modifier '-62' to the procedure code. In this situation, the modifier '-62' may be appended to the procedure code(s) 22800-22819 as long as both surgeons continue to work together as primary surgeons.

22800   Arthrodesis, posterior, for spinal deformity, with or without cast; up to 6 vertebral segments

(22801 has been deleted. To report, use 22800)

22802   7 to 12 vertebral segments

(22803 has been deleted. To report, use 22802)

22804   13 or more vertebral segments

22808   Arthrodesis, anterior, for spinal deformity, with or without cast; 2 to 3 vertebral segments

22810   4 to 7 vertebral segments

22812   8 or more vertebral segments

22818   Kyphectomy, circumferential exposure of spine and resection of vertebral segment(s) (including body and posterior elements); single or 2 segments

22819   3 or more segments

(To report arthrodesis, see 22800-22804 and add modifier '-51')

Exploration

(22820 has been deleted. To report, see 20930-20938)

22830   Exploration of spinal fusion

Spinal Instrumentation

Segmental instrumentation is defined as fixation at each end of the construct and at least one additional interposed bony attachment.

Non-segmental instrumentation is defined as fixation at each end of the construct and may span several vertebral segments without attachment to the intervening segments.

Insertion of spinal instrumentation is reported separately and in addition to arthrodesis. Instrumentation procedure codes 22840-22848, 22851 are reported in addition to the definitive procedure(s) without modifier '-51'. Do not append modifier '-62' to spinal instrumentation codes 22840-▶22848 and 22850-22852.◀

To report bone graft procedures, see codes 20930-20938. (Report in addition to code(s) for definitive procedure(s) without modifier '-51'.) Do not append modifier '-62' to bone graft codes 20900-20938.

A vertebral segment describes the basic constituent part into which the spine may be divided. It represents a single complete vertebral bone with its associated articular processes and laminae. A vertebral interspace is the non-bony compartment between two adjacent vertebral bodies, which contains the intervertebral disk, and includes the nucleus pulposus, annulus fibrosus, and two cartilagenous endplates.

(List codes 22840-22848, 22851 separately, in addition to code for fracture, dislocation, or arthrodesis of the spine, 22325, 22326, 22327, 22548-22812)

⊘ **22840**   Posterior non-segmental instrumentation (eg, Harrington rod technique, pedicle fixation across one interspace, atlantoaxial transarticular screw fixation, sublaminar wiring at C1, facet screw fixation)

⊘ **22841**   Internal spinal fixation by wiring of spinous processes

⊘ **22842**   Posterior segmental instrumentation (eg, pedicle fixation, dual rods with multiple hooks and sublaminar wires); 3 to 6 vertebral segments

⊘ **22843**   7 to 12 vertebral segments

⊘ **22844**   13 or more vertebral segments

⊘ **22845**   Anterior instrumentation; 2 to 3 vertebral segments

⊘ **22846**   4 to 7 vertebral segments

⊘ **22847**   8 or more vertebral segments

⊘ **22848**   Pelvic fixation (attachment of caudal end of instrumentation to pelvic bony structures) other than sacrum

22849   Reinsertion of spinal fixation device

22850   Removal of posterior nonsegmental instrumentation (eg, Harrington rod)

⊘ **22851**   Application of intervertebral biomechanical device(s) (eg, synthetic cage(s), threaded bone dowel(s), methylmethacrylate) to vertebral defect or interspace

22852   Removal of posterior segmental instrumentation

22855   Removal of anterior instrumentation

Other Procedures

22899   Unlisted procedure, spine

Abdomen

Excision

22900   Excision, abdominal wall tumor, subfascial (eg, desmoid)

(22910 has been deleted. To report, use 22999)

Other Procedures

22999   Unlisted procedure, abdomen, musculoskeletal system

Shoulder

Clavicle, scapula, humerus head and neck, sterno-clavicular joint, acromioclavicular joint and shoulder joint.

Incision

23000   Removal of subdeltoid calcareous deposits, open

▶(For arthroscopic removal of bursal deposits, use 29999)◀

23020   Capsular contracture release (eg, Sever type procedure)

(For incision and drainage procedures, superficial, see 10040-10160)

23030   Incision and drainage, shoulder area; deep abscess or hematoma

23031   infected bursa

23035   Incision, bone cortex (eg, osteomyelitis or bone abscess), shoulder area

(23036 has been deleted)

23040   Arthrotomy, glenohumeral joint, including exploration, drainage, or removal of foreign body

(23042 has been deleted)

23044   Arthrotomy, acromioclavicular, sternoclavicular joint, including exploration, drainage, or removal of foreign body

Surgery: Musculoskeletal System

Excision

23065 Biopsy, soft tissue of shoulder area; superficial

23066 deep

(For needle biopsy of soft tissue, use 20206)

23075 Excision, soft tissue tumor, shoulder area; subcutaneous

23076 deep, subfascial, or intramuscular

23077 Radical resection of tumor (eg, malignant neoplasm), soft tissue of shoulder area

23100 Arthrotomy, glenohumeral joint, including biopsy

23101 Arthrotomy, acromioclavicular joint or sternoclavicular joint, including biopsy and/or excision of torn cartilage

23105 Arthrotomy; glenohumeral joint, with synovectomy, with or without biopsy

23106 sternoclavicular joint, with synovectomy, with or without biopsy

23107 Arthrotomy, glenohumeral joint, with joint exploration, with or without removal of loose or foreign body

(23110 has been deleted. To report, use 23929)

23120 Claviculectomy; partial

(For arthroscopic procedure, use 29824)

23125 total

23130 Acromioplasty or acromionectomy, partial, with or without coracoacromial ligament release

23140 Excision or curettage of bone cyst or benign tumor of clavicle or scapula;

23145 with autograft (includes obtaining graft)

23146 with allograft

23150 Excision or curettage of bone cyst or benign tumor of proximal humerus;

23155 with autograft (includes obtaining graft)

23156 with allograft

23170 Sequestrectomy (eg, for osteomyelitis or bone abscess), clavicle

(23171 has been deleted)

23172 Sequestrectomy (eg, for osteomyelitis or bone abscess), scapula

(23173 has been deleted)

23174 Sequestrectomy (eg, for osteomyelitis or bone abscess), humeral head to surgical neck

(23175 has been deleted)

23180 Partial excision (craterization, saucerization, or diaphysectomy) bone (eg, osteomyelitis), clavicle

(23181 has been deleted)

23182 Partial excision (craterization, saucerization, or diaphysectomy) bone (eg, osteomyelitis), scapula

(23183 has been deleted)

23184 Partial excision (craterization, saucerization, or diaphysectomy) bone (eg, osteomyelitis), proximal humerus

(23185 has been deleted)

23190 Ostectomy of scapula, partial (eg, superior medial angle)

23195 Resection, humeral head

(For replacement with implant, use 23470)

23200 Radical resection for tumor; clavicle

23210 scapula

23220 Radical resection of bone tumor, proximal humerus;

23221 with autograft (includes obtaining graft)

23222 with prosthetic replacement

Introduction or Removal

(For arthrocentesis or needling of bursa, use 20610)

(For K-wire or pin insertion or removal, see 20650, 20670, 20680)

23330 Removal of foreign body, shoulder; subcutaneous

23331 deep (eg, Neer hemiarthroplasty removal)

23332 complicated (eg, total shoulder)

23350 Injection procedure for shoulder arthrography or enhanced CT/MRI shoulder arthrography

(For radiographic arthrography, radiological supervision and interpretation, use 73040. Fluoroscopy (76003) is inclusive of radiographic arthrography)

(When fluoroscopic guided injection is performed for enhanced CT arthrography, use codes 23350, 76003, and 73201 or 73202)

(When fluoroscopic guided injection is performed for enhanced MR arthrography, use codes 23350, 76003, and 73222 or 73223)

(For enhanced CT or enhanced MRI arthrography, use 76003 and either 73201, 73202, 73222 or 73223)

(23355-23358 have been deleted. To report, see 29805-29826)

Repair, Revision, and/or Reconstruction

23395 Muscle transfer, any type, shoulder or upper arm; single

23397 multiple

23400 Scapulopexy (eg, Sprengels deformity or for paralysis)

23405 Tenotomy, shoulder area; single tendon

23406 multiple tendons through same incision

▲ **23410**   Repair of ruptured musculotendinous cuff (eg, rotator cuff) open; acute

23412   chronic

        ▶(For arthroscopic procedure, use 29827)◀

23415   Coracoacromial ligament release, with or without acromioplasty

        (For arthroscopic procedure, use 29826)

23420   Reconstruction of complete shoulder (rotator) cuff avulsion, chronic (includes acromioplasty)

23430   Tenodesis of long tendon of biceps

23440   Resection or transplantation of long tendon of biceps

23450   Capsulorrhaphy, anterior; Putti-Platt procedure or Magnuson type operation

        (To report arthroscopic thermal capsulorrhaphy, use 29999)

23455   with labral repair (eg, Bankart procedure)

        (For arthroscopic procedure, use 29807)

23460   Capsulorrhaphy, anterior, any type; with bone block

23462   with coracoid process transfer

        (To report open thermal capsulorrhaphy, use 23929)

23465   Capsulorrhaphy, glenohumeral joint, posterior, with or without bone block

        (For sternoclavicular and acromioclavicular reconstruction, see 23530, 23550)

23466   Capsulorrhaphy, glenohumeral joint, any type multi-directional instability

23470   Arthroplasty, glenohumeral joint; hemiarthroplasty

23472   total shoulder (glenoid and proximal humeral replacement (eg, total shoulder))

        (For removal of total shoulder implants, see 23331, 23332)

        (For osteotomy, proximal humerus, use 24400)

23480   Osteotomy, clavicle, with or without internal fixation;

23485   with bone graft for nonunion or malunion (includes obtaining graft and/or necessary fixation)

23490   Prophylactic treatment (nailing, pinning, plating or wiring) with or without methylmethacrylate; clavicle

23491   proximal humerus

Fracture and/or Dislocation

23500   Closed treatment of clavicular fracture; without manipulation

23505   with manipulation

        (23510 has been deleted. To report, see 23500, 23505, 23515)

23515   Open treatment of clavicular fracture, with or without internal or external fixation

23520   Closed treatment of sternoclavicular dislocation; without manipulation

23525   with manipulation

23530   Open treatment of sternoclavicular dislocation, acute or chronic;

23532   with fascial graft (includes obtaining graft)

23540   Closed treatment of acromioclavicular dislocation; without manipulation

23545   with manipulation

23550   Open treatment of acromioclavicular dislocation, acute or chronic;

23552   with fascial graft (includes obtaining graft)

23570   Closed treatment of scapular fracture; without manipulation

23575   with manipulation, with or without skeletal traction (with or without shoulder joint involvement)

        (23580 has been deleted. To report, see 23570, 23575, 23585)

23585   Open treatment of scapular fracture (body, glenoid or acromion) with or without internal fixation

23600   Closed treatment of proximal humeral (surgical or anatomical neck) fracture; without manipulation

23605   with manipulation, with or without skeletal traction

        (23610 has been deleted. To report, see 23600, 23605, 23615)

23615   Open treatment of proximal humeral (surgical or anatomical neck) fracture, with or without internal or external fixation, with or without repair of tuberosity(s);

23616   with proximal humeral prosthetic replacement

23620   Closed treatment of greater humeral tuberosity fracture; without manipulation

23625   with manipulation

23630   Open treatment of greater humeral tuberosity fracture, with or without internal or external fixation

23650   Closed treatment of shoulder dislocation, with manipulation; without anesthesia

23655   requiring anesthesia

        (23658 has been deleted. To report, see 23650, 23655, 23660, 23665, 23670)

23660   Open treatment of acute shoulder dislocation

        (Repairs for recurrent dislocations, see 23450-23466)

23665   Closed treatment of shoulder dislocation, with fracture of greater humeral tuberosity, with manipulation

23670   Open treatment of shoulder dislocation, with fracture of greater humeral tuberosity, with or without internal or external fixation

Surgery: Musculoskeletal System

23675 Closed treatment of shoulder dislocation, with surgical or anatomical neck fracture, with manipulation

23680 Open treatment of shoulder dislocation, with surgical or anatomical neck fracture, with or without internal or external fixation

Manipulation

23700* Manipulation under anesthesia, shoulder joint, including application of fixation apparatus (dislocation excluded)

Arthrodesis

23800 Arthrodesis, glenohumeral joint;

23802 with autogenous graft (includes obtaining graft)

Amputation

23900 Interthoracoscapular amputation (forequarter)

23920 Disarticulation of shoulder;

23921 secondary closure or scar revision

Other Procedures

23929 Unlisted procedure, shoulder

Humerus (Upper Arm) and Elbow

Elbow area includes head and neck of radius and olecranon process.

Incision

(For incision and drainage procedures, superficial, see 10040-10160)

23930 Incision and drainage, upper arm or elbow area; deep abscess or hematoma

23931 bursa

23935 Incision, deep, with opening of bone cortex (eg, for osteomyelitis or bone abscess), humerus or elbow

(23936 has been deleted)

24000 Arthrotomy, elbow, including exploration, drainage, or removal of foreign body

(24001 has been deleted)

24006 Arthrotomy of the elbow, with capsular excision for capsular release (separate procedure)

Excision

24065 Biopsy, soft tissue of upper arm or elbow area; superficial

24066 deep (subfascial or intramuscular)

(For needle biopsy of soft tissue, use 20206)

24075 Excision, tumor, soft tissue of upper arm or elbow area; subcutaneous

24076 deep (subfascial or intramuscular)

24077 Radical resection of tumor (eg, malignant neoplasm), soft tissue of upper arm or elbow area

24100 Arthrotomy, elbow; with synovial biopsy only

24101 with joint exploration, with or without biopsy, with or without removal of loose or foreign body

24102 with synovectomy

24105 Excision, olecranon bursa

24110 Excision or curettage of bone cyst or benign tumor, humerus;

24115 with autograft (includes obtaining graft)

24116 with allograft

24120 Excision or curettage of bone cyst or benign tumor of head or neck of radius or olecranon process;

24125 with autograft (includes obtaining graft)

24126 with allograft

24130 Excision, radial head

(For replacement with implant, use 24366)

24134 Sequestrectomy (eg, for osteomyelitis or bone abscess), shaft or distal humerus

(24135 has been deleted)

24136 Sequestrectomy (eg, for osteomyelitis or bone abscess), radial head or neck

(24137 has been deleted)

24138 Sequestrectomy (eg, for osteomyelitis or bone abscess), olecranon process

(24139 has been deleted)

24140 Partial excision (craterization, saucerization, or diaphysectomy) bone (eg, osteomyelitis), humerus

(24144 has been deleted)

24145 Partial excision (craterization, saucerization, or diaphysectomy) bone (eg, osteomyelitis), radial head or neck

(24146 has been deleted)

24147 Partial excision (craterization, saucerization, or diaphysectomy) bone (eg, osteomyelitis), olecranon process

(24148 has been deleted)

24149 Radical resection of capsule, soft tissue, and heterotopic bone, elbow, with contracture release (separate procedure)

(For capsular and soft tissue release only, use 24006)

24150 Radical resection for tumor, shaft or distal humerus;

24151 with autograft (includes obtaining graft)

Surgery: Musculoskeletal System

24152 Radical resection for tumor, radial head or neck;

24153   with autograft (includes obtaining graft)

24155 Resection of elbow joint (arthrectomy)

Introduction or Removal

(For K-wire or pin insertion or removal, see 20650, 20670, 20680)

(For arthrocentesis or needling of bursa or joint, use 20605)

24160 Implant removal; elbow joint

24164   radial head

24200 Removal of foreign body, upper arm or elbow area; subcutaneous

24201   deep (subfascial or intramuscular)

24220 Injection procedure for elbow arthrography

(For radiological supervision and interpretation, use 73085. Do not report 76003 in addition to 73085)

(For injection of tennis elbow, use 20550)

Repair, Revision, and/or Reconstruction

24300 Manipulation, elbow, under anesthesia

(For application of external fixation, see 20690 or 20692)

24301 Muscle or tendon transfer, any type, upper arm or elbow, single (excluding 24320-24331)

24305 Tendon lengthening, upper arm or elbow, each tendon

24310 Tenotomy, open, elbow to shoulder, each tendon

24320 Tenoplasty, with muscle transfer, with or without free graft, elbow to shoulder, single (Seddon-Brookes type procedure)

24330 Flexor-plasty, elbow (eg, Steindler type advancement);

24331   with extensor advancement

24332 Tenolysis, triceps

24340 Tenodesis of biceps tendon at elbow (separate procedure)

24341 Repair, tendon or muscle, upper arm or elbow, each tendon or muscle, primary or secondary (excludes rotator cuff)

24342 Reinsertion of ruptured biceps or triceps tendon, distal, with or without tendon graft

24343 Repair lateral collateral ligament, elbow, with local tissue

24344 Reconstruction lateral collateral ligament, elbow, with tendon graft (includes harvesting of graft)

24345 Repair medial collateral ligament, elbow, with local tissue

24346 Reconstruction medial collateral ligament, elbow, with tendon graft (includes harvesting of graft)

24350 Fasciotomy, lateral or medial (eg, tennis elbow or epicondylitis);

24351   with extensor origin detachment

24352   with annular ligament resection

24354   with stripping

24356   with partial ostectomy

24360 Arthroplasty, elbow; with membrane (eg, fascial)

24361   with distal humeral prosthetic replacement

24362   with implant and fascia lata ligament reconstruction

24363   with distal humerus and proximal ulnar prosthetic replacement (eg, total elbow)

24365 Arthroplasty, radial head;

24366   with implant

24400 Osteotomy, humerus, with or without internal fixation

24410 Multiple osteotomies with realignment on intramedullary rod, humeral shaft (Sofield type procedure)

24420 Osteoplasty, humerus (eg, shortening or lengthening) (excluding 64876)

24430 Repair of nonunion or malunion, humerus; without graft (eg, compression technique)

24435   with iliac or other autograft (includes obtaining graft)

(For proximal radius and/or ulna, see 25400-25420)

24470 Hemiepiphyseal arrest (eg, cubitus varus or valgus, distal humerus)

24495 Decompression fasciotomy, forearm, with brachial artery exploration

24498 Prophylactic treatment (nailing, pinning, plating or wiring), with or without methylmethacrylate, humeral shaft

Fracture and/or Dislocation

24500 Closed treatment of humeral shaft fracture; without manipulation

24505   with manipulation, with or without skeletal traction

(24506 has been deleted. To report, use 24516)

(24510 has been deleted. To report, see 24500, 24505, 24515, 24516)

24515 Open treatment of humeral shaft fracture with plate/screws, with or without cerclage

▲ **24516** Treatment of humeral shaft fracture, with insertion of intramedullary implant, with or without cerclage and/or locking screws

Surgery: Musculoskeletal System

24530 Closed treatment of supracondylar or transcondylar humeral fracture, with or without intercondylar extension; without manipulation

(24531 has been deleted. To report, use 24535)

24535   with manipulation, with or without skin or skeletal traction

(24536 has been deleted. To report, use 24535)

24538 Percutaneous skeletal fixation of supracondylar or transcondylar humeral fracture, with or without intercondylar extension

(24540 and 24542 have been deleted. To report, see 24530, 24535, 24538, 24545, 24546)

24545 Open treatment of humeral supracondylar or transcondylar fracture, with or without internal or external fixation; without intercondylar extension

24546   with intercondylar extension

24560 Closed treatment of humeral epicondylar fracture, medial or lateral; without manipulation

24565   with manipulation

24566 Percutaneous skeletal fixation of humeral epicondylar fracture, medial or lateral, with manipulation

(24570 has been deleted. To report, see 24560, 24565, 24575)

24575 Open treatment of humeral epicondylar fracture, medial or lateral, with or without internal or external fixation

24576 Closed treatment of humeral condylar fracture, medial or lateral; without manipulation

24577   with manipulation

(24578 has been deleted. To report, see 24576, 24577, 24579)

24579 Open treatment of humeral condylar fracture, medial or lateral, with or without internal or external fixation

(24580 has been deleted. To report, see 24530, 24560, 24576, 24650, 24670)

(24581 has been deleted. To report, see 24535, 24565, 24577, 24675)

24582 Percutaneous skeletal fixation of humeral condylar fracture, medial or lateral, with manipulation

(24583 has been deleted. To report, see 24535, 24538, 24545, 24560, 24565, 24577)

(24585 has been deleted. To report, see 24538, 24545, 24575, 24579, 24665, 24666, 24685)

24586 Open treatment of periarticular fracture and/or dislocation of the elbow (fracture distal humerus and proximal ulna and/ or proximal radius);

24587   with implant arthroplasty

(See also 24361)

(24588 has been deleted. To report, see 24586, 24587)

24600 Treatment of closed elbow dislocation; without anesthesia

24605   requiring anesthesia

(24610 has been deleted. To report, see 24586, 24600, 24605, 24615)

24615 Open treatment of acute or chronic elbow dislocation

24620 Closed treatment of Monteggia type of fracture dislocation at elbow (fracture proximal end of ulna with dislocation of radial head), with manipulation

(24625 has been deleted. To report, see 24620, 24635)

24635 Open treatment of Monteggia type of fracture dislocation at elbow (fracture proximal end of ulna with dislocation of radial head), with or without internal or external fixation

24640* Closed treatment of radial head subluxation in child, nursemaid elbow, with manipulation

24650 Closed treatment of radial head or neck fracture; without manipulation

24655   with manipulation

(24660 has been deleted. To report, see 24650, 24655, 24665, 24666)

24665 Open treatment of radial head or neck fracture, with or without internal fixation or radial head excision;

24666   with radial head prosthetic replacement

24670 Closed treatment of ulnar fracture, proximal end (olecranon process); without manipulation

24675   with manipulation

(24680 has been deleted. To report, see 24670, 24675, 24685)

24685 Open treatment of ulnar fracture proximal end (olecranon process), with or without internal or external fixation

(24700 has been deleted. To report, use 24999)

Arthrodesis

24800 Arthrodesis, elbow joint; local

24802   with autogenous graft (includes obtaining graft)

Amputation

24900 Amputation, arm through humerus; with primary closure

24920   open, circular (guillotine)

24925   secondary closure or scar revision

24930   re-amputation

24931   with implant

24935 Stump elongation, upper extremity

24940 Cineplasty, upper extremity, complete procedure

Surgery: Musculoskeletal System

Other Procedures

24999   Unlisted procedure, humerus or elbow

Forearm and Wrist

Radius, ulna, carpal bones and joints.

Incision

25000   Incision, extensor tendon sheath, wrist (eg, deQuervains disease)

(For decompression median nerve or for carpal tunnel syndrome, use 64721)

(25005 has been deleted. To report, use 25000)

25001   Incision, flexor tendon sheath, wrist (eg, flexor carpi radialis)

25020   Decompression fasciotomy, forearm and/or wrist, flexor OR extensor compartment; without debridement of nonviable muscle and/or nerve

25023   with debridement of nonviable muscle and/or nerve

(For decompression fasciotomy with brachial artery exploration, use 24495)

(For incision and drainage procedures, superficial, see 10040-10160)

(For debridement, see also 11000-11044)

25024   Decompression fasciotomy, forearm and/or wrist, flexor AND extensor compartment; without debridement of nonviable muscle and/or nerve

25025   with debridement of nonviable muscle and/or nerve

25028   Incision and drainage, forearm and/or wrist; deep abscess or hematoma

25031   bursa

25035   Incision, deep, bone cortex, forearm and/or wrist (eg, osteomyelitis or bone abscess)

(25036 has been deleted)

25040   Arthrotomy, radiocarpal or midcarpal joint, with exploration, drainage, or removal of foreign body

(25041 has been deleted)

Excision

25065   Biopsy, soft tissue of forearm and/or wrist; superficial

25066   deep (subfascial or intramuscular)

(For needle biopsy of soft tissue, use 20206)

25075   Excision, tumor, soft tissue of forearm and/or wrist area; subcutaneous

25076   deep (subfascial or intramuscular)

25077   Radical resection of tumor (eg, malignant neoplasm), soft tissue of forearm and/or wrist area

25085   Capsulotomy, wrist (eg, contracture)

25100   Arthrotomy, wrist joint; with biopsy

25101   with joint exploration, with or without biopsy, with or without removal of loose or foreign body

25105   with synovectomy

25107   Arthrotomy, distal radioulnar joint including repair of triangular cartilage, complex

25110   Excision, lesion of tendon sheath, forearm and/or wrist

25111   Excision of ganglion, wrist (dorsal or volar); primary

25112   recurrent

(For hand or finger, use 26160)

25115   Radical excision of bursa, synovia of wrist, or forearm tendon sheaths (eg, tenosynovitis, fungus, Tbc, or other granulomas, rheumatoid arthritis); flexors

25116   extensors, with or without transposition of dorsal retinaculum

(For finger synovectomies, use 26145)

25118   Synovectomy, extensor tendon sheath, wrist, single compartment;

25119   with resection of distal ulna

25120   Excision or curettage of bone cyst or benign tumor of radius or ulna (excluding head or neck of radius and olecranon process);

(For head or neck of radius or olecranon process, see 24120-24126)

25125   with autograft (includes obtaining graft)

25126   with allograft

25130   Excision or curettage of bone cyst or benign tumor of carpal bones;

25135   with autograft (includes obtaining graft)

25136   with allograft

25145   Sequestrectomy (eg, for osteomyelitis or bone abscess), forearm and/or wrist

(25146 has been deleted)

25150   Partial excision (craterization, saucerization, or diaphysectomy) of bone (eg, for osteomyelitis); ulna

25151   radius

(25153 has been deleted)

(For head or neck of radius or olecranon process, see 24145, 24147)

25170   Radical resection for tumor, radius or ulna

25210   Carpectomy; one bone

(For carpectomy with implant, see 25441-25445)

25215   all bones of proximal row

25230   Radial styloidectomy (separate procedure)

Surgery: Musculoskeletal System

25240 Excision distal ulna partial or complete (eg, Darrach type or matched resection)

(For implant replacement, distal ulna, use 25442)

(For obtaining fascia for interposition, see 20920, 20922)

Introduction or Removal

(For K-wire, pin or rod insertion or removal, see 20650, 20670, 20680)

25246 Injection procedure for wrist arthrography

(For radiological supervision and interpretation, use 73115. Do not report 76003 in addition to 73115)

(For foreign body removal, superficial use 20520)

25248 Exploration with removal of deep foreign body, forearm or wrist

25250 Removal of wrist prosthesis; (separate procedure)

25251 complicated, including total wrist

25259 Manipulation, wrist, under anesthesia

(For application of external fixation, see 20690 or 20692)

Repair, Revision, and/or Reconstruction

25260 Repair, tendon or muscle, flexor, forearm and/or wrist; primary, single, each tendon or muscle

25263 secondary, single, each tendon or muscle

25265 secondary, with free graft (includes obtaining graft), each tendon or muscle

25270 Repair, tendon or muscle, extensor, forearm and/or wrist; primary, single, each tendon or muscle

25272 secondary, single, each tendon or muscle

25274 secondary, with free graft (includes obtaining graft), each tendon or muscle

25275 Repair, tendon sheath, extensor, forearm and/or wrist, with free graft (includes obtaining graft) (eg, for extensor carpi ulnaris subluxation)

25280 Lengthening or shortening of flexor or extensor tendon, forearm and/or wrist, single, each tendon

25290 Tenotomy, open, flexor or extensor tendon, forearm and/or wrist, single, each tendon

25295 Tenolysis, flexor or extensor tendon, forearm and/or wrist, single, each tendon

25300 Tenodesis at wrist; flexors of fingers

25301 extensors of fingers

25310 Tendon transplantation or transfer, flexor or extensor, forearm and/or wrist, single; each tendon

25312 with tendon graft(s) (includes obtaining graft), each tendon

25315 Flexor origin slide (eg, for cerebral palsy, Volkmann contracture), forearm and/or wrist;

25316 with tendon(s) transfer

(25317, 25318 have been deleted. To report, see 25315, 25316)

▲ **25320** Capsulorrhaphy or reconstruction, wrist, open (eg, capsulodesis, ligament repair, tendon transfer or graft) (includes synovectomy, capsulotomy and open reduction) for carpal instability

(25330, 25331 have been deleted. To report, see 25332 and 25441-25446)

25332 Arthroplasty, wrist, with or without interposition, with or without external or internal fixation

(For obtaining fascia for interposition, see 20920, 20922)

(For prosthetic replacement arthroplasty, see 25441-25446)

25335 Centralization of wrist on ulna (eg, radial club hand)

25337 Reconstruction for stabilization of unstable distal ulna or distal radioulnar joint, secondary by soft tissue stabilization (eg, tendon transfer, tendon graft or weave, or tenodesis) with or without open reduction of distal radioulnar joint

(For harvesting of fascia lata graft, see 20920, 20922)

25350 Osteotomy, radius; distal third

25355 middle or proximal third

25360 Osteotomy; ulna

25365 radius AND ulna

25370 Multiple osteotomies, with realignment on intramedullary rod (Sofield type procedure); radius OR ulna

25375 radius AND ulna

25390 Osteoplasty, radius OR ulna; shortening

25391 lengthening with autograft

25392 Osteoplasty, radius AND ulna; shortening (excluding 64876)

25393 lengthening with autograft

25394 Osteoplasty, carpal bone, shortening

25400 Repair of nonunion or malunion, radius OR ulna; without graft (eg, compression technique)

25405 with autograft (includes obtaining graft)

25415 Repair of nonunion or malunion, radius AND ulna; without graft (eg, compression technique)

25420 with autograft (includes obtaining graft)

25425 Repair of defect with autograft; radius OR ulna

25426 radius AND ulna

25430 Insertion of vascular pedicle into carpal bone (eg, Hori procedure)

Surgery: Musculoskeletal System

25431   Repair of nonunion of carpal bone (excluding carpal scaphoid (navicular)) (includes obtaining graft and necessary fixation), each bone

25440   Repair of nonunion, scaphoid carpal (navicular) bone, with or without radial styloidectomy (includes obtaining graft and necessary fixation)

25441   Arthroplasty with prosthetic replacement; distal radius

25442   distal ulna

25443   scaphoid carpal (navicular)

25444   lunate

25445   trapezium

25446   distal radius and partial or entire carpus (total wrist)

25447   Arthroplasty, interposition, intercarpal or carpometacarpal joints

(For wrist arthroplasty, use 25332)

25449   Revision of arthroplasty, including removal of implant, wrist joint

25450   Epiphyseal arrest by epiphysiodesis or stapling; distal radius OR ulna

25455   distal radius AND ulna

25490   Prophylactic treatment (nailing, pinning, plating or wiring) with or without methylmethacrylate; radius

25491   ulna

25492   radius AND ulna

Fracture and/or Dislocation

25500   Closed treatment of radial shaft fracture; without manipulation

25505   with manipulation

(25510 has been deleted. To report, see 25500, 25505, 25515)

25515   Open treatment of radial shaft fracture, with or without internal or external fixation

25520   Closed treatment of radial shaft fracture and closed treatment of dislocation of distal radioulnar joint (Galeazzi fracture/dislocation)

25525   Open treatment of radial shaft fracture, with internal and/ or external fixation and closed treatment of dislocation of distal radioulnar joint (Galeazzi fracture/dislocation), with or without percutaneous skeletal fixation

25526   Open treatment of radial shaft fracture, with internal and/or external fixation and open treatment, with or without internal or external fixation of distal radioulnar joint (Galeazzi fracture/dislocation), includes repair of triangular fibrocartilage complex

25530   Closed treatment of ulnar shaft fracture; without manipulation

25535   with manipulation

(25540 has been deleted. To report, see 25530, 25535, 25545)

25545   Open treatment of ulnar shaft fracture, with or without internal or external fixation

25560   Closed treatment of radial and ulnar shaft fractures; without manipulation

25565   with manipulation

(25570 has been deleted. To report, see 25560, 25565, 25574, 25575)

25574   Open treatment of radial AND ulnar shaft fractures, with internal or external fixation; of radius OR ulna

25575   of radius AND ulna

25600   Closed treatment of distal radial fracture (eg, Colles or Smith type) or epiphyseal separation, with or without fracture of ulnar styloid; without manipulation

25605   with manipulation

(25610 has been deleted. To report, use 25605)

25611   Percutaneous skeletal fixation of distal radial fracture (eg, Colles or Smith type) or epiphyseal separation, with or without fracture of ulnar styloid, requiring manipulation, with or without external fixation

(25615 has been deleted. To report, see 25600, 25605, 25611, 25620)

25620   Open treatment of distal radial fracture (eg, Colles or Smith type) or epiphyseal separation, with or without fracture of ulnar styloid, with or without internal or external fixation

25622   Closed treatment of carpal scaphoid (navicular) fracture; without manipulation

25624   with manipulation

(25626 has been deleted. To report, see 25622, 25624, 25628)

25628   Open treatment of carpal scaphoid (navicular) fracture, with or without internal or external fixation

25630   Closed treatment of carpal bone fracture (excluding carpal scaphoid (navicular)); without manipulation, each bone

25635   with manipulation, each bone

(25640 has been deleted. To report, see 25630, 25635, 25645)

25645   Open treatment of carpal bone fracture (other than carpal scaphoid (navicular)), each bone

25650   Closed treatment of ulnar styloid fracture

25651   Percutaneous skeletal fixation of ulnar styloid fracture

25652   Open treatment of ulnar styloid fracture

25660 Closed treatment of radiocarpal or intercarpal dislocation, one or more bones, with manipulation

(25665 has been deleted. To report, see 25650, 25660, 25670)

25670 Open treatment of radiocarpal or intercarpal dislocation, one or more bones

25671 Percutaneous skeletal fixation of distal radioulnar dislocation

25675 Closed treatment of distal radioulnar dislocation with manipulation

25676 Open treatment of distal radioulnar dislocation, acute or chronic

25680 Closed treatment of trans-scaphoperilunar type of fracture dislocation, with manipulation

25685 Open treatment of trans-scaphoperilunar type of fracture dislocation

25690 Closed treatment of lunate dislocation, with manipulation

25695 Open treatment of lunate dislocation

(25700 has been deleted. To report, use 25999)

Arthrodesis

25800 Arthrodesis, wrist; complete, without bone graft (includes radiocarpal and/or intercarpal and/or carpometacarpal joints)

25805 with sliding graft

25810 with iliac or other autograft (includes obtaining graft)

(25815 has been deleted. To report, see 25820, 25825)

25820 Arthrodesis, wrist; limited, without bone graft (eg, intercarpal or radiocarpal)

25825 with autograft (includes obtaining graft)

25830 Arthrodesis, distal radioulnar joint with segmental resection of ulna, with or without bone graft (eg, Sauve-Kapandji procedure)

Amputation

25900 Amputation, forearm, through radius and ulna;

25905 open, circular (guillotine)

25907 secondary closure or scar revision

25909 re-amputation

25915 Krukenberg procedure

25920 Disarticulation through wrist;

25922 secondary closure or scar revision

25924 re-amputation

25927 Transmetacarpal amputation;

25929 secondary closure or scar revision

25931 re-amputation

Other Procedures

25999 Unlisted procedure, forearm or wrist

Hand and Fingers

Incision

26010* Drainage of finger abscess; simple

26011* complicated (eg, felon)

26020 Drainage of tendon sheath, digit and/or palm, each

26025 Drainage of palmar bursa; single, bursa

26030 multiple bursa

(26032 has been deleted)

26034 Incision, bone cortex, hand or finger (eg, osteomyelitis or bone abscess)

26035 Decompression fingers and/or hand, injection injury (eg, grease gun)

26037 Decompressive fasciotomy, hand (excludes 26035)

(For injection injury, use 26035)

26040 Fasciotomy, palmar (eg, Dupuytren's contracture); percutaneous

26045 open, partial

(For fasciectomy, see 26121-26125)

26055 Tendon sheath incision (eg, for trigger finger)

26060 Tenotomy, percutaneous, single, each digit

26070 Arthrotomy, with exploration, drainage, or removal of loose or foreign body; carpometacarpal joint

26075 metacarpophalangeal joint, each

26080 interphalangeal joint, each

Excision

26100 Arthrotomy with biopsy; carpometacarpal joint, each

26105 metacarpophalangeal joint, each

26110 interphalangeal joint, each

26115 Excision, tumor or vascular malformation, soft tissue of hand or finger; subcutaneous

26116 deep (subfascial or intramuscular)

26117 Radical resection of tumor (eg, malignant neoplasm), soft tissue of hand or finger

(26120 has been deleted. To report, see 26121-26125)

26121 Fasciectomy, palm only, with or without Z-plasty, other local tissue rearrangement, or skin grafting (includes obtaining graft)

(26122 has been deleted. To report, use 26121-26125)

26123 Fasciectomy, partial palmar with release of single digit including proximal interphalangeal joint, with or without Z-plasty, other local tissue rearrangement, or skin grafting (includes obtaining graft);

(26124 has been deleted. To report, use 26121-26125)

+ 26125 each additional digit (List separately in addition to code for primary procedure)

(Use 26125 in conjunction with code 26123)

(26126, 26128 have been deleted. To report, use 26121-26125)

(For fasciotomy, see 26040, 26045)

26130 Synovectomy, carpometacarpal joint

26135 Synovectomy, metacarpophalangeal joint including intrinsic release and extensor hood reconstruction, each digit

26140 Synovectomy, proximal interphalangeal joint, including extensor reconstruction, each interphalangeal joint

26145 Synovectomy, tendon sheath, radical (tenosynovectomy), flexor tendon, palm and/or finger, each tendon

(For tendon sheath synovectomies at wrist, see 25115, 25116)

26160 Excision of lesion of tendon sheath or joint capsule (eg, cyst, mucous cyst, or ganglion), hand or finger

(For wrist ganglion, see 25111, 25112)

(For trigger digit, use 26055)

26170 Excision of tendon, palm, flexor, single (separate procedure), each

26180 Excision of tendon, finger, flexor (separate procedure), each tendon

26185 Sesamoidectomy, thumb or finger (separate procedure)

26200 Excision or curettage of bone cyst or benign tumor of metacarpal;

26205 with autograft (includes obtaining graft)

(26206 has been deleted. To report, use 26989)

26210 Excision or curettage of bone cyst or benign tumor of proximal, middle, or distal phalanx of finger;

26215 with autograft (includes obtaining graft)

(26216 has been deleted. To report, use 26989)

26230 Partial excision (craterization, saucerization, or diaphysectomy) bone (eg, osteomyelitis); metacarpal

26235 proximal or middle phalanx of finger

26236 distal phalanx of finger

26250 Radical resection, metacarpal (eg, tumor);

26255 with autograft (includes obtaining graft)

26260 Radical resection, proximal or middle phalanx of finger (eg, tumor);

26261 with autograft (includes obtaining graft)

26262 Radical resection, distal phalanx of finger (eg, tumor)

Introduction or Removal

26320 Removal of implant from finger or hand

(For removal of foreign body in hand or finger, see 20520, 20525)

Repair, Revision, and/or Reconstruction

26340 Manipulation, finger joint, under anesthesia, each joint

(For application of external fixation, see 20690 or 20692)

26350 Repair or advancement, flexor tendon, not in zone 2 digital flexor tendon sheath (eg, no man's land); primary or secondary without free graft, each tendon

26352 secondary with free graft (includes obtaining graft), each tendon

26356 Repair or advancement, flexor tendon, in zone 2 digital flexor tendon sheath (eg, no man's land); primary or secondary without free graft, each tendon

26357 secondary, each tendon

26358 secondary with free graft (includes obtaining graft), each tendon

26370 Repair or advancement of profundus tendon, with intact superficialis tendon; primary, each tendon

26372 secondary with free graft (includes obtaining graft), each tendon

26373 secondary without free graft, each tendon

26390 Excision flexor tendon, with implantation of synthetic rod for delayed tendon graft, hand or finger, each rod

26392 Removal of synthetic rod and insertion of flexor tendon graft, hand or finger (includes obtaining graft), each rod

26410 Repair, extensor tendon, hand, primary or secondary; without free graft, each tendon

26412 with free graft (includes obtaining graft), each tendon

26415 Excision of extensor tendon, with implantation of synthetic rod for delayed tendon graft, hand or finger, each rod

26416 Removal of synthetic rod and insertion of extensor tendon graft (includes obtaining graft), hand or finger, each rod

26418 Repair, extensor tendon, finger, primary or secondary; without free graft, each tendon

26420 with free graft (includes obtaining graft) each tendon

26426 Repair of extensor tendon, central slip, secondary (eg, boutonniere deformity); using local tissue(s), including lateral band(s), each finger

26428 with free graft (includes obtaining graft), each finger

26432 Closed treatment of distal extensor tendon insertion, with or without percutaneous pinning (eg, mallet finger)

▲=Revised Code   ●=New Code   ✻=Service Includes Surgical Procedure Only

26433   Repair of extensor tendon, distal insertion, primary or secondary; without graft (eg, mallet finger)

26434   with free graft (includes obtaining graft)

(For tenovaginotomy for trigger finger, use 26055)

26437   Realignment of extensor tendon, hand, each tendon

26440   Tenolysis, flexor tendon; palm OR finger, each tendon

26442   palm AND finger, each tendon

26445   Tenolysis, extensor tendon, hand OR finger; each tendon

26449   Tenolysis, complex, extensor tendon, finger, including forearm, each tendon

26450   Tenotomy, flexor, palm, open, each tendon

26455   Tenotomy, flexor, finger, open, each tendon

26460   Tenotomy, extensor, hand or finger, open, each tendon

26471   Tenodesis; of proximal interphalangeal joint, each joint

26474   of distal joint, each joint

26476   Lengthening of tendon, extensor, hand or finger, each tendon

26477   Shortening of tendon, extensor, hand or finger, each tendon

26478   Lengthening of tendon, flexor, hand or finger, each tendon

26479   Shortening of tendon, flexor, hand or finger, each tendon

26480   Transfer or transplant of tendon, carpometacarpal area or dorsum of hand; without free graft, each tendon

26483   with free tendon graft (includes obtaining graft), each tendon

26485   Transfer or transplant of tendon, palmar; without free tendon graft, each tendon

26489   with free tendon graft (includes obtaining graft), each tendon

26490   Opponensplasty; superficialis tendon transfer type, each tendon

26492   tendon transfer with graft (includes obtaining graft), each tendon

26494   hypothenar muscle transfer

26496   other methods

(For thumb fusion in opposition, use 26820)

26497   Transfer of tendon to restore intrinsic function; ring and small finger

26498   all four fingers

26499   Correction claw finger, other methods

26500   Reconstruction of tendon pulley, each tendon; with local tissues (separate procedure)

26502   with tendon or fascial graft (includes obtaining graft) (separate procedure)

26504   with tendon prosthesis (separate procedure)

26508   Release of thenar muscle(s) (eg, thumb contracture)

26510   Cross intrinsic transfer, each tendon

26516   Capsulodesis, metacarpophalangeal joint; single digit

26517   two digits

26518   three or four digits

26520   Capsulectomy or capsulotomy; metacarpophalangeal joint, each joint

26525   interphalangeal joint, each joint

(26527 has been deleted. To report, use 25447)

26530   Arthroplasty, metacarpophalangeal joint; each joint

26531   with prosthetic implant, each joint

26535   Arthroplasty, interphalangeal joint; each joint

26536   with prosthetic implant, each joint

26540   Repair of collateral ligament, metacarpophalangeal or interphalangeal joint

26541   Reconstruction, collateral ligament, metacarpophalangeal joint, single; with tendon or fascial graft (includes obtaining graft)

26542   with local tissue (eg, adductor advancement)

26545   Reconstruction, collateral ligament, interphalangeal joint, single, including graft, each joint

26546   Repair non-union, metacarpal or phalanx, (includes obtaining bone graft with or without external or internal fixation)

26548   Repair and reconstruction, finger, volar plate, interphalangeal joint

26550   Pollicization of a digit

26551   Transfer, toe-to-hand with microvascular anastomosis; great toe wrap-around with bone graft

(For great toe with web space, use 20973)

(26552 has been deleted. To report, see 20973 or 26551, 26553, 26554)

26553   other than great toe, single

26554   other than great toe, double

(Do not report code 69990 in addition to codes 26551-26554)

26555   Transfer, finger to another position without microvascular anastomosis

26556   Transfer, free toe joint, with microvascular anastomosis

(Do not report code 69990 in addition to code 26556)

(26557-26559 have been deleted. To report, see 20973 or 26551, 26553, 26554)

26560   Repair of syndactyly (web finger) each web space; with skin flaps

26561   with skin flaps and grafts

26562   complex (eg, involving bone, nails)

26565   Osteotomy; metacarpal, each

26567   phalanx of finger, each

26568   Osteoplasty, lengthening, metacarpal or phalanx

(26570, 26574 have been deleted. To report, use 26989)

26580   Repair cleft hand

(26585 has been deleted. To report, use 26587)

26587   Reconstruction of polydactylous digit, soft tissue and bone

(For excision of polydactylous digit, soft tissue only, use 11200)

26590   Repair macrodactylia, each digit

26591   Repair, intrinsic muscles of hand, each muscle

26593   Release, intrinsic muscles of hand, each muscle

26596   Excision of constricting ring of finger, with multiple Z-plasties

(26597 has been deleted. To report, see 11041-11042, 14040-14041, or 15120, 15240)

Fracture and/or Dislocation

26600   Closed treatment of metacarpal fracture, single; without manipulation, each bone

26605   with manipulation, each bone

26607   Closed treatment of metacarpal fracture, with manipulation, with external fixation, each bone

26608   Percutaneous skeletal fixation of metacarpal fracture, each bone

(26610 has been deleted. To report, see 26605, 26607, 26608)

26615   Open treatment of metacarpal fracture, single, with or without internal or external fixation, each bone

26641   Closed treatment of carpometacarpal dislocation, thumb, with manipulation

26645   Closed treatment of carpometacarpal fracture dislocation, thumb (Bennett fracture), with manipulation

26650   Percutaneous skeletal fixation of carpometacarpal fracture dislocation, thumb (Bennett fracture), with manipulation, with or without external fixation

(26655 has been deleted. To report, see 26645, 26650, 26665)

(26660 has been deleted. To report, see 26650, 26665)

26665   Open treatment of carpometacarpal fracture dislocation, thumb (Bennett fracture), with or without internal or external fixation

26670   Closed treatment of carpometacarpal dislocation, other than thumb, with manipulation, each joint; without anesthesia

26675   requiring anesthesia

26676   Percutaneous skeletal fixation of carpometacarpal dislocation, other than thumb, with manipulation, each joint

(26680 has been deleted. To report, see 26670, 26675, 26676, 26685)

26685   Open treatment of carpometacarpal dislocation, other than thumb; with or without internal or external fixation, each joint

26686   complex, multiple or delayed reduction

26700   Closed treatment of metacarpophalangeal dislocation, single, with manipulation; without anesthesia

26705   requiring anesthesia

26706   Percutaneous skeletal fixation of metacarpophalangeal dislocation, single, with manipulation

(26710 has been deleted. To report, see 26700, 26705, 26706, 26715)

26715   Open treatment of metacarpophalangeal dislocation, single, with or without internal or external fixation

26720   Closed treatment of phalangeal shaft fracture, proximal or middle phalanx, finger or thumb; without manipulation, each

26725   with manipulation, with or without skin or skeletal traction, each

26727   Percutaneous skeletal fixation of unstable phalangeal shaft fracture, proximal or middle phalanx, finger or thumb, with manipulation, each

(26730 has been deleted. To report, see 26720, 26725, 26727, 26735)

26735   Open treatment of phalangeal shaft fracture, proximal or middle phalanx, finger or thumb, with or without internal or external fixation, each

26740   Closed treatment of articular fracture, involving metacarpophalangeal or interphalangeal joint; without manipulation, each

26742   with manipulation, each

(26743 has been deleted. To report, use 26989)

(26744 has been deleted. To report, see 26740, 26742, 26746)

26746   Open treatment of articular fracture, involving metacarpophalangeal or interphalangeal joint, with or without internal or external fixation, each

26750   Closed treatment of distal phalangeal fracture, finger or thumb; without manipulation, each

26755   with manipulation, each

26756   Percutaneous skeletal fixation of distal phalangeal fracture, finger or thumb, each

(26760 has been deleted. To report, see 26750, 26755, 26756, 26765)

26765   Open treatment of distal phalangeal fracture, finger or thumb, with or without internal or external fixation, each

Surgery: Musculoskeletal System

Surgery: Musculoskeletal System

26770 Closed treatment of interphalangeal joint dislocation, single, with manipulation; without anesthesia

26775 requiring anesthesia

26776 Percutaneous skeletal fixation of interphalangeal joint dislocation, single, with manipulation

(26780 has been deleted. To report, see 26770, 26775, 26776, 26785)

26785 Open treatment of interphalangeal joint dislocation, with or without internal or external fixation, single

Arthrodesis

26820 Fusion in opposition, thumb, with autogenous graft (includes obtaining graft)

26841 Arthrodesis, carpometacarpal joint, thumb, with or without internal fixation;

26842 with autograft (includes obtaining graft)

26843 Arthrodesis, carpometacarpal joint, digit, other than thumb, each;

26844 with autograft (includes obtaining graft)

26850 Arthrodesis, metacarpophalangeal joint, with or without internal fixation;

26852 with autograft (includes obtaining graft)

26860 Arthrodesis, interphalangeal joint, with or without internal fixation;

+ 26861 each additional interphalangeal joint (List separately in addition to code for primary procedure)

(Use 26861 in conjunction with code 26860)

26862 with autograft (includes obtaining graft)

+ 26863 with autograft (includes obtaining graft), each additional joint (List separately in addition to code for primary procedure)

(Use 26863 in conjunction with code 26862)

Amputation

(For hand through metacarpal bones, use 25927)

26910 Amputation, metacarpal, with finger or thumb (ray amputation), single, with or without interosseous transfer

(For repositioning, see 26550, 26555)

26951 Amputation, finger or thumb, primary or secondary, any joint or phalanx, single, including neurectomies; with direct closure

26952 with local advancement flaps (V-Y, hood)

(For repair of soft tissue defect requiring split or full thickness graft or other pedicle flaps, see 15050-15758)

Other Procedures

26989 Unlisted procedure, hands or fingers

Pelvis and Hip Joint

Including head and neck of femur.

Incision

(For incision and drainage procedures, superficial, see 10040-10160)

26990 Incision and drainage, pelvis or hip joint area; deep abscess or hematoma

26991 infected bursa

26992 Incision, bone cortex, pelvis and/or hip joint (eg, osteomyelitis or bone abscess)

(26995 has been deleted)

27000 Tenotomy, adductor of hip, percutaneous (separate procedure)

27001 Tenotomy, adductor of hip, open

(27002 has been deleted. To report, use 27001 with modifier '-50')

27003 Tenotomy, adductor, subcutaneous, open, with obturator neurectomy

(27004 has been deleted. To report, use 27003 with modifier '-50')

27005 Tenotomy, hip flexor(s), open (separate procedure)

27006 Tenotomy, abductors and/or extensor(s) of hip, open (separate procedure)

(27010, 27015 have been deleted. To report, use 27025)

27025 Fasciotomy, hip or thigh, any type

(27026 has been deleted. To report, use 27025 with modifier '-50')

27030 Arthrotomy, hip, with drainage (eg, infection)

(27031 has been deleted)

27033 Arthrotomy, hip, including exploration or removal of loose or foreign body

27035 Denervation, hip joint, intrapelvic or extrapelvic intra-articular branches of sciatic, femoral, or obturator nerves

(For obturator neurectomy, see 64763, 64766)

27036 Capsulectomy or capsulotomy, hip, with or without excision of heterotopic bone, with release of hip flexor muscles (ie, gluteus medius, gluteus minimus, tensor fascia latae, rectus femoris, sartorius, iliopsoas)

Excision

27040 Biopsy, soft tissue of pelvis and hip area; superficial

27041 deep, subfascial or intramuscular

(For needle biopsy of soft tissue, use 20206)

27047 Excision, tumor, pelvis and hip area; subcutaneous tissue

27048 deep, subfascial, intramuscular

27049   Radical resection of tumor, soft tissue of pelvis and hip area (eg, malignant neoplasm)

27050   Arthrotomy, with biopsy; sacroiliac joint

27052   hip joint

27054   Arthrotomy with synovectomy, hip joint

27060   Excision; ischial bursa

27062   trochanteric bursa or calcification

          (For arthrocentesis or needling of bursa, use 20610)

27065   Excision of bone cyst or benign tumor; superficial (wing of ilium, symphysis pubis, or greater trochanter of femur) with or without autograft

27066   deep, with or without autograft

27067   with autograft requiring separate incision

27070   Partial excision (craterization, saucerization) (eg, osteomyelitis or bone abscess); superficial (eg, wing of ilium, symphysis pubis, or greater trochanter of femur)

27071   deep (subfascial or intramuscular)

27075   Radical resection of tumor or infection; wing of ilium, one pubic or ischial ramus or symphysis pubis

27076   ilium, including acetabulum, both pubic rami, or ischium and acetabulum

27077   innominate bone, total

27078   ischial tuberosity and greater trochanter of femur

27079   ischial tuberosity and greater trochanter of femur, with skin flaps

27080   Coccygectomy, primary

          (For pressure (decubitus) ulcer, see 15920, 15922 and 15931-15958)

Introduction or Removal

27086*   Removal of foreign body, pelvis or hip; subcutaneous tissue

27087   deep (subfascial or intramuscular)

          (27088 has been deleted. To report, use 27087)

27090   Removal of hip prosthesis; (separate procedure)

27091   complicated, including total hip prosthesis, methylmethacrylate with or without insertion of spacer

27093   Injection procedure for hip arthrography; without anesthesia

          (For radiological supervision and interpretation, use 73525. Do not report 76003 in addition to 73525)

27095   with anesthesia

          (For radiological supervision and interpretation, use 73525. Do not report 76003 in addition to 73525)

27096   Injection procedure for sacroiliac joint, arthrography and/or anesthetic/steroid

          (27096 is to be used only with imaging confirmation of intra-articular needle positioning)

          (For radiological supervision and interpretation of sacroiliac joint arthrography, use 73542)

          (For fluoroscopic guidance without formal arthrography, use 76005)

          (Code 27096 is a unilateral procedure. For bilateral procedure, use modifier '-50')

Repair, Revision, and/or Reconstruction

27097   Release or recession, hamstring, proximal

27098   Transfer, adductor to ischium

27100   Transfer external oblique muscle to greater trochanter including fascial or tendon extension (graft)

27105   Transfer paraspinal muscle to hip (includes fascial or tendon extension graft)

27110   Transfer iliopsoas; to greater trochanter of femur

27111   to femoral neck

          (27115 has been deleted. To report, use 27299)

27120   Acetabuloplasty; (eg, Whitman, Colonna, Haygroves, or cup type)

27122   resection, femoral head (eg, Girdlestone procedure)

27125   Hemiarthroplasty, hip, partial (eg, femoral stem prosthesis, bipolar arthroplasty)

          (For prosthetic replacement following fracture of the hip, use 27236)

          (27126, 27127 have been deleted. To report, use 27120)

27130   Arthroplasty, acetabular and proximal femoral prosthetic replacement (total hip arthroplasty), with or without autograft or allograft

          (27131 has been deleted. To report, use 27132)

27132   Conversion of previous hip surgery to total hip arthroplasty, with or without autograft or allograft

27134   Revision of total hip arthroplasty; both components, with or without autograft or allograft

          (27135 has been deleted. To report, see 27134, 27137, 27138)

27137   acetabular component only, with or without autograft or allograft

27138   femoral component only, with or without allograft

27140   Osteotomy and transfer of greater trochanter of femur (separate procedure)

Surgery: Musculoskeletal System

Surgery: Musculoskeletal System

27146   Osteotomy, iliac, acetabular or innominate bone;

27147   with open reduction of hip

27151   with femoral osteotomy

27156   with femoral osteotomy and with open reduction of hip

             (27157 has been deleted)

27158   Osteotomy, pelvis, bilateral (eg, congenital malformation)

27161   Osteotomy, femoral neck (separate procedure)

27165   Osteotomy, intertrochanteric or subtrochanteric including internal or external fixation and/or cast

27170   Bone graft, femoral head, neck, intertrochanteric or subtrochanteric area (includes obtaining bone graft)

27175   Treatment of slipped femoral epiphysis; by traction, without reduction

27176   by single or multiple pinning, in situ

27177   Open treatment of slipped femoral epiphysis; single or multiple pinning or bone graft (includes obtaining graft)

27178   closed manipulation with single or multiple pinning

27179   osteoplasty of femoral neck (Heyman type procedure)

27181   osteotomy and internal fixation

27185   Epiphyseal arrest by epiphysiodesis or stapling, greater trochanter of femur

27187   Prophylactic treatment (nailing, pinning, plating or wiring) with or without methylmethacrylate, femoral neck and proximal femur

Fracture and/or Dislocation

             (27190, 27191 have been deleted. To report, see 27193, 27194)

             (27192 has been deleted. To report, see 27215, 27216)

27193   Closed treatment of pelvic ring fracture, dislocation, diastasis or subluxation; without manipulation

27194   with manipulation, requiring more than local anesthesia

             (27195 has been deleted. To report, use 27193)

             (27196 has been deleted. To report, use 27194)

27200   Closed treatment of coccygeal fracture

             (27201 has been deleted. To report, see 27200, 27202)

27202   Open treatment of coccygeal fracture

             (27210, 27211, 27212 have been deleted. To report, see 27193, 27194, 27215, 27216, 27217, 27218)

             (27214 has been deleted. To report, see 27215, 27216, 27217, 27218)

27215   Open treatment of iliac spine(s), tuberosity avulsion, or iliac wing fracture(s) (eg, pelvic fracture(s) which do not disrupt the pelvic ring), with internal fixation

27216   Percutaneous skeletal fixation of posterior pelvic ring fracture and/or dislocation (includes ilium, sacroiliac joint and/or sacrum)

27217   Open treatment of anterior ring fracture and/or dislocation with internal fixation (includes pubic symphysis and/or rami)

27218   Open treatment of posterior ring fracture and/or dislocation with internal fixation (includes ilium, sacroiliac joint and/or sacrum)

27220   Closed treatment of acetabulum (hip socket) fracture(s); without manipulation

27222   with manipulation, with or without skeletal traction

             (27224 has been deleted. To report, see 27226, 27227)

             (27225 has been deleted. To report, see 27227, 27228)

27226   Open treatment of posterior or anterior acetabular wall fracture, with internal fixation

27227   Open treatment of acetabular fracture(s) involving anterior or posterior (one) column, or a fracture running transversely across the acetabulum, with internal fixation

27228   Open treatment of acetabular fracture(s) involving anterior and posterior (two) columns, includes T-fracture and both column fracture with complete articular detachment, or single column or transverse fracture with associated acetabular wall fracture, with internal fixation

27230   Closed treatment of femoral fracture, proximal end, neck; without manipulation

27232   with manipulation, with or without skeletal traction

             (27234 has been deleted. To report, see 27230, 27232, 27235, 27236)

▲**27235**   Percutaneous skeletal fixation of femoral fracture, proximal end, neck

27236   Open treatment of femoral fracture, proximal end, neck, internal fixation or prosthetic replacement

27238   Closed treatment of intertrochanteric, pertrochanteric, or subtrochanteric femoral fracture; without manipulation

27240   with manipulation, with or without skin or skeletal traction

             (27242 has been deleted. To report, see 27238, 27240, 27244, 27245)

▲**27244**   Treatment of intertrochanteric, pertrochanteric, or subtrochanteric femoral fracture; with plate/screw type implant, with or without cerclage

27245   with intramedullary implant, with or without interlocking screws and/or cerclage

27246   Closed treatment of greater trochanteric fracture, without manipulation

27248 Open treatment of greater trochanteric fracture, with or without internal or external fixation

27250 Closed treatment of hip dislocation, traumatic; without anesthesia

27252   requiring anesthesia

27253 Open treatment of hip dislocation, traumatic, without internal fixation

27254 Open treatment of hip dislocation, traumatic, with acetabular wall and femoral head fracture, with or without internal or external fixation

(27255 has been deleted. To report, see 27226, 27227, 27253, 27254)

27256* Treatment of spontaneous hip dislocation (developmental, including congenital or pathological), by abduction, splint or traction; without anesthesia, without manipulation

27257*   with manipulation, requiring anesthesia

27258 Open treatment of spontaneous hip dislocation (developmental, including congenital or pathological), replacement of femoral head in acetabulum (including tenotomy, etc);

27259   with femoral shaft shortening

27265 Closed treatment of post hip arthroplasty dislocation; without anesthesia

27266   requiring regional or general anesthesia

Manipulation

27275* Manipulation, hip joint, requiring general anesthesia

Arthrodesis

27280 Arthrodesis, sacroiliac joint (including obtaining graft)

(27281 has been deleted. To report, use 27280 with modifier '-50')

27282 Arthrodesis, symphysis pubis (including obtaining graft)

27284 Arthrodesis, hip joint (including obtaining graft);

27286   with subtrochanteric osteotomy

Amputation

27290 Interpelviabdominal amputation (hindquarter amputation)

27295 Disarticulation of hip

Other Procedures

27299 Unlisted procedure, pelvis or hip joint

Femur (Thigh Region) and Knee Joint

Including tibial plateaus.

Incision

(For incision and drainage of abscess or hematoma, superficial, see 10040-10160)

27301 Incision and drainage, deep abscess, bursa, or hematoma, thigh or knee region

27303 Incision, deep, with opening of bone cortex, femur or knee (eg, osteomyelitis or bone abscess)

(27304 has been deleted)

27305 Fasciotomy, iliotibial (tenotomy), open

(For combined Ober-Yount fasciotomy, use 27025)

27306 Tenotomy, percutaneous, adductor or hamstring; single tendon (separate procedure)

27307   multiple tendons

27310 Arthrotomy, knee, with exploration, drainage, or removal of foreign body (eg, infection)

(27311 has been deleted)

27315 Neurectomy, hamstring muscle

27320 Neurectomy, popliteal (gastrocnemius)

Excision

27323 Biopsy, soft tissue of thigh or knee area; superficial

27324   deep (subfascial or intramuscular)

(For needle biopsy of soft tissue, use 20206)

27327 Excision, tumor, thigh or knee area; subcutaneous

27328   deep, subfascial, or intramuscular

27329 Radical resection of tumor (eg, malignant neoplasm), soft tissue of thigh or knee area

27330 Arthrotomy, knee; with synovial biopsy only

27331   including joint exploration, biopsy, or removal of loose or foreign bodies

27332 Arthrotomy, with excision of semilunar cartilage (meniscectomy) knee; medial OR lateral

27333   medial AND lateral

27334 Arthrotomy, with synovectomy, knee; anterior OR posterior

27335   anterior AND posterior including popliteal area

27340 Excision, prepatellar bursa

27345 Excision of synovial cyst of popliteal space (eg, Baker's cyst)

27347 Excision of lesion of meniscus or capsule (eg, cyst, ganglion), knee

Surgery: Musculoskeletal System

27350	Patellectomy or hemipatellectomy
27355	Excision or curettage of bone cyst or benign tumor of femur;
27356	with allograft
27357	with autograft (includes obtaining graft)
+ 27358	with internal fixation (List in addition to code for primary procedure)

(Use 27358 in conjunction with codes 27355, 27356, or 27357)

27360	Partial excision (craterization, saucerization, or diaphysectomy) bone, femur, proximal tibia and/or fibula (eg, osteomyelitis or bone abscess)

(27361 has been deleted)

27365	Radical resection of tumor, bone, femur or knee

(For radical resection of tumor, soft tissue, use 27329)

Introduction or Removal

27370	Injection procedure for knee arthrography

(For radiological supervision and interpretation, use 73580. Do not report 76003 in addition to 73580)

27372	Removal of foreign body, deep, thigh region or knee area

(For removal of knee prosthesis including "total knee," use 27488)

(27373-27379 have been deleted. To report, see 29870-29887)

Repair, Revision, and/or Reconstruction

27380	Suture of infrapatellar tendon; primary
27381	secondary reconstruction, including fascial or tendon graft
27385	Suture of quadriceps or hamstring muscle rupture; primary
27386	secondary reconstruction, including fascial or tendon graft
27390	Tenotomy, open, hamstring, knee to hip; single tendon
27391	multiple tendons, one leg
27392	multiple tendons, bilateral
27393	Lengthening of hamstring tendon; single tendon
27394	multiple tendons, one leg
27395	multiple tendons, bilateral
27396	Transplant, hamstring tendon to patella; single tendon
27397	multiple tendons
27400	Transfer, tendon or muscle, hamstrings to femur (eg, Egger's type procedure)

27403	Arthrotomy with meniscus repair, knee

(For arthroscopic repair, use 29882)

27405	Repair, primary, torn ligament and/or capsule, knee; collateral
27407	cruciate

(27408 has been deleted. To report, use 27427)

27409	collateral and cruciate ligaments

(27410-27416 have been deleted. To report, see 27427-27429)

27418	Anterior tibial tubercleplasty (eg, Maquet type procedure)
27420	Reconstruction of dislocating patella; (eg, Hauser type procedure)
27422	with extensor realignment and/or muscle advancement or release (eg, Campbell, Goldwaite type procedure)
27424	with patellectomy
▲ 27425	Lateral retinacular release open

▶(For arthroscopic lateral release, use 29873)◀

27427	Ligamentous reconstruction (augmentation), knee; extra-articular
27428	intra-articular (open)
27429	intra-articular (open) and extra-articular

(For primary repair of ligament(s) performed in addition to reconstruction, report 27405, 27407 or 27409 in addition to code 27427, 27428 or 27429)

27430	Quadricepsplasty (eg, Bennett or Thompson type)
27435	Capsulotomy, posterior capsular release, knee

(27436 has been deleted. To report, use 29887)

27437	Arthroplasty, patella; without prosthesis
27438	with prosthesis
27440	Arthroplasty, knee, tibial plateau;
27441	with debridement and partial synovectomy
27442	Arthroplasty, femoral condyles or tibial plateau(s), knee;
27443	with debridement and partial synovectomy

(27444 has been deleted. To report, see 27445-27447)

27445	Arthroplasty, knee, hinge prosthesis (eg, Walldius type)
27446	Arthroplasty, knee, condyle and plateau; medial OR lateral compartment
27447	medial AND lateral compartments with or without patella resurfacing (total knee arthroplasty)

(For revision of total knee arthroplasty, use 27487)

(For removal of total knee prosthesis, use 27488)

27448   Osteotomy, femur, shaft or supracondylar; without fixation

(27449 has been deleted. To report, use 27448 with modifier '-50')

27450   with fixation

(27452 has been deleted. To report, use 27450 with modifier '-50')

27454   Osteotomy, multiple, with realignment on intramedullary rod, femoral shaft (eg, Sofield type procedure)

27455   Osteotomy, proximal tibia, including fibular excision or osteotomy (includes correction of genu varus (bowleg) or genu valgus (knock-knee)); before epiphyseal closure

27457   after epiphyseal closure

(27460 has been deleted. To report, use 27455 with modifier '-50')

(27462 has been deleted. To report, use 27457 with modifier '-50')

27465   Osteoplasty, femur; shortening (excluding 64876)

27466   lengthening

27468   combined, lengthening and shortening with femoral segment transfer

27470   Repair, nonunion or malunion, femur, distal to head and neck; without graft (eg, compression technique)

27472   with iliac or other autogenous bone graft (includes obtaining graft)

27475   Arrest, epiphyseal, any method (eg, epiphysiodesis); distal femur

27477   tibia and fibula, proximal

27479   combined distal femur, proximal tibia and fibula

27485   Arrest, hemiepiphyseal, distal femur or proximal tibia or fibula (eg, genu varus or valgus)

27486   Revision of total knee arthroplasty, with or without allograft; one component

27487   femoral and entire tibial component

27488   Removal of prosthesis, including total knee prosthesis, methylmethacrylate with or without insertion of spacer, knee

(27490 has been deleted. To report, use 29882)

27495   Prophylactic treatment (nailing, pinning, plating or wiring) with or without methylmethacrylate, femur

27496   Decompression fasciotomy, thigh and/or knee, one compartment (flexor or extensor or adductor);

27497   with debridement of nonviable muscle and/or nerve

27498   Decompression fasciotomy, thigh and/or knee, multiple compartments;

27499   with debridement of nonviable muscle and/or nerve

Fracture and/or Dislocation

(For arthroscopic treatment of intercondylar spine(s) and tuberosity fracture(s) of the knee, see 29850, 29851)

(For arthroscopic treatment of tibial fracture, see 29855, 29856)

27500   Closed treatment of femoral shaft fracture, without manipulation

27501   Closed treatment of supracondylar or transcondylar femoral fracture with or without intercondylar extension, without manipulation

27502   Closed treatment of femoral shaft fracture, with manipulation, with or without skin or skeletal traction

27503   Closed treatment of supracondylar or transcondylar femoral fracture with or without intercondylar extension, with manipulation, with or without skin or skeletal traction

(27504 has been deleted. To report, see 27500, 27501, 27502, 27503, 27506, 27507, 27509, 27511, 27513)

27506   Open treatment of femoral shaft fracture, with or without external fixation, with insertion of intramedullary implant, with or without cerclage and/or locking screws

27507   Open treatment of femoral shaft fracture with plate/screws, with or without cerclage

27508   Closed treatment of femoral fracture, distal end, medial or lateral condyle, without manipulation

27509   Percutaneous skeletal fixation of femoral fracture, distal end, medial or lateral condyle, or supracondylar or transcondylar, with or without intercondylar extension, or distal femoral epiphyseal separation

27510   Closed treatment of femoral fracture, distal end, medial or lateral condyle, with manipulation

27511   Open treatment of femoral supracondylar or transcondylar fracture without intercondylar extension, with or without internal or external fixation

(27512 has been deleted. To report, see 27508, 27510, 27514)

27513   Open treatment of femoral supracondylar or transcondylar fracture with intercondylar extension, with or without internal or external fixation

27514   Open treatment of femoral fracture, distal end, medial or lateral condyle, with or without internal or external fixation

27516   Closed treatment of distal femoral epiphyseal separation; without manipulation

27517   with manipulation, with or without skin or skeletal traction

(27518 has been deleted. To report, see 27516, 27517, 27519)

Surgery: Musculoskeletal System

▲=Revised Code   ●=New Code   ✳=Service Includes Surgical Procedure Only   American Medical Association   **91**

27519 Open treatment of distal femoral epiphyseal separation, with or without internal or external fixation

27520 Closed treatment of patellar fracture, without manipulation

(27522 has been deleted. To report, see 27520, 27524)

27524 Open treatment of patellar fracture, with internal fixation and/or partial or complete patellectomy and soft tissue repair

27530 Closed treatment of tibial fracture, proximal (plateau); without manipulation

27532 with or without manipulation, with skeletal traction

(27534 has been deleted. To report, see 27530, 27532, 27535, 27536)

(For arthroscopic treatment, see 29855, 29856)

27535 Open treatment of tibial fracture, proximal (plateau); unicondylar, with or without internal or external fixation

27536 bicondylar, with or without internal fixation

(For arthroscopic treatment, see 29855, 29856)

(27537 has been deleted. To report, see 27535, 27536)

27538 Closed treatment of intercondylar spine(s) and/or tuberosity fracture(s) of knee, with or without manipulation

(For arthroscopic treatment, see 29850, 29851)

27540 Open treatment of intercondylar spine(s) and/or tuberosity fracture(s) of the knee, with or without internal or external fixation

27550 Closed treatment of knee dislocation; without anesthesia

27552 requiring anesthesia

(27554 has been deleted. To report, see 27550, 27552, 27556, 27557, 27558)

27556 Open treatment of knee dislocation, with or without internal or external fixation; without primary ligamentous repair or augmentation/reconstruction

27557 with primary ligamentous repair

27558 with primary ligamentous repair, with augmentation/reconstruction

27560 Closed treatment of patellar dislocation; without anesthesia

(For recurrent dislocation, see 27420-27424)

27562 requiring anesthesia

(27564 has been deleted. To report, see 27560, 27562, 27566)

27566 Open treatment of patellar dislocation, with or without partial or total patellectomy

Manipulation

27570* Manipulation of knee joint under general anesthesia (includes application of traction or other fixation devices)

Arthrodesis

27580 Arthrodesis, knee, any technique

Amputation

27590 Amputation, thigh, through femur, any level;

27591 immediate fitting technique including first cast

27592 open, circular (guillotine)

27594 secondary closure or scar revision

27596 re-amputation

27598 Disarticulation at knee

Other Procedures

27599 Unlisted procedure, femur or knee

Leg (Tibia and Fibula) and Ankle Joint

Incision

27600 Decompression fasciotomy, leg; anterior and/or lateral compartments only

27601 posterior compartment(s) only

27602 anterior and/or lateral, and posterior compartment(s)

(For incision and drainage procedures, superficial, see 10040-10160)

(For decompression fasciotomy with debridement, see 27892-27894)

27603 Incision and drainage, leg or ankle; deep abscess or hematoma

27604 infected bursa

27605* Tenotomy, percutaneous, Achilles tendon (separate procedure); local anesthesia

27606 general anesthesia

27607 Incision (eg, osteomyelitis or bone abscess), leg or ankle

(27608 has been deleted)

27610 Arthrotomy, ankle, including exploration, drainage, or removal of foreign body

(27611 has been deleted)

27612 Arthrotomy, posterior capsular release, ankle, with or without Achilles tendon lengthening

(See also 27685)

Excision

27613   Biopsy, soft tissue of leg or ankle area; superficial

27614   deep (subfascial or intramuscular)

(For needle biopsy of soft tissue, use 20206)

27615   Radical resection of tumor (eg, malignant neoplasm), soft tissue of leg or ankle area

27618   Excision, tumor, leg or ankle area; subcutaneous tissue

27619   deep (subfascial or intramuscular)

27620   Arthrotomy, ankle, with joint exploration, with or without biopsy, with or without removal of loose or foreign body

27625   Arthrotomy, with synovectomy, ankle;

27626   including tenosynovectomy

27630   Excision of lesion of tendon sheath or capsule (eg, cyst or ganglion), leg and/or ankle

27635   Excision or curettage of bone cyst or benign tumor, tibia or fibula;

27637   with autograft (includes obtaining graft)

27638   with allograft

27640   Partial excision (craterization, saucerization, or diaphysectomy) bone (eg, osteomyelitis or exostosis); tibia

27641   fibula

27645   Radical resection of tumor, bone; tibia

27646   fibula

27647   talus or calcaneus

Introduction or Removal

27648   Injection procedure for ankle arthrography

(For radiological supervision and interpretation, use 73615. Do not report 76003 in addition to 73615)

(For ankle arthroscopy, see 29894-29898)

Repair, Revision, and/or Reconstruction

27650   Repair, primary, open or percutaneous, ruptured Achilles tendon;

27652   with graft (includes obtaining graft)

27654   Repair, secondary, Achilles tendon, with or without graft

27656   Repair, fascial defect of leg

27658   Repair, flexor tendon, leg; primary, without graft, each tendon

27659   secondary, with or without graft, each tendon

27664   Repair, extensor tendon, leg; primary, without graft, each tendon

27665   secondary, with or without graft, each tendon

27675   Repair, dislocating peroneal tendons; without fibular osteotomy

27676   with fibular osteotomy

27680   Tenolysis, flexor or extensor tendon, leg and/or ankle; single, each tendon

27681   multiple tendons (through separate incision(s))

27685   Lengthening or shortening of tendon, leg or ankle; single tendon (separate procedure)

27686   multiple tendons (through same incision), each

27687   Gastrocnemius recession (eg, Strayer procedure)

(Toe extensors are considered as a group to be a single tendon when transplanted into midfoot)

27690   Transfer or transplant of single tendon (with muscle redirection or rerouting); superficial (eg, anterior tibial extensors into midfoot)

27691   deep (eg, anterior tibial or posterior tibial through interosseous space, flexor digitorum longus, flexor hallucis longus, or peroneal tendon to midfoot or hindfoot)

+ 27692   each additional tendon (List separately in addition to code for primary procedure)

(Use 27692 in conjunction with codes 27690, 27691)

27695   Repair, primary, disrupted ligament, ankle; collateral

27696   both collateral ligaments

27698   Repair, secondary, disrupted ligament, ankle, collateral (eg, Watson-Jones procedure)

27700   Arthroplasty, ankle;

27702   with implant (total ankle)

27703   revision, total ankle

27704   Removal of ankle implant

27705   Osteotomy; tibia

27707   fibula

27709   tibia and fibula

27712   multiple, with realignment on intramedullary rod (eg, Sofield type procedure)

(For osteotomy to correct genu varus (bowleg) or genu valgus (knock-knee), see 27455-27457)

27715   Osteoplasty, tibia and fibula, lengthening or shortening

27720   Repair of nonunion or malunion, tibia; without graft, (eg, compression technique)

27722   with sliding graft

27724   with iliac or other autograft (includes obtaining graft)

27725   by synostosis, with fibula, any method

27727   Repair of congenital pseudarthrosis, tibia

Surgery: Musculoskeletal System

▲ **27730**   Arrest, epiphyseal (epiphysiodesis), open; distal tibia

27732   distal fibula

27734   distal tibia and fibula

27740   Arrest, epiphyseal (epiphysiodesis), any method, combined, proximal and distal tibia and fibula;

27742   and distal femur

        (For epiphyseal arrest of proximal tibia and fibula, use 27477)

27745   Prophylactic treatment (nailing, pinning, plating or wiring) with or without methylmethacrylate, tibia

---

Fracture and/or Dislocation

27750   Closed treatment of tibial shaft fracture (with or without fibular fracture); without manipulation

27752   with manipulation, with or without skeletal traction

        (27754 has been deleted. To report, see 27750, 27752, 27756, 27758)

27756   Percutaneous skeletal fixation of tibial shaft fracture (with or without fibular fracture) (eg, pins or screws)

27758   Open treatment of tibial shaft fracture, (with or without fibular fracture) with plate/screws, with or without cerclage

▲ **27759**   Treatment of tibial shaft fracture (with or without fibular fracture) by intramedullary implant, with or without interlocking screws and/or cerclage

27760   Closed treatment of medial malleolus fracture; without manipulation

27762   with manipulation, with or without skin or skeletal traction

        (27764 has been deleted. To report, see 27762, 27766)

27766   Open treatment of medial malleolus fracture, with or without internal or external fixation

27780   Closed treatment of proximal fibula or shaft fracture; without manipulation

27781   with manipulation

        (27782 has been deleted. To report, see 27780, 27781, 27784)

27784   Open treatment of proximal fibula or shaft fracture, with or without internal or external fixation

27786   Closed treatment of distal fibular fracture (lateral malleolus); without manipulation

27788   with manipulation

        (27790 has been deleted. To report, see 27786, 27788, 27792)

27792   Open treatment of distal fibular fracture (lateral malleolus), with or without internal or external fixation

        (27800 has been deleted. To report, use 27750)

        (27802 has been deleted. To report, use 27752)

        (27804 has been deleted. To report, see 27750, 27752, 27756, 27758, 27759)

        (27806 has been deleted. To report, see 27756, 27758, 27759)

27808   Closed treatment of bimalleolar ankle fracture, (including Potts); without manipulation

27810   with manipulation

        (27812 has been deleted. To report, see 27808, 27810, 27814)

27814   Open treatment of bimalleolar ankle fracture, with or without internal or external fixation

27816   Closed treatment of trimalleolar ankle fracture; without manipulation

27818   with manipulation

        (27820 has been deleted. To report, see 27816, 27818, 27822, 27823)

27822   Open treatment of trimalleolar ankle fracture, with or without internal or external fixation, medial and/or lateral malleolus; without fixation of posterior lip

27823   with fixation of posterior lip

27824   Closed treatment of fracture of weight bearing articular portion of distal tibia (eg, pilon or tibial plafond), with or without anesthesia; without manipulation

27825   with skeletal traction and/or requiring manipulation

27826   Open treatment of fracture of weight bearing articular surface/portion of distal tibia (eg, pilon or tibial plafond), with internal or external fixation; of fibula only

27827   of tibia only

27828   of both tibia and fibula

27829   Open treatment of distal tibiofibular joint (syndesmosis) disruption, with or without internal or external fixation

27830   Closed treatment of proximal tibiofibular joint dislocation; without anesthesia

27831   requiring anesthesia

27832   Open treatment of proximal tibiofibular joint dislocation, with or without internal or external fixation, or with excision of proximal fibula

27840   Closed treatment of ankle dislocation; without anesthesia

27842   requiring anesthesia, with or without percutaneous skeletal fixation

        (27844 has been deleted. To report, see 27840, 27842, 27846, 27848)

27846   Open treatment of ankle dislocation, with or without percutaneous skeletal fixation; without repair or internal fixation

27848   with repair or internal or external fixation

        (27850-27853 have been deleted. To report, see 29894-29898)

Manipulation

27860*   Manipulation of ankle under general anesthesia (includes application of traction or other fixation apparatus)

Arthrodesis

▲ **27870**   Arthrodesis, ankle, open

     ►(For arthroscopic ankle arthrodesis, use 29899)◄

27871   Arthrodesis, tibiofibular joint, proximal or distal

Amputation

27880   Amputation, leg, through tibia and fibula;

27881   with immediate fitting technique including application of first cast

27882   open, circular (guillotine)

27884   secondary closure or scar revision

27886   re-amputation

27888   Amputation, ankle, through malleoli of tibia and fibula (eg, Syme, Pirogoff type procedures), with plastic closure and resection of nerves

27889   Ankle disarticulation

Other Procedures

27892   Decompression fasciotomy, leg; anterior and/or lateral compartments only, with debridement of nonviable muscle and/or nerve

     (For decompression fasciotomy of the leg without debridement, use 27600)

27893   posterior compartment(s) only, with debridement of nonviable muscle and/or nerve

     (For decompression fasciotomy of the leg without debridement, use 27601)

27894   anterior and/or lateral, and posterior compartment(s), with debridement of nonviable muscle and/or nerve

     (For decompression fasciotomy of the leg without debridement, use 27602)

27899   Unlisted procedure, leg or ankle

Foot and Toes

Incision

     (For incision and drainage procedures, superficial, see 10040-10160)

28001*   Incision and drainage, bursa, foot

28002*   Incision and drainage below fascia, with or without tendon sheath involvement, foot; single bursal space

28003   multiple areas

     (28004 has been deleted)

28005   Incision, bone cortex (eg, osteomyelitis or bone abscess), foot

     (28006 has been deleted)

28008   Fasciotomy, foot and/or toe

     (See also 28060, 28062, 28250)

28010   Tenotomy, percutaneous, toe; single tendon

28011   multiple tendons

     (For open tenotomy, see 28230-28234)

28020   Arthrotomy, including exploration, drainage, or removal of loose or foreign body; intertarsal or tarsometatarsal joint

28022   metatarsophalangeal joint

28024   interphalangeal joint

28030   Neurectomy, intrinsic musculature of foot

28035   Release, tarsal tunnel (posterior tibial nerve decompression)

     (For other nerve entrapments, see 64704, 64722)

Excision

28043   Excision, tumor, foot; subcutaneous tissue

28045   deep, subfascial, intramuscular

28046   Radical resection of tumor (eg, malignant neoplasm), soft tissue of foot

28050   Arthrotomy with biopsy; intertarsal or tarsometatarsal joint

28052   metatarsophalangeal joint

28054   interphalangeal joint

28060   Fasciectomy, plantar fascia; partial (separate procedure)

28062   radical (separate procedure)

     (For plantar fasciotomy, see 28008, 28250)

28070   Synovectomy; intertarsal or tarsometatarsal joint, each

28072   metatarsophalangeal joint, each

28080   Excision, interdigital (Morton) neuroma, single, each

28086   Synovectomy, tendon sheath, foot; flexor

28088   extensor

28090   Excision of lesion, tendon, tendon sheath, or capsule (including synovectomy) (eg, cyst or ganglion); foot

28092   toe(s), each

28100   Excision or curettage of bone cyst or benign tumor, talus or calcaneus;

28102   with iliac or other autograft (includes obtaining graft)

28103   with allograft

28104   Excision or curettage of bone cyst or benign tumor, tarsal or metatarsal, except talus or calcaneus;

28106   with iliac or other autograft (includes obtaining graft)

28107   with allograft

Surgery: Musculoskeletal System

Surgery: Musculoskeletal System

28108 Excision or curettage of bone cyst or benign tumor, phalanges of foot

(For ostectomy, partial (eg, hallux valgus, Silver type procedure), use 28290)

(28109 has been deleted. To report, use 28899)

28110 Ostectomy, partial excision, fifth metatarsal head (bunionette) (separate procedure)

28111 Ostectomy, complete excision; first metatarsal head

28112 other metatarsal head (second, third or fourth)

28113 fifth metatarsal head

28114 all metatarsal heads, with partial proximal phalangectomy, excluding first metatarsal (eg, Clayton type procedure)

28116 Ostectomy, excision of tarsal coalition

28118 Ostectomy, calcaneus;

28119 for spur, with or without plantar fascial release

28120 Partial excision (craterization, saucerization, sequestrectomy, or diaphysectomy) bone (eg, osteomyelitis or bossing); talus or calcaneus

(28121 has been deleted)

28122 tarsal or metatarsal bone, except talus or calcaneus

(For partial excision of talus or calcaneus, use 28120)

(For cheilectomy for hallux rigidus, use 28289)

(28123 has been deleted)

28124 phalanx of toe

28126 Resection, partial or complete, phalangeal base, each toe

28130 Talectomy (astragalectomy)

(28135 has been deleted. To report, use 28118)

28140 Metatarsectomy

28150 Phalangectomy, toe, each toe

28153 Resection, condyle(s), distal end of phalanx, each toe

28160 Hemiphalangectomy or interphalangeal joint excision, toe, proximal end of phalanx, each

28171 Radical resection of tumor, bone; tarsal (except talus or calcaneus)

28173 metatarsal

28175 phalanx of toe

(For talus or calcaneus, use 27647)

Introduction or Removal

28190* Removal of foreign body, foot; subcutaneous

28192 deep

28193 complicated

Repair, Revision, and/or Reconstruction

28200 Repair, tendon, flexor, foot; primary or secondary, without free graft, each tendon

28202 secondary with free graft, each tendon (includes obtaining graft)

28208 Repair, tendon, extensor, foot; primary or secondary, each tendon

28210 secondary with free graft, each tendon (includes obtaining graft)

28220 Tenolysis, flexor, foot; single tendon

28222 multiple tendons

28225 Tenolysis, extensor, foot; single tendon

28226 multiple tendons

28230 Tenotomy, open, tendon flexor; foot, single or multiple tendon(s) (separate procedure)

28232 toe, single tendon (separate procedure)

28234 Tenotomy, open, extensor, foot or toe, each tendon

(28236 has been deleted. To report, see 27690, 27691)

28238 Reconstruction (advancement), posterior tibial tendon with excision of accessory tarsal navicular bone (eg, Kidner type procedure)

(For subcutaneous tenotomy, see 28010, 28011)

(For transfer or transplant of tendon with muscle redirection or rerouting, see 27690-27692)

(For extensor hallucis longus transfer with great toe IP fusion (Jones procedure), use 28760)

28240 Tenotomy, lengthening, or release, abductor hallucis muscle

28250 Division of plantar fascia and muscle (eg, Steindler stripping) (separate procedure)

28260 Capsulotomy, midfoot; medial release only (separate procedure)

28261 with tendon lengthening

28262 extensive, including posterior talotibial capsulotomy and tendon(s) lengthening (eg, resistant clubfoot deformity)

28264 Capsulotomy, midtarsal (eg, Heyman type procedure)

28270 Capsulotomy; metatarsophalangeal joint, with or without tenorrhaphy, each joint (separate procedure)

28272 interphalangeal joint, each joint (separate procedure)

28280 Syndactylization, toes (eg, webbing or Kelikian type procedure)

28285 Correction, hammertoe (eg, interphalangeal fusion, partial or total phalangectomy)

28286 Correction, cock-up fifth toe, with plastic skin closure (eg, Ruiz-Mora type procedure)

28288 Ostectomy, partial, exostectomy or condylectomy, metatarsal head, each metatarsal head

28289 Hallux rigidus correction with cheilectomy, debridement and capsular release of the first metatarsophalangeal joint

28290 Correction, hallux valgus (bunion), with or without sesamoidectomy; simple exostectomy (eg, Silver type procedure)

28292   Keller, McBride, or Mayo type procedure

28293   resection of joint with implant

28294   with tendon transplants (eg, Joplin type procedure)

28296   with metatarsal osteotomy (eg, Mitchell, Chevron, or concentric type procedures)

28297   Lapidus type procedure

28298   by phalanx osteotomy

28299   by double osteotomy

28300 Osteotomy; calcaneus (eg, Dwyer or Chambers type procedure), with or without internal fixation

28302   talus

28304 Osteotomy, tarsal bones, other than calcaneus or talus;

28305   with autograft (includes obtaining graft) (eg, Fowler type)

28306 Osteotomy, with or without lengthening, shortening or angular correction, metatarsal; first metatarsal

28307   first metatarsal with autograft (other than first toe)

28308   other than first metatarsal, each

28309   multiple (eg, Swanson type cavus foot procedure)

28310 Osteotomy, shortening, angular or rotational correction; proximal phalanx, first toe (separate procedure)

28312   other phalanges, any toe

28313 Reconstruction, angular deformity of toe, soft tissue procedures only (eg, overlapping second toe, fifth toe, curly toes)

28315 Sesamoidectomy, first toe (separate procedure)

28320 Repair, nonunion or malunion; tarsal bones

28322   metatarsal, with or without bone graft (includes obtaining graft)

28340 Reconstruction, toe, macrodactyly; soft tissue resection

28341   requiring bone resection

28344 Reconstruction, toe(s); polydactyly

28345   syndactyly, with or without skin graft(s), each web

28360 Reconstruction, cleft foot

Fracture and/or Dislocation

28400 Closed treatment of calcaneal fracture; without manipulation

28405   with manipulation

28406 Percutaneous skeletal fixation of calcaneal fracture, with manipulation

(28410 has been deleted. To report, see 28400, 28405, 28406, 28415, 28420)

28415 Open treatment of calcaneal fracture, with or without internal or external fixation;

28420   with primary iliac or other autogenous bone graft (includes obtaining graft)

28430 Closed treatment of talus fracture; without manipulation

28435   with manipulation

28436 Percutaneous skeletal fixation of talus fracture, with manipulation

(28440 has been deleted. To report, see 28430, 28435, 28436, 28445)

28445 Open treatment of talus fracture, with or without internal or external fixation

28450 Treatment of tarsal bone fracture (except talus and calcaneus); without manipulation, each

28455   with manipulation, each

28456 Percutaneous skeletal fixation of tarsal bone fracture (except talus and calcaneus), with manipulation, each

(28460 has been deleted. To report, see 28450, 28455, 28456, 28465)

28465 Open treatment of tarsal bone fracture (except talus and calcaneus), with or without internal or external fixation, each

28470 Closed treatment of metatarsal fracture; without manipulation, each

28475   with manipulation, each

28476 Percutaneous skeletal fixation of metatarsal fracture, with manipulation, each

(28480 has been deleted. To report, see 28470, 28475, 28476, 28485)

28485 Open treatment of metatarsal fracture, with or without internal or external fixation, each

28490 Closed treatment of fracture great toe, phalanx or phalanges; without manipulation

28495   with manipulation

28496 Percutaneous skeletal fixation of fracture great toe, phalanx or phalanges, with manipulation

(28500 has been deleted. To report, see 28490, 28495, 28496, 28505)

28505   Open treatment of fracture great toe, phalanx or phalanges, with or without internal or external fixation

28510   Closed treatment of fracture, phalanx or phalanges, other than great toe; without manipulation, each

28515   with manipulation, each

(28520 has been deleted. To report, see 28510, 28515, 28525)

28525   Open treatment of fracture, phalanx or phalanges, other than great toe, with or without internal or external fixation, each

28530   Closed treatment of sesamoid fracture

28531   Open treatment of sesamoid fracture, with or without internal fixation

28540   Closed treatment of tarsal bone dislocation, other than talotarsal; without anesthesia

28545   requiring anesthesia

28546   Percutaneous skeletal fixation of tarsal bone dislocation, other than talotarsal, with manipulation

(28550 has been deleted. To report, see 28540, 28545, 28546, 28555)

28555   Open treatment of tarsal bone dislocation, with or without internal or external fixation

28570   Closed treatment of talotarsal joint dislocation; without anesthesia

28575   requiring anesthesia

28576   Percutaneous skeletal fixation of talotarsal joint dislocation, with manipulation

(28580 has been deleted. To report, see 28570, 28575, 28576, 28585)

28585   Open treatment of talotarsal joint dislocation, with or without internal or external fixation

28600   Closed treatment of tarsometatarsal joint dislocation; without anesthesia

28605   requiring anesthesia

28606   Percutaneous skeletal fixation of tarsometatarsal joint dislocation, with manipulation

(28610 has been deleted. To report, see 28600, 28605, 28606, 28615)

28615   Open treatment of tarsometatarsal joint dislocation, with or without internal or external fixation

28630*   Closed treatment of metatarsophalangeal joint dislocation; without anesthesia

28635*   requiring anesthesia

28636   Percutaneous skeletal fixation of metatarsophalangeal joint dislocation, with manipulation

(28640 has been deleted. To report, see 28630, 28635, 28636, 28645)

28645   Open treatment of metatarsophalangeal joint dislocation, with or without internal or external fixation

28660*   Closed treatment of interphalangeal joint dislocation; without anesthesia

28665*   requiring anesthesia

28666   Percutaneous skeletal fixation of interphalangeal joint dislocation, with manipulation

(28670 has been deleted. To report, see 28660, 28665, 28666, 28675)

28675   Open treatment of interphalangeal joint dislocation, with or without internal or external fixation

Arthrodesis

28705   Arthrodesis; pantalar

28715   triple

28725   subtalar

28730   Arthrodesis, midtarsal or tarsometatarsal, multiple or transverse;

28735   with osteotomy (eg, flatfoot correction)

28737   Arthrodesis, with tendon lengthening and advancement, midtarsal, tarsal navicular-cuneiform (eg, Miller type procedure)

28740   Arthrodesis, midtarsal or tarsometatarsal, single joint

28750   Arthrodesis, great toe; metatarsophalangeal joint

28755   interphalangeal joint

28760   Arthrodesis, with extensor hallucis longus transfer to first metatarsal neck, great toe, interphalangeal joint (eg, Jones type procedure)

(For hammertoe operation or interphalangeal fusion, use 28285)

Amputation

28800   Amputation, foot; midtarsal (eg, Chopart type procedure)

28805   transmetatarsal

28810   Amputation, metatarsal, with toe, single

28820   Amputation, toe; metatarsophalangeal joint

28825   interphalangeal joint

(For amputation of tuft of distal phalanx, use 11752)

Other Procedures

(For extracorporeal shock wave therapy involving musculoskeletal system, or plantar fascia, see Category III codes 0019T, 0020T)

28899   Unlisted procedure, foot or toes

Application of Casts and Strapping

The listed procedures apply when the cast application or strapping is a replacement procedure used during or after the period of follow-up care, or when the cast application or strapping is an initial service performed without a restorative treatment or procedure(s) to stabilize or protect a fracture, injury, or dislocation and/or to afford comfort to a patient. Restorative treatment or procedure(s) rendered by another physician following the application of the initial cast/splint/strap may be reported with a treatment of fracture and/or dislocation code.

A physician who applies the initial cast, strap or splint and also assumes all of the subsequent fracture, dislocation, or injury care cannot use the application of casts and strapping codes as an initial service, since the first cast/splint or strap application is included in the treatment of fracture and/or dislocation codes. (See notes under Musculoskeletal System, page 61). A temporary cast/splint/strap is not considered to be part of the preoperative care, and the use of the modifier '-56' is not applicable. Additional evaluation and management services are reportable only if significant identifiable further services are provided at the time of the cast application or strapping.

If cast application or strapping is provided as an initial service (eg, casting of a sprained ankle or knee) in which no other procedure or treatment (eg, surgical repair, reduction of a fracture or joint dislocation) is performed or is expected to be performed by a physician rendering the initial care only, use the casting, strapping and/or supply code (99070) in addition to an evaluation and management code as appropriate.

Listed procedures include removal of cast or strapping.

(For orthotics fitting and training, use 97504)

Body and Upper Extremity

Casts

29000	Application of halo type body cast (see 20661-20663 for insertion)
29010	Application of Risser jacket, localizer, body; only
29015	including head
29020	Application of turnbuckle jacket, body; only
29025	including head
29035	Application of body cast, shoulder to hips;
29040	including head, Minerva type
29044	including one thigh
29046	including both thighs

29049	Application, cast; figure-of-eight
29055	shoulder spica
29058	plaster Velpeau
29065	shoulder to hand (long arm)
29075	elbow to finger (short arm)
29085	hand and lower forearm (gauntlet)
29086	finger (eg, contracture)

Splints

29105	Application of long arm splint (shoulder to hand)
29125	Application of short arm splint (forearm to hand); static
29126	dynamic
29130	Application of finger splint; static
29131	dynamic

Strapping—Any Age

29200	Strapping; thorax
29220	low back
29240	shoulder (eg, Velpeau)
29260	elbow or wrist
29280	hand or finger

Lower Extremity

Casts

29305	Application of hip spica cast; one leg
29325	one and one-half spica or both legs

(For hip spica (body) cast, including thighs only, use 29046)

29345	Application of long leg cast (thigh to toes);
29355	walker or ambulatory type
29358	Application of long leg cast brace
29365	Application of cylinder cast (thigh to ankle)
29405	Application of short leg cast (below knee to toes);
29425	walking or ambulatory type
29435	Application of patellar tendon bearing (PTB) cast
29440	Adding walker to previously applied cast
29445	Application of rigid total contact leg cast
29450	Application of clubfoot cast with molding or manipulation, long or short leg

(29455 has been deleted. To report, use 29450 with modifier '-50')

Surgery: Musculoskeletal System

Splints

29505	Application of long leg splint (thigh to ankle or toes)
29515	Application of short leg splint (calf to foot)

Strapping—Any Age

29520	Strapping; hip
29530	knee
▲ 29540	ankle and/or foot
29550	toes
29580	Unna boot
29590	Denis-Browne splint strapping

Removal or Repair

Codes for cast removals should be employed only for casts applied by another physician.

29700	Removal or bivalving; gauntlet, boot or body cast
29705	full arm or full leg cast
29710	shoulder or hip spica, Minerva, or Risser jacket, etc.
29715	turnbuckle jacket
29720	Repair of spica, body cast or jacket
29730	Windowing of cast
29740	Wedging of cast (except clubfoot casts)
29750	Wedging of clubfoot cast

(29751 has been deleted. To report, use 29750 with modifier '-50')

Other Procedures

29799	Unlisted procedure, casting or strapping

Endoscopy/Arthroscopy

Surgical endoscopy/arthroscopy always includes a diagnostic endoscopy/arthroscopy.

When arthroscopy is performed in conjunction with arthrotomy, add modifier '-51'.

29800	Arthroscopy, temporomandibular joint, diagnostic, with or without synovial biopsy (separate procedure)
29804	Arthroscopy, temporomandibular joint, surgical

(For open procedure, use 21010)

29805	Arthroscopy, shoulder, diagnostic, with or without synovial biopsy (separate procedure)

(For open procedure, see 23065-23066, 23100-23101)

29806	Arthroscopy, shoulder, surgical; capsulorrhaphy

(For open procedure, see 23450-23466)

(To report thermal capsulorrhaphy, use 29999)

29807	repair of slap lesion

(29815 has been deleted. To report, use 29805)

29819	with removal of loose body or foreign body

(For open procedure, see 23040-23044, 23107)

29820	synovectomy, partial

(For open procedure, see 23105)

29821	synovectomy, complete

(For open procedure, see 23105)

29822	debridement, limited

(For open procedure, see specific open shoulder procedure performed)

29823	debridement, extensive

(For open procedure, see specific open shoulder procedure performed)

29824	distal claviculectomy including distal articular surface (Mumford procedure)

(For open procedure, use 23120)

29825	with lysis and resection of adhesions, with or without manipulation

(For open procedure, see specific open shoulder procedure performed)

29826	decompression of subacromial space with partial acromioplasty, with or without coracoacromial release

(For open procedure, use 23130 or 23415)

● 29827	with rotator cuff repair

►(For open or mini-open rotator cuff repair, use 23412)◄

►(When arthroscopic subacromial decompression is performed at the same setting, use 29826 and append modifier '-51')◄

►(When arthroscopic distal clavicle resection is performed at the same setting, use 29824 and append modifier '-51')◄

29830	Arthroscopy, elbow, diagnostic, with or without synovial biopsy (separate procedure)
29834	Arthroscopy, elbow, surgical; with removal of loose body or foreign body
29835	synovectomy, partial
29836	synovectomy, complete
29837	debridement, limited
29838	debridement, extensive

29840   Arthroscopy, wrist, diagnostic, with or without synovial biopsy (separate procedure)

29843   Arthroscopy, wrist, surgical; for infection, lavage and drainage

29844   synovectomy, partial

29845   synovectomy, complete

29846   excision and/or repair of triangular fibrocartilage and/or joint debridement

29847   internal fixation for fracture or instability

29848   Endoscopy, wrist, surgical, with release of transverse carpal ligament

(For open procedure, use 64721)

29850   Arthroscopically aided treatment of intercondylar spine(s) and/or tuberosity fracture(s) of the knee, with or without manipulation; without internal or external fixation (includes arthroscopy)

29851   with internal or external fixation (includes arthroscopy)

(For bone graft, use 20900, 20902)

29855   Arthroscopically aided treatment of tibial fracture, proximal (plateau); unicondylar, with or without internal or external fixation (includes arthroscopy)

29856   bicondylar, with or without internal or external fixation (includes arthroscopy)

(For bone graft, use 20900, 20902)

29860   Arthroscopy, hip, diagnostic with or without synovial biopsy (separate procedure)

29861   Arthroscopy, hip, surgical; with removal of loose body or foreign body

29862   with debridement/shaving of articular cartilage (chondroplasty), abrasion arthroplasty, and/or resection of labrum

29863   with synovectomy

29870   Arthroscopy, knee, diagnostic, with or without synovial biopsy (separate procedure)

(For surgical arthroscopy of the knee with implantation of osteochondral graft for treatment of articular surface defect, see Category III codes 0012T, 0013T)

(For meniscal transplantation, medial or lateral, knee, use Category III code 0014T)

29871   Arthroscopy, knee, surgical; for infection, lavage and drainage

(29872 has been deleted)

● **29873**   with lateral release

▶(For open lateral release, use 27425)◀

29874   for removal of loose body or foreign body (eg, osteochondritis dissecans fragmentation, chondral fragmentation)

29875   synovectomy, limited (eg, plica or shelf resection) (separate procedure)

29876   synovectomy, major, two or more compartments (eg, medial or lateral)

29877   debridement/shaving of articular cartilage (chondroplasty)

29879   abrasion arthroplasty (includes chondroplasty where necessary) or multiple drilling or microfracture

29880   with meniscectomy (medial AND lateral, including any meniscal shaving)

29881   with meniscectomy (medial OR lateral, including any meniscal shaving)

29882   with meniscus repair (medial OR lateral)

29883   with meniscus repair (medial AND lateral)

29884   with lysis of adhesions, with or without manipulation (separate procedure)

29885   drilling for osteochondritis dissecans with bone grafting, with or without internal fixation (including debridement of base of lesion)

29886   drilling for intact osteochondritis dissecans lesion

29887   drilling for intact osteochondritis dissecans lesion with internal fixation

29888   Arthroscopically aided anterior cruciate ligament repair/augmentation or reconstruction

29889   Arthroscopically aided posterior cruciate ligament repair/augmentation or reconstruction

(Procedures 29888 and 29889 should not be used with reconstruction procedures 27427-27429)

(29890 has been deleted)

29891   Arthroscopy, ankle, surgical; excision of osteochondral defect of talus and/or tibia, including drilling of the defect

29892   Arthroscopically aided repair of large osteochondritis dissecans lesion, talar dome fracture, or tibial plafond fracture, with or without internal fixation (includes arthroscopy)

29893   Endoscopic plantar fasciotomy

29894   Arthroscopy, ankle (tibiotalar and fibulotalar joints), surgical; with removal of loose body or foreign body

29895   synovectomy, partial

(29896 has been deleted)

29897   debridement, limited

29898   debridement, extensive

● **29899**   with ankle arthrodesis

▶(For open ankle arthrodesis, use 27870)◀

Surgery: Musculoskeletal System

29900   Arthroscopy, metacarpophalangeal joint, diagnostic, includes synovial biopsy

(Do not report 29900 with 29901, 29902)

29901   Arthroscopy, metacarpophalangeal joint, surgical; with debridement

29902   with reduction of displaced ulnar collateral ligament (eg, Stenar lesion)

(29909 has been deleted. To report, use 29999)

29999   Unlisted procedure, arthroscopy

Respiratory System

Nose

Incision

30000*   Drainage abscess or hematoma, nasal, internal approach

      (For external approach, see 10060, 10140)

30020*   Drainage abscess or hematoma, nasal septum

      (For lateral rhinotomy, see specific application (eg, 30118, 30320))

Excision

30100   Biopsy, intranasal

      (For biopsy skin of nose, see 11100, 11101)

30110   Excision, nasal polyp(s), simple

      (30110 would normally be completed in an office setting)

      (30111 has been deleted. To report, use 30110 with modifier '-50')

30115   Excision, nasal polyp(s), extensive

      (30115 would normally require the facilities available in a hospital setting)

      (30116 has been deleted. To report, use 30115 with modifier '-50')

30117   Excision or destruction (eg, laser), intranasal lesion; internal approach

30118   external approach (lateral rhinotomy)

30120   Excision or surgical planing of skin of nose for rhinophyma

30124   Excision dermoid cyst, nose; simple, skin, subcutaneous

30125   complex, under bone or cartilage

30130   Excision turbinate, partial or complete, any method

30140   Submucous resection turbinate, partial or complete, any method

      (For submucous resection of nasal septum, use 30520)

      (For reduction of turbinates, use 30140 with modifier '-52')

30150   Rhinectomy; partial

30160   total

      (For closure and/or reconstruction, primary or delayed, see **Integumentary System,** 13150-13160, 14060-14300, 15120, 15121, 15260, 15261, 15760, 20900-20912)

Introduction

30200*   Injection into turbinate(s), therapeutic

30210*   Displacement therapy (Proetz type)

30220   Insertion, nasal septal prosthesis (button)

Removal of Foreign Body

30300*   Removal foreign body, intranasal; office type procedure

30310   requiring general anesthesia

30320   by lateral rhinotomy

Repair

      (For obtaining tissues for graft, see 20900-20926, 21210)

30400   Rhinoplasty, primary; lateral and alar cartilages and/or elevation of nasal tip

      (For columellar reconstruction, see 13150 et seq)

30410   complete, external parts including bony pyramid, lateral and alar cartilages, and/or elevation of nasal tip

30420   including major septal repair

30430   Rhinoplasty, secondary; minor revision (small amount of nasal tip work)

30435   intermediate revision (bony work with osteotomies)

30450   major revision (nasal tip work and osteotomies)

30460   Rhinoplasty for nasal deformity secondary to congenital cleft lip and/or palate, including columellar lengthening; tip only

30462   tip, septum, osteotomies

      (30500 has been deleted. To report, use 30520)

30465   Repair of nasal vestibular stenosis (eg, spreader grafting, lateral nasal wall reconstruction)

      (30465 excludes obtaining graft. For graft procedure, see 20900-20926, 21210)

      (30465 is used to report a bilateral procedure. For unilateral procedure, use modifier '-52')

30520   Septoplasty or submucous resection, with or without cartilage scoring, contouring or replacement with graft

      (For submucous resection of turbinates, use 30140)

30540   Repair choanal atresia; intranasal

30545   transpalatine

      ▶(Do not report modifier '-63' in conjunction with 30540, 30545)◀

30560*   Lysis intranasal synechia

30580   Repair fistula; oromaxillary (combine with 31030 if antrotomy is included)

30600   oronasal

Surgery: Respiratory System

30620   Septal or other intranasal dermatoplasty (does not include obtaining graft)

30630   Repair nasal septal perforations

Destruction

(30800 has been deleted. To report, see 30801 and 30802)

30801*   Cautery and/or ablation, mucosa of turbinates, unilateral or bilateral, any method, (separate procedure); superficial

30802   intramural

(30805, 30820 have been deleted. To report, see 30801 and 30802)

Other Procedures

(30900 has been deleted. To report, see 30901, 30903)

30901*   Control nasal hemorrhage, anterior, simple (limited cautery and/or packing) any method

(30902 has been deleted. To report, use 30901 with modifier '-50')

30903*   Control nasal hemorrhage, anterior, complex (extensive cautery and/or packing) any method

(30904 has been deleted. To report, use 30903 with modifier '-50')

30905*   Control nasal hemorrhage, posterior, with posterior nasal packs and/or cautery, any method; initial

30906*   subsequent

30915   Ligation arteries; ethmoidal

30920   internal maxillary artery, transantral

(For ligation external carotid artery, use 37600)

30930   Fracture nasal turbinate(s), therapeutic

30999   Unlisted procedure, nose

Accessory Sinuses

Incision

31000*   Lavage by cannulation; maxillary sinus (antrum puncture or natural ostium)

(31001 has been deleted. To report, use 31000 with modifier '-50')

31002*   sphenoid sinus

31020   Sinusotomy, maxillary (antrotomy); intranasal

(31021 has been deleted. To report, use 31020 with modifier '-50')

31030   radical (Caldwell-Luc) without removal of antrochoanal polyps

(31031 has been deleted. To report, use 31030 with modifier '-50')

31032   radical (Caldwell-Luc) with removal of antrochoanal polyps

(31033 has been deleted. To report, use 31032 with modifier '-50')

31040   Pterygomaxillary fossa surgery, any approach

(For transantral ligation of internal maxillary artery, use 30920)

31050   Sinusotomy, sphenoid, with or without biopsy;

31051   with mucosal stripping or removal of polyp(s)

31070   Sinusotomy frontal; external, simple (trephine operation)

(31071 has been deleted. To report, use 31276)

31075   transorbital, unilateral (for mucocele or osteoma, Lynch type)

31080   obliterative without osteoplastic flap, brow incision (includes ablation)

31081   obliterative, without osteoplastic flap, coronal incision (includes ablation)

31084   obliterative, with osteoplastic flap, brow incision

31085   obliterative, with osteoplastic flap, coronal incision

31086   nonobliterative, with osteoplastic flap, brow incision

31087   nonobliterative, with osteoplastic flap, coronal incision

31090   Sinusotomy, unilateral, three or more paranasal sinuses (frontal, maxillary, ethmoid, sphenoid)

Excision

31200   Ethmoidectomy; intranasal, anterior

31201   intranasal, total

31205   extranasal, total

31225   Maxillectomy; without orbital exenteration

31230   with orbital exenteration (en bloc)

(For orbital exenteration only, see 65110 et seq)

(For skin grafts, see 15120 et seq)

Endoscopy

A surgical sinus endoscopy includes a sinusotomy (when appropriate) and diagnostic endoscopy.

Codes 31231-31294 are used to report unilateral procedures unless otherwise specified.

The codes 31231-31235 for diagnostic evaluation refer to employing a nasal/sinus endoscope to inspect the interior of the nasal cavity and the middle and superior meatus, the turbinates, and the spheno-ethmoid recess. Any time a diagnostic evaluation is performed all these areas would be inspected and a separate code is not reported for each area.

31231   Nasal endoscopy, diagnostic, unilateral or bilateral (separate procedure)

31233   Nasal/sinus endoscopy, diagnostic with maxillary sinusoscopy (via inferior meatus or canine fossa puncture)

31235   Nasal/sinus endoscopy, diagnostic with sphenoid sinusoscopy (via puncture of sphenoidal face or cannulation of ostium)

31237   Nasal/sinus endoscopy, surgical; with biopsy, polypectomy or debridement (separate procedure)

31238   with control of nasal hemorrhage

31239   with dacryocystorhinostomy

31240   with concha bullosa resection

(31245 has been deleted. To report, use 31254)

(31246 has been deleted. To report, use 31254 and 31256)

(31247 has been deleted. To report, use 31254 and 31267)

(31248 has been deleted. To report, use 31254 and 31276)

(31249 has been deleted. To report, use 31254, 31256, and 31276)

(31250 has been deleted. To report, see 31231-31235)

(31251 has been deleted. To report, use 31254, 31267, and 31276)

(31252 has been deleted. To report, use 31237)

31254   Nasal/sinus endoscopy, surgical; with ethmoidectomy, partial (anterior)

31255   with ethmoidectomy, total (anterior and posterior)

31256   Nasal/sinus endoscopy, surgical, with maxillary antrostomy;

(31258 has been deleted. To report, use 31237)

(31260 has been deleted. To report, use 31233)

(31261 has been deleted. To report, use 31255)

(31262 has been deleted. To report, use 31255 and 31256)

(31263 has been deleted. To report, use 31267)

(31264 has been deleted. To report, use 31255 and 31267)

(31265 has been deleted. To report, use 31267)

(31266 has been deleted. To report, use 31255 and 31276)

31267   with removal of tissue from maxillary sinus

(31268 has been deleted. To report, use 31267)

(31269 has been deleted. To report, use 31255, 31256, and 31276)

(31270 has been deleted. To report, use 31235)

(31271 has been deleted. To report, use 31255, 31267, and 31276)

(31275 has been deleted. To report, use 31287)

31276   Nasal/sinus endoscopy, surgical with frontal sinus exploration, with or without removal of tissue from frontal sinus

(31277 has been deleted. To report, use 31288)

(31280 has been deleted. To report, use 31255, and 31287 or 31288)

(31281 has been deleted. To report, use 31255, 31256, and 31287 or 31288)

(31282 has been deleted. To report, use 31255, 31267, and 31287 or 31288)

(31283 has been deleted. To report, use 31255, 31287 or 31288, and 31276)

(31284 has been deleted. To report, use 31255, 31256, 31287 or 31288, and 31276)

(31285 has been deleted. To report, see 31231-31235)

(31286 has been deleted. To report, use 31255, 31267, 31287 or 31288, and 31276)

31287   Nasal/sinus endoscopy, surgical, with sphenoidotomy;

31288   with removal of tissue from the sphenoid sinus

31290   Nasal/sinus endoscopy, surgical, with repair of cerebrospinal fluid leak; ethmoid region

31291   sphenoid region

31292   Nasal/sinus endoscopy, surgical; with medial or inferior orbital wall decompression

31293   with medial orbital wall and inferior orbital wall decompression

31294   with optic nerve decompression

Other Procedures

(For hypophysectomy, transantral or transeptal approach, use 61548)

(For transcranial hypophysectomy, use 61546)

31299   Unlisted procedure, accessory sinuses

Larynx

Excision

31300   Laryngotomy (thyrotomy, laryngofissure); with removal of tumor or laryngocele, cordectomy

31320   diagnostic

31360   Laryngectomy; total, without radical neck dissection

31365   total, with radical neck dissection

31367   subtotal supraglottic, without radical neck dissection

31368   subtotal supraglottic, with radical neck dissection

Surgery: Respiratory System

31370 Partial laryngectomy (hemilaryngectomy); horizontal

31375 laterovertical

31380 anterovertical

31382 antero-latero-vertical

31390 Pharyngolaryngectomy, with radical neck dissection; without reconstruction

31395 with reconstruction

31400 Arytenoidectomy or arytenoidopexy, external approach

(For endoscopic arytenoidectomy, use 31560)

31420 Epiglottidectomy

Introduction

⊘ **31500** Intubation, endotracheal, emergency procedure

(For injection procedure for bronchography, see 31656, 31708, 31710)

31502 Tracheotomy tube change prior to establishment of fistula tract

Endoscopy

For endoscopic procedures, code appropriate endoscopy of each anatomic site examined.

31505 Laryngoscopy, indirect; diagnostic (separate procedure)

31510 with biopsy

31511 with removal of foreign body

31512 with removal of lesion

31513 with vocal cord injection

31515 Laryngoscopy direct, with or without tracheoscopy; for aspiration

31520 diagnostic, newborn

▶(Do not report modifier '-63' in conjunction with 31520)◀

31525 diagnostic, except newborn

31526 diagnostic, with operating microscope

(Do not report code 69990 in addition to code 31526)

31527 with insertion of obturator

31528 with dilation, initial

31529 with dilation, subsequent

31530 Laryngoscopy, direct, operative, with foreign body removal;

31531 with operating microscope

(Do not report code 69990 in addition to code 31531)

31535 Laryngoscopy, direct, operative, with biopsy;

31536 with operating microscope

(Do not report code 69990 in addition to code 31536)

31540 Laryngoscopy, direct, operative, with excision of tumor and/or stripping of vocal cords or epiglottis;

31541 with operating microscope

(Do not report code 69990 in addition to code 31541)

31560 Laryngoscopy, direct, operative, with arytenoidectomy;

31561 with operating microscope

(Do not report code 69990 in addition to code 31561)

31570 Laryngoscopy, direct, with injection into vocal cord(s), therapeutic;

31571 with operating microscope

(Do not report code 69990 in addition to code 31571)

31575 Laryngoscopy, flexible fiberoptic; diagnostic

31576 with biopsy

31577 with removal of foreign body

31578 with removal of lesion

▶(To report flexible fiberoptic endoscopic evaluation of swallowing, see 92612-92613)◀

▶(To report flexible fiberoptic endoscopic evaluation with sensory testing, see 92614-92615)◀

▶(To report flexible fiberoptic endoscopic evaluation of swallowing with sensory testing, see 92616-92617)◀

31579 Laryngoscopy, flexible or rigid fiberoptic, with stroboscopy

Repair

31580 Laryngoplasty; for laryngeal web, two stage, with keel insertion and removal

31582 for laryngeal stenosis, with graft or core mold, including tracheotomy

31584 with open reduction of fracture

31585 Treatment of closed laryngeal fracture; without manipulation

31586 with closed manipulative reduction

31587 Laryngoplasty, cricoid split

31588 Laryngoplasty, not otherwise specified (eg, for burns, reconstruction after partial laryngectomy)

31590 Laryngeal reinnervation by neuromuscular pedicle

Destruction

31595 Section recurrent laryngeal nerve, therapeutic (separate procedure), unilateral

Other Procedures

31599 Unlisted procedure, larynx

Trachea and Bronchi

Incision

31600 Tracheostomy, planned (separate procedure);

31601   under two years

31603 Tracheostomy, emergency procedure; transtracheal

31605   cricothyroid membrane

31610 Tracheostomy, fenestration procedure with skin flaps

(For endotracheal intubation, use 31500)

(For tracheal aspiration under direct vision, use 31515)

31611 Construction of tracheoesophageal fistula and subsequent insertion of an alaryngeal speech prosthesis (eg, voice button, Blom-Singer prosthesis)

31612 Tracheal puncture, percutaneous with transtracheal aspiration and/or injection

31613 Tracheostoma revision; simple, without flap rotation

31614   complex, with flap rotation

Endoscopy

For endoscopy procedures, code appropriate endoscopy of each anatomic site examined. Surgical bronchoscopy always includes diagnostic bronchoscopy when performed by the same physician. Codes 31622-31646 include fluoroscopic guidance, when performed.

(For tracheoscopy, see laryngoscopy codes 31515-31578)

31615 Tracheobronchoscopy through established tracheostomy incision

(31620, 31621 have been deleted. To report, use 31622)

31622 Bronchoscopy (rigid or flexible); diagnostic, with or without cell washing (separate procedure)

31623   with brushing or protected brushings

31624   with bronchial alveolar lavage

31625   with biopsy

(31626 has been deleted. To report, use 31625)

(31627 has been deleted. To report, use 31622)

31628   with transbronchial lung biopsy, with or without fluoroscopic guidance

31629   with transbronchial needle aspiration biopsy

31630   with tracheal or bronchial dilation or closed reduction of fracture

31631   with tracheal dilation and placement of tracheal stent

31635   with removal of foreign body

31640   with excision of tumor

31641 Bronchoscopy, (rigid or flexible); with destruction of tumor or relief of stenosis by any method other than excision (eg, laser therapy, cryotherapy)

(For bronchoscopic photodynamic therapy, report 31641 in addition to 96570, 96571 as appropriate)

31643   with placement of catheter(s) for intracavitary radioelement application

(For intracavitary radioelement application, see 77761-77763, 77781-77784)

31645   with therapeutic aspiration of tracheobronchial tree, initial (eg, drainage of lung abscess)

31646   with therapeutic aspiration of tracheobronchial tree, subsequent

(For catheter aspiration of tracheobronchial tree at bedside, use 31725)

(31650, 31651 have been deleted. To report, see 31645, 31646)

31656   with injection of contrast material for segmental bronchography (fiberscope only)

(For radiological supervision and interpretation, see 71040, 71060)

(31659 has been deleted)

Introduction

(For endotracheal intubation, use 31500)

(For tracheal aspiration under direct vision, see 31515)

31700 Catheterization, transglottic (separate procedure)

31708 Instillation of contrast material for laryngography or bronchography, without catheterization

(For radiological supervision and interpretation, see 70373, 71040, 71060)

31710 Catheterization for bronchography, with or without instillation of contrast material

(For bronchoscopic catheterization for bronchography, fiberscope only, use 31656)

(For radiological supervision and interpretation, see 71040, 71060)

31715 Transtracheal injection for bronchography

(For radiological supervision and interpretation, see 71040, 71060)

(For prolonged services, see 99354-99360)

31717 Catheterization with bronchial brush biopsy

(31719 has been deleted. To report, use 31730)

Surgery: Respiratory System

31720 Catheter aspiration (separate procedure); nasotracheal

31725 tracheobronchial with fiberscope, bedside

31730 Transtracheal (percutaneous) introduction of needle wire dilator/stent or indwelling tube for oxygen therapy

Repair

31750 Tracheoplasty; cervical

31755 tracheopharyngeal fistulization, each stage

31760 intrathoracic

31766 Carinal reconstruction

31770 Bronchoplasty; graft repair

31775 excision stenosis and anastomosis

(For lobectomy and bronchoplasty, use 32501)

31780 Excision tracheal stenosis and anastomosis; cervical

31781 cervicothoracic

31785 Excision of tracheal tumor or carcinoma; cervical

31786 thoracic

31800 Suture of tracheal wound or injury; cervical

31805 intrathoracic

31820 Surgical closure tracheostomy or fistula; without plastic repair

31825 with plastic repair

(For repair tracheoesophageal fistula, see 43305, 43312)

31830 Revision of tracheostomy scar

Other Procedures

31899 Unlisted procedure, trachea, bronchi

Lungs and Pleura

Incision

⊘ **32000*** Thoracentesis, puncture of pleural cavity for aspiration, initial or subsequent

(If imaging guidance is performed, see 76003, 76360, 76942)

(32001 has been deleted. To report, use 32997)

⊘ **32002** Thoracentesis with insertion of tube with or without water seal (eg, for pneumothorax) (separate procedure)

(If imaging guidance is performed, see 76003, 76360, 76942)

32005 Chemical pleurodesis (eg, for recurrent or persistent pneumothorax)

⊘ **32020** Tube thoracostomy with or without water seal (eg, for abscess, hemothorax, empyema) (separate procedure)

(If imaging guidance is performed, use 75989)

32035 Thoracostomy; with rib resection for empyema

32036 with open flap drainage for empyema

32095 Thoracotomy, limited, for biopsy of lung or pleura

(To report wound exploration due to penetrating trauma without thoractomy, use 20102)

32100 Thoracotomy, major; with exploration and biopsy

32110 with control of traumatic hemorrhage and/or repair of lung tear

32120 for postoperative complications

32124 with open intrapleural pneumonolysis

32140 with cyst(s) removal, with or without a pleural procedure

32141 with excision-plication of bullae, with or without any pleural procedure

(For lung volume reduction, use 32491)

32150 with removal of intrapleural foreign body or fibrin deposit

32151 with removal of intrapulmonary foreign body

32160 with cardiac massage

(For segmental or other resections of lung, see 32480-32525)

32200 Pneumonostomy; with open drainage of abscess or cyst

32201 with percutaneous drainage of abscess or cyst

(For radiological supervision and interpretation, use 75989)

32215 Pleural scarification for repeat pneumothorax

32220 Decortication, pulmonary (separate procedure); total

32225 partial

Excision

32310 Pleurectomy, parietal (separate procedure)

(32315 has been deleted. To report, use 32310)

32320 Decortication and parietal pleurectomy

32400* Biopsy, pleura; percutaneous needle

(If imaging guidance is performed, see 76003, 76360, 76393, 76942)

(For fine needle aspiration, use 10021 or 10022)

(For evaluation of fine needle aspirate, see 88172, 88173)

32402 open

32405　Biopsy, lung or mediastinum, percutaneous needle

(For radiological supervision and interpretation, see 76003, 76360, 76393, 76942)

(For fine needle aspiration, use 10022)

(For evaluation of fine needle aspirate, see 88172, 88173)

32420*　Pneumocentesis, puncture of lung for aspiration

32440　Removal of lung, total pneumonectomy;

32442　　with resection of segment of trachea followed by broncho-tracheal anastomosis (sleeve pneumonectomy)

32445　　extrapleural

(32450 has been deleted. To report, use 32445 and 32540)

32480　Removal of lung, other than total pneumonectomy; single lobe (lobectomy)

32482　　two lobes (bilobectomy)

32484　　single segment (segmentectomy)

(32485 has been deleted. To report, use 32501)

32486　　with circumferential resection of segment of bronchus followed by broncho-bronchial anastomosis (sleeve lobectomy)

32488　　all remaining lung following previous removal of a portion of lung (completion pneumonectomy)

(32490 has been deleted. To report, use 32320 and the appropriate removal of lung code)

32491　　excision-plication of emphysematous lung(s) (bullous or non-bullous) for lung volume reduction, sternal split or transthoracic approach, with or without any pleural procedure

32500　　wedge resection, single or multiple

+ 32501　Resection and repair of portion of bronchus (bronchoplasty) when performed at time of lobectomy or segmentectomy (List separately in addition to code for primary procedure)

(Use 32501 in conjunction with codes 32480, 32482, 32484)

(32501 is to be used when a portion of the bronchus to preserved lung is removed and requires plastic closure to preserve function of that preserved lung. It is not to be used for closure for the proximal end of a resected bronchus.)

32520　Resection of lung; with resection of chest wall

32522　　with reconstruction of chest wall, without prosthesis

32525　　with major reconstruction of chest wall, with prosthesis

32540　Extrapleural enucleation of empyema (empyemectomy)

(32545 has been deleted. To report, use 32540 and the appropriate removal of lung code)

Endoscopy

Surgical thoracoscopy always includes diagnostic thoracoscopy.

For endoscopic procedures, code appropriate endoscopy of each anatomic site examined.

32601　Thoracoscopy, diagnostic (separate procedure); lungs and pleural space, without biopsy

32602　　lungs and pleural space, with biopsy

32603　　pericardial sac, without biopsy

32604　　pericardial sac, with biopsy

32605　　mediastinal space, without biopsy

32606　　mediastinal space, with biopsy

(Surgical thoracoscopy always includes diagnostic thoracoscopy)

32650　Thoracoscopy, surgical; with pleurodesis (eg, mechanical or chemical)

32651　　with partial pulmonary decortication

32652　　with total pulmonary decortication, including intrapleural pneumonolysis

32653　　with removal of intrapleural foreign body or fibrin deposit

32654　　with control of traumatic hemorrhage

32655　　with excision-plication of bullae, including any pleural procedure

32656　　with parietal pleurectomy

32657　　with wedge resection of lung, single or multiple

32658　　with removal of clot or foreign body from pericardial sac

32659　　with creation of pericardial window or partial resection of pericardial sac for drainage

32660　　with total pericardiectomy

32661　　with excision of pericardial cyst, tumor, or mass

32662　　with excision of mediastinal cyst, tumor, or mass

32663　　with lobectomy, total or segmental

32664　　with thoracic sympathectomy

32665　　with esophagomyotomy (Heller type)

(32700 and 32705 have been deleted. To report, see 32601-32606)

Repair

32800　Repair lung hernia through chest wall

32810　Closure of chest wall following open flap drainage for empyema (Clagett type procedure)

32815　Open closure of major bronchial fistula

32820　Major reconstruction, chest wall (posttraumatic)

Surgery: Respiratory System

Lung Transplantation

32850 Donor pneumonectomy(ies) with preparation and maintenance of allograft (cadaver)

32851 Lung transplant, single; without cardiopulmonary bypass

32852 with cardiopulmonary bypass

32853 Lung transplant, double (bilateral sequential or en bloc); without cardiopulmonary bypass

32854 with cardiopulmonary bypass

Surgical Collapse Therapy; Thoracoplasty

(See also 32520-32525)

32900 Resection of ribs, extrapleural, all stages

32905 Thoracoplasty, Schede type or extrapleural (all stages);

32906 with closure of bronchopleural fistula

(For open closure of major bronchial fistula, use 32815)

(For resection of first rib for thoracic outlet compression, see 21615, 21616)

32940 Pneumonolysis, extraperiosteal, including filling or packing procedures

32960* Pneumothorax, therapeutic, intrapleural injection of air

Other Procedures

32997 Total lung lavage (unilateral)

(For bronchoscopic bronchial alveolar lavage, use 31624)

32999 Unlisted procedure, lungs and pleura

Cardiovascular System

Selective vascular catheterizations should be coded to include introduction and all lesser order selective catheterizations used in the approach (eg, the description for a selective right middle cerebral artery catheterization includes the introduction and placement catheterization of the right common and internal carotid arteries).

Additional second and/or third order arterial catheterizations within the same family of arteries supplied by a single first order artery should be expressed by 36218 or 36248. Additional first order or higher catheterizations in vascular families supplied by a first order vessel different from a previously selected and coded family should be separately coded using the conventions described above.

(For monitoring, operation of pump and other nonsurgical services, see 99190-99192, 99291, 99292, 99354-99360)

(For other medical or laboratory related services, see appropriate section)

(For radiological supervision and interpretation, see 75600-75978)

Heart and Pericardium

Pericardium

33010*   Pericardiocentesis; initial

(For radiological supervision and interpretation, use 76930)

33011*   subsequent

(For radiological supervision and interpretation, use 76930)

33015   Tube pericardiostomy

33020   Pericardiotomy for removal of clot or foreign body (primary procedure)

33025   Creation of pericardial window or partial resection for drainage

33030   Pericardiectomy, subtotal or complete; without cardiopulmonary bypass

33031   with cardiopulmonary bypass

(33035 has been deleted. To report, use 33031)

33050   Excision of pericardial cyst or tumor

(33100 has been deleted. To report, see 33030, 33031)

Cardiac Tumor

33120   Excision of intracardiac tumor, resection with cardiopulmonary bypass

33130   Resection of external cardiac tumor

Transmyocardial Revascularization

33140   Transmyocardial laser revascularization, by thoracotomy; (separate procedure)

+ 33141   performed at the time of other open cardiac procedure(s) (List separately in addition to code for primary procedure)

(Use 33141 in conjunction with codes 33400-33496,33510-33536, ►33542)◄

Pacemaker or Pacing Cardioverter-Defibrillator

A pacemaker system includes a pulse generator containing electronics and a battery, and one or more electrodes (leads). Pulse generators are placed in a subcutaneous "pocket" created in either a subclavicular site or underneath the abdominal muscles just below the ribcage. Electrodes may be inserted through a vein (transvenous) or they may be placed on the surface of the heart (epicardial). The epicardial location of electrodes requires a thoracotomy for electrode insertion.

A single chamber pacemaker system includes a pulse generator and one electrode inserted in either the atrium or ventricle. A dual chamber pacemaker system includes a pulse generator and one electrode inserted in the right atrium and one electrode inserted in the right ventricle. ►In certain circumstances, an additional electrode may be required to achieve pacing of the left ventricle (bi-ventricular pacing). In this event, transvenous (cardiac vein) placement of the electrode should be separately reported using code 33224 or 33225.◄

Like a pacemaker system, a pacing cardioverter-defibrillator system includes a pulse generator and electrodes, although pacing cardioverter-defibrillators may require multiple leads, even when only a single chamber is being paced. A pacing cardioverter-defibrillator system may be inserted in a single chamber (pacing in the ventricle) or in dual chambers (pacing in atrium and ventricle). These devices use a combination of antitachycardia pacing, low energy cardioversion or defibrillating shocks to treat ventricular tachycardia or ventricular fibrillation.

Pacing cardioverter-defibrillator pulse generators may be implanted in a subcutaneous infraclavicular pocket or in an abdominal pocket. Removal of a pacing cardioverter-defibrillator pulse generator requires opening of the existing subcutaneous pocket and disconnection of the pulse generator from its electrode(s). A thoracotomy (or laparotomy in the case of abdominally placed pulse generators) is not required to remove the pulse generator.

The electrodes (leads) of a pacing cardioverter-defibrillator system are positioned in the heart via the venous system (transvenously), in most circumstances. ►In certain circumstances, an additional electrode may be required to achieve pacing of the left ventricle (bi-ventricular pacing). In this event, transvenous (cardiac vein) placement of the electrode should be separately reported using code 33224 or 33225.◄

Electrode positioning on the epicardial surface of the heart requires a thoracotomy (codes 33245-33246). Removal of electrode(s) may first be attempted by transvenous extraction (code 33244). However, if transvenous extraction is unsuccessful, a thoracotomy may be required to remove the electrodes (code 33243).

When the "battery" of a pacemaker or pacing cardioverter-defibrillator is changed, it is actually the pulse generator that is changed. Replacement of a pulse generator should be reported with a code for removal of the pulse generator and another code for insertion of a pulse generator.

►Repositioning of a pacemaker electrode, pacing cardioverter-defibrillator electrode(s), or a left ventricular pacing electrode is reported using 33215 or 33226, as appropriate. Replacement of a pacemaker electrode, pacing cardioverter-defibrillator electrode(s), of a left ventricular pacing electrode is reported using 33206-33208, 33210-33213, or 33224, as appropriate.◄

(For electronic, telephonic analysis of internal pacemaker system, see 93731-93736)

(For radiological supervision and interpretation with insertion of pacemaker, use 71090)

33200 Insertion of permanent pacemaker with epicardial electrode(s); by thoracotomy

33201 by xiphoid approach

(33205 has been deleted. To report, see 33206-33208)

33206 Insertion or replacement of permanent pacemaker with transvenous electrode(s); atrial

33207 ventricular

33208 atrial and ventricular

(Codes 33206-33208 include subcutaneous insertion of the pulse generator and transvenous placement of electrode(s))

33210 Insertion or replacement of temporary transvenous single chamber cardiac electrode or pacemaker catheter (separate procedure)

33211 Insertion or replacement of temporary transvenous dual chamber pacing electrodes (separate procedure)

33212 Insertion or replacement of pacemaker pulse generator only; single chamber, atrial or ventricular

33213 dual chamber

33214 Upgrade of implanted pacemaker system, conversion of single chamber system to dual chamber system (includes removal of previously placed pulse generator, testing of existing lead, insertion of new lead, insertion of new pulse generator)

●**33215** Repositioning of previously implanted transvenous pacemaker or pacing cardioverter-defibrillator (right atrial or right ventricular) electrode

▲**33216** Insertion of a transvenous electrode; single chamber (one electrode) permanent pacemaker or single chamber pacing cardioverter-defibrillator

33217 dual chamber (two electrodes) permanent pacemaker or dual chamber pacing cardioverter-defibrillator

(Do not report 33216-33217 in conjunction with code 33214)

33218 Repair of single transvenous electrode for a single chamber, permanent pacemaker or single chamber pacing cardioverter-defibrillator

(33219 has been deleted. To report, see 33212 or 33213 and 33218 or 33220)

33220 Repair of two transvenous electrodes for a dual chamber permanent pacemaker or dual chamber pacing cardioverter-defibrillator

33222 Revision or relocation of skin pocket for pacemaker

33223 Revision of skin pocket for single or dual chamber pacing cardioverter-defibrillator

●**33224** Insertion of pacing electrode, cardiac venous system, for left ventricular pacing, with attachment to previously placed pacemaker or pacing cardioverter-defibrillator pulse generator (including revision of pocket, removal, insertion and/or replacement of generator)

+●**33225** Insertion of pacing electrode, cardiac venous system, for left ventricular pacing, at time of insertion of pacing cardioverter-defibrillator or pacemaker pulse generator (including upgrade to dual chamber system) (List separately in addition to code for primary procedure)

►(Use 33225 in conjunction with 33206, 33207, 33208, 33212, 33213, 33214, 33216, 33217, 33222, 33233, 33234, 33235, 33240, 33249)◄

●**33226** Repositioning of previously implanted cardiac venous system (left ventricular) electrode (including removal, insertion and/or replacement of generator)

(33232 has been deleted. To report, see 33233, 33234, 33236)

33233 Removal of permanent pacemaker pulse generator

33234 Removal of transvenous pacemaker electrode(s); single lead system, atrial or ventricular

33235 dual lead system

33236 Removal of permanent epicardial pacemaker and electrodes by thoracotomy; single lead system, atrial or ventricular

33237 dual lead system

33238 Removal of permanent transvenous electrode(s) by thoracotomy

33240 Insertion of single or dual chamber pacing cardioverter-defibrillator pulse generator

33241   Subcutaneous removal of single or dual chamber pacing cardioverter-defibrillator pulse generator

(For removal of electrode(s) by thoracotomy, use 33243 in conjunction with code 33241)

(For removal of electrode(s) by transvenous extraction, use 33244 in conjunction with code 33241)

(For removal and reinsertion of a pacing cardioverter-defibrillator system (pulse generator and electrodes), report 33241 and 33243 or 33244 and 33249)

(33242 has been deleted. To report, see 33218, 33220)

33243   Removal of single or dual chamber pacing cardioverter-defibrillator electrode(s); by thoracotomy

33244   by transvenous extraction

(For subcutaneous removal of the pulse generator, use 33241 in conjunction with code 33243 or 33244)

33245   Insertion of epicardial single or dual chamber pacing cardioverter-defibrillator electrodes by thoracotomy;

33246   with insertion of pulse generator

(33247 has been deleted. To report, use 33216)

(33248 has been deleted. To report, see 33242, 33243, 33244)

33249   Insertion or repositioning of electrode lead(s) for single or dual chamber pacing cardioverter-defibrillator and insertion of pulse generator

(For removal and reinsertion of a pacing cardioverter-defibrillator system (pulse generator and electrodes), report 33241 and 33243 or 33244 and 33249)

Electrophysiologic Operative Procedures

33250   Operative ablation of supraventricular arrhythmogenic focus or pathway (eg, Wolff-Parkinson-White, atrioventricular node re-entry), tract(s) and/or focus (foci); without cardiopulmonary bypass

33251   with cardiopulmonary bypass

33253   Operative incisions and reconstruction of atria for treatment of atrial fibrillation or atrial flutter (eg, maze procedure)

(33260 has been deleted. To report, use 33261)

33261   Operative ablation of ventricular arrhythmogenic focus with cardiopulmonary bypass

Patient-Activated Event Recorder

33282   Implantation of patient-activated cardiac event recorder

(Initial implantation includes programming. For subsequent electronic analysis and/or reprogramming, use 93727)

33284   Removal of an implantable, patient-activated cardiac event recorder

Wounds of the Heart and Great Vessels

33300   Repair of cardiac wound; without bypass

33305   with cardiopulmonary bypass

33310   Cardiotomy, exploratory (includes removal of foreign body); without bypass

33315   with cardiopulmonary bypass

33320   Suture repair of aorta or great vessels; without shunt or cardiopulmonary bypass

33321   with shunt bypass

33322   with cardiopulmonary bypass

33330   Insertion of graft, aorta or great vessels; without shunt, or cardiopulmonary bypass

33332   with shunt bypass

33335   with cardiopulmonary bypass

(33350 has been deleted)

Cardiac Valves

Aortic Valve

33400   Valvuloplasty, aortic valve; open, with cardiopulmonary bypass

33401   open, with inflow occlusion

33403   using transventricular dilation, with cardiopulmonary bypass

▶(Do not report modifier '-63' in conjunction with 33401, 33403)◀

33404   Construction of apical-aortic conduit

33405   Replacement, aortic valve, with cardiopulmonary bypass; with prosthetic valve other than homograft or stentless valve

33406   with allograft valve (freehand)

(33407 has been deleted. To report, use 33403)

(33408 has been deleted. To report, use 33401)

33410   with stentless tissue valve

33411   Replacement, aortic valve; with aortic annulus enlargement, noncoronary cusp

33412   with transventricular aortic annulus enlargement (Konno procedure)

33413   by translocation of autologous pulmonary valve with allograft replacement of pulmonary valve (Ross procedure)

33414   Repair of left ventricular outflow tract obstruction by patch enlargement of the outflow tract

33415   Resection or incision of subvalvular tissue for discrete subvalvular aortic stenosis

Surgery: Cardiovascular System

33416 Ventriculomyotomy (-myectomy) for idiopathic hypertrophic subaortic stenosis (eg, asymmetric septal hypertrophy)

33417 Aortoplasty (gusset) for supravalvular stenosis

Mitral Valve

33420 Valvotomy, mitral valve; closed heart

33422 open heart, with cardiopulmonary bypass

33425 Valvuloplasty, mitral valve, with cardiopulmonary bypass;

33426 with prosthetic ring

33427 radical reconstruction, with or without ring

33430 Replacement, mitral valve, with cardiopulmonary bypass

Tricuspid Valve

(33450 has been deleted. To report, see 33463, 33464)

(33452 has been deleted. To report, see 33463, 33464)

33460 Valvectomy, tricuspid valve, with cardiopulmonary bypass

33463 Valvuloplasty, tricuspid valve; without ring insertion

33464 with ring insertion

33465 Replacement, tricuspid valve, with cardiopulmonary bypass

33468 Tricuspid valve repositioning and plication for Ebstein anomaly

Pulmonary Valve

33470 Valvotomy, pulmonary valve, closed heart; transventricular

►(Do not report modifier '-63' in conjunction with 33470)◄

33471 via pulmonary artery

(To report percutaneous valvuloplasty of pulmonary valve, use 92990)

33472 Valvotomy, pulmonary valve, open heart; with inflow occlusion

►(Do not report modifier '-63' in conjunction with 33472)◄

33474 with cardiopulmonary bypass

33475 Replacement, pulmonary valve

33476 Right ventricular resection for infundibular stenosis, with or without commissurotomy

33478 Outflow tract augmentation (gusset), with or without commissurotomy or infundibular resection

(33480-33492 have been deleted. To report, see 33400-33478 and add modifier '-51' to the secondary valve procedure code when multiple valve procedures are performed.)

Other Valvular Procedures

33496 Repair of non-structural prosthetic valve dysfunction with cardiopulmonary bypass (separate procedure)

(For reoperation, use 33530 in addition to 33496)

Coronary Artery Anomalies

Basic procedures include endarterectomy or angioplasty.

33500 Repair of coronary arteriovenous or arteriocardiac chamber fistula; with cardiopulmonary bypass

33501 without cardiopulmonary bypass

33502 Repair of anomalous coronary artery; by ligation

33503 by graft, without cardiopulmonary bypass

►(Do not report modifier '-63' in conjunction with 33502, 33503)◄

33504 by graft, with cardiopulmonary bypass

33505 with construction of intrapulmonary artery tunnel (Takeuchi procedure)

33506 by translocation from pulmonary artery to aorta

►(Do not report modifier '-63' in conjunction with 33505, 33506)◄

►Endoscopy◄

►Surgical vascular endoscopy always includes diagnostic endoscopy.◄

✚ ● **33508** Endoscopy, surgical, including video-assisted harvest of vein(s) for coronary artery bypass procedure (List separately in addition to code for primary procedure)

►(Use 33508 in conjunction with code 33510-33523)◄

►(For open harvest of upper extremity vein procedure, use 35500)◄

Venous Grafting Only for Coronary Artery Bypass

The following codes are used to report coronary artery bypass procedures using venous grafts only. These codes should NOT be used to report the performance of coronary artery bypass procedures using arterial grafts and venous grafts during the same procedure. See 33517-33523 and 33533-33536 for reporting combined arterial-venous grafts.

Procurement of the saphenous vein graft is included in the description of the work for 33510-33516 and should not be reported as a separate service or co-surgery. ►To report harvesting of an upper extremity vein, use 35500 in addition to the bypass procedure. To report harvesting of a femoropopliteal vein segment, report 35572 in addition to the bypass procedure. When surgical assistant performs graft procurement,◀ add modifier '-80' to 33510-33516.

33510   Coronary artery bypass, vein only; single coronary venous graft

33511   two coronary venous grafts

33512   three coronary venous grafts

33513   four coronary venous grafts

33514   five coronary venous grafts

33516   six or more coronary venous grafts

Combined Arterial-Venous Grafting for Coronary Bypass

The following codes are used to report coronary artery bypass procedures using venous grafts and arterial grafts during the same procedure. These codes may NOT be used alone.

To report combined arterial-venous grafts it is necessary to report two codes: 1) the appropriate combined arterial-venous graft code (33517-33523); and 2) the appropriate arterial graft code (33533-33536).

Procurement of the saphenous vein graft is included in the description of the work for 33517-33523 and should not be reported as a separate service or co-surgery. Procurement of the artery for grafting is included in the description of the work for 33533-33536 and should not be reported as a separate service or co-surgery, except when an upper extremity artery (eg, radial artery) is procured. To report harvesting of an upper extremity artery, use 35600 in addition to the bypass procedure. ▶To report harvesting of an upper extremity vein, use 35500 in addition to the bypass procedure. To report harvesting of a femoropopliteal vein segment, report 35572 in addition to the bypass procedure.◀ When ▶surgical assistant performs◀ arterial and/or venous graft procurement, add modifier '-80' to 33517-33523, 33533-33536, as appropriate.

⊘ **33517**   Coronary artery bypass, using venous graft(s) and arterial graft(s); single vein graft (List separately in addition to code for arterial graft)

⊘ **33518**   two venous grafts (List separately in addition to code for arterial graft)

⊘ **33519**   three venous grafts (List separately in addition to code for arterial graft)

           (33520 has been deleted)

⊘ **33521**   four venous grafts (List separately in addition to code for arterial graft)

⊘ **33522**   five venous grafts (List separately in addition to code for arterial graft)

⊘ **33523**   six or more venous grafts (List separately in addition to code for arterial graft)

           (33525, 33528 have been deleted)

+ **33530**   Reoperation, coronary artery bypass procedure or valve procedure, more than one month after original operation (List separately in addition to code for primary procedure)

           (Use 33530 in conjunction with codes 33400-33496; 33510-33536, 33863)

           (33532 has been deleted. To report, use 33999)

Arterial Grafting for Coronary Artery Bypass

The following codes are used to report coronary artery bypass procedures using either arterial grafts only or a combination of arterial-venous grafts. The codes include the use of the internal mammary artery, gastroepiploic artery, epigastric artery, radial artery, and arterial conduits procured from other sites.

To report combined arterial-venous grafts it is necessary to report two codes: 1) the appropriate arterial graft code (33533-33536); and 2) the appropriate combined arterial-venous graft code (33517-33523).

Procurement of the artery for grafting is included in the description of the work for 33533-33536 and should not be reported as a separate service or co-surgery, except when an upper extremity artery (eg, radial artery) is procured. To report harvesting of an upper extremity artery, use 35600 in addition to the bypass procedure. ▶To report harvesting of an upper extremity vein, use 35500 in addition to the bypass procedure. To report harvesting of a femoropopliteal vein segment, report 35572 in addition to the bypass procedure.◀ When ▶surgical assistant performs◀ arterial and/or venous graft procurement, add modifier '-80' to 33517-33523, 33533-33536, as appropriate.

33533   Coronary artery bypass, using arterial graft(s); single arterial graft

33534   two coronary arterial grafts

33535   three coronary arterial grafts

33536   four or more coronary arterial grafts

33542   Myocardial resection (eg, ventricular aneurysmectomy)

33545   Repair of postinfarction ventricular septal defect, with or without myocardial resection

           (33560 has been deleted)

Surgery: Cardiovascular System

Coronary Endarterectomy

(33570 has been deleted. To report, see 33510-33536 and 33572)

+ 33572 Coronary endarterectomy, open, any method, of left anterior descending, circumflex, or right coronary artery performed in conjunction with coronary artery bypass graft procedure, each vessel (List separately in addition to primary procedure)

(Use 33572 in conjunction with 33510-33516, 33533-33536)

(33575 has been deleted. To report, see 33510-33536 and 33572)

Single Ventricle and Other Complex Cardiac Anomalies

33600 Closure of atrioventricular valve (mitral or tricuspid) by suture or patch

33602 Closure of semilunar valve (aortic or pulmonary) by suture or patch

33606 Anastomosis of pulmonary artery to aorta (Damus-Kaye-Stansel procedure)

33608 Repair of complex cardiac anomaly other than pulmonary atresia with ventricular septal defect by construction or replacement of conduit from right or left ventricle to pulmonary artery

(For repair of pulmonary atresia with ventricular septal defect, see 33918, 33919, 33920)

33610 Repair of complex cardiac anomalies (eg, single ventricle with subaortic obstruction) by surgical enlargement of ventricular septal defect

▶(Do not report modifier '-63' in conjunction with 33610)◀

33611 Repair of double outlet right ventricle with intraventricular tunnel repair;

▶(Do not report modifier '-63' in conjunction with 33611)◀

33612 with repair of right ventricular outflow tract obstruction

33615 Repair of complex cardiac anomalies (eg, tricuspid atresia) by closure of atrial septal defect and anastomosis of atria or vena cava to pulmonary artery (simple Fontan procedure)

33617 Repair of complex cardiac anomalies (eg, single ventricle) by modified Fontan procedure

33619 Repair of single ventricle with aortic outflow obstruction and aortic arch hypoplasia (hypoplastic left heart syndrome) (eg, Norwood procedure)

▶(Do not report modifier '-63' in conjunction with 33619)◀

Septal Defect

(33640 has been deleted. To report, use 33641)

33641 Repair atrial septal defect, secundum, with cardiopulmonary bypass, with or without patch

(33643 has been deleted. To report, use 33641)

33645 Direct or patch closure, sinus venosus, with or without anomalous pulmonary venous drainage

33647 Repair of atrial septal defect and ventricular septal defect, with direct or patch closure

▶(Do not report modifier '-63' in conjunction with 33647)◀

(33649 has been deleted. To report, use 33615)

33660 Repair of incomplete or partial atrioventricular canal (ostium primum atrial septal defect), with or without atrioventricular valve repair

33665 Repair of intermediate or transitional atrioventricular canal, with or without atrioventricular valve repair

33670 Repair of complete atrioventricular canal, with or without prosthetic valve

▶(Do not report modifier '-63' in conjunction with 33670)◀

33681 Closure of ventricular septal defect, with or without patch;

(33682 has been deleted. To report, use 33681)

33684 with pulmonary valvotomy or infundibular resection (acyanotic)

33688 with removal of pulmonary artery band, with or without gusset

33690 Banding of pulmonary artery

▶(Do not report modifier '-63' in conjunction with 33690)◀

33692 Complete repair tetralogy of Fallot without pulmonary atresia;

33694 with transannular patch

▶(Do not report modifier '-63' in conjunction with 33694)◀

(33696 has been deleted. To report, use 33924)

33697 Complete repair tetralogy of Fallot with pulmonary atresia including construction of conduit from right ventricle to pulmonary artery and closure of ventricular septal defect

(33698 has been deleted. To report, use 33924)

Sinus of Valsalva

33702   Repair sinus of Valsalva fistula, with cardiopulmonary bypass;

33710   with repair of ventricular septal defect

33720   Repair sinus of Valsalva aneurysm, with cardiopulmonary bypass

33722   Closure of aortico-left ventricular tunnel

Total Anomalous Pulmonary Venous Drainage

33730   Complete repair of anomalous venous return (supracardiac, intracardiac, or infracardiac types)

▶(Do not report modifier '-63' in conjunction with 33730)◀

(For partial anomalous return, see atrial septal defect)

33732   Repair of cor triatriatum or supravalvular mitral ring by resection of left atrial membrane

▶(Do not report modifier '-63' in conjunction with 33732)◀

Shunting Procedures

33735   Atrial septectomy or septostomy; closed heart (Blalock-Hanlon type operation)

33736   open heart with cardiopulmonary bypass

▶(Do not report modifier '-63' in conjunction with 33735, 33736)◀

33737   open heart, with inflow occlusion

(33738 has been deleted. To report, use 92992)

(33739 has been deleted. To report, use 92993)

33750   Shunt; subclavian to pulmonary artery (Blalock-Taussig type operation)

33755   ascending aorta to pulmonary artery (Waterston type operation)

33762   descending aorta to pulmonary artery (Potts-Smith type operation)

▶(Do not report modifier '-63' in conjunction with 33750, 33755, 33762)◀

33764   central, with prosthetic graft

33766   superior vena cava to pulmonary artery for flow to one lung (classical Glenn procedure)

33767   superior vena cava to pulmonary artery for flow to both lungs (bidirectional Glenn procedure)

Transposition of the Great Vessels

33770   Repair of transposition of the great arteries with ventricular septal defect and subpulmonary stenosis; without surgical enlargement of ventricular septal defect

33771   with surgical enlargement of ventricular septal defect

33774   Repair of transposition of the great arteries, atrial baffle procedure (eg, Mustard or Senning type) with cardiopulmonary bypass;

33775   with removal of pulmonary band

33776   with closure of ventricular septal defect

33777   with repair of subpulmonic obstruction

33778   Repair of transposition of the great arteries, aortic pulmonary artery reconstruction (eg, Jatene type);

▶(Do not report modifier '-63' in conjunction with 33778)◀

33779   with removal of pulmonary band

33780   with closure of ventricular septal defect

33781   with repair of subpulmonic obstruction

(33782, 33783, 33784, 33785 have been deleted. To report, see 33774-33781)

Truncus Arteriosus

33786   Total repair, truncus arteriosus (Rastelli type operation)

▶(Do not report modifier '-63' in conjunction with 33786)◀

33788   Reimplantation of an anomalous pulmonary artery

(For pulmonary artery band, use 33690)

Aortic Anomalies

33800   Aortic suspension (aortopexy) for tracheal decompression (eg, for tracheomalacia) (separate procedure)

33802   Division of aberrant vessel (vascular ring);

33803   with reanastomosis

(33810, 33812 have been deleted)

33813   Obliteration of aortopulmonary septal defect; without cardiopulmonary bypass

33814   with cardiopulmonary bypass

33820   Repair of patent ductus arteriosus; by ligation

33822   by division, under 18 years

33824   by division, 18 years and older

(33830 has been deleted. To report, see 33820-33824)

Surgery: Cardiovascular System

33840 Excision of coarctation of aorta, with or without associated patent ductus arteriosus; with direct anastomosis

33845   with graft

(33850 has been deleted. To report, use 33999)

33851   repair using either left subclavian artery or prosthetic material as gusset for enlargement

33852 Repair of hypoplastic or interrupted aortic arch using autogenous or prosthetic material; without cardiopulmonary bypass

33853   with cardiopulmonary bypass

(33855 has been deleted. To report, use 33619)

Thoracic Aortic Aneurysm

33860 Ascending aorta graft, with cardiopulmonary bypass, with or without valve suspension;

33861   with coronary reconstruction

33863   with aortic root replacement using composite prosthesis and coronary reconstruction

(33865 has been deleted. To report, see 33860 or 33861 and 33405 or 33406)

33870 Transverse arch graft, with cardiopulmonary bypass

33875 Descending thoracic aorta graft, with or without bypass

33877 Repair of thoracoabdominal aortic aneurysm with graft, with or without cardiopulmonary bypass

Pulmonary Artery

33910 Pulmonary artery embolectomy; with cardiopulmonary bypass

33915   without cardiopulmonary bypass

33916 Pulmonary endarterectomy, with or without embolectomy, with cardiopulmonary bypass

33917 Repair of pulmonary artery stenosis by reconstruction with patch or graft

33918 Repair of pulmonary atresia with ventricular septal defect, by unifocalization of pulmonary arteries; without cardiopulmonary bypass

33919   with cardiopulmonary bypass

►(Do not report modifier '-63' in conjunction with 33918, 33919)◄

33920 Repair of pulmonary atresia with ventricular septal defect, by construction or replacement of conduit from right or left ventricle to pulmonary artery

(For repair of other complex cardiac anomalies by construction or replacement of right or left ventricle to pulmonary artery conduit, use 33608)

33922 Transection of pulmonary artery with cardiopulmonary bypass

►(Do not report modifier '-63' in conjunction with 33922)◄

+ 33924 Ligation and takedown of a systemic-to-pulmonary artery shunt, performed in conjunction with a congenital heart procedure (List separately in addition to code for primary procedure)

(Use 33924 in conjunction with 33470-33475, 33600-33619, 33684-33688, 33692-33697, 33735-33767, 33770-33781, 33786, 33918-33922)

Heart/Lung Transplantation

33930 Donor cardiectomy-pneumonectomy, with preparation and maintenance of allograft

33935 Heart-lung transplant with recipient cardiectomy-pneumonectomy

33940 Donor cardiectomy, with preparation and maintenance of allograft

33945 Heart transplant, with or without recipient cardiectomy

(33950 has been deleted. To report, see 33940, 33945)

Cardiac Assist

33960 Prolonged extracorporeal circulation for cardiopulmonary insufficiency; initial 24 hours

+ 33961   each additional 24 hours (List separately in addition to code for primary procedure)

►(Do not report modifier '-63' in conjunction with 33960, 33961)◄

(Use 33961 in conjunction with code 33960)

(For insertion of cannula for prolonged extracorporeal circulation, use 36822)

33967 Insertion of intra-aortic balloon assist device, percutaneous

33968 Removal of intra-aortic balloon assist device, percutaneous

33970 Insertion of intra-aortic balloon assist device through the femoral artery, open approach

33971 Removal of intra-aortic balloon assist device including repair of femoral artery, with or without graft

(33972 has been deleted. To report, use appropriate E/M code)

33973 Insertion of intra-aortic balloon assist device through the ascending aorta

33974 Removal of intra-aortic balloon assist device from the ascending aorta, including repair of the ascending aorta, with or without graft

33975   Insertion of ventricular assist device; extracorporeal, single ventricle

33976   extracorporeal, biventricular

33977   Removal of ventricular assist device; extracorporeal, single ventricle

33978   extracorporeal, biventricular

33979   Insertion of ventricular assist device, implantable intracorporeal, single ventricle

33980   Removal of ventricular assist device, implantable intracorporeal, single ventricle

Other Procedures

33999   Unlisted procedure, cardiac surgery

Arteries and Veins

Primary vascular procedure listings include establishing both inflow and outflow by whatever procedures necessary. Also included is that portion of the operative arteriogram performed by the surgeon, as indicated. Sympathectomy, when done, is included in the listed aortic procedures. For unlisted vascular procedure, use 37799.

Embolectomy/Thrombectomy

Arterial, With or Without Catheter

34001   Embolectomy or thrombectomy, with or without catheter; carotid, subclavian or innominate artery, by neck incision

34051   innominate, subclavian artery, by thoracic incision

34101   axillary, brachial, innominate, subclavian artery, by arm incision

34111   radial or ulnar artery, by arm incision

34151   renal, celiac, mesentery, aortoiliac artery, by abdominal incision

34201   femoropopliteal, aortoiliac artery, by leg incision

34203   popliteal-tibio-peroneal artery, by leg incision

Venous, Direct or With Catheter

34401   Thrombectomy, direct or with catheter; vena cava, iliac vein, by abdominal incision

34421   vena cava, iliac, femoropopliteal vein, by leg incision

34451   vena cava, iliac, femoropopliteal vein, by abdominal and leg incision

34471   subclavian vein, by neck incision

34490   axillary and subclavian vein, by arm incision

Venous Reconstruction

34501   Valvuloplasty, femoral vein

34502   Reconstruction of vena cava, any method

34510   Venous valve transposition, any vein donor

34520   Cross-over vein graft to venous system

34530   Saphenopopliteal vein anastomosis

Endovascular Repair of Abdominal Aortic Aneurysm

Codes 34800-34826 represent a family of component procedures to report placement of an endovascular graft for abdominal aortic aneurysm repair. These codes describe open femoral or iliac artery exposure, device manipulation and deployment, and closure of the arteriotomy sites. Balloon angioplasty and/or stent deployment within the target treatment zone for the endoprosthesis, either before or after endograft deployment, are not separately reportable. Introduction of guidewires and catheters should be reported separately (eg, 36200, 36245-36248, 36140). Extensive repair or replacement of an artery should be additionally reported (eg, 35226 or 35286).

For fluoroscopic guidance in conjunction with endovascular aneurysm repair, see code 75952 or 75953, as appropriate. Code 75952 includes angiography of the aorta and its branches for diagnostic imaging prior to deployment of the endovascular device (including all routine components of modular devices), fluoroscopic guidance in the delivery of the endovascular components, and intraprocedural arterial angiography (eg, confirm position, detect endoleak, evaluate runoff). Code 75953 includes the analogous services for placement of additional extension prostheses (not for routine components of modular devices).

Other interventional procedures performed at the time of endovascular abdominal aortic aneurysm repair should be additionally reported (eg, renal transluminal angioplasty, arterial embolization, intravascular ultrasound, balloon angioplasty or stenting of native artery(s) outside the endoprosthesis target zone, when done before or after deployment of graft).

34800   Endovascular repair of infrarenal abdominal aortic aneurysm or dissection; using aorto-aortic tube prosthesis

34802   using modular bifurcated prosthesis (one docking limb)

         (For endovascular repair of infrarenal abdominal aortic aneurysm or dissection using a modular bifurcated prosthesis (two docking limbs), use Category III code 0001T)

Surgery: Cardiovascular System

Surgery: Cardiovascular System

34804 using unibody bifurcated prosthesis

(For endovascular repair of infrarenal adbominal aortic aneurysm or dissection using an aorto-uniiliac or aorto-unifemoral prosthesis, use Category III code 0002T)

+ 34808 Endovascular placement of iliac artery occlusion device (List separately in addition to code for primary procedure)

(Use 34808 in conjunction with codes 34800, 34813, 34825, 34826)

(For radiological supervision and interpretation, use 75952 in conjunction with 34800, 34802, 34804, 34808)

(For open approach, report codes 34812-34820 in addition to codes 34800, 34802, 34804, 34808 as appropriate)

▲ 34812 Open femoral artery exposure for delivery of endovascular prosthesis, by groin incision, unilateral

(For bilateral procedure, use modifier '-50')

+ 34813 Placement of femoral-femoral prosthetic graft during endovascular aortic aneurysm repair (List separately in addition to code for primary procedure)

(Use 34813 in conjunction with code 34812)

(For femoral artery grafting, see 35521, 35533, 35546, 35551-35558, 35566, 35621, 35646, 35651-35661, 35666, 35700)

34820 Open iliac artery exposure for delivery of endovascular prosthesis or iliac occlusion during endovascular therapy, by abdominal or retroperitoneal incision, unilateral

(For bilateral procedure, use modifier '-50')

▲ 34825 Placement of proximal or distal extension prosthesis for endovascular repair of infrarenal abdominal aortic or iliac aneurysm, false aneurysm, or dissection; initial vessel

+ 34826 each additional vessel (List separately in addition to code for primary procedure)

(Use 34826 in conjunction with code 34825)

(Use 34825, 34826 in addition to codes 34800-34808, ►34900◄ as appropriate)

(For staged procedure, use modifier '-58')

(For radiological supervision and interpretation, use 75953)

34830 Open repair of infrarenal aortic aneurysm or dissection, plus repair of associated arterial trauma, following unsuccessful endovascular repair; tube prosthesis

34831 aorto-bi-iliac prosthesis

34832 aorto-bifemoral prosthesis

● 34833 Open iliac artery exposure with creation of conduit for delivery of infrarenal aortic or iliac endovascular prosthesis, by abdominal or retroperitoneal incision, unilateral

►(For bilateral procedure, use modifier '-50')◄

►(Do not report 34833 in addition to 34820)◄

● 34834 Open brachial artery exposure to assist in the deployment of infrarenal aortic or iliac endovascular prosthesis by arm incision, unilateral

►(For bilateral procedure, use modifier '-50')◄

►Endovascular Repair of Iliac Aneurysm◄

►Code 34900 represents a procedure to report introduction, positioning, and deployment of an endovascular graft for treatment of aneurysm, pseudoaneurysm, or arteriovenous malformation or trauma of the iliac artery (common, hypogastric, external). All balloon angioplasty and/or stent deployments within the target treatment zone for the endoprosthesis, either before or after endograft deployment, are included in the work of 34900 and are not separately reportable. Open femoral or iliac artery exposure (eg, 34812, 34820), introduction of guidewires and catheters (eg, 36200, 36215-36218), and extensive repair or replacement of an artery (eg 35206-35286) should be additionally reported.

For fluoroscopic guidance in conjunction with endovascular iliac aneurysm repair, see code 75954. Code 75954 includes angiography of the aorta and iliac arteries for diagnostic imaging prior to deployment of the endovascular device (including all routine components), fluoroscopic guidance in the delivery of the endovascular components, and intraprocedural arterial angiography to confirm appropriate position of the graft, detect endoleaks, and evaluate the status of the runoff vessels (eg, evaluation for dissection, stenosis, thrombosis, distal embolization, or iatrogenic injury).

Other interventional procedures performed at the time of endovascular aortic aneurysm repair should be additionally reported (eg, transluminal angioplasty outside the aneurysm target zone, arterial embolization, intravascular ultrasound).◄

● 34900 Endovascular graft replacement for repair of iliac artery (eg, aneurysm, pseudoaneurysm, arteriovenous malformation, trauma)

►(For radiological supervision and interpretation, use 75954)◄

►(For placement of extension prosthesis during endovascular iliac artery repair, use 34825)◄

►(For bilateral procedure, use modifier '-50')◄

Direct Repair of Aneurysm or Excision (Partial or Total) and Graft Insertion for Aneurysm, Pseudoaneurysm, Ruptured Aneurysm, and Associated Occlusive Disease

Procedures 35001-35162 include preparation of artery for anastomosis including endarterectomy.

(For direct repairs associated with occlusive disease only, see 35201-35286)

(For intracranial aneurysm, see 61700 et seq)

▶(For endovascular repair of abdominal aortic aneurysm, see 34800-34826)◀

▶(For endovascular repair of iliac artery aneurysm, see 34900)◀

(For thoracic aortic aneurysm, see 33860-33875)

▶(For endovascular repair of thoracic aortic aneurysm, see Category III codes 0033T-0034T)◀

35001   Direct repair of aneurysm, pseudoaneurysm, or excision (partial or total) and graft insertion, with or without patch graft; for aneurysm and associated occlusive disease, carotid, subclavian artery, by neck incision

35002   for ruptured aneurysm, carotid, subclavian artery, by neck incision

35005   for aneurysm, pseudoaneurysm, and associated occlusive disease, vertebral artery

35011   for aneurysm and associated occlusive disease, axillary-brachial artery, by arm incision

35013   for ruptured aneurysm, axillary-brachial artery, by arm incision

35021   for aneurysm, pseudoaneurysm, and associated occlusive disease, innominate, subclavian artery, by thoracic incision

35022   for ruptured aneurysm, innominate, subclavian artery, by thoracic incision

35045   for aneurysm, pseudoaneurysm, and associated occlusive disease, radial or ulnar artery

35081   for aneurysm, pseudoaneurysm, and associated occlusive disease, abdominal aorta

35082   for ruptured aneurysm, abdominal aorta

35091   for aneurysm, pseudoaneurysm, and associated occlusive disease, abdominal aorta involving visceral vessels (mesenteric, celiac, renal)

35092   for ruptured aneurysm, abdominal aorta involving visceral vessels (mesenteric, celiac, renal)

35102   for aneurysm, pseudoaneurysm, and associated occlusive disease, abdominal aorta involving iliac vessels (common, hypogastric, external)

35103   for ruptured aneurysm, abdominal aorta involving iliac vessels (common, hypogastric, external)

35111   for aneurysm, pseudoaneurysm, and associated occlusive disease, splenic artery

35112   for ruptured aneurysm, splenic artery

35121   for aneurysm, pseudoaneurysm, and associated occlusive disease, hepatic, celiac, renal, or mesenteric artery

35122   for ruptured aneurysm, hepatic, celiac, renal, or mesenteric artery

35131   for aneurysm, pseudoaneurysm, and associated occlusive disease, iliac artery (common, hypogastric, external)

35132   for ruptured aneurysm, iliac artery (common, hypogastric, external)

35141   for aneurysm, pseudoaneurysm, and associated occlusive disease, common femoral artery (profunda femoris, superficial femoral)

35142   for ruptured aneurysm, common femoral artery (profunda femoris, superficial femoral)

35151   for aneurysm, pseudoaneurysm, and associated occlusive disease, popliteal artery

35152   for ruptured aneurysm, popliteal artery

35161   for aneurysm, pseudoaneurysm, and associated occlusive disease, other arteries

35162   for ruptured aneurysm, other arteries

Repair Arteriovenous Fistula

35180   Repair, congenital arteriovenous fistula; head and neck

35182   thorax and abdomen

35184   extremities

35188   Repair, acquired or traumatic arteriovenous fistula; head and neck

35189   thorax and abdomen

35190   extremities

Repair Blood Vessel Other Than for Fistula, With or Without Patch Angioplasty

(For AV fistula repair, see 35180-35190)

35201   Repair blood vessel, direct; neck

35206   upper extremity

35207   hand, finger

35211	intrathoracic, with bypass
35216	intrathoracic, without bypass
35221	intra-abdominal
35226	lower extremity
35231	Repair blood vessel with vein graft; neck
35236	upper extremity
35241	intrathoracic, with bypass
35246	intrathoracic, without bypass
35251	intra-abdominal
35256	lower extremity
35261	Repair blood vessel with graft other than vein; neck
35266	upper extremity
35271	intrathoracic, with bypass
35276	intrathoracic, without bypass
35281	intra-abdominal
35286	lower extremity

Thromboendarterectomy

(For coronary artery, see 33510-33536 and 33572)

35301	Thromboendarterectomy, with or without patch graft; carotid, vertebral, subclavian, by neck incision
35311	subclavian, innominate, by thoracic incision
35321	axillary-brachial
35331	abdominal aorta
35341	mesenteric, celiac, or renal
35351	iliac
35355	iliofemoral
35361	combined aortoiliac
35363	combined aortoiliofemoral
35371	common femoral
35372	deep (profunda) femoral
35381	femoral and/or popliteal, and/or tibioperoneal
+ 35390	Reoperation, carotid, thromboendarterectomy, more than one month after original operation (List separately in addition to code for primary procedure)

(Use 35390 in conjunction with code 35301)

Angioscopy

+ 35400	Angioscopy (non-coronary vessels or grafts) during therapeutic intervention (List separately in addition to code for primary procedure)

Transluminal Angioplasty

If done as part of another operation, use modifier '-51' or use modifier '-52'.

(For radiological supervision and interpretation, see 75962-75968 and 75978)

Open

35450	Transluminal balloon angioplasty, open; renal or other visceral artery
35452	aortic
35454	iliac
35456	femoral-popliteal
35458	brachiocephalic trunk or branches, each vessel
35459	tibioperoneal trunk and branches
35460	venous

Percutaneous

Codes for catheter placement and the radiologic supervision and interpretation should also be reported, in addition to the code(s) for the therapeutic aspect of the procedure.

35470	Transluminal balloon angioplasty, percutaneous; tibioperoneal trunk or branches, each vessel
35471	renal or visceral artery
35472	aortic
35473	iliac
35474	femoral-popliteal
35475	brachiocephalic trunk or branches, each vessel
35476	venous

(For radiological supervision and interpretation, use 75978)

Transluminal Atherectomy

If done as part of another operation, use modifier '-51' or use modifier '-52'.

(For radiological supervision and interpretation, see 75992-75996)

Open

35480	Transluminal peripheral atherectomy, open; renal or other visceral artery
35481	aortic
35482	iliac

35483	femoral-popliteal
35484	brachiocephalic trunk or branches, each vessel
35485	tibioperoneal trunk and branches

Percutaneous

Codes for catheter placement and the radiologic supervision and interpretation should also be reported, in addition to the code(s) for the therapeutic aspect of the procedure.

35490	Transluminal peripheral atherectomy, percutaneous; renal or other visceral artery
35491	aortic
35492	iliac
35493	femoral-popliteal
35494	brachiocephalic trunk or branches, each vessel
35495	tibioperoneal trunk and branches

Bypass Graft

Vein

►Procurement of the saphenous vein graft is included in the description of the work for 35501-35587 and should not be reported as a separate service or co-surgery. To report harvesting of an upper extremity vein, use 35500 in addition to the bypass procedure. To report harvesting of a femoropopliteal vein segment, use 35572 in addition to the bypass procedure. To report harvesting and construction of an autogenous composite graft of two segments from two distant locations, report 35682 in addition to the bypass procedure, for autogenous composite of three or more segments from distant sites, report 35683.◄

+ 35500 Harvest of upper extremity vein, one segment, for lower extremity or coronary artery bypass procedure (List separately in addition to code for primary procedure)

(Use 35500 in conjunction with codes 33510-33536, 35556, 35566, 35571, 35583-35587)

(For harvest of more than one vein segment, see 35682, 35683)

►(For endoscopic procedure, use 33508)◄

35501	Bypass graft, with vein; carotid
35506	carotid-subclavian
35507	subclavian-carotid
35508	carotid-vertebral
35509	carotid-carotid
35511	subclavian-subclavian
35515	subclavian-vertebral

35516	subclavian-axillary
35518	axillary-axillary
35521	axillary-femoral

(For bypass graft performed with synthetic graft, use 35621)

35526	aortosubclavian or carotid

(For bypass graft performed with synthetic graft, use 35626)

35531	aortoceliac or aortomesenteric
35533	axillary-femoral-femoral

(For bypass graft performed with synthetic graft, use 35654)

35536	splenorenal
35541	aortoiliac or bi-iliac

(For bypass graft performed with synthetic graft, use 35641)

35546	aortofemoral or bifemoral

(For bypass graft performed with synthetic graft, use 35646)

35548	aortoiliofemoral, unilateral

(For bypass graft performed with synthetic graft, use 37799)

35549	aortoiliofemoral, bilateral

(For bypass graft performed with synthetic graft, use 37799)

35551	aortofemoral-popliteal
35556	femoral-popliteal
35558	femoral-femoral
35560	aortorenal
35563	ilioiliac
35565	iliofemoral
35566	femoral-anterior tibial, posterior tibial, peroneal artery or other distal vessels
35571	popliteal-tibial, -peroneal artery or other distal vessels

+ ● 35572 Harvest of femoropopliteal vein, one segment, for vascular reconstruction procedure (eg, aortic, vena caval, coronary, peripheral artery) (List separately in addition to code for primary procedure)

►(Use 35572 in conjunction with codes 33510-33516, 33517-33523, 34502, 34520, 35001-35002, 35011-35022, 35102-35103, 35121-35152, 35231-35256, 35501-35587, 35879-35881, 35901-35907)◄

In-Situ Vein

35582   In-situ vein bypass; aortofemoral-popliteal (only femoral-popliteal portion in-situ)

35583   femoral-popliteal

35585   femoral-anterior tibial, posterior tibial, or peroneal artery

35587   popliteal-tibial, peroneal

Other Than Vein

⊘ 35600   Harvest of upper extremity artery, one segment, for coronary artery bypass procedure

35601   Bypass graft, with other than vein; carotid

35606   carotid-subclavian

▶(For open subclavian to carotid artery transposition performed in conjunction with endovascular thoracic aneurysm repair, use Category III code 0037T)◀

35612   subclavian-subclavian

35616   subclavian-axillary

35621   axillary-femoral

35623   axillary-popliteal or -tibial

35626   aortosubclavian or carotid

35631   aortoceliac, aortomesenteric, aortorenal

35636   splenorenal (splenic to renal arterial anastomosis)

(35637 has been deleted. To report, use 35691)

(35638 has been deleted. To report, use 35693)

35641   aortoiliac or bi-iliac

▶(For open placement of aorto-bi-iliac prosthesis following unsuccessful endovascular repair, use 34831)◀

35642   carotid-vertebral

35645   subclavian-vertebral

35646   aortobifemoral

▶(For open placement of aortobifemoral prosthesis following unsuccessful endovascular repair, use 34832)◀

35647   aortofemoral

35650   axillary-axillary

35651   aortofemoral-popliteal

35654   axillary-femoral-femoral

35656   femoral-popliteal

35661   femoral-femoral

35663   ilioiliac

35665   iliofemoral

35666   femoral-anterior tibial, posterior tibial, or peroneal artery

35671   popliteal-tibial or -peroneal artery

Composite Grafts

Codes 35682-35683 are used to report harvest and anastomosis of multiple vein segments from distant sites for use as arterial bypass graft conduits. These codes are intended for use when the two or more vein segments are harvested from a limb other than that undergoing bypass. Add-on codes 35682 and 35683 may be reported in addition to codes 35556, 35566, 35571, 35583-35587, as appropriate.

+ 35681   Bypass graft; composite, prosthetic and vein (List separately in addition to code for primary procedure)

(Do not report 35681 in addition to 35682, 35683)

+ 35682   autogenous composite, two segments of veins from two locations (List separately in addition to code for primary procedure)

(Do not report 35682 in addition to 35681, 35683)

+ 35683   autogenous composite, three or more segments of vein from two or more locations (List separately in addition to code for primary procedure)

(Do not report 35683 in addition to 35681, 35682)

Adjuvant Techniques

Adjuvant (additional) technique(s) may be required at the time a bypass graft is created to improve patency of the lower extremity autogenous or synthetic bypass graft (eg, femoral-popliteal, femoral-tibial, or popliteal-tibial arteries). Code 35685 should be reported in addition to the primary synthetic bypass graft procedure, when an interposition of venous tissue (vein patch or cuff) is placed at the anastomosis between the synthetic bypass conduit and the involved artery (includes harvest).

Code 35686 should be reported in addition to the primary bypass graft procedure, when autogenous vein is used to create a fistula between the tibial or peroneal artery and vein at or beyond the distal bypass anastomosis site of the involved artery.

(For composite graft(s), see 35681-35683)

+ 35685   Placement of vein patch or cuff at distal anastomosis of bypass graft, synthetic conduit (List separately in addition to code for primary procedure)

(Use 35685 in conjunction with codes 35656, 35666, or 35671)

+ 35686   Creation of distal arteriovenous fistula during lower extremity bypass surgery (non-hemodialysis) (List separately in addition to code for primary procedure)

(Use 35686 in conjunction with codes 35556, 35566, 35571, 35583-35587, 35623, 35656, 35666, 35671)

Arterial Transposition

35691   Transposition and/or reimplantation; vertebral to carotid artery

35693   vertebral to subclavian artery

35694   subclavian to carotid artery

▶(For open subclavian to carotid artery transposition performed in conjunction with endovascular thoracic aneurysm repair, use Category III code 0037T)◀

35695   carotid to subclavian artery

Exploration/Revision

+ **35700**   Reoperation, femoral-popliteal or femoral (popliteal)-anterior tibial, posterior tibial, peroneal artery or other distal vessels, more than one month after original operation (List separately in addition to code for primary procedure)

(Use 35700 in conjunction with codes 35556, 35566, 35571, 35583, 35585, 35587, 35656, 35666, 35671)

35701   Exploration (not followed by surgical repair), with or without lysis of artery; carotid artery

35721   femoral artery

35741   popliteal artery

35761   other vessels

35800   Exploration for postoperative hemorrhage, thrombosis or infection; neck

35820   chest

35840   abdomen

35860   extremity

35870   Repair of graft-enteric fistula

35875   Thrombectomy of arterial or venous graft (other than hemodialysis graft or fistula);

35876   with revision of arterial or venous graft

(For thrombectomy of hemodialysis graft or fistula, see 36831, 36833)

(35880 has been deleted. To report, use 35875)

(35900 has been deleted. To report, see 35901-35907 and appropriate revascularization code)

Codes 35879 and 35881 describe open revision of graft-threatening stenoses of lower extremity arterial bypass graft(s) (previously constructed with autogenous vein conduit) using vein patch angioplasty or segmental vein interposition techniques. For thrombectomy with revision of any non-coronary arterial or venous graft, including those of the lower extremity, (other than

hemodialysis graft or fistula), use 35876. For direct repair (other than for fistula) of a lower extremity blood vessel (with or without patch angioplasty), use 35226. For repair (other than for fistula) of a lower extremity blood vessel using a vein graft, use 35256.

35879   Revision, lower extremity arterial bypass, without thrombectomy, open; with vein patch angioplasty

35881   with segmental vein interposition

35901   Excision of infected graft; neck

35903   extremity

35905   thorax

35907   abdomen

(35910 has been deleted. To report, see 35901-35907 and appropriate revascularization code)

Vascular Injection Procedures

Listed services for injection procedures include necessary local anesthesia, introduction of needles or catheter, injection of contrast media with or without automatic power injection, and/or necessary pre- and postinjection care specifically related to the injection procedure.

Catheters, drugs, and contrast media are not included in the listed service for the injection procedures.

Selective vascular catheterization should be coded to include introduction and all lesser order selective catheterization used in the approach (eg, the description for a selective right middle cerebral artery catheterization includes the introduction and placement catheterization of the right common and internal carotid arteries).

Additional second and/or third order arterial catheterization within the same family of arteries or veins supplied by a single first order vessel should be expressed by 36012, 36218 or 36248.

Additional first order or higher catheterization in vascular families supplied by a first order vessel different from a previously selected and coded family should be separately coded using the conventions described above.

(For radiological supervision and interpretation, see **Radiology**)

(For injection procedures in conjunction with cardiac catheterization, see 93541-93545)

(For chemotherapy of malignant disease, see 96400-96549)

Intravenous

An intracatheter is a sheathed combination of needle and short catheter.

36000* Introduction of needle or intracatheter, vein

(36001 has been deleted. To report, use 36000 with modifier '-50')

36002 Injection procedures (eg, thrombin) for percutaneous treatment of extremity pseudoaneurysm

(For imaging guidance, see 76003, 76360, 76393, or 76942)

(For ultrasound guided compression repair of pseudoaneurysms, use 76936)

(Do not report 36002 for vascular sealant of an arteriotomy site)

36005 Injection procedure for extremity venography (including introduction of needle or intracatheter)

(For radiological supervision and interpretation, see 75820, 75822)

36010 Introduction of catheter, superior or inferior vena cava

36011 Selective catheter placement, venous system; first order branch (eg, renal vein, jugular vein)

36012 second order, or more selective, branch (eg, left adrenal vein, petrosal sinus)

36013 Introduction of catheter, right heart or main pulmonary artery

36014 Selective catheter placement, left or right pulmonary artery

36015 Selective catheter placement, segmental or subsegmental pulmonary artery

(For insertion of flow directed catheter (eg, Swan-Ganz), use 93503)

(For venous catheterization for selective organ blood sampling, use 36500)

Intra-Arterial—Intra-Aortic

(For radiological supervision and interpretation, see **Radiology**)

36100 Introduction of needle or intracatheter, carotid or vertebral artery

(36101 has been deleted. To report, use 36100 with modifier '-50')

36120 Introduction of needle or intracatheter; retrograde brachial artery

36140 extremity artery

36145 arteriovenous shunt created for dialysis (cannula, fistula, or graft)

(For insertion of arteriovenous cannula, see 36810-36821)

36160 Introduction of needle or intracatheter, aortic, translumbar

36200 Introduction of catheter, aorta

(36210 has been deleted. To report, see 36215-36218)

36215 Selective catheter placement, arterial system; each first order thoracic or brachiocephalic branch, within a vascular family

(For catheter placement for coronary angiography, use 93508)

36216 initial second order thoracic or brachiocephalic branch, within a vascular family

36217 initial third order or more selective thoracic or brachiocephalic branch, within a vascular family

+ 36218 additional second order, third order, and beyond, thoracic or brachiocephalic branch, within a vascular family (List in addition to code for initial second or third order vessel as appropriate)

(Use 36218 in conjunction with codes 36216, 36217)

(For angiography, see 75600-75790)

(For angioplasty, see 35470-35475)

(For transcatheter therapies, see 37200-37208, 61624, 61626)

(36220 has been deleted. To report, see 36215-36218)

(36230 has been deleted. When coronary artery, arterial conduit (eg, internal mammary, inferior epigastric or free radial artery) or venous bypass graft angiography is performed in conjunction with cardiac catheterization, see the appropriate cardiac catheterization code(s) (93501-93556) in the **Medicine** section of *CPT*. When coronary artery, arterial coronary conduit or venous bypass graft angiography is performed without concomitant left heart cardiac catheterization, use 93508. When internal mammary artery angiography only is performed without a concomitant left heart cardiac catheterization, use 36216 or 36217 as appropriate.)

(36240 has been deleted. To report, use 36248)

36245 Selective catheter placement, arterial system; each first order abdominal, pelvic, or lower extremity artery branch, within a vascular family

36246 initial second order abdominal, pelvic, or lower extremity artery branch, within a vascular family

36247 initial third order or more selective abdominal, pelvic, or lower extremity artery branch, within a vascular family

+ 36248 additional second order, third order, and beyond, abdominal, pelvic, or lower extremity artery branch, within a vascular family (List in addition to code for initial second or third order vessel as appropriate)

(Use 36248 in conjunction with codes 36246, 36247)

(36250 has been deleted. To report, use 36248)

36260   Insertion of implantable intra-arterial infusion pump (eg, for chemotherapy of liver)

36261   Revision of implanted intra-arterial infusion pump

36262   Removal of implanted intra-arterial infusion pump

36299   Unlisted procedure, vascular injection

Venous

Venipuncture, needle or catheter for diagnostic study or intravenous therapy, percutaneous.

36400   Venipuncture, under age 3 years; femoral or jugular

36405*   scalp vein

36406   other vein

36410*   Venipuncture, child over age 3 years or adult, necessitating physician's skill (separate procedure), for diagnostic or therapeutic purposes. Not to be used for routine venipuncture.

▲36415*   Collection of venous blood by venipuncture

▶(Do not report modifier '-63' in conjunction with 36415)◀

●36416   Collection of capillary blood specimen (eg, finger, heel, ear stick)

36420   Venipuncture, cutdown; under age 1 year

▶(Do not report modifier '-63' in conjunction with 36420)◀

36425   age 1 or over

36430   Transfusion, blood or blood components

(36431 has been deleted)

36440*   Push transfusion, blood, 2 years or under

36450   Exchange transfusion, blood; newborn

▶(Do not report modifier '-63' in conjunction with 36450)◀

36455   other than newborn

36460   Transfusion, intrauterine, fetal

▶(Do not report modifier '-63' in conjunction with 36460)◀

(For radiological supervision and interpretation, use 76941)

36468   Single or multiple injections of sclerosing solutions, spider veins (telangiectasia); limb or trunk

36469   face

36470*   Injection of sclerosing solution; single vein

36471*   multiple veins, same leg

(36480 has been deleted. To report, use 36488 or 36489)

36481   Percutaneous portal vein catheterization by any method

(For radiological supervision and interpretation, see 75885, 75887)

(36485 has been deleted. To report, use 36490 or 36491)

⊘36488*   Placement of central venous catheter (subclavian, jugular, or other vein) (eg, for central venous pressure, hyperalimentation, hemodialysis, or chemotherapy); percutaneous, age 2 years or under

⊘36489*   percutaneous, over age 2

(If imaging guidance is performed, see 76000, 76003, 76942)

⊘36490*   cutdown, age 2 years or under

⊘36491*   cutdown, over age 2

(For examination of patient and instruction to patient, review of prescription of fluids for long-term or permanent hyperalimentation, use **Evaluation and Management** codes for office or hospital inpatient category or follow-up inpatient consultation codes as appropriate)

36493   Repositioning of previously placed central venous catheter under fluoroscopic guidance

(For fluoroscopic guidance use 76000)

(36495-36497 have been deleted. To report, see 36530-36535)

36500   Venous catheterization for selective organ blood sampling

(For catheterization in superior or inferior vena cava, use 36010)

(For radiological supervision and interpretation, use 75893)

36510*   Catheterization of umbilical vein for diagnosis or therapy, newborn

▶(Do not report modifier '-63' in conjunction with 36510)◀

●36511   Therapeutic apheresis; for white blood cells

●36512   for red blood cells

●36513   for platelets

●36514   for plasma pheresis

●36515   with extracorporeal immunoadsorption and plasma reinfusion

●36516   with extracorporeal selective adsorption or selective filtration and plasma reinfusion

▶(36520 has been deleted. To report see 36511-36512)◀

▶(36521 has been deleted. To report, use 36516)◀

36522   Photopheresis, extracorporeal

36530   Insertion of implantable intravenous infusion pump

(If imaging guidance is performed, see 76000, 76003, 76942)

36531   Revision of implantable intravenous infusion pump

36532   Removal of implantable intravenous infusion pump

(If imaging guidance is performed, use 76000)

36533   Insertion of implantable venous access device, with or without subcutaneous reservoir

(For removal, use 36535)

(If imaging guidance is performed, see 76000, 76003, 76942)

(For refilling and maintenance of an implantable pump or reservoir for ►intravenous or intra-arterial drug delivery,◄ use 96530)

36534   Revision of implantable venous access device, and/or subcutaneous reservoir

(For removal, use 36535)

36535   Removal of implantable venous access device, and/or subcutaneous reservoir

(Use 36535 in conjunction with codes 36533, 36534, as appropriate)

(Do not use 36535 in conjunction with codes 36488-36491)

(If imaging guidance is performed, use 76000)

● **36536**   Mechanical removal of pericatheter obstructive material (eg, fibrin sheath) from central venous device via separate venous access

►(Do not report 36550 in addition to 36536)◄

►For venous catheterization, see 36010-36012)◄

►For radiological supervision and interpretation , use 75901)◄

● **36537**   Mechanical removal of intraluminal (intracatheter) obstructive material from central venous device through device lumen

►(Do not report 36550 in addition to 36537)◄

►(For venous catheterization, see 36010-36012)◄

►(For radiological supervision and interpretation , use 75902)◄

▲ **36540**   Collection of blood specimen from a completely implantable venous access device

►(Do not report 36540 in conjunction with 36415, 36416)◄

►(For collection of venous blood specimen by venipuncture, use 36415)◄

►(For collection of capillary blood specimen, use 36416)◄

36550   Declotting by thrombolytic agent of implanted vascular access device or catheter

Arterial

36600*   Arterial puncture, withdrawal of blood for diagnosis

⊘ **36620**   Arterial catheterization or cannulation for sampling, monitoring or transfusion (separate procedure); percutaneous

36625   cutdown

36640   Arterial catheterization for prolonged infusion therapy (chemotherapy), cutdown

(See also 96420-96425)

(For arterial catheterization for occlusion therapy, see 75894)

⊘ **36660***   Catheterization, umbilical artery, newborn, for diagnosis or therapy

►(Do not report modifier '-63' in conjunction with 36660)◄

Intraosseous

36680   Placement of needle for intraosseous infusion

Hemodialysis Access, Intervascular Cannulation for Extracorporeal Circulation, or Shunt Insertion

36800   Insertion of cannula for hemodialysis, other purpose (separate procedure); vein to vein

36810   arteriovenous, external (Scribner type)

36815   arteriovenous, external revision, or closure

(36820 has been deleted. To report, use 36821)

36819   Arteriovenous anastomosis, open; by upper arm basilic vein transposition

36820   by forearm vein transposition

36821   direct, any site (eg, Cimino type) (separate procedure)

36822   Insertion of cannula(s) for prolonged extracorporeal circulation for cardiopulmonary insufficiency (ECMO) (separate procedure)

(For maintenance of prolonged extracorporeal circulation, see 33960, ►33961◄)

36823   Insertion of arterial and venous cannula(s) for isolated extracorporeal circulation including regional chemotherapy perfusion to an extremity, with or without hyperthermia, with removal of cannula(s) and repair of arteriotomy and venotomy sites

(36823 includes chemotherapy perfusion supported by a membrane oxygenator/perfusion pump. Do not report 96408-96425 in conjunction with 36823)

36825   Creation of arteriovenous fistula by other than direct arteriovenous anastomosis (separate procedure); autogenous graft

(For direct arteriovenous anastomosis, use 36821)

▲**36830**   nonautogenous graft (eg, biological collagen, thermoplastic graft)

(For direct arteriovenous anastomosis, use 36821)

36831   Thrombectomy, open, arteriovenous fistula without revision, autogenous or nonautogenous dialysis graft (separate procedure)

36832   Revision, open, arteriovenous fistula; without thrombectomy, autogenous or nonautogenous dialysis graft (separate procedure)

36833   with thrombectomy, autogenous or nonautogenous dialysis graft (separate procedure)

36834   Plastic repair of arteriovenous aneurysm (separate procedure)

36835   Insertion of Thomas shunt (separate procedure)

(36840 has been deleted)

(36845 has been deleted)

36860   External cannula declotting (separate procedure); without balloon catheter

36861   with balloon catheter

(If imaging guidance is performed, use 76000)

36870   Thrombectomy, percutaneous, arteriovenous fistula, autogenous or nonautogenous graft (includes mechanical thrombus extraction and intra-graft thrombolysis)

(Do not report 36550 in conjunction with code 36870)

(For catheterization, use 36145)

(For radiological supervision and interpretation, use 75790)

Portal Decompression Procedures

▲**37140**   Venous anastomosis, open; portocaval

(For peritoneal-venous shunt, use 49425)

37145   renoportal

37160   caval-mesenteric

37180   splenorenal, proximal

37181   splenorenal, distal (selective decompression of esophagogastric varices, any technique)

►(For percutaneous procedure, use 37182)◄

(37190 has been deleted. To report, use 36834)

●**37182**   Insertion of transvenous intrahepatic portosystemic shunt(s) (TIPS) (includes venous access, hepatic and portal vein catheterization, portography with hemodynamic evaluation, intrahepatic tract formation/ dilatation, stent placement and all associated imaging guidance and documentation)

►(Do not report 75885 or 75887 in conjunction with code 37182)◄

►(For open procedure, use 37140)◄

●**37183**   Revision of transvenous intrahepatic portosystemic shunt(s) (TIPS) (includes venous access, hepatic and portal vein catheterization, portography with hemodynamic evaluation, intrahepatic tract recanulization/dilatation, stent placement and all associated imaging guidance and documentation)

►(Do not report 75885 or 75887 in conjunction with code 37183)◄

Transcatheter Procedures

Codes for catheter placement and the radiologic supervision and interpretation should also be reported, in addition to the code(s) for the therapeutic aspect of the procedure.

37195   Thrombolysis, cerebral, by intravenous infusion

37200   Transcatheter biopsy

(For radiological supervision and interpretation, use 75970)

37201   Transcatheter therapy, infusion for thrombolysis other than coronary

(For radiological supervision and interpretation, use 75896)

37202   Transcatheter therapy, infusion other than for thrombolysis, any type (eg, spasmolytic, vasoconstrictive)

(For thrombolysis of coronary vessels, see 92975, 92977)

(For radiological supervision and interpretation, use 75896)

37203   Transcatheter retrieval, percutaneous, of intravascular foreign body (eg, fractured venous or arterial catheter)

(For radiological supervision and interpretation, use 75961)

37204   Transcatheter occlusion or embolization (eg, for tumor destruction, to achieve hemostasis, to occlude a vascular malformation), percutaneous, any method, non-central nervous system, non-head or neck

(See also 61624, 61626)

(For radiological supervision and interpretation, use 75894)

37205 Transcatheter placement of an intravascular stent(s), (non-coronary vessel), percutaneous; initial vessel

(For radiological supervision and interpretation, use 75960)

+ 37206 each additional vessel (List separately in addition to code for primary procedure)

(Use 37206 in conjunction with code 37205)

(For transcatheter placement of extracranial cerebrovascular artery stent(s), see Category III codes 0005T, 0006T)

(For radiological supervision and interpretation, use 75960)

37207 Transcatheter placement of an intravascular stent(s), (non-coronary vessel), open; initial vessel

+ 37208 each additional vessel (List separately in addition to code for primary procedure)

(Use 37208 in conjunction with code 37207)

(For radiological supervision and interpretation, use 75960)

(For catheterizations, see 36215-36248)

(For transcatheter placement of intracoronary stent(s), see 92980, 92981)

37209 Exchange of a previously placed arterial catheter during thrombolytic therapy

(For radiological supervision and interpretation, use 75900)

Intravascular Ultrasound Services

Intravascular ultrasound services include all transducer manipulations and repositioning within the specific vessel being examined, both before and after therapeutic intervention (eg, stent placement).

Vascular access for intravascular ultrasound performed during a therapeutic intervention is not reported separately.

+ 37250 Intravascular ultrasound (non-coronary vessel) during diagnostic evaluation and/or therapeutic intervention; initial vessel (List separately in addition to code for primary procedure)

+ 37251 each additional vessel (List separately in addition to code for primary procedure)

(Use 37251 in conjunction with code 37250)

(For catheterizations, see 36215-36248)

(For transcatheter therapies, see 37200-37208, 61624, 61626)

(For radiological supervision and interpretation see 75945, 75946)

►Endoscopy◄

►Surgical vascular endoscopy always includes diagnostic endoscopy.◄

● **37500** Vascular endoscopy, surgical, with ligation of perforator veins, subfascial (SEPS)

►(For open procedure, use 37760)◄

● **37501** Unlisted vascular endoscopy procedure

Ligation and Other Procedures

(37400-37560 have been deleted. To report, see 35201-35286)

37565 Ligation, internal jugular vein

37600 Ligation; external carotid artery

37605 internal or common carotid artery

37606 internal or common carotid artery, with gradual occlusion, as with Selverstone or Crutchfield clamp

►(For transcatheter permanent arterial occlusion or embolization, see 61624-61626)◄

►(For endovascular temporary arterial balloon occlusion, use 61623)◄

(For ligation treatment of intracranial aneurysm, use 61703)

37607 Ligation or banding of angioaccess arteriovenous fistula

37609 Ligation or biopsy, temporal artery

37615 Ligation, major artery (eg, post-traumatic, rupture); neck

37616 chest

37617 abdomen

37618 extremity

37620 Interruption, partial or complete, of inferior vena cava by suture, ligation, plication, clip, extravascular, intravascular (umbrella device)

(For radiological supervision and interpretation, use 75940)

37650 Ligation of femoral vein

(37651 has been deleted. To report, use 37650 with modifier '-50')

37660 Ligation of common iliac vein

37700 Ligation and division of long saphenous vein at saphenofemoral junction, or distal interruptions

(37701 has been deleted. To report, use 37700 with modifier '-50')

37720   Ligation and division and complete stripping of long or short saphenous veins

(37721 has been deleted. To report, use 37720 with modifier '-50')

37730   Ligation and division and complete stripping of long and short saphenous veins

(37731 has been deleted. To report, use 37730 with modifier '-50')

37735   Ligation and division and complete stripping of long or short saphenous veins with radical excision of ulcer and skin graft and/or interruption of communicating veins of lower leg, with excision of deep fascia

(37737 has been deleted. To report, use 37735 with modifier '-50')

▲ **37760**   Ligation of perforator veins, subfascial, radical (Linton type), with or without skin graft, open

►(For endoscopic procedure, use 37500)◄

37780   Ligation and division of short saphenous vein at saphenopopliteal junction (separate procedure)

(37781 has been deleted. To report, use 37780 with modifier '-50')

37785   Ligation, division, and/or excision of recurrent or secondary varicose veins (clusters), one leg

(37787 has been deleted. To report, use 37785 with modifier '-50')

37788   Penile revascularization, artery, with or without vein graft

37790   Penile venous occlusive procedure

37799   Unlisted procedure, vascular surgery

Hemic and Lymphatic Systems

Spleen

Excision

(38090 has been deleted. To report, use 38999)

38100   Splenectomy; total (separate procedure)

38101   partial (separate procedure)

+ **38102**   total, en bloc for extensive disease, in conjunction with other procedure (List in addition to code for primary procedure)

Repair

38115   Repair of ruptured spleen (splenorrhaphy) with or without partial splenectomy

Laparoscopy

Surgical laparoscopy always includes diagnostic laparoscopy. To report a diagnostic laparoscopy (peritoneoscopy) (separate procedure), use 49320.

38120   Laparoscopy, surgical, splenectomy

38129   Unlisted laparoscopy procedure, spleen

Introduction

38200   Injection procedure for splenoportography

(For radiological supervision and interpretation, use 75810)

General

Bone Marrow or Stem Cell Services/Procedures

● **38204**   Management of recipient hematopoietic progenitor cell donor search and cell acquisition

● **38205**   Blood-derived hematopoietic progenitor cell harvesting for transplantation, per collection; allogenic

● **38206**   autologous

● **38207**   Transplant preparation of hematopoietic progenitor cells; cryopreservation and storage

►(For diagnostic cryopreservation and storage, see 88240)◄

● **38208**   thawing of previously frozen harvest

►(For diagnostic thawing and expansion of frozen cells, see 88241)◄

● **38209**   washing of harvest

● **38210**   specific cell depletion within harvest, T-cell depletion

● **38211**   tumor cell depletion

● **38212**   red blood cell removal

● **38213**   platelet depletion

● **38214**   plasma (volume) depletion

● **38215**   cell concentration in plasma, mononuclear, or buffy coat layer

▲ **38220**   Bone marrow; aspiration only

▲ **38221**   biopsy, needle or trocar

(For bone marrow biopsy interpretation, use 88305)

38230 Bone marrow harvesting for transplantation

▶(38231 has been deleted. To report, use 38205-38206)◀

38240 Bone marrow or blood-derived peripheral stem cell transplantation; allogenic

38241 autologous

● **38242** allogeneic donor lymphocyte infusions

(For bone marrow aspiration, use 38220)

(For modification, treatment, and processing of bone marrow or blood-derived stem cell specimens for transplantation, use 86915)

(For cryopreservation, freezing and storage of blood-derived stem cells for transplantation, use 88240)

(For thawing and expansion of blood-derived stem cells for transplantation, use 88241)

(For compatibility studies, see 86812-86822)

Lymph Nodes and Lymphatic Channels

Incision

38300* Drainage of lymph node abscess or lymphadenitis; simple

38305 extensive

38308 Lymphangiotomy or other operations on lymphatic channels

38380 Suture and/or ligation of thoracic duct; cervical approach

38381 thoracic approach

38382 abdominal approach

Excision

(For injection for sentinel node identification, use 38792)

38500 Biopsy or excision of lymph node(s); open, superficial

(Do not report 38500 with 38700-38780)

38505 by needle, superficial (eg, cervical, inguinal, axillary)

(If imaging guidance is performed, see 76360, 76393, 76942)

(For fine needle aspiration, use 10021 or 10022)

(For evaluation of fine needle aspirate, see 88172, 88173)

38510 open, deep cervical node(s)

38520 open, deep cervical node(s) with excision scalene fat pad

38525 open, deep axillary node(s)

38530 open, internal mammary node(s)

(Do not report 38530 with 38720-38746)

(For percutaneous needle biopsy, retroperitoneal lymph node or mass, use 49180. For fine needle aspiration, use 10022)

(38540 has been deleted. To report, see 38510, 38520)

38542 Dissection, deep jugular node(s)

(For radical cervical neck dissection, use 38720)

38550 Excision of cystic hygroma, axillary or cervical; without deep neurovascular dissection

38555 with deep neurovascular dissection

Limited Lymphadenectomy for Staging

38562 Limited lymphadenectomy for staging (separate procedure); pelvic and para-aortic

(When combined with prostatectomy, use 55812 or 55842)

(When combined with insertion of radioactive substance into prostate, use 55862)

38564 retroperitoneal (aortic and/or splenic)

Laparoscopy

Surgical laparoscopy always includes diagnostic laparoscopy. To report a diagnostic laparoscopy (peritoneoscopy) (separate procedure), use 49320.

38570 Laparoscopy, surgical; with retroperitoneal lymph node sampling (biopsy), single or multiple

38571 with bilateral total pelvic lymphadenectomy

38572 with bilateral total pelvic lymphadenectomy and peri-aortic lymph node sampling (biopsy), single or multiple

(For drainage of lymphocele to peritoneal cavity, use 49323)

38589 Unlisted laparoscopy procedure, lymphatic system

Radical Lymphadenectomy (Radical Resection of Lymph Nodes)

(For limited pelvic and retroperitoneal lymphadenectomies, see 38562, 38564)

38700 Suprahyoid lymphadenectomy

(38701 has been deleted. To report, use 38700 with modifier '-50')

38720 Cervical lymphadenectomy (complete)

(38721 has been deleted. To report, use 38720 with modifier '-50')

38724	Cervical lymphadenectomy (modified radical neck dissection)
38740	Axillary lymphadenectomy; superficial
38745	complete
+ 38746	Thoracic lymphadenectomy, regional, including mediastinal and peritracheal nodes (List separately in addition to code for primary procedure)
+ 38747	Abdominal lymphadenectomy, regional, including celiac, gastric, portal, peripancreatic, with or without para-aortic and vena caval nodes (List separately in addition to code for primary procedure)
38760	Inguinofemoral lymphadenectomy, superficial, including Cloquets node (separate procedure)

(38761 has been deleted. To report, use 38760 with modifier '-50')

38765	Inguinofemoral lymphadenectomy, superficial, in continuity with pelvic lymphadenectomy, including external iliac, hypogastric, and obturator nodes (separate procedure)

(38766 has been deleted. To report, use 38765 with modifier '-50')

38770	Pelvic lymphadenectomy, including external iliac, hypogastric, and obturator nodes (separate procedure)

(38771 has been deleted. To report, use 38770 with modifier '-50')

38780	Retroperitoneal transabdominal lymphadenectomy, extensive, including pelvic, aortic, and renal nodes (separate procedure)

(For excision and repair of lymphedematous skin and subcutaneous tissue, see 15000, 15570-15650)

Introduction

38790	Injection procedure; lymphangiography

(For radiological supervision and interpretation, see 75801-75807)

(38791 has been deleted. To report, use 38790 with modifier '-50')

⊘ 38792	for identification of sentinel node

(For excision of sentinel node, see 38500-38542)

(For nuclear medicine lymphatics and lymph gland imaging, use 78195)

38794	Cannulation, thoracic duct

Other Procedures

38999	Unlisted procedure, hemic or lymphatic system

Mediastinum and Diaphragm

Mediastinum

Incision

39000	Mediastinotomy with exploration, drainage, removal of foreign body, or biopsy; cervical approach
39010	transthoracic approach, including either transthoracic or median sternotomy

(39020 has been deleted. To report, use 39010)

(39050-39070 have been deleted. To report, see 39000-39010)

Excision

39200	Excision of mediastinal cyst
39220	Excision of mediastinal tumor

(For substernal thyroidectomy, use 60270)

(For thymectomy, use 60520)

Endoscopy

39400	Mediastinoscopy, with or without biopsy

Other Procedures

39499	Unlisted procedure, mediastinum

Diaphragm

Repair

(39500 has been deleted. To report, see 43324, 43325)

39501	Repair, laceration of diaphragm, any approach
39502	Repair, paraesophageal hiatus hernia, transabdominal, with or without fundoplasty, vagotomy, and/or pyloroplasty, except neonatal
39503	Repair, neonatal diaphragmatic hernia, with or without chest tube insertion and with or without creation of ventral hernia

▶(Do not report modifier '-63' in conjunction with 39503)◀

(39510 has been deleted. To report, see 43324, 43325)

39520	Repair, diaphragmatic hernia (esophageal hiatal); transthoracic
39530	combined, thoracoabdominal
39531	combined, thoracoabdominal, with dilation of stricture (with or without gastroplasty)

39540 Repair, diaphragmatic hernia (other than neonatal), traumatic; acute

39541 chronic

39545 Imbrication of diaphragm for eventration, transthoracic or transabdominal, paralytic or nonparalytic

(39547 has been deleted. To report, use 39545)

39560 Resection, diaphragm; with simple repair (eg, primary suture)

39561 with complex repair (eg, prosthetic material, local muscle flap)

Other Procedures

39599 Unlisted procedure, diaphragm

Digestive System

Lips

(For procedures on skin of lips, see 10040 et seq)

Excision

40490   Biopsy of lip

40500   Vermilionectomy (lip shave), with mucosal advancement

40510   Excision of lip; transverse wedge excision with primary closure

40520   V-excision with primary direct linear closure

    (For excision of mucous lesions, see 40810-40816)

40525   full thickness, reconstruction with local flap (eg, Estlander or fan)

40527   full thickness, reconstruction with cross lip flap (Abbe-Estlander)

40530   Resection of lip, more than one-fourth, without reconstruction

    (For reconstruction, see 13131 et seq)

Repair (Cheiloplasty)

40650   Repair lip, full thickness; vermilion only

40652   up to half vertical height

40654   over one-half vertical height, or complex

40700   Plastic repair of cleft lip/nasal deformity; primary, partial or complete, unilateral

40701   primary bilateral, one stage procedure

40702   primary bilateral, one of two stages

40720   secondary, by recreation of defect and reclosure

    (To report rhinoplasty only for nasal deformity secondary to congenital cleft lip, see 30460, 30462)

    (40740 has been deleted. To report, use 40720 with modifier '-50')

    (40760 has been deleted. To report, use 40527)

40761   with cross lip pedicle flap (Abbe-Estlander type), including sectioning and inserting of pedicle

    (For repair cleft palate, see 42200 et seq)

    (For other reconstructive procedures, see 14060, 14061, 15120-15261, 15574, 15576, 15630)

Other Procedures

40799   Unlisted procedure, lips

Vestibule of Mouth

The vestibule is the part of the oral cavity outside the dentoalveolar structures; it includes the mucosal and submucosal tissue of lips and cheeks.

Incision

40800*   Drainage of abscess, cyst, hematoma, vestibule of mouth; simple

40801   complicated

40804*   Removal of embedded foreign body, vestibule of mouth; simple

40805   complicated

40806   Incision of labial frenum (frenotomy)

Excision, Destruction

40808   Biopsy, vestibule of mouth

40810   Excision of lesion of mucosa and submucosa, vestibule of mouth; without repair

40812   with simple repair

40814   with complex repair

40816   complex, with excision of underlying muscle

40818   Excision of mucosa of vestibule of mouth as donor graft

40819   Excision of frenum, labial or buccal (frenumectomy, frenulectomy, frenectomy)

40820   Destruction of lesion or scar of vestibule of mouth by physical methods (eg, laser, thermal, cryo, chemical)

Repair

40830   Closure of laceration, vestibule of mouth; 2.5 cm or less

40831   over 2.5 cm or complex

40840   Vestibuloplasty; anterior

40842   posterior, unilateral

40843   posterior, bilateral

40844   entire arch

40845   complex (including ridge extension, muscle repositioning)

    (For skin grafts, see 15000 et seq)

Other Procedures

40899   Unlisted procedure, vestibule of mouth

Surgery: Digestive System

Tongue and Floor of Mouth

Incision

41000* Intraoral incision and drainage of abscess, cyst, or hematoma of tongue or floor of mouth; lingual

41005* sublingual, superficial

41006 sublingual, deep, supramylohyoid

41007 submental space

41008 submandibular space

41009 masticator space

41010 Incision of lingual frenum (frenotomy)

41015 Extraoral incision and drainage of abscess, cyst, or hematoma of floor of mouth; sublingual

41016 submental

41017 submandibular

41018 masticator space

(For frenoplasty, use 41520)

Excision

41100 Biopsy of tongue; anterior two-thirds

41105 posterior one-third

41108 Biopsy of floor of mouth

41110 Excision of lesion of tongue without closure

41112 Excision of lesion of tongue with closure; anterior two-thirds

41113 posterior one-third

41114 with local tongue flap

(List 41114 in addition to code 41112 or 41113)

41115 Excision of lingual frenum (frenectomy)

41116 Excision, lesion of floor of mouth

41120 Glossectomy; less than one-half tongue

41130 hemiglossectomy

41135 partial, with unilateral radical neck dissection

41140 complete or total, with or without tracheostomy, without radical neck dissection

41145 complete or total, with or without tracheostomy, with unilateral radical neck dissection

41150 composite procedure with resection floor of mouth and mandibular resection, without radical neck dissection

41153 composite procedure with resection floor of mouth, with suprahyoid neck dissection

41155 composite procedure with resection floor of mouth, mandibular resection, and radical neck dissection (Commando type)

Repair

41250* Repair of laceration 2.5 cm or less; floor of mouth and/or anterior two-thirds of tongue

41251* posterior one-third of tongue

41252* Repair of laceration of tongue, floor of mouth, over 2.6 cm or complex

Other Procedures

41500 Fixation of tongue, mechanical, other than suture (eg, K-wire)

41510 Suture of tongue to lip for micrognathia (Douglas type procedure)

41520 Frenoplasty (surgical revision of frenum, eg, with Z-plasty)

(For frenotomy, see 40806, 41010)

41599 Unlisted procedure, tongue, floor of mouth

Dentoalveolar Structures

Incision

41800* Drainage of abscess, cyst, hematoma from dentoalveolar structures

41805 Removal of embedded foreign body from dentoalveolar structures; soft tissues

41806 bone

Excision, Destruction

41820 Gingivectomy, excision gingiva, each quadrant

41821 Operculectomy, excision pericoronal tissues

41822 Excision of fibrous tuberosities, dentoalveolar structures

41823 Excision of osseous tuberosities, dentoalveolar structures

41825 Excision of lesion or tumor (except listed above), dentoalveolar structures; without repair

41826 with simple repair

41827 with complex repair

(For nonexcisional destruction, use 41850)

41828 Excision of hyperplastic alveolar mucosa, each quadrant (specify)

41830 Alveolectomy, including curettage of osteitis or sequestrectomy

41850 Destruction of lesion (except excision), dentoalveolar structures

Other Procedures

41870 Periodontal mucosal grafting

41872 Gingivoplasty, each quadrant (specify)

41874	Alveoloplasty, each quadrant (specify)
	(For closure of lacerations, see 40830, 40831)
	(For segmental osteotomy, use 21206)
	(For reduction of fractures, see 21421-21490)
41899	Unlisted procedure, dentoalveolar structures

Palate and Uvula

Incision

42000* Drainage of abscess of palate, uvula

Excision, Destruction

42100	Biopsy of palate, uvula
42104	Excision, lesion of palate, uvula; without closure
42106	with simple primary closure
42107	with local flap closure
	(For skin graft, see 14040-14300)
	(For mucosal graft, use 40818)
42120	Resection of palate or extensive resection of lesion
	(For reconstruction of palate with extraoral tissue, see 14040-14300, 15050, 15120, 15240, 15576)
42140	Uvulectomy, excision of uvula
42145	Palatopharyngoplasty (eg, uvulopalatopharyngoplasty, uvulopharyngoplasty)
	(42150 has been deleted. To report, see 21031, 21032)
42160	Destruction of lesion, palate or uvula (thermal, cryo or chemical)

Repair

42180	Repair, laceration of palate; up to 2 cm
42182	over 2 cm or complex
42200	Palatoplasty for cleft palate, soft and/or hard palate only
42205	Palatoplasty for cleft palate, with closure of alveolar ridge; soft tissue only
42210	with bone graft to alveolar ridge (includes obtaining graft)
42215	Palatoplasty for cleft palate; major revision
42220	secondary lengthening procedure
42225	attachment pharyngeal flap
42226	Lengthening of palate, and pharyngeal flap
42227	Lengthening of palate, with island flap
42235	Repair of anterior palate, including vomer flap
	(42250 has been deleted. To report, use 30600)

42260	Repair of nasolabial fistula
	(For repair of cleft lip, see 40700 et seq)
42280	Maxillary impression for palatal prosthesis
42281	Insertion of pin-retained palatal prosthesis

Other Procedures

42299 Unlisted procedure, palate, uvula

Salivary Gland and Ducts

Incision

42300*	Drainage of abscess; parotid, simple
42305	parotid, complicated
42310*	Drainage of abscess; submaxillary or sublingual, intraoral
42320*	submaxillary, external
42325	Fistulization of sublingual salivary cyst (ranula);
42326	with prosthesis
42330	Sialolithotomy; submandibular (submaxillary), sublingual or parotid, uncomplicated, intraoral
42335	submandibular (submaxillary), complicated, intraoral
42340	parotid, extraoral or complicated intraoral

Excision

42400*	Biopsy of salivary gland; needle
	▶(For fine needle aspiration, see 10021, 10022)◀
	▶(For evaluation of fine needle aspirate, see 88172, 88173)◀
	(If imaging guidance is performed, see 76003, 76360, 76393, 76942)
42405	incisional
	(If imaging guidance is performed, see 76003, 76360, 76393, 76942)
42408	Excision of sublingual salivary cyst (ranula)
42409	Marsupialization of sublingual salivary cyst (ranula)
	(For fistulization of sublingual salivary cyst, use 42325)
42410	Excision of parotid tumor or parotid gland; lateral lobe, without nerve dissection
42415	lateral lobe, with dissection and preservation of facial nerve
42420	total, with dissection and preservation of facial nerve
42425	total, en bloc removal with sacrifice of facial nerve
42426	total, with unilateral radical neck dissection
	(For suture or grafting of facial nerve, see 64864, 64865, 69740, 69745)

42440 Excision of submandibular (submaxillary) gland

42450 Excision of sublingual gland

Repair

42500 Plastic repair of salivary duct, sialodochoplasty; primary or simple

42505 secondary or complicated

42507 Parotid duct diversion, bilateral (Wilke type procedure);

42508 with excision of one submandibular gland

42509 with excision of both submandibular glands

42510 with ligation of both submandibular (Wharton's) ducts

Other Procedures

42550 Injection procedure for sialography

(For radiological supervision and interpretation, use 70390)

42600 Closure salivary fistula

42650* Dilation salivary duct

42660* Dilation and catheterization of salivary duct, with or without injection

42665 Ligation salivary duct, intraoral

42699 Unlisted procedure, salivary glands or ducts

Pharynx, Adenoids, and Tonsils

Incision

42700* Incision and drainage abscess; peritonsillar

42720 retropharyngeal or parapharyngeal, intraoral approach

42725 retropharyngeal or parapharyngeal, external approach

Excision, Destruction

42800 Biopsy; oropharynx

42802 hypopharynx

42804 nasopharynx, visible lesion, simple

42806 nasopharynx, survey for unknown primary lesion

(For laryngoscopic biopsy, see 31510, 31535, 31536)

42808 Excision or destruction of lesion of pharynx, any method

42809 Removal of foreign body from pharynx

42810 Excision branchial cleft cyst or vestige, confined to skin and subcutaneous tissues

42815 Excision branchial cleft cyst, vestige, or fistula, extending beneath subcutaneous tissues and/or into pharynx

42820 Tonsillectomy and adenoidectomy; under age 12

42821 age 12 or over

42825 Tonsillectomy, primary or secondary; under age 12

42826 age 12 or over

42830 Adenoidectomy, primary; under age 12

42831 age 12 or over

42835 Adenoidectomy, secondary; under age 12

42836 age 12 or over

42842 Radical resection of tonsil, tonsillar pillars, and/or retromolar trigone; without closure

42844 closure with local flap (eg, tongue, buccal)

42845 closure with other flap

(For closure with other flap(s), use appropriate number for flap(s))

(When combined with radical neck dissection, use also 38720)

42860 Excision of tonsil tags

42870 Excision or destruction lingual tonsil, any method (separate procedure)

(42880 has been deleted. For resection of the nasopharynx (eg, juvenile angiofibroma) by bicoronal and/or transzygomatic approach, see 61586 and 61600)

42890 Limited pharyngectomy

42892 Resection of lateral pharyngeal wall or pyriform sinus, direct closure by advancement of lateral and posterior pharyngeal walls

(When combined with radical neck dissection, use also 38720)

42894 Resection of pharyngeal wall requiring closure with myocutaneous flap

(When combined with radical neck dissection, use also 38720)

(42895 has been deleted. To report, use 38720 with 42890)

Repair

42900 Suture pharynx for wound or injury

42950 Pharyngoplasty (plastic or reconstructive operation on pharynx)

(For pharyngeal flap, use 42225)

42953 Pharyngoesophageal repair

(For closure with myocutaneous or other flap, use appropriate number in addition)

Surgery: Digestive System

Other Procedures

42955 Pharyngostomy (fistulization of pharynx, external for feeding)

42960 Control oropharyngeal hemorrhage, primary or secondary (eg, post-tonsillectomy); simple

42961 complicated, requiring hospitalization

42962 with secondary surgical intervention

42970 Control of nasopharyngeal hemorrhage, primary or secondary (eg, postadenoidectomy); simple, with posterior nasal packs, with or without anterior packs and/or cautery

42971 complicated, requiring hospitalization

42972 with secondary surgical intervention

42999 Unlisted procedure, pharynx, adenoids, or tonsils

Esophagus

Incision

(For esophageal intubation with laparotomy, use 43510)

(43000 has been deleted)

43020 Esophagotomy, cervical approach, with removal of foreign body

43030 Cricopharyngeal myotomy

(43040 has been deleted)

43045 Esophagotomy, thoracic approach, with removal of foreign body

Excision

(For gastrointestinal reconstruction for previous esophagectomy, see 43360, 43361)

43100 Excision of lesion, esophagus, with primary repair; cervical approach

43101 thoracic or abdominal approach

(43105 has been deleted. To report, see 43107, 43116, 43124, and 31360)

(43106 has been deleted. To report, see 43107, 43116, 43124, and 31365)

43107 Total or near total esophagectomy, without thoracotomy; with pharyngogastrostomy or cervical esophagogastrostomy, with or without pyloroplasty (transhiatal)

43108 with colon interposition or small intestine reconstruction, including intestine mobilization, preparation and anastomosis(es)

(43110 has been deleted. To report, see 43107-43113)

(43111 has been deleted. To report, see 43107-43113)

43112 Total or near total esophagectomy, with thoracotomy; with pharyngogastrostomy or cervical esophagogastrostomy, with or without pyloroplasty

43113 with colon interposition or small intestine reconstruction, including intestine mobilization, preparation, and anastomosis(es)

(43115 has been deleted. To report, see 43116-43118)

43116 Partial esophagectomy, cervical, with free intestinal graft, including microvascular anastomosis, obtaining the graft and intestinal reconstruction

(Do not report code 69990 in addition to code 43116)

(Report 43116 with the modifier '-52' appended if intestinal or free jejunal graft with microvascular anastomosis is performed by another physician)

(For free jejunal graft with microvascular anastomosis performed by another physician, use 43496)

43117 Partial esophagectomy, distal two-thirds, with thoracotomy and separate abdominal incision, with or without proximal gastrectomy; with thoracic esophagogastrostomy, with or without pyloroplasty (Ivor Lewis)

43118 with colon interposition or small intestine reconstruction, including intestine mobilization, preparation, and anastomosis(es)

(43119 has been deleted. To report, see 43107, 43124)

(43120 has been deleted. To report, use 43122)

43121 Partial esophagectomy, distal two-thirds, with thoracotomy only, with or without proximal gastrectomy, with thoracic esophagogastrostomy, with or without pyloroplasty

43122 Partial esophagectomy, thoracoabdominal or abdominal approach, with or without proximal gastrectomy; with esophagogastrostomy, with or without pyloroplasty

43123 with colon interposition or small intestine reconstruction, including intestine mobilization, preparation, and anastomosis(es)

43124 Total or partial esophagectomy, without reconstruction (any approach), with cervical esophagostomy

43130 Diverticulectomy of hypopharynx or esophagus, with or without myotomy; cervical approach

43135 thoracic approach

(43136 has been deleted. To report, use 43499)

Surgery: Digestive System

Endoscopy

For endoscopic procedures, code appropriate endoscopy of each anatomic site examined.

Surgical endoscopy always includes diagnostic endoscopy.

43200   Esophagoscopy, rigid or flexible; diagnostic, with or without collection of specimen(s) by brushing or washing (separate procedure)

●**43201**   with directed submucosal injection(s), any substance

▶(For injection sclerosis of esophageal varices, use 43204)◀

43202   with biopsy, single or multiple

43204   with injection sclerosis of esophageal varices

43205   with band ligation of esophageal varices

43215   with removal of foreign body

(For radiological supervision and interpretation, use 74235)

43216   with removal of tumor(s), polyp(s), or other lesion(s) by hot biopsy forceps or bipolar cautery

43217   with removal of tumor(s), polyp(s), or other lesion(s) by snare technique

(43218 has been deleted. To report, use 43499)

43219   with insertion of plastic tube or stent

43220   with balloon dilation (less than 30 mm diameter)

(If imaging guidance is performed, use 74360)

(For endoscopic dilation with balloon 30 mm diameter or larger, use 43458)

(For dilation without visualization, use 43450-43453)

(43221 has been deleted. To report, use 43200 or 43235)

(43222 has been deleted. To report, use 43200, 43202, 43235, or 43239)

(43223 has been deleted. To report, use 43215 or 43247)

(43224 has been deleted. To report, use 43217 or 43251)

(43225 has been deleted. To report, use 43499)

43226   with insertion of guide wire followed by dilation over guide wire

(For radiological supervision and interpretation, use 74360)

43227   with control of bleeding (eg, injection, bipolar cautery, unipolar cautery, laser, heater probe, stapler, plasma coagulator)

43228   with ablation of tumor(s), polyp(s), or other lesion(s), not amenable to removal by hot biopsy forceps, bipolar cautery or snare technique

(For esophagoscopic photodynamic therapy, report 43228 in addition to 96570, 96571 as appropriate)

43231   with endoscopic ultrasound examination

43232   with transendoscopic ultrasound-guided intramural or transmural fine needle aspiration/biopsy(s)

(Do not report 76975 in conjunction with 43231, 43232)

(For interpretation of specimen, see 88172-88173)

43234   Upper gastrointestinal endoscopy, simple primary examination (eg, with small diameter flexible endoscope) (separate procedure)

43235   Upper gastrointestinal endoscopy including esophagus, stomach, and either the duodenum and/or jejunum as appropriate; diagnostic, with or without collection of specimen(s) by brushing or washing (separate procedure)

●**43236**   with directed submucosal injection(s), any substance

▶(For injection sclerosis of esophageal and/or gastric varices, use 43243)◀

43239   with biopsy, single or multiple

(For upper gastrointestinal endoscopy with suturing of the esophagogastric junction, use Category III code 0008T)

43240   with transmural drainage of pseudocyst

43241   with transendoscopic intraluminal tube or catheter placement

43242   with transendoscopic ultrasound-guided intramural or transmural fine needle aspiration/biopsy(s)

(Do not report 76975 in conjunction with 43242)

(For interpretation of specimen, see 88172-88173)

43243   with injection sclerosis of esophageal and/or gastric varices

43244   with band ligation of esophageal and/or gastric varices

43245   with dilation of gastric outlet for obstruction (eg, balloon, guide wire, bougie)

▶(Do not report 43245 in conjunction with 43256)◀

43246   with directed placement of percutaneous gastrostomy tube

(For radiological supervision and interpretation, use 74350)

43247   with removal of foreign body

(For radiological supervision and interpretation, use 74235)

43248   with insertion of guide wire followed by dilation of esophagus over guide wire

43249   with balloon dilation of esophagus (less than 30 mm diameter)

43250   with removal of tumor(s), polyp(s), or other lesion(s) by hot biopsy forceps or bipolar cautery

43251   with removal of tumor(s), polyp(s), or other lesion(s) by snare technique

43255   with control of bleeding, any method

43256   with transendoscopic stent placement (includes predilation)

43258   with ablation of tumor(s), polyp(s), or other lesion(s) not amenable to removal by hot biopsy forceps, bipolar cautery or snare technique

(For injection sclerosis of esophageal varices, use 43204 or 43243)

43259   with endoscopic ultrasound examination

(For radiological supervision and interpretation, use 76975)

43260   Endoscopic retrograde cholangiopancreatography (ERCP); diagnostic, with or without collection of specimen(s) by brushing or washing (separate procedure)

(For radiological supervision and interpretation, see 74328, 74329, 74330)

43261   with biopsy, single or multiple

43262   with sphincterotomy/papillotomy

(For radiological supervision and interpretation, see 74328, 74329, 74330)

43263   with pressure measurement of sphincter of Oddi (pancreatic duct or common bile duct)

(For radiological supervision and interpretation, see 74328, 74329, 74330)

43264   with endoscopic retrograde removal of calculus/calculi from biliary and/or pancreatic ducts

(When done with sphincterotomy, also use 43262)

(For radiological supervision and interpretation, see 74328, 74329, 74330)

43265   with endoscopic retrograde destruction, lithotripsy of calculus/calculi, any method

(When done with sphincterotomy, also use 43262)

(For radiological supervision and interpretation, see 74328, 74329, 74330)

43267   with endoscopic retrograde insertion of nasobiliary or nasopancreatic drainage tube

(When done with sphincterotomy, also use 43262)

(For radiological supervision and interpretation, see 74328, 74329, 74330)

43268   with endoscopic retrograde insertion of tube or stent into bile or pancreatic duct

(When done with sphincterotomy, also use 43262)

(For radiological supervision and interpretation, see 74328, 74329, 74330)

43269   with endoscopic retrograde removal of foreign body and/or change of tube or stent

(When done with sphincterotomy, also use 43262)

(For radiological supervision and interpretation, see 74328, 74329, 74330)

43271   with endoscopic retrograde balloon dilation of ampulla, biliary and/or pancreatic duct(s)

(When done with sphincterotomy, also use 43262)

(For radiological supervision and interpretation, see 74328, 74329, 74330)

43272   with ablation of tumor(s), polyp(s), or other lesion(s) not amenable to removal by hot biopsy forceps, bipolar cautery or snare technique

(For radiological supervision and interpretation, see 74328, 74329, 74330)

Laparoscopy

Surgical laparoscopy always includes diagnostic laparoscopy. To report a diagnostic laparoscopy (peritoneoscopy) (separate procedure), use 49320.

43280   Laparoscopy, surgical, esophagogastric fundoplasty (eg, Nissen, Toupet procedures)

(For open approach, use 43324)

43289   Unlisted laparoscopy procedure, esophagus

Repair

43300   Esophagoplasty (plastic repair or reconstruction), cervical approach; without repair of tracheoesophageal fistula

43305   with repair of tracheoesophageal fistula

43310   Esophagoplasty (plastic repair or reconstruction), thoracic approach; without repair of tracheoesophageal fistula

43312   with repair of tracheoesophageal fistula

43313   Esophagoplasty for congenital defect (plastic repair or reconstruction), thoracic approach; without repair of congenital tracheoesophageal fistula

43314   with repair of congenital tracheoesophageal fistula

▶(Do not report modifier '-63' in conjunction with 43313, 43314)◄

43320   Esophagogastrostomy (cardioplasty), with or without vagotomy and pyloroplasty, transabdominal or transthoracic approach

(43321 has been deleted. To report, use 43320)

43324   Esophagogastric fundoplasty (eg, Nissen, Belsey IV, Hill procedures)

(For laparoscopic procedure, use 43280)

43325   Esophagogastric fundoplasty; with fundic patch (Thal-Nissen procedure)

(For cricopharyngeal myotomy, use 43030)

43326   with gastroplasty (eg, Collis)

43330   Esophagomyotomy (Heller type); abdominal approach

43331   thoracic approach

(For thoracoscopic esophagomyotomy, use 32665)

Surgery: Digestive System

43340 Esophagojejunostomy (without total gastrectomy); abdominal approach

43341   thoracic approach

43350 Esophagostomy, fistulization of esophagus, external; abdominal approach

43351   thoracic approach

43352   cervical approach

43360 Gastrointestinal reconstruction for previous esophagectomy, for obstructing esophageal lesion or fistula, or for previous esophageal exclusion; with stomach, with or without pyloroplasty

43361   with colon interposition or small intestine reconstruction, including intestine mobilization, preparation, and anastomosis(es)

43400 Ligation, direct, esophageal varices

43401 Transection of esophagus with repair, for esophageal varices

43405 Ligation or stapling at gastroesophageal junction for pre-existing esophageal perforation

43410 Suture of esophageal wound or injury; cervical approach

43415   transthoracic or transabdominal approach

43420 Closure of esophagostomy or fistula; cervical approach

43425   transthoracic or transabdominal approach

(For repair of esophageal hiatal hernia, see 39520 et seq)

Manipulation

(For associated esophagogram, use 74220)

43450* Dilation of esophagus, by unguided sound or bougie, single or multiple passes

(43451 has been deleted. To report, use 43450)

43453 Dilation of esophagus, over guide wire

(For dilation with direct visualization, use 43220)

(43455 has been deleted. To report, see 43220, 43458, 74360)

43456 Dilation of esophagus, by balloon or dilator, retrograde

43458 Dilation of esophagus with balloon (30 mm diameter or larger) for achalasia

(For dilation with balloon less than 30 mm diameter, use 43220)

(For radiological supervision and interpretation, use 74360)

43460 Esophagogastric tamponade, with balloon (Sengstaaken type)

(For removal of esophageal foreign body by balloon catheter, see 43215, 43247, 74235)

Other Procedures

43496 Free jejunum transfer with microvascular anastomosis

(Do not report code 69990 in addition to code 43496)

43499 Unlisted procedure, esophagus

Stomach

Incision

43500 Gastrotomy; with exploration or foreign body removal

43501   with suture repair of bleeding ulcer

43502   with suture repair of pre-existing esophagogastric laceration (eg, Mallory-Weiss)

43510   with esophageal dilation and insertion of permanent intraluminal tube (eg, Celestin or Mousseaux-Barbin)

43520 Pyloromyotomy, cutting of pyloric muscle (Fredet-Ramstedt type operation)

▶(Do not report modifier '-63' in conjunction with 43520)◀

Excision

43600 Biopsy of stomach; by capsule, tube, peroral (one or more specimens)

43605   by laparotomy

43610 Excision, local; ulcer or benign tumor of stomach

43611   malignant tumor of stomach

43620 Gastrectomy, total; with esophagoenterostomy

43621   with Roux-en-Y reconstruction

43622   with formation of intestinal pouch, any type

(43625 has been deleted. To report, use 43622)

(43630 has been deleted. To report, see 43631-43634)

43631 Gastrectomy, partial, distal; with gastroduodenostomy

43632   with gastrojejunostomy

43633   with Roux-en-Y reconstruction

43634   with formation of intestinal pouch

✛ 43635 Vagotomy when performed with partial distal gastrectomy (List separately in addition to code(s) for primary procedure)

(Use 43635 in conjunction with codes 43631, 43632, 43633, 43634)

43638 Gastrectomy, partial, proximal, thoracic or abdominal approach including esophagogastrostomy, with vagotomy;

43639   with pyloroplasty or pyloromyotomy

(For regional thoracic lymphadenectomy, use 38746)

(For regional abdominal lymphadenectomy, use 38747)

43640   Vagotomy including pyloroplasty, with or without gastrostomy; truncal or selective

(For pyloroplasty, use 43800)

(For vagotomy, see 64752-64760)

43641   parietal cell (highly selective)

(For upper gastrointestinal endoscopy, see 43234-43259)

(43700 has been deleted. To report, use 43235)

(43702 has been deleted. To report, use 43239)

(43709 has been deleted. To report, use 43247)

(43711 has been deleted. To report, use 43251)

(43712 has been deleted. To report, use 43255)

(43714 has been deleted. To report, use 43258)

Laparoscopy

Surgical laparoscopy always includes diagnostic laparoscopy. To report a diagnostic laparoscopy (peritoneoscopy) (separate procedure), use 49320.

43651   Laparoscopy, surgical; transection of vagus nerves, truncal

43652   transection of vagus nerves, selective or highly selective

43653   gastrostomy, without construction of gastric tube (eg, Stamm procedure) (separate procedure)

43659   Unlisted laparoscopy procedure, stomach

Introduction

43750   Percutaneous placement of gastrostomy tube

(For radiological supervision and interpretation, use 74350)

43752   Naso- or oro-gastric tube placement, necessitating physician's skill

(If imaging guidance is performed, use 76000)

(For enteric tube placement, see 44500, 74340)

(Do not report 43752 in conjunction with critical care codes 99291-99292, or neonatal intensive care codes, 99295-99298)

43760*   Change of gastrostomy tube

(For endoscopic placement of gastrostomy tube, use 43246)

(For radiological supervision and interpretation, use 75984)

43761   Repositioning of the gastric feeding tube, any method, through the duodenum for enteric nutrition

(If imaging guidance is performed, use 75984)

(43765 has been deleted. To report, use 43760)

Other Procedures

43800   Pyloroplasty

(For pyloroplasty and vagotomy, use 43640)

43810   Gastroduodenostomy

43820   Gastrojejunostomy; without vagotomy

43825   with vagotomy, any type

43830   Gastrostomy, open; without construction of gastric tube (eg, Stamm procedure) (separate procedure)

43831   neonatal, for feeding

(For change of gastrostomy tube, use 43760)

▶(Do not report modifier '-63' in conjunction with 43831)◀

43832   with construction of gastric tube (eg, Janeway procedure)

(43834 has been deleted. To report, use 43246)

43840   Gastrorrhaphy, suture of perforated duodenal or gastric ulcer, wound, or injury

43842   Gastric restrictive procedure, without gastric bypass, for morbid obesity; vertical-banded gastroplasty

43843   other than vertical-banded gastroplasty

(43844 has been deleted. To report, use 43847)

(43845 has been deleted. To report, see 43842, 43843)

43846   Gastric restrictive procedure, with gastric bypass for morbid obesity; with short limb (less than 100 cm) Roux-en-Y gastroenterostomy

43847   with small intestine reconstruction to limit absorption

43848   Revision of gastric restrictive procedure for morbid obesity (separate procedure)

43850   Revision of gastroduodenal anastomosis (gastroduodenostomy) with reconstruction; without vagotomy

43855   with vagotomy

43860   Revision of gastrojejunal anastomosis (gastrojejunostomy) with reconstruction, with or without partial gastrectomy or intestine resection; without vagotomy

43865   with vagotomy

43870   Closure of gastrostomy, surgical

43880   Closure of gastrocolic fistula

(43885 has been deleted)

43999   Unlisted procedure, stomach

Surgery: Digestive System

Intestines (Except Rectum)

Incision

(44000 has been deleted)

44005 Enterolysis (freeing of intestinal adhesion) (separate procedure)

(Do not report 44005 in addition to 45136)

(For laparoscopic approach, use 44200)

44010 Duodenotomy, for exploration, biopsy(s), or foreign body removal

+ 44015 Tube or needle catheter jejunostomy for enteral alimentation, intraoperative, any method (List separately in addition to primary procedure)

44020 Enterotomy, small intestine, other than duodenum; for exploration, biopsy(s), or foreign body removal

44021 for decompression (eg, Baker tube)

44025 Colotomy, for exploration, biopsy(s), or foreign body removal

(44040 has been deleted. To report, see 44602-44605)

44050 Reduction of volvulus, intussusception, internal hernia, by laparotomy

44055 Correction of malrotation by lysis of duodenal bands and/or reduction of midgut volvulus (eg, Ladd procedure)

►(Do not report modifier '-63' in conjunction with 44055)◄

(44060 has been deleted. To report, use 44799)

Excision

44100 Biopsy of intestine by capsule, tube, peroral (one or more specimens)

44110 Excision of one or more lesions of small or large intestine not requiring anastomosis, exteriorization, or fistulization; single enterotomy

44111 multiple enterotomies

(44115 has been deleted. To report, use 44799)

44120 Enterectomy, resection of small intestine; single resection and anastomosis

(Do not report 44120 in addition to 45136)

+ 44121 each additional resection and anastomosis (List separately in addition to code for primary procedure)

(Use 44121 in conjunction with code 44120)

44125 with enterostomy

44126 Enterectomy, resection of small intestine for congenital atresia, single resection and anastomosis of proximal segment of intestine; without tapering

44127 with tapering

+ 44128 each additional resection and anastomosis (List separately in addition to code for primary procedure)

(Use 44128 in conjunction with codes 44126, 44127)

►(Do not report modifier '-63' in conjunction with 44126, 44127, 44128)◄

44130 Enteroenterostomy, anastomosis of intestine, with or without cutaneous enterostomy (separate procedure)

(44131 has been deleted)

44132 Donor enterectomy, open, with preparation and maintenance of allograft; from cadaver donor

44133 partial, from living donor

44135 Intestinal allotransplantation; from cadaver donor

44136 from living donor

+ 44139 Mobilization (take-down) of splenic flexure performed in conjunction with partial colectomy (List separately in addition to primary procedure)

(Use 44139 in conjunction with codes 44140-44147)

44140 Colectomy, partial; with anastomosis

(For laparoscopic procedure, use 44204)

44141 with skin level cecostomy or colostomy

44143 with end colostomy and closure of distal segment (Hartmann type procedure)

►(For laparoscopic procedure, use 44206)◄

44144 with resection, with colostomy or ileostomy and creation of mucofistula

44145 with coloproctostomy (low pelvic anastomosis)

►(For laparoscopic procedure, use 44207)◄

44146 with coloproctostomy (low pelvic anastomosis), with colostomy

►(For laparoscopic procedure, use 44208)◄

44147 abdominal and transanal approach

44150 Colectomy, total, abdominal, without proctectomy; with ileostomy or ileoproctostomy

►(For laparoscopic procedure, use 44210)◄

44151 with continent ileostomy

44152 with rectal mucosectomy, ileoanal anastomosis, with or without loop ileostomy

►(For laparoscopic procedure, use 44211)◄

44153 with rectal mucosectomy, ileoanal anastomosis, creation of ileal reservoir (S or J), with or without loop ileostomy

►(For laparoscopic procedure, use 44211)◄

44155 Colectomy, total, abdominal, with proctectomy; with ileostomy

►(For laparoscopic procedure, use 44212)◄

44156 with continent ileostomy

44160   Colectomy, partial, with removal of terminal ileum with ileocolostomy

(For laparoscopic procedure, use 44205)

Laparoscopy

Surgical laparoscopy always includes diagnostic laparoscopy. To report a diagnostic laparoscopy (peritoneoscopy) (separate procedure), use 49320.

44200   Laparoscopy, surgical; enterolysis (freeing of intestinal adhesion) (separate procedure)

(For laparoscopy with salpingolysis, ovariolysis, use 58660)

44201   jejunostomy (eg, for decompression or feeding)

44202   enterectomy, resection of small intestine, single resection and anastomosis

+ 44203   each additional small intestine resection and anastomosis (List separately in addition to code for primary procedure)

(Use 44203 in conjunction with code 44202)

(For open procedure, see 44120, 44121)

44204   colectomy, partial, with anastomosis

(For open procedure, use 44140)

44205   colectomy, partial, with removal of terminal ileum with ileocolostomy

(For open procedure, use 44160)

● **44206**   colectomy, partial, with end colostomy and closure of distal segment (Hartmann type procedure)

►(For open procedure, use 44143)◄

● **44207**   colectomy, partial, with anastomosis, with coloproctostomy (low pelvic anastomosis)

►(For open procedure, use 44145)◄

● **44208**   colectomy, partial, with anastomosis, with coloproctostomy (low pelvic anastomosis) with colostomy

►(For open procedure, use 44146)◄

►(44209 has been deleted. To report, use 44238)◄

● **44210**   colectomy, total, abdominal, without proctectomy, with ileostomy or ileoproctostomy

►(For open procedure, use 44150)◄

● **44211**   colectomy, total, abdominal, with proctectomy, with ileoanal anastomosis, creation of ileal reservoir (S or J), with loop ileostomy, with or without rectal mucosectomy

►(For open procedure, see 44152, 44153)◄

● **44212**   colectomy, total, abdominal, with proctectomy, with ileostomy

►(For open procedure, use 44155)◄

● **44238**   Unlisted laparoscopy procedure, intestine (except rectum)

● **44239**   Unlisted laparoscopy procedure, rectum

Enterostomy—External Fistulization of Intestines

44300   Enterostomy or cecostomy, tube (eg, for decompression or feeding) (separate procedure)

(44305 has been deleted)

(44308 has been deleted. To report, use 44799)

44310   Ileostomy or jejunostomy, non-tube (separate procedure)

(Do not report 44310 in addition to 45136)

44312   Revision of ileostomy; simple (release of superficial scar) (separate procedure)

44314   complicated (reconstruction in-depth) (separate procedure)

44316   Continent ileostomy (Kock procedure) (separate procedure)

(For fiberoptic evaluation, use 44385)

44320   Colostomy or skin level cecostomy; (separate procedure)

44322   with multiple biopsies (eg, for congenital megacolon) (separate procedure)

44340   Revision of colostomy; simple (release of superficial scar) (separate procedure)

44345   complicated (reconstruction in-depth) (separate procedure)

44346   with repair of paracolostomy hernia (separate procedure)

Endoscopy, Small Intestine and Stomal

Surgical endoscopy always includes diagnostic endoscopy.

(For upper gastrointestinal endoscopy, see 43234-43258)

44360   Small intestinal endoscopy, enteroscopy beyond second portion of duodenum, not including ileum; diagnostic, with or without collection of specimen(s) by brushing or washing (separate procedure)

44361   with biopsy, single or multiple

44363   with removal of foreign body

44364   with removal of tumor(s), polyp(s), or other lesion(s) by snare technique

44365   with removal of tumor(s), polyp(s), or other lesion(s) by hot biopsy forceps or bipolar cautery

44366   with control of bleeding (eg, injection, bipolar cautery, unipolar cautery, laser, heater probe, stapler, plasma coagulator)

44369   with ablation of tumor(s), polyp(s), or other lesion(s) not amenable to removal by hot biopsy forceps, bipolar cautery or snare technique

Surgery: Digestive System

44370   with transendoscopic stent placement (includes predilation)

44372   with placement of percutaneous jejunostomy tube

44373   with conversion of percutaneous gastrostomy tube to percutaneous jejunostomy tube

(44375 has been deleted. To report, use 43235)

44376   Small intestinal endoscopy, enteroscopy beyond second portion of duodenum, including ileum; diagnostic, with or without collection of specimen(s) by brushing or washing (separate procedure)

44377   with biopsy, single or multiple

44378   with control of bleeding (eg, injection, bipolar cautery, unipolar cautery, laser, heater probe, stapler, plasma coagulator)

44379   with transendoscopic stent placement (includes predilation)

44380   Ileoscopy, through stoma; diagnostic, with or without collection of specimen(s) by brushing or washing (separate procedure)

44382   with biopsy, single or multiple

44383   with transendoscopic stent placement (includes predilation)

44385   Endoscopic evaluation of small intestinal (abdominal or pelvic) pouch; diagnostic, with or without collection of specimen(s) by brushing or washing (separate procedure)

44386   with biopsy, single or multiple

44388   Colonoscopy through stoma; diagnostic, with or without collection of specimen(s) by brushing or washing (separate procedure)

44389   with biopsy, single or multiple

44390   with removal of foreign body

44391   with control of bleeding (eg, injection, bipolar cautery, unipolar cautery, laser, heater probe, stapler, plasma coagulator)

44392   with removal of tumor(s), polyp(s), or other lesion(s) by hot biopsy forceps or bipolar cautery

44393   with ablation of tumor(s), polyp(s), or other lesion(s) not amenable to removal by hot biopsy forceps, bipolar cautery or snare technique

44394   with removal of tumor(s), polyp(s), or other lesion(s) by snare technique

(For colonoscopy per rectum, see 45330-45385)

(44400, 44405 have been deleted. To report, use 44799)

44397   with transendoscopic stent placement (includes predilation)

Introduction

⊘ **44500**   Introduction of long gastrointestinal tube (eg, Miller-Abbott) (separate procedure)

(For radiological supervision and interpretation, use 74340)

(For naso- or oro-gastric tube placement, use 43752)

Repair

(44600 has been deleted. To report, see 44602, 44604)

44602   Suture of small intestine (enterorrhaphy) for perforated ulcer, diverticulum, wound, injury or rupture; single perforation

44603   multiple perforations

44604   Suture of large intestine (colorrhaphy) for perforated ulcer, diverticulum, wound, injury or rupture (single or multiple perforations); without colostomy

44605   with colostomy

(44610 has been deleted. To report, see 44603, 44604)

44615   Intestinal stricturoplasty (enterotomy and enterorrhaphy) with or without dilation, for intestinal obstruction

44620   Closure of enterostomy, large or small intestine;

44625   with resection and anastomosis other than colorectal

44626   with resection and colorectal anastomosis (eg, closure of Hartmann type procedure)

44640   Closure of intestinal cutaneous fistula

44650   Closure of enteroenteric or enterocolic fistula

44660   Closure of enterovesical fistula; without intestinal or bladder resection

44661   with intestine and/or bladder resection

(For closure of renocolic fistula, see 50525, 50526)

(For closure of gastrocolic fistula, use 43880)

(For closure of rectovesical fistula, see 45800, 45805)

44680   Intestinal plication (separate procedure)

Other Procedures

44700   Exclusion of small intestine from pelvis by mesh or other prosthesis, or native tissue (eg, bladder or omentum)

(For therapeutic radiation clinical treatment, see **Radiation Oncology** section)

+ ● **44701**   Intraoperative colonic lavage (List separately in addition to code for primary procedure)

▶(Use 44701 in conjunction with codes 44140, 44145, 44150, or 44604 as appropriate)◀

▶(Do not report 44701 in conjunction with 44300, 44950-44960)◀

44799   Unlisted procedure, intestine

▶(For unlisted laparoscopic procedure, intestine except rectum, use 44238)◀

Meckel's Diverticulum and the Mesentery

Excision

44800   Excision of Meckel's diverticulum (diverticulectomy) or omphalomesenteric duct

44820   Excision of lesion of mesentery (separate procedure)

(With intestine resection, see 44120 or 44140 et seq)

Suture

44850   Suture of mesentery (separate procedure)

(For reduction and repair of internal hernia, use 44050)

Other Procedures

44899   Unlisted procedure, Meckels diverticulum and the mesentery

Appendix

Incision

44900   Incision and drainage of appendiceal abscess; open

44901   percutaneous

(For radiological supervision and interpretation, use 75989)

Excision

44950   Appendectomy;

(Incidental appendectomy during intra-abdominal surgery does not usually warrant a separate identification. If necessary to report, add modifier '-52')

+ 44955   when done for indicated purpose at time of other major procedure (not as separate procedure) (List separately in addition to code for primary procedure)

44960   for ruptured appendix with abscess or generalized peritonitis

Laparoscopy

Surgical laparoscopy always includes diagnostic laparoscopy. To report a diagnostic laparoscopy (peritoneoscopy) (separate procedure), use 49320.

44970   Laparoscopy, surgical, appendectomy

44979   Unlisted laparoscopy procedure, appendix

Rectum

Incision

45000   Transrectal drainage of pelvic abscess

45005   Incision and drainage of submucosal abscess, rectum

45020   Incision and drainage of deep supralevator, pelvirectal, or retrorectal abscess

(See also 46050, 46060)

Excision

45100   Biopsy of anorectal wall, anal approach (eg, congenital megacolon)

(45105 has been deleted. To report, use 45100)

(For endoscopic biopsy, use 45305)

45108   Anorectal myomectomy

45110   Proctectomy; complete, combined abdominoperineal, with colostomy

45111   partial resection of rectum, transabdominal approach

45112   Proctectomy, combined abdominoperineal, pull-through procedure (eg, colo-anal anastomosis)

(For colo-anal anastomosis with colonic reservoir or pouch, use 45119)

45113   Proctectomy, partial, with rectal mucosectomy, ileoanal anastomosis, creation of ileal reservoir (S or J), with or without loop ileostomy

45114   Proctectomy, partial, with anastomosis; abdominal and transsacral approach

45116   transsacral approach only (Kraske type)

45119   Proctectomy, combined abdominoperineal pull-through procedure (eg, colo-anal anastomosis), with creation of colonic reservoir (eg, J-pouch), with or without proximal diverting ostomy

45120   Proctectomy, complete (for congenital megacolon), abdominal and perineal approach; with pull-through procedure and anastomosis (eg, Swenson, Duhamel, or Soave type operation)

45121   with subtotal or total colectomy, with multiple biopsies

45123   Proctectomy, partial, without anastomosis, perineal approach

45126   Pelvic exenteration for colorectal malignancy, with proctectomy (with or without colostomy), with removal of bladder and ureteral transplantations, and/or hysterectomy, or cervicectomy, with or without removal of tube(s), with or without removal of ovary(s), or any combination thereof

45130   Excision of rectal procidentia, with anastomosis; perineal approach

45135   abdominal and perineal approach

Surgery: Digestive System

45136   Excision of ileoanal reservoir with ileostomy

(Do not report 45136 in addition to 44005, 44120, 44310)

45150   Division of stricture of rectum

45160   Excision of rectal tumor by proctotomy, transsacral or transcoccygeal approach

45170   Excision of rectal tumor, transanal approach

(45180, 45181 have been deleted. To report, see 45170, 45190)

Destruction

45190   Destruction of rectal tumor (eg, electrodessication, electrosurgery, laser ablation, laser resection, cryosurgery) transanal approach

Endoscopy

Definitions

Proctosigmoidoscopy is the examination of the rectum and sigmoid colon.

Sigmoidoscopy is the examination of the entire rectum, sigmoid colon and may include examination of a portion of the descending colon.

Colonoscopy is the examination of the entire colon, from the rectum to the cecum, and may include the examination of the terminal ileum.

For an incomplete colonoscopy, with full preparation for a colonoscopy, use a colonoscopy code with the modifier '-52' and provide documentation.

Surgical endoscopy always includes diagnostic endoscopy.

45300   Proctosigmoidoscopy, rigid; diagnostic, with or without collection of specimen(s) by brushing or washing (separate procedure)

(45302 has been deleted. To report, use 45300)

45303   with dilation (eg, balloon, guide wire, bougie)

(For radiological supervision and interpretation, use 74360)

45305   with biopsy, single or multiple

45307   with removal of foreign body

45308   with removal of single tumor, polyp, or other lesion by hot biopsy forceps or bipolar cautery

45309   with removal of single tumor, polyp, or other lesion by snare technique

(45310 has been deleted. To report, see 45308, 45309)

45315   with removal of multiple tumors, polyps, or other lesions by hot biopsy forceps, bipolar cautery or snare technique

45317   with control of bleeding (eg, injection, bipolar cautery, unipolar cautery, laser, heater probe, stapler, plasma coagulator)

(45319 has been deleted. To report, use 45999)

45320   with ablation of tumor(s), polyp(s), or other lesion(s) not amenable to removal by hot biopsy forceps, bipolar cautery or snare technique (eg, laser)

45321   with decompression of volvulus

(45325 colonoscopy has been renumbered 45355 without change in terminology)

45327   with transendoscopic stent placement (includes predilation)

45330   Sigmoidoscopy, flexible; diagnostic, with or without collection of specimen(s) by brushing or washing (separate procedure)

45331   with biopsy, single or multiple

45332   with removal of foreign body

45333   with removal of tumor(s), polyp(s), or other lesion(s) by hot biopsy forceps or bipolar cautery

45334   with control of bleeding (eg, injection, bipolar cautery, unipolar cautery, laser, heater probe, stapler, plasma coagulator)

● **45335**   with directed submucosal injection(s), any substance

(45336 has been deleted. To report, use 45339)

45337   with decompression of volvulus, any method

45338   with removal of tumor(s), polyp(s), or other lesion(s) by snare technique

45339   with ablation of tumor(s), polyp(s), or other lesion(s) not amenable to removal by hot biopsy forceps, bipolar cautery or snare technique

● **45340**   with dilation by balloon, 1 or more strictures

▶(Do not report 45340 in conjunction with 45345)◀

45341   with endoscopic ultrasound examination

45342   with transendoscopic ultrasound guided intramural or transmural fine needle aspiration/biopsy(s)

(Do not report 76975 in conjunction with codes 45341, 45342)

(For interpretation of specimen, see 88172-88173)

(For transrectal ultrasound utilizing rigid probe device, use 76872)

45345   with transendoscopic stent placement (includes predilation)

45355   Colonoscopy, rigid or flexible, transabdominal via colotomy, single or multiple

(45360-45372 have been deleted. To report, see 45330-45337)

45378   Colonoscopy, flexible, proximal to splenic flexure; diagnostic, with or without collection of specimen(s) by brushing or washing, with or without colon decompression (separate procedure)

45379   with removal of foreign body

45380   with biopsy, single or multiple

● **45381**   with directed submucosal injection(s), any substance

45382   with control of bleeding (eg, injection, bipolar cautery, unipolar cautery, laser, heater probe, stapler, plasma coagulator)

45383   with ablation of tumor(s), polyp(s), or other lesion(s) not amenable to removal by hot biopsy forceps, bipolar cautery or snare technique

45384   with removal of tumor(s), polyp(s), or other lesion(s) by hot biopsy forceps or bipolar cautery

45385   with removal of tumor(s), polyp(s), or other lesion(s) by snare technique

(45386 has been deleted. To report, use 44799)

(For small intestine and stomal endoscopy, see 44360-44393)

● **45386**   with dilation by balloon, 1 or more strictures

▶(Do not report 45386 in conjunction with 45387)◀

45387   with transendoscopic stent placement (includes predilation)

Repair

45500   Proctoplasty; for stenosis

45505   for prolapse of mucous membrane

45520   Perirectal injection of sclerosing solution for prolapse

(45521 has been deleted)

45540   Proctopexy for prolapse; abdominal approach

45541   perineal approach

45550   Proctopexy combined with sigmoid resection, abdominal approach

45560   Repair of rectocele (separate procedure)

(For repair of rectocele with posterior colporrhaphy, use 57250)

45562   Exploration, repair, and presacral drainage for rectal injury;

45563   with colostomy

45800   Closure of rectovesical fistula;

45805   with colostomy

45820   Closure of rectourethral fistula;

45825   with colostomy

(For rectovaginal fistula closure, see 57300-57308)

Manipulation

45900*   Reduction of procidentia (separate procedure) under anesthesia

45905*   Dilation of anal sphincter (separate procedure) under anesthesia other than local

45910   Dilation of rectal stricture (separate procedure) under anesthesia other than local

45915*   Removal of fecal impaction or foreign body (separate procedure) under anesthesia

Other Procedures

45999   Unlisted procedure, rectum

▶(For unlisted laparoscopic procedure, rectum, use 44239)◀

Anus

Incision

(46000 has been deleted. To report, use 46270)

46020   Placement of seton

(Do not report 46020 in addition to 46060, 46280, 46600)

46030*   Removal of anal seton, other marker

(46032 has been deleted. To report, use 46999)

46040   Incision and drainage of ischiorectal and/or perirectal abscess (separate procedure)

46045   Incision and drainage of intramural, intramuscular, or submucosal abscess, transanal, under anesthesia

46050*   Incision and drainage, perianal abscess, superficial

(See also 45020, 46060)

46060   Incision and drainage of ischiorectal or intramural abscess, with fistulectomy or fistulotomy, submuscular, with or without placement of seton

(Do not report 46060 in addition to 46020)

(See also 45020)

46070   Incision, anal septum (infant)

(For anoplasty, see 46700-46705)

▶(Do not report modifier '-63' in conjunction with 46070)◀

46080*   Sphincterotomy, anal, division of sphincter (separate procedure)

46083   Incision of thrombosed hemorrhoid, external

Excision

46200   Fissurectomy, with or without sphincterotomy

46210   Cryptectomy; single

46211   multiple (separate procedure)

46220   Papillectomy or excision of single tag, anus (separate procedure)

46221   Hemorrhoidectomy, by simple ligature (eg, rubber band)

46230   Excision of external hemorrhoid tags and/or multiple papillae

46250   Hemorrhoidectomy, external, complete

46255   Hemorrhoidectomy, internal and external, simple;

46257   with fissurectomy

46258   with fistulectomy, with or without fissurectomy

46260   Hemorrhoidectomy, internal and external, complex or extensive;

46261   with fissurectomy

46262   with fistulectomy, with or without fissurectomy

46270   Surgical treatment of anal fistula (fistulectomy/fistulotomy); subcutaneous

46275   submuscular

46280   complex or multiple, with or without placement of seton

(Do not report 46280 in addition to 46020)

(46281 has been renumbered to 46288 without change in terminology)

46285   second stage

46288   Closure of anal fistula with rectal advancement flap

46320*   Enucleation or excision of external thrombotic hemorrhoid

Introduction

46500*   Injection of sclerosing solution, hemorrhoids

(46510, 46530 have been deleted. To report, use 46999)

Endoscopy

Surgical endoscopy always includes diagnostic endoscopy.

46600   Anoscopy; diagnostic, with or without collection of specimen(s) by brushing or washing (separate procedure)

(Do not report 46600 in addition to 46020)

(46602 has been deleted. To report, use 46600)

46604   with dilation (eg, balloon, guide wire, bougie)

46606   with biopsy, single or multiple

46608   with removal of foreign body

46610   with removal of single tumor, polyp, or other lesion by hot biopsy forceps or bipolar cautery

46611   with removal of single tumor, polyp, or other lesion by snare technique

46612   with removal of multiple tumors, polyps, or other lesions by hot biopsy forceps, bipolar cautery or snare technique

46614   with control of bleeding (eg, injection, bipolar cautery, unipolar cautery, laser, heater probe, stapler, plasma coagulator)

46615   with ablation of tumor(s), polyp(s), or other lesion(s) not amenable to removal by hot biopsy forceps, bipolar cautery or snare technique

Repair

46700   Anoplasty, plastic operation for stricture; adult

46705   infant

(For simple incision of anal septum, use 46070)

►(Do not report modifier '-63' in conjunction with 46705)◄

● **46706**   Repair of anal fistula with fibrin glue

46715   Repair of low imperforate anus; with anoperineal fistula (cut-back procedure)

46716   with transposition of anoperineal or anovestibular fistula

►(Do not report modifier '-63' in conjunction with 46715, 46716)◄

46730   Repair of high imperforate anus without fistula; perineal or sacroperineal approach

46735   combined transabdominal and sacroperineal approaches

►(Do not report modifier '-63' in conjunction with 46730, 46735)◄

46740   Repair of high imperforate anus with rectourethral or rectovaginal fistula; perineal or sacroperineal approach

46742   combined transabdominal and sacroperineal approaches

►(Do not report modifier '-63' in conjunction with 46740, 46742)◄

46744   Repair of cloacal anomaly by anorectovaginoplasty and urethroplasty, sacroperineal approach

►(Do not report modifier '-63' in conjunction with 46744)◄

46746   Repair of cloacal anomaly by anorectovaginoplasty and urethroplasty, combined abdominal and sacroperineal approach;

46748   with vaginal lengthening by intestinal graft or pedicle flaps

46750	Sphincteroplasty, anal, for incontinence or prolapse; adult
46751	child
46753	Graft (Thiersch operation) for rectal incontinence and/or prolapse
46754	Removal of Thiersch wire or suture, anal canal
46760	Sphincteroplasty, anal, for incontinence, adult; muscle transplant
46761	levator muscle imbrication (Park posterior anal repair)
46762	implantation artificial sphincter

Destruction

46900*	Destruction of lesion(s), anus (eg, condyloma, papilloma, molluscum contagiosum, herpetic vesicle), simple; chemical
46910*	electrodesiccation
46916	cryosurgery
46917	laser surgery

(46920 has been deleted. To report, use 46922)

46922	surgical excision
46924	Destruction of lesion(s), anus (eg, condyloma, papilloma, molluscum contagiosum, herpetic vesicle), extensive (eg, laser surgery, electrosurgery, cryosurgery, chemosurgery)

(46930 has been deleted. To report, use 46924)

(46932 has been deleted. To report, use 46916)

(46933 has been deleted. To report, use 46924)

46934	Destruction of hemorrhoids, any method; internal
46935	external
46936	internal and external
46937	Cryosurgery of rectal tumor; benign
46938	malignant
46940	Curettage or cautery of anal fissure, including dilation of anal sphincter (separate procedure); initial
46942	subsequent

Suture

46945	Ligation of internal hemorrhoids; single procedure
46946	multiple procedures

Other Procedures

46999	Unlisted procedure, anus

Liver

Incision

47000*	Biopsy of liver, needle; percutaneous

(If imaging guidance is performed, see 76003, 76360, 76393, 76942)

+ 47001	when done for indicated purpose at time of other major procedure (List separately in addition to code for primary procedure)

(If imaging guidance is performed, see 76003, 76942)

(For fine needle aspiration in conjunction with 47000, 47001, see 10021, 10022)

(For evaluation of fine needle aspirate in conjunction with 47000, 47001, see 88172, 88173)

47010	Hepatotomy; for open drainage of abscess or cyst, one or two stages
47011	for percutaneous drainage of abscess or cyst, one or two stages

(For radiological supervision and interpretation, use 75989)

47015	Laparotomy, with aspiration and/or injection of hepatic parasitic (eg, amoebic or echinococcal) cyst(s) or abscess(es)

Excision

47100	Biopsy of liver, wedge
47120	Hepatectomy, resection of liver; partial lobectomy
47122	trisegmentectomy
47125	total left lobectomy
47130	total right lobectomy
47133	Donor hepatectomy, with preparation and maintenance of allograft; from cadaver donor
47134	partial, from living donor
47135	Liver allotransplantation; orthotopic, partial or whole, from cadaver or living donor, any age
47136	heterotopic, partial or whole, from cadaver or living donor, any age

Repair

47300	Marsupialization of cyst or abscess of liver
47350	Management of liver hemorrhage; simple suture of liver wound or injury

(47355 has been deleted)

47360	complex suture of liver wound or injury, with or without hepatic artery ligation

Surgery: Digestive System

47361   exploration of hepatic wound, extensive debridement, coagulation and/or suture, with or without packing of liver

47362   re-exploration of hepatic wound for removal of packing

Laparoscopy

Surgical laparoscopy always includes diagnostic laparoscopy. To report a diagnostic laparoscopy (peritoneoscopy) (separate procedure), use 49320

47370   Laparoscopy, surgical, ablation of one or more liver tumor(s); radiofrequency

(For imaging guidance, use 76490)

47371   cryosurgical

(For imaging guidance, use 76490)

47379   Unlisted laparoscopic procedure, liver

Other Procedures

47380   Ablation, open, of one or more liver tumor(s); radiofrequency

(For imaging guidance, use 76490)

47381   cryosurgical

(For imaging guidance, use 76490)

47382   Ablation, one or more liver tumor(s), percutaneous, radiofrequency

(For imaging guidance and monitoring, see code 76362, 76394, or 76490)

47399   Unlisted procedure, liver

Biliary Tract

Incision

47400   Hepaticotomy or hepaticostomy with exploration, drainage, or removal of calculus

47420   Choledochotomy or choledochostomy with exploration, drainage, or removal of calculus, with or without cholecystotomy; without transduodenal sphincterotomy or sphincteroplasty

47425   with transduodenal sphincterotomy or sphincteroplasty

(47440 has been deleted)

47460   Transduodenal sphincterotomy or sphincteroplasty, with or without transduodenal extraction of calculus (separate procedure)

47480   Cholecystotomy or cholecystostomy with exploration, drainage, or removal of calculus (separate procedure)

47490   Percutaneous cholecystostomy

(For radiological supervision and interpretation, use 75989)

Introduction

47500   Injection procedure for percutaneous transhepatic cholangiography

(For radiological supervision and interpretation, use 74320)

47505   Injection procedure for cholangiography through an existing catheter (eg, percutaneous transhepatic or T-tube)

(For radiological supervision and interpretation, use 74305)

47510   Introduction of percutaneous transhepatic catheter for biliary drainage

(For radiological supervision and interpretation, use 75980)

47511   Introduction of percutaneous transhepatic stent for internal and external biliary drainage

(For radiological supervision and interpretation, use 75982)

47525   Change of percutaneous biliary drainage catheter

(For radiological supervision and interpretation, use 75984)

47530   Revision and/or reinsertion of transhepatic tube

(For radiological supervision and interpretation, use 75984)

Endoscopy

Surgical endoscopy always includes diagnostic endoscopy.

+ 47550   Biliary endoscopy, intraoperative (choledochoscopy) (List separately in addition to code for primary procedure)

47552   Biliary endoscopy, percutaneous via T-tube or other tract; diagnostic, with or without collection of specimen(s) by brushing and/or washing (separate procedure)

47553   with biopsy, single or multiple

47554   with removal of calculus/calculi

47555   with dilation of biliary duct stricture(s) without stent

(For ERCP, see 43260-43272, 74363)

(If imaging guidance is performed, see 74363, 75982)

47556   with dilation of biliary duct stricture(s) with stent

(If imaging guidance is performed, see 74363, 75982)

Surgery: Digestive System

Laparoscopy

Surgical laparoscopy always includes diagnostic laparoscopy. To report a diagnostic laparoscopy (peritoneoscopy) (separate procedure), use 49320.

47560   Laparoscopy, surgical; with guided transhepatic cholangiography, without biopsy

47561   with guided transhepatic cholangiography with biopsy

47562   cholecystectomy

47563   cholecystectomy with cholangiography

47564   cholecystectomy with exploration of common duct

47570   cholecystoenterostomy

47579   Unlisted laparoscopy procedure, biliary tract

Excision

47600   Cholecystectomy;

47605   with cholangiography

(For laparoscopic approach, see 47562-47564)

47610   Cholecystectomy with exploration of common duct;

(47611 has been deleted. To report, use 47610 and 47550)

47612   with choledochoenterostomy

47620   with transduodenal sphincterotomy or sphincteroplasty, with or without cholangiography

47630   Biliary duct stone extraction, percutaneous via T-tube tract, basket, or snare (eg, Burhenne technique)

(For radiological supervision and interpretation, use 74327)

47700   Exploration for congenital atresia of bile ducts, without repair, with or without liver biopsy, with or without cholangiography

▶(Do not report modifier '-63' in conjunction with 47700)◀

47701   Portoenterostomy (eg, Kasai procedure)

▶(Do not report modifier '-63' in conjunction with 47701)◀

(47710 has been deleted. To report, see 47711, 47712)

47711   Excision of bile duct tumor, with or without primary repair of bile duct; extrahepatic

47712   intrahepatic

(For anastomosis, see 47760-47800)

47715   Excision of choledochal cyst

47716   Anastomosis, choledochal cyst, without excision

Repair

47720   Cholecystoenterostomy; direct

(For laparoscopic approach, use 47570)

47721   with gastroenterostomy

47740   Roux-en-Y

47741   Roux-en-Y with gastroenterostomy

47760   Anastomosis, of extrahepatic biliary ducts and gastrointestinal tract

47765   Anastomosis, of intrahepatic ducts and gastrointestinal tract

47780   Anastomosis, Roux-en-Y, of extrahepatic biliary ducts and gastrointestinal tract

47785   Anastomosis, Roux-en-Y, of intrahepatic biliary ducts and gastrointestinal tract

47800   Reconstruction, plastic, of extrahepatic biliary ducts with end-to-end anastomosis

47801   Placement of choledochal stent

47802   U-tube hepaticoenterostomy

(47810 has been deleted. To report, use 47999)

(47850, 47855 have been deleted. To report, use 47999)

47900   Suture of extrahepatic biliary duct for pre-existing injury (separate procedure)

Other Procedures

47999   Unlisted procedure, biliary tract

Pancreas

(For peroral pancreatic endoscopic procedures, see 43260-43272)

Incision

48000   Placement of drains, peripancreatic, for acute pancreatitis;

48001   with cholecystostomy, gastrostomy, and jejunostomy

48005   Resection or debridement of pancreas and peripancreatic tissue for acute necrotizing pancreatitis

48020   Removal of pancreatic calculus

Surgery: Digestive System

Surgery: Digestive System

Excision

48100 Biopsy of pancreas, open (eg, fine needle aspiration, needle core biopsy, wedge biopsy)

48102* Biopsy of pancreas, percutaneous needle

(For radiological supervision and interpretation, see 76003, 76360, 76393, 76942)

(For fine needle aspiration, use 10022)

(For evaluation of fine needle aspirate, see 88172, 88173)

48120 Excision of lesion of pancreas (eg, cyst, adenoma)

48140 Pancreatectomy, distal subtotal, with or without splenectomy; without pancreaticojejunostomy

48145   with pancreaticojejunostomy

48146 Pancreatectomy, distal, near-total with preservation of duodenum (Child-type procedure)

48148 Excision of ampulla of Vater

48150 Pancreatectomy, proximal subtotal with total duodenectomy, partial gastrectomy, choledochoenterostomy and gastrojejunostomy (Whipple-type procedure); with pancreatojejunostomy

(48151 has been deleted. To report, use 48146)

48152   without pancreatojejunostomy

48153 Pancreatectomy, proximal subtotal with near-total duodenectomy, choledochoenterostomy and duodenojejunostomy (pylorus-sparing, Whipple-type procedure); with pancreatojejunostomy

48154   without pancreatojejunostomy

48155 Pancreatectomy, total

48160 Pancreatectomy, total or subtotal, with autologous transplantation of pancreas or pancreatic islet cells

48180 Pancreaticojejunostomy, side-to-side anastomosis (Puestow-type operation)

Introduction

+ 48400 Injection procedure for intraoperative pancreatography (List separately in addition to code for primary procedure)

(For radiological supervision and interpretation, see 74300-74305)

Repair

48500 Marsupialization of pancreatic cyst

48510 External drainage, pseudocyst of pancreas; open

48511   percutaneous

(For radiological supervision and interpretation, use 75989)

48520 Internal anastomosis of pancreatic cyst to gastrointestinal tract; direct

48540   Roux-en-Y

48545 Pancreatorrhaphy for injury

48547 Duodenal exclusion with gastrojejunostomy for pancreatic injury

Pancreas Transplantation

48550 Donor pancreatectomy, with preparation and maintenance of allograft from cadaver donor, with or without duodenal segment for transplantation

48554 Transplantation of pancreatic allograft

48556 Removal of transplanted pancreatic allograft

Other Procedures

48999 Unlisted procedure, pancreas

Abdomen, Peritoneum, and Omentum

Incision

49000 Exploratory laparotomy, exploratory celiotomy with or without biopsy(s) (separate procedure)

(To report wound exploration due to penetrating trauma without laparotomy, use 20102)

49002 Reopening of recent laparotomy

(To report re-exploration of hepatic wound for removal of packing, use 47362)

49010 Exploration, retroperitoneal area with or without biopsy(s) (separate procedure)

(To report wound exploration due to penetrating trauma without laparotomy, use 20102)

49020 Drainage of peritoneal abscess or localized peritonitis, exclusive of appendiceal abscess; open

(For appendiceal abscess, use 44900)

49021   percutaneous

(For radiological supervision and interpretation, use 75989)

49040 Drainage of subdiaphragmatic or subphrenic abscess; open

49041   percutaneous

(For radiological supervision and interpretation, use 75989)

49060 Drainage of retroperitoneal abscess; open

49061   percutaneous

(For laparoscopic drainage, use 49323)

(For radiological supervision and interpretation, use 75989)

49062 Drainage of extraperitoneal lymphocele to peritoneal cavity, open

49080* Peritoneocentesis, abdominal paracentesis, or peritoneal lavage (diagnostic or therapeutic); initial

49081* subsequent

(If imaging guidance is performed, see 76360, 76942)

49085 Removal of peritoneal foreign body from peritoneal cavity

(For lysis of intestinal adhesions, use 44005)

Excision, Destruction

49180* Biopsy, abdominal or retroperitoneal mass, percutaneous needle

(If imaging guidance is performed, see 76003, 76360, 76393, 76942)

(For fine needle aspiration, use 10021 or 10022)

(For evaluation of fine needle aspirate, see 88172, 88173)

▲ **49200** Excision or destruction, open, intra-abdominal or retroperitoneal tumors or cysts or endometriomas;

49201 extensive

49215 Excision of presacral or sacrococcygeal tumor

▶(Do not report modifier '-63' in conjunction with 49215)◀

49220 Staging laparotomy for Hodgkins disease or lymphoma (includes splenectomy, needle or open biopsies of both liver lobes, possibly also removal of abdominal nodes, abdominal node and/or bone marrow biopsies, ovarian repositioning)

49250 Umbilectomy, omphalectomy, excision of umbilicus (separate procedure)

49255 Omentectomy, epiploectomy, resection of omentum (separate procedure)

(49300 has been deleted. To report, use 49320)

(49301 has been deleted. To report, use 49321)

(49302 has been deleted. To report, use 47560)

(49303 has been deleted. To report, use 47561)

(49310 has been deleted. To report, use 47562)

(49311 has been deleted. To report, use 47563)

(49315 has been deleted. To report, use 44970)

Laparoscopy

Surgical laparoscopy always includes diagnostic laparoscopy. To report a diagnostic laparoscopy (peritoneoscopy), (separate procedure), use 49320.

For laparoscopic fulguration or excision of lesions of the ovary, pelvic viscera, or peritoneal surface use 58662.

49320 Laparoscopy, abdomen, peritoneum, and omentum, diagnostic, with or without collection of specimen(s) by brushing or washing (separate procedure)

49321 Laparoscopy, surgical; with biopsy (single or multiple)

49322 with aspiration of cavity or cyst (eg, ovarian cyst) (single or multiple)

49323 with drainage of lymphocele to peritoneal cavity

(For percutaneous or open drainage, see 49060, 49061)

49329 Unlisted laparoscopy procedure, abdomen, peritoneum and omentum

Introduction, Revision, and/or Removal

49400* Injection of air or contrast into peritoneal cavity (separate procedure)

(For radiological supervision and interpretation, use 74190)

(49401 has been deleted. To report, use 49400)

● **49419** Insertion of intraperitoneal cannula or catheter, with subcutaneous reservoir, permanent (ie, totally implantable)

▶(For removal, use 49422)◀

49420* Insertion of intraperitoneal cannula or catheter for drainage or dialysis; temporary

49421 permanent

49422 Removal of permanent intraperitoneal cannula or catheter

(For removal of a temporary catheter/cannula, use appropriate E/M code)

49423 Exchange of previously placed abscess or cyst drainage catheter under radiological guidance (separate procedure)

(For radiological supervision and interpretation, use 75984)

49424 Contrast injection for assessment of abscess or cyst via previously placed drainage catheter or tube (separate procedure)

(For radiological supervision and interpretation, use 76080)

49425 Insertion of peritoneal-venous shunt

49426 Revision of peritoneal-venous shunt

(For shunt patency test, use 78291)

49427 Injection procedure (eg, contrast media) for evaluation of previously placed peritoneal-venous shunt

(For radiological supervision and interpretation, see 75809, 78291)

49428 Ligation of peritoneal-venous shunt

49429 Removal of peritoneal-venous shunt

(49430, 49440 have been deleted. To report, use 49999)

Surgery: Digestive System

Repair

Hernioplasty, Herniorrhaphy, Herniotomy

The hernia repair codes in this section are categorized primarily by the type of hernia (inguinal, femoral, incisional, etc.).

Some types of hernias are further categorized as "initial" or "recurrent" based on whether or not the hernia has required previous repair(s).

Additional variables accounted for by some of the codes include patient age and clinical presentation (reducible vs. incarcerated or strangulated).

With the exception of the incisional hernia repairs (see 49560-49566) the use of mesh or other prostheses is not separately reported.

The excision/repair of strangulated organs or structures such as testicle(s), intestine, ovaries are reported by using the appropriate code for the excision/repair (eg, 44120, 54520, and 58940) in addition to the appropriate code for the repair of the strangulated hernia.

(For reduction and repair of intra-abdominal hernia, use 44050)

(For debridement of abdominal wall, see 11042, 11043)

(All codes for bilateral procedures in hernia repair have been deleted. To report, add modifier '-50')

49491   Repair, initial inguinal hernia, preterm infant (less than 37 weeks gestation at birth), performed from birth up to 50 weeks postconception age, with or without hydrocelectomy; reducible

49492   incarcerated or strangulated

▶(Do not report modifier '-63' in conjunction with 49491, 49492)◀

(Postconception age equals gestational age at birth plus age of infant in weeks at the time of the hernia repair. Initial inguinal hernia repairs that are performed on preterm infants who are over 50 weeks postconception age and under age 6 months at the time of surgery, should be reported using codes 49495, 49496)

49495   Repair, initial inguinal hernia, full term infant under age 6 months, or preterm infant over 50 weeks postconception age and under age 6 months at the time of surgery, with or without hydrocelectomy; reducible

49496   incarcerated or strangulated

(Postconception age equals gestational age at birth plus age in weeks at the time of the hernia repair. Initial inguinal hernia repairs that are performed on preterm infants who are under or up to 50 weeks postconception age but under 6 months of age since birth, should be reported using codes 49491, 49492. Inguinal hernia repairs on infants age 6 months to under 5 years should be reported using codes 49500-49501)

▶(Do not report modifier '-63' in conjunction with 49495, 49496)◀

49500   Repair initial inguinal hernia, age 6 months to under 5 years, with or without hydrocelectomy; reducible

49501   incarcerated or strangulated

49505   Repair initial inguinal hernia, age 5 years or over; reducible

49507   incarcerated or strangulated

(49510 has been deleted. To report, see 49505 or 49507 and 54520)

(49515 has been deleted. To report, see 49505 or 49507 and 54840 or 55040)

49520   Repair recurrent inguinal hernia, any age; reducible

49521   incarcerated or strangulated

49525   Repair inguinal hernia, sliding, any age

(49530 has been deleted. To report, see 49496, 49501, 49507, 49521)

(49535 has been deleted. To report, see 49496, 49501, 49507, 49521)

49540   Repair lumbar hernia

49550   Repair initial femoral hernia, any age; reducible

(49552 has been deleted. To report, see 49550 or 49553)

49553   incarcerated or strangulated

49555   Repair recurrent femoral hernia; reducible

49557   incarcerated or strangulated

49560   Repair initial incisional or ventral hernia; reducible

49561   incarcerated or strangulated

49565   Repair recurrent incisional or ventral hernia; reducible

49566   incarcerated or strangulated

+ 49568   Implantation of mesh or other prosthesis for incisional or ventral hernia repair (List separately in addition to code for the incisional or ventral hernia repair)

49570   Repair epigastric hernia (eg, preperitoneal fat); reducible (separate procedure)

49572   incarcerated or strangulated

(49575 has been deleted. To report, use 49572)

49580   Repair umbilical hernia, under age 5 years; reducible

(49581 has been deleted. To report, see 49585 or 49587)

49582   incarcerated or strangulated

49585   Repair umbilical hernia, age 5 years or over; reducible

49587   incarcerated or strangulated

49590   Repair spigelian hernia

49600   Repair of small omphalocele, with primary closure

▶(Do not report modifier '-63' in conjunction with 49600)◀

49605   Repair of large omphalocele or gastroschisis; with or without prosthesis

49606   with removal of prosthesis, final reduction and closure, in operating room

▶(Do not report modifier '-63' in conjunction with 49605, 49606)◀

49610   Repair of omphalocele (Gross type operation); first stage

49611   second stage

▶(Do not report modifier '-63' in conjunction with 49610, 49611)◀

(For diaphragmatic or hiatal hernia repair, see 39502-39541)

(49630-49640 have been deleted. For surgical repair of omentum, use 49999)

Laparoscopy

Surgical laparoscopy always includes diagnostic laparoscopy. To report a diagnostic laparoscopy (peritoneoscopy) (separate procedure), use 49320.

49650   Laparoscopy, surgical; repair initial inguinal hernia

49651   repair recurrent inguinal hernia

49659   Unlisted laparoscopy procedure, hernioplasty, herniorrhaphy, herniotomy

Suture

49900   Suture, secondary, of abdominal wall for evisceration or dehiscence

(For suture of ruptured diaphragm, see 39540, 39541)

(For debridement of abdominal wall, see 11042, 11043)

Other Procedures

● 49904   Omental flap, extra-abdominal (eg, for reconstruction of sternal and chest wall defects)

▶(Code 49904 includes harvest and transfer. If a second surgeon harvests the omental flap, then the two surgeons should code 49904 as co-surgeons, using modifier '-62')◀

+ ▲ 49905   Omental flap, intra-abdominal (List separately in addition to code for primary procedure)

▶(Do not report 49905 in conjunction with 47700)◀

(49910 has been deleted. To report, use 49999)

49906   Free omental flap with microvascular anastomosis

(Do not report code 69990 in addition to 49906)

49999   Unlisted procedure, abdomen, peritoneum and omentum

Surgery: Digestive System

Notes

 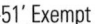=Modifier '-51' Exempt   ▶ ◀ or ▶ ◀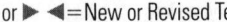=New or Revised Text   ✚=Add-on Code

Surgery: Digestive System

Urinary System

(For provision of chemotherapeutic agents, use 96545 in addition to code for primary procedure)

Kidney

Incision

(For retroperitoneal exploration, abscess, tumor, or cyst, see 49010, 49060, 49200, 49201)

50010   Renal exploration, not necessitating other specific procedures

▶(For laparoscopic ablation of renal mass lesion(s), use 50542)◀

50020   Drainage of perirenal or renal abscess; open

50021   percutaneous

(For radiological supervision and interpretation, use 75989)

50040   Nephrostomy, nephrotomy with drainage

50045   Nephrotomy, with exploration

(For renal endoscopy performed in conjunction with this procedure, see 50570-50580)

50060   Nephrolithotomy; removal of calculus

50065   secondary surgical operation for calculus

50070   complicated by congenital kidney abnormality

50075   removal of large staghorn calculus filling renal pelvis and calyces (including anatrophic pyelolithotomy)

50080   Percutaneous nephrostolithotomy or pyelostolithotomy, with or without dilation, endoscopy, lithotripsy, stenting, or basket extraction; up to 2 cm

50081   over 2 cm

(For establishment of nephrostomy without nephrostolithotomy, see 50040, 50395, 52334)

(For fluoroscopic guidance, see 76000, 76001)

50100   Transection or repositioning of aberrant renal vessels (separate procedure)

50120   Pyelotomy; with exploration

(For renal endoscopy performed in conjunction with this procedure, see 50570-50580)

50125   with drainage, pyelostomy

50130   with removal of calculus (pyelolithotomy, pelviolithotomy, including coagulum pyelolithotomy)

50135   complicated (eg, secondary operation, congenital kidney abnormality)

(For supply of anticarcinogenic agents, use 99070 in addition to code for primary procedure)

Excision

(For excision of retroperitoneal tumor or cyst, see 49200, 49201)

▶(For laparoscopic ablation of renal mass lesion(s), use 50542)◀

50200*   Renal biopsy; percutaneous, by trocar or needle

(For radiological supervision and interpretation, see 76003, 76360, 76393, 76942)

(For fine needle aspiration, use 10022)

(For evaluation of fine needle aspirate, see 88172, 88173)

50205   by surgical exposure of kidney

50220   Nephrectomy, including partial ureterectomy, any open approach including rib resection;

50225   complicated because of previous surgery on same kidney

50230   radical, with regional lymphadenectomy and/or vena caval thrombectomy

(When vena caval resection with reconstruction is necessary, use 37799)

50234   Nephrectomy with total ureterectomy and bladder cuff; through same incision

50236   through separate incision

50240   Nephrectomy, partial

▶(For laparoscopic partial nephrectomy, use 50543)◀

50280   Excision or unroofing of cyst(s) of kidney

(For laparoscopic ablation of renal cysts, use 50541)

50290   Excision of perinephric cyst

Renal Transplantation

(For dialysis, see 90935-90999)

(For laparoscopic donor nephrectomy, use 50547)

(For laparoscopic drainage of lymphocele to peritoneal cavity, use 49323)

50300   Donor nephrectomy, with preparation and maintenance of allograft, from cadaver donor, unilateral or bilateral

50320   Donor nephrectomy, open from living donor (excluding preparation and maintenance of allograft)

50340   Recipient nephrectomy (separate procedure)

(50341 has been deleted. To report, use 50340 with modifier '-50')

50360   Renal allotransplantation, implantation of graft; excluding donor and recipient nephrectomy

50365   with recipient nephrectomy

(50366 has been deleted. To report, use 50365 with modifier '-50')

Surgery: Urinary System

50370 Removal of transplanted renal allograft

50380 Renal autotransplantation, reimplantation of kidney

(For extra-corporeal "bench" surgery, use autotransplantation as the primary procedure and add the secondary procedure (eg, partial nephrectomy, nephrolithotomy), and use the modifier '-51')

Introduction

50390* Aspiration and/or injection of renal cyst or pelvis by needle, percutaneous

(For radiological supervision and interpretation, see 74425, 74470, 76003, 76360, 76393, 76942)

(For evaluation of fine needle aspirate, see 88172, 88173)

50392 Introduction of intracatheter or catheter into renal pelvis for drainage and/or injection, percutaneous

(For radiological supervision and interpretation, see 74475, 76360, 76942)

50393 Introduction of ureteral catheter or stent into ureter through renal pelvis for drainage and/or injection, percutaneous

(For radiological supervision and interpretation, see 74480, 76003, 76360, 76942)

50394 Injection procedure for pyelography (as nephrostogram, pyelostogram, antegrade pyeloureterograms) through nephrostomy or pyelostomy tube, or indwelling ureteral catheter

(For radiological supervision and interpretation, use 74425)

50395 Introduction of guide into renal pelvis and/or ureter with dilation to establish nephrostomy tract, percutaneous

(For radiological supervision and interpretation, see 74475, 74480, 74485)

(For nephrostolithotomy, see 50080, 50081)

(For retrograde percutaneous nephrostomy, use 52334)

(For endoscopic surgery, see 50551-50561)

50396 Manometric studies through nephrostomy or pyelostomy tube, or indwelling ureteral catheter

(For radiological supervision and interpretation, see 74425, 74475, 74480)

50398* Change of nephrostomy or pyelostomy tube

(For radiological supervision and interpretation, use 75984)

Repair

50400 Pyeloplasty (Foley Y-pyeloplasty), plastic operation on renal pelvis, with or without plastic operation on ureter, nephropexy, nephrostomy, pyelostomy, or ureteral splinting; simple

50405 complicated (congenital kidney abnormality, secondary pyeloplasty, solitary kidney, calycoplasty)

(For laparoscopic approach, use 50544)

(50420 has been deleted)

50500 Nephrorrhaphy, suture of kidney wound or injury

50520 Closure of nephrocutaneous or pyelocutaneous fistula

50525 Closure of nephrovisceral fistula (eg, renocolic), including visceral repair; abdominal approach

50526 thoracic approach

50540 Symphysiotomy for horseshoe kidney with or without pyeloplasty and/or other plastic procedure, unilateral or bilateral (one operation)

Laparoscopy

Surgical laparoscopy always includes diagnostic laparoscopy. To report a diagnostic laparoscopy (peritoneoscopy) (separate procedure), use 49320.

50541 Laparoscopy, surgical; ablation of renal cysts

● **50542** ablation of renal mass lesion(s)

►(For open procedure, see 50220-50240)◄

● **50543** partial nephrectomy

►(For open procedure, use 50240)◄

50544 pyeloplasty

50545 radical nephrectomy (includes removal of Gerota's fascia and surrounding fatty tissue, removal of regional lymph nodes, and adrenalectomy)

(For open procedure, use 50230)

50546 nephrectomy, including partial ureterectomy

50547 donor nephrectomy from living donor (excluding preparation and maintenance of allograft)

(For open procedure, use 50320)

50548 nephrectomy with total ureterectomy

(For open procedure, see 50234, 50236)

50549 Unlisted laparoscopy procedure, renal

(For laparoscopic drainage of lymphocele to peritoneal cavity, use 49323)

Endoscopy

(For supplies and materials, use 99070)

(References to office and hospital have been deleted)

50551   Renal endoscopy through established nephrostomy or pyelostomy, with or without irrigation, instillation, or ureteropyelography, exclusive of radiologic service;

50553   with ureteral catheterization, with or without dilation of ureter

50555   with biopsy

50557   with fulguration and/or incision, with or without biopsy

50559   with insertion of radioactive substance with or without biopsy and/or fulguration

50561   with removal of foreign body or calculus

● 50562   with resection of tumor

(When procedures 50570-50580 provide a significant identifiable service, they may be added to 50045 and 50120)

50570   Renal endoscopy through nephrotomy or pyelotomy, with or without irrigation, instillation, or ureteropyelography, exclusive of radiologic service;

(For nephrotomy, use 50045)

(For pyelotomy, use 50120)

50572   with ureteral catheterization, with or without dilation of ureter

50574   with biopsy

50575   with endopyelotomy (includes cystoscopy, ureteroscopy, dilation of ureter and ureteral pelvic junction, incision of ureteral pelvic junction and insertion of endopyelotomy stent)

50576   with fulguration and/or incision, with or without biopsy

50578   with insertion of radioactive substance, with or without biopsy and/or fulguration

50580   with removal of foreign body or calculus

Other Procedures

50590   Lithotripsy, extracorporeal shock wave

Ureter

Incision

50600   Ureterotomy with exploration or drainage (separate procedure)

(For ureteral endoscopy performed in conjunction with this procedure, see 50970-50980)

50605   Ureterotomy for insertion of indwelling stent, all types

50610   Ureterolithotomy; upper one-third of ureter

50620   middle one-third of ureter

50630   lower one-third of ureter

(For laparoscopic approach, use 50945)

(For transvesical ureterolithotomy, use 51060)

(For cystotomy with stone basket extraction of ureteral calculus, use 51065)

(For endoscopic extraction or manipulation of ureteral calculus, see 50080, 50081, 50561, 50961, 50980, 52320-52330, 52352, 52353)

Excision

(For ureterocele, see 51535, 52300)

50650   Ureterectomy, with bladder cuff (separate procedure)

50660   Ureterectomy, total, ectopic ureter, combination abdominal, vaginal and/or perineal approach

Introduction

50684   Injection procedure for ureterography or ureteropyelography through ureterostomy or indwelling ureteral catheter

(For radiological supervision and interpretation, use 74425)

50686   Manometric studies through ureterostomy or indwelling ureteral catheter

50688* Change of ureterostomy tube

(If imaging guidance is performed, use 75984)

50690   Injection procedure for visualization of ileal conduit and/or ureteropyelography, exclusive of radiologic service

(For radiological supervision and interpretation, use 74425)

Repair

50700   Ureteroplasty, plastic operation on ureter (eg, stricture)

50715   Ureterolysis, with or without repositioning of ureter for retroperitoneal fibrosis

(50716 has been deleted. To report, use 50715 with modifier '-50')

50722   Ureterolysis for ovarian vein syndrome

50725   Ureterolysis for retrocaval ureter, with reanastomosis of upper urinary tract or vena cava

50727   Revision of urinary-cutaneous anastomosis (any type urostomy);

50728   with repair of fascial defect and hernia

50740   Ureteropyelostomy, anastomosis of ureter and renal pelvis

Surgery: Urinary System

▲=Revised Code   ●=New Code   ✱=Service Includes Surgical Procedure Only

Surgery: Urinary System

50750   Ureterocalycostomy, anastomosis of ureter to renal calyx

50760   Ureteroureterostomy

50770   Transureteroureterostomy, anastomosis of ureter to contralateral ureter

(Codes 50780-50785 include minor procedures to prevent vesicoureteral reflux)

50780   Ureteroneocystostomy; anastomosis of single ureter to bladder

(50781 has been deleted. To report, use 50780 with modifier '-50')

(When combined with cystourethroplasty or vesical neck revision, use 51820)

50782   anastomosis of duplicated ureter to bladder

50783   with extensive ureteral tailoring

50785   with vesico-psoas hitch or bladder flap

(50786 has been deleted. To report, use 50785 with modifier '-50')

50800   Ureteroenterostomy, direct anastomosis of ureter to intestine

(50801 has been deleted. To report, use 50800 with modifier '-50')

50810   Ureterosigmoidostomy, with creation of sigmoid bladder and establishment of abdominal or perineal colostomy, including intestine anastomosis

50815   Ureterocolon conduit, including intestine anastomosis

(50816 has been deleted. To report, use 50815 with modifier '-50')

50820   Ureteroileal conduit (ileal bladder), including intestine anastomosis (Bricker operation)

(For combination of 50800-50820 with cystectomy, see 51580-51595)

(50821 has been deleted. To report, use 50820 with modifier '-50')

50825   Continent diversion, including intestine anastomosis using any segment of small and/or large intestine (Kock pouch or Camey enterocystoplasty)

50830   Urinary undiversion (eg, taking down of ureteroileal conduit, ureterosigmoidostomy or ureteroenterostomy with ureteroureterostomy or ureteroneocystostomy)

50840   Replacement of all or part of ureter by intestine segment, including intestine anastomosis

(50841 has been deleted. To report, use 50840 with modifier '-50')

50845   Cutaneous appendico-vesicostomy

50860   Ureterostomy, transplantation of ureter to skin

(50861 has been deleted. To report, use 50860 with modifier '-50')

50900   Ureterorrhaphy, suture of ureter (separate procedure)

50920   Closure of ureterocutaneous fistula

50930   Closure of ureterovisceral fistula (including visceral repair)

50940   Deligation of ureter

(For ureteroplasty, ureterolysis, see 50700-50860)

Laparoscopy

Surgical laparoscopy always includes diagnostic laparoscopy. To report a diagnostic laparoscopy (peritoneoscopy) (separate procedure), use 49320.

50945   Laparoscopy, surgical; ureterolithotomy

50947   ureteroneocystostomy with cystoscopy and ureteral stent placement

50948   ureteroneocystostomy without cystoscopy and ureteral stent placement

(For open ureteroneocystostomy, see 50780-50785)

50949   Unlisted laparoscopy procedure, ureter

Endoscopy

(References to office and hospital have been deleted)

50951   Ureteral endoscopy through established ureterostomy, with or without irrigation, instillation, or ureteropyelography, exclusive of radiologic service;

50953   with ureteral catheterization, with or without dilation of ureter

50955   with biopsy

50957   with fulguration and/or incision, with or without biopsy

50959   with insertion of radioactive substance, with or without biopsy and/or fulguration (not including provision of material)

50961   with removal of foreign body or calculus

(When procedures 50970-50980 provide a significant identifiable service, they may be added to 50600)

50970   Ureteral endoscopy through ureterotomy, with or without irrigation, instillation, or ureteropyelography, exclusive of radiologic service;

(For ureterotomy, use 50600)

50972   with ureteral catheterization, with or without dilation of ureter

50974   with biopsy

50976   with fulguration and/or incision, with or without biopsy

50978   with insertion of radioactive substance, with or without biopsy and/or fulguration (not including provision of material)

50980   with removal of foreign body or calculus

Bladder

Incision

51000*   Aspiration of bladder by needle

51005*   Aspiration of bladder; by trocar or intracatheter

51010   with insertion of suprapubic catheter

              (If imaging guidance is performed, see 76003, 76360, 76942)

51020   Cystotomy or cystostomy; with fulguration and/or insertion of radioactive material

51030   with cryosurgical destruction of intravesical lesion

51040   Cystostomy, cystotomy with drainage

51045   Cystotomy, with insertion of ureteral catheter or stent (separate procedure)

51050   Cystolithotomy, cystotomy with removal of calculus, without vesical neck resection

51060   Transvesical ureterolithotomy

51065   Cystotomy, with calculus basket extraction and/or ultrasonic or electrohydraulic fragmentation of ureteral calculus

51080   Drainage of perivesical or prevesical space abscess

Excision

51500   Excision of urachal cyst or sinus, with or without umbilical hernia repair

51520   Cystotomy; for simple excision of vesical neck (separate procedure)

51525   for excision of bladder diverticulum, single or multiple (separate procedure)

51530   for excision of bladder tumor

              (For transurethral resection, see 52234-52240, 52305)

51535   Cystotomy for excision, incision, or repair of ureterocele

              (For transurethral excision, use 52300)

              (51536 has been deleted. To report, use 51535 with modifier '-50')

51550   Cystectomy, partial; simple

51555   complicated (eg, postradiation, previous surgery, difficult location)

51565   Cystectomy, partial, with reimplantation of ureter(s) into bladder (ureteroneocystostomy)

51570   Cystectomy, complete; (separate procedure)

51575   with bilateral pelvic lymphadenectomy, including external iliac, hypogastric, and obturator nodes

51580   Cystectomy, complete, with ureterosigmoidostomy or ureterocutaneous transplantations;

51585   with bilateral pelvic lymphadenectomy, including external iliac, hypogastric, and obturator nodes

51590   Cystectomy, complete, with ureteroileal conduit or sigmoid bladder, including intestine anastomosis;

51595   with bilateral pelvic lymphadenectomy, including external iliac, hypogastric, and obturator nodes

51596   Cystectomy, complete, with continent diversion, any open technique, using any segment of small and/or large intestine to construct neobladder

51597   Pelvic exenteration, complete, for vesical, prostatic or urethral malignancy, with removal of bladder and ureteral transplantations, with or without hysterectomy and/or abdominoperineal resection of rectum and colon and colostomy, or any combination thereof

              (For pelvic exenteration for gynecologic malignancy, use 58240)

Introduction

51600*   Injection procedure for cystography or voiding urethrocystography

              (For radiological supervision and interpretation, see 74430, 74455)

51605   Injection procedure and placement of chain for contrast and/or chain urethrocystography

              (For radiological supervision and interpretation, use 74430)

51610   Injection procedure for retrograde urethrocystography

              (For radiological supervision and interpretation, use 74450)

51700*   Bladder irrigation, simple, lavage and/or instillation

              ►(Codes 51701-51702 are reported only when performed independently. Do not report 51701-51702 when catheter insertion is an inclusive component of another procedure.)◄

● **51701**   Insertion of non-indwelling bladder catheter (eg, straight catheterization for residual urine)

● **51702**   Insertion of temporary indwelling bladder catheter; simple (eg, Foley)

● **51703**   complicated (eg, altered anatomy, fractured catheter/balloon)

51705*   Change of cystostomy tube; simple

51710*   complicated

              (If imaging guidance is performed, use 75984)

51715   Endoscopic injection of implant material into the submucosal tissues of the urethra and/or bladder neck

51720   Bladder instillation of anticarcinogenic agent (including detention time)

Surgery: Urinary System

Urodynamics

The following section (51725-51797) lists procedures that may be used separately or in many and varied combinations.

When multiple procedures are performed in the same investigative session, modifier '-51' should be employed.

All procedures in this section imply that these services are performed by, or are under the direct supervision of, a physician and that all instruments, equipment, fluids, gases, probes, catheters, technician's fees, medications, gloves, trays, tubing and other sterile supplies be provided by the physician. When the physician only interprets the results and/or operates the equipment, a professional component, modifier '-26', should be used to identify physicians' services.

51725   Simple cystometrogram (CMG) (eg, spinal manometer)

51726   Complex cystometrogram (eg, calibrated electronic equipment)

(51727-51733 have been deleted. To report, use 51726)

51736   Simple uroflowmetry (UFR) (eg, stop-watch flow rate, mechanical uroflowmeter)

(51737, 51738 have been deleted. To report, use 51736)

(51739 has been deleted)

51741   Complex uroflowmetry (eg, calibrated electronic equipment)

(51742-51749 have been deleted. To report, use 51741)

(51751-51769 have been deleted. To report, use 53899)

51772   Urethral pressure profile studies (UPP) (urethral closure pressure profile), any technique

(51773-51783 have been deleted. To report, use 51772)

51784   Electromyography studies (EMG) of anal or urethral sphincter, other than needle, any technique

51785   Needle electromyography studies (EMG) of anal or urethral sphincter, any technique

(51786-51791 have been deleted. To report, use 51785)

51792   Stimulus evoked response (eg, measurement of bulbocavernosus reflex latency time)

51795   Voiding pressure studies (VP); bladder voiding pressure, any technique

(51796 has been deleted. To report, use 51795)

51797   intra-abdominal voiding pressure (AP) (rectal, gastric, intraperitoneal)

● **51798**   Measurement of post-voiding residual urine and/or bladder capacity by ultrasound, non-imaging

Repair

51800   Cystoplasty or cystourethroplasty, plastic operation on bladder and/or vesical neck (anterior Y-plasty, vesical fundus resection), any procedure, with or without wedge resection of posterior vesical neck

51820   Cystourethroplasty with unilateral or bilateral ureteroneocystostomy

51840   Anterior vesicourethropexy, or urethropexy (eg, Marshall-Marchetti-Krantz, Burch); simple

51841   complicated (eg, secondary repair)

(For urethropexy (Pereyra type), use 57289)

51845   Abdomino-vaginal vesical neck suspension, with or without endoscopic control (eg, Stamey, Raz, modified Pereyra)

51860   Cystorrhaphy, suture of bladder wound, injury or rupture; simple

51865   complicated

51880   Closure of cystostomy (separate procedure)

51900   Closure of vesicovaginal fistula, abdominal approach

(For vaginal approach, see 57320-57330)

51920   Closure of vesicouterine fistula;

51925   with hysterectomy

(For closure of vesicoenteric fistula, see 44660, 44661)

(For closure of rectovesical fistula, see 45800-45805)

51940   Closure, exstrophy of bladder

(See also 54390)

51960   Enterocystoplasty, including intestinal anastomosis

51980   Cutaneous vesicostomy

Laparoscopy

Surgical laparoscopy always includes diagnostic laparoscopy. To report a diagnostic laparoscopy (peritoneoscopy) (separate procedure), use 49320.

51990   Laparoscopy, surgical; urethral suspension for stress incontinence

51992   sling operation for stress incontinence (eg, fascia or synthetic)

(For open sling operation for stress incontinence, use 57288)

(For reversal or removal of sling operation for stress incontinence, use 57287)

Endoscopy—Cystoscopy, Urethroscopy, Cystourethroscopy

Endoscopic descriptions are listed so that the main procedure can be identified without having to list all the minor related functions performed at the same time. For example: meatotomy, urethral calibration and/or dilation, urethro-scopy, and cystoscopy prior to a transurethral resection of prostate; ureteral catheterization following extraction of ureteral calculus; internal urethrotomy and bladder neck fulguration when performing a cystourethroscopy for the female urethral syndrome. When the secondary procedure requires significant additional time and effort, it may be identified by the addition of modifier '-22'.

For example: urethrotomy performed for a documented pre-existing stricture or bladder neck contracture.

(References to office and hospital have been deleted)

52000　Cystourethroscopy (separate procedure)

▲**52001**　Cystourethroscopy with irrigation and evacuation of multiple obstructing clots

(Do not report 52001 in addition to 52000)

52005　Cystourethroscopy, with ureteral catheterization, with or without irrigation, instillation, or ureteropyelography, exclusive of radiologic service;

52007　　with brush biopsy of ureter and/or renal pelvis

52010　Cystourethroscopy, with ejaculatory duct catheterization, with or without irrigation, instillation, or duct radiography, exclusive of radiologic service

(For radiological supervision and interpretation, use 74440)

(52190 has been deleted)

Transurethral Surgery

Urethra and Bladder

(References to office and hospital have been deleted)

52204　Cystourethroscopy, with biopsy

52214　Cystourethroscopy, with fulguration (including cryosurgery or laser surgery) of trigone, bladder neck, prostatic fossa, urethra, or periurethral glands

52224　Cystourethroscopy, with fulguration (including cryosurgery or laser surgery) or treatment of MINOR (less than 0.5 cm) lesion(s) with or without biopsy

52234　Cystourethroscopy, with fulguration (including cryosurgery or laser surgery) and/or resection of; SMALL bladder tumor(s) (0.5 to 2.0 cm)

52235　　MEDIUM bladder tumor(s) (2.0 to 5.0 cm)

52240　　LARGE bladder tumor(s)

52250　Cystourethroscopy with insertion of radioactive substance, with or without biopsy or fulguration

52260　Cystourethroscopy, with dilation of bladder for interstitial cystitis; general or conduction (spinal) anesthesia

52265　　local anesthesia

52270　Cystourethroscopy, with internal urethrotomy; female

52275　　male

52276　Cystourethroscopy with direct vision internal urethrotomy

52277　Cystourethroscopy, with resection of external sphincter (sphincterotomy)

52281　Cystourethroscopy, with calibration and/or dilation of urethral stricture or stenosis, with or without meatotomy, with or without injection procedure for cystography, male or female

52282　Cystourethroscopy, with insertion of urethral stent

52283　Cystourethroscopy, with steroid injection into stricture

52285　Cystourethroscopy for treatment of the female urethral syndrome with any or all of the following: urethral meatotomy, urethral dilation, internal urethrotomy, lysis of urethrovaginal septal fibrosis, lateral incisions of the bladder neck, and fulguration of polyp(s) of urethra, bladder neck, and/or trigone

52290　Cystourethroscopy; with ureteral meatotomy, unilateral or bilateral

52300　　with resection or fulguration of orthotopic ureterocele(s), unilateral or bilateral

52301　　with resection or fulguration of ectopic ureterocele(s), unilateral or bilateral

52305　　with incision or resection of orifice of bladder diverticulum, single or multiple

52310　Cystourethroscopy, with removal of foreign body, calculus, or ureteral stent from urethra or bladder (separate procedure); simple

52315　　complicated

52317　Litholapaxy: crushing or fragmentation of calculus by any means in bladder and removal of fragments; simple or small (less than 2.5 cm)

52318　　complicated or large (over 2.5 cm)

Ureter and Pelvis

Surgical cystourethroscopy always includes diagnostic cystourethroscopy. To report a diagnostic cystourethroscopy, use 52351.

Do not report 52351 in conjunction with 52341-52346, 52352-52355.

The insertion and removal of a temporary stent during diagnostic or therapeutic cystourethroscopic intervention(s) is included in 52320-52355 and should not be reported separately.

To report insertion of a self-retaining, indwelling stent performed during cystourethroscopic diagnostic or therapeutic intervention(s), use code 52332, in addition to primary procedure(s) performed, and append the modifier '-51'. Code 52332 is used to report a unilateral procedure unless otherwise specified.

For bilateral insertion of self-retaining, indwelling ureteral stents, use code 52332, and append the modifier '-50'.

To report cystourethroscopic removal of a self-retaining, indwelling ureteral stent, see codes 52310, 52315, and append the modifier '-58'.

52320 Cystourethroscopy (including ureteral catheterization); with removal of ureteral calculus

52325 with fragmentation of ureteral calculus (eg, ultrasonic or electro-hydraulic technique)

52327 with subureteric injection of implant material

52330 with manipulation, without removal of ureteral calculus

52332 Cystourethroscopy, with insertion of indwelling ureteral stent (eg, Gibbons or double-J type)

52334 Cystourethroscopy with insertion of ureteral guide wire through kidney to establish a percutaneous nephrostomy, retrograde

(For percutaneous nephrostolithotomy, see 50080, 50081; for establishment of nephrostomy tract only, use 50395)

(52335 has been deleted. To report, use 52351)

(52336 has been deleted. To report, use 52352)

(52337 has been deleted. To report, use 52353)

(52338 has been deleted. To report, use 52354)

(52339 has been deleted. To report, use 52355)

(52340 has been deleted. To report, use 52400)

52341 Cystourethroscopy; with treatment of ureteral stricture (eg, balloon dilation, laser, electrocautery, and incision)

52342 with treatment of ureteropelvic junction stricture (eg, balloon dilation, laser, electrocautery, and incision)

52343 with treatment of intra-renal stricture (eg, balloon dilation, laser, electrocautery, and incision)

52344 Cystourethroscopy with ureteroscopy; with treatment of ureteral stricture (eg, balloon dilation, laser, electrocautery, and incision)

52345 with treatment of ureteropelvic junction stricture (eg, balloon dilation, laser, electrocautery, and incision)

52346 with treatment of intra-renal stricture (eg, balloon dilation, laser, electrocautery, and incision)

52347 Cystourethroscopy with transurethral resection or incision of ejaculatory ducts

52351 Cystourethroscopy, with ureteroscopy and/or pyeloscopy; diagnostic

(For radiological supervision and interpretation, use 74485)

(Do not report 52351 in conjunction with 52341-52346, 52352-52355)

52352 with removal or manipulation of calculus (ureteral catheterization is included)

52353 with lithotripsy (ureteral catheterization is included)

▲ **52354** with biopsy and/or fulguration of ureteral or renal pelvic lesion

▲ **52355** with resection of ureteral or renal pelvic tumor

Vesical Neck and Prostate

52400 Cystourethroscopy with incision, fulguration, or resection of congenital posterior urethral valves, or congenital obstructive hypertrophic mucosal folds

52450 Transurethral incision of prostate

52500 Transurethral resection of bladder neck (separate procedure)

52510 Transurethral balloon dilation of the prostatic urethra

52601 Transurethral electrosurgical resection of prostate, including control of postoperative bleeding, complete (vasectomy, meatotomy, cystourethroscopy, urethral calibration and/or dilation, and internal urethrotomy are included)

(For other approaches, see 55801-55845)

(52605 has been deleted. To report, use 52606)

52606 Transurethral fulguration for postoperative bleeding occurring after the usual follow-up time

52612 Transurethral resection of prostate; first stage of two-stage resection (partial resection)

52614 second stage of two-stage resection (resection completed)

52620 Transurethral resection; of residual obstructive tissue after 90 days postoperative

52630 of regrowth of obstructive tissue longer than one year postoperative

52640 of postoperative bladder neck contracture

52647 Non-contact laser coagulation of prostate, including control of postoperative bleeding, complete (vasectomy, meatotomy, cystourethroscopy, urethral calibration and/or dilation, and internal urethrotomy are included)

52648 Contact laser vaporization with or without transurethral resection of prostate, including control of postoperative bleeding, complete (vasectomy, meatotomy, cystourethroscopy, urethral calibration and/or dilation, and internal urethrotomy are included)

(52650 has been deleted)

Surgery: Urinary System

52700 Transurethral drainage of prostatic abscess

(52800, 52805 have been deleted. To report, see 52317, 52318)

Urethra

(For endoscopy, see cystoscopy, urethroscopy, cystourethroscopy, 52000-52700)

(For injection procedure for urethrocystography, see 51600-51610)

Incision

53000 Urethrotomy or urethrostomy, external (separate procedure); pendulous urethra

53010   perineal urethra, external

53020 Meatotomy, cutting of meatus (separate procedure); except infant

(53021 has been deleted. To report, use 53020)

53025   infant

▶(Do not report modifier '-63' in conjunction with 53025)◀

53040 Drainage of deep periurethral abscess

(For subcutaneous abscess, see 10060, 10061)

53060 Drainage of Skene's gland abscess or cyst

53080 Drainage of perineal urinary extravasation; uncomplicated (separate procedure)

53085   complicated

Excision

53200 Biopsy of urethra

53210 Urethrectomy, total, including cystostomy; female

53215   male

53220 Excision or fulguration of carcinoma of urethra

53230 Excision of urethral diverticulum (separate procedure); female

53235   male

53240 Marsupialization of urethral diverticulum, male or female

53250 Excision of bulbourethral gland (Cowper's gland)

53260 Excision or fulguration; urethral polyp(s), distal urethra

(For endoscopic approach, see 52214, 52224)

53265   urethral caruncle

53270   Skene's glands

53275   urethral prolapse

Repair

(For hypospadias, see 54300-54352)

53400 Urethroplasty; first stage, for fistula, diverticulum, or stricture (eg, Johannsen type)

53405   second stage (formation of urethra), including urinary diversion

53410 Urethroplasty, one-stage reconstruction of male anterior urethra

53415 Urethroplasty, transpubic or perineal, one stage, for reconstruction or repair of prostatic or membranous urethra

53420 Urethroplasty, two-stage reconstruction or repair of prostatic or membranous urethra; first stage

53425   second stage

53430 Urethroplasty, reconstruction of female urethra

53431 Urethroplasty with tubularization of posterior urethra and/or lower bladder for incontinence (eg, Tenago, Leadbetter procedure)

▲ **53440** Sling operation for correction of male urinary incontinence (eg, fascia or synthetic)

▲ **53442** Removal or revision of sling for male urinary incontinence (eg, fascia or synthetic)

(53443 has been deleted. To report, use 53431)

53444 Insertion of tandem cuff (dual cuff)

53445 Insertion of inflatable urethral/bladder neck sphincter, including placement of pump, reservoir, and cuff

53446 Removal of inflatable urethral/bladder neck sphincter, including pump, reservoir, and cuff

53447 Removal and replacement of inflatable urethral/bladder neck sphincter including pump, reservoir, and cuff at the same operative session

53448 Removal and replacement of inflatable urethral/bladder neck sphincter including pump, reservoir, and cuff through an infected field at the same operative session including irrigation and debridement of infected tissue

(Do not report 11040-11043 in addition to 53448)

53449 Repair of inflatable urethral/bladder neck sphincter, including pump, reservoir, and cuff

53450 Urethromeatoplasty, with mucosal advancement

(For meatotomy, see 53020, 53025)

53460 Urethromeatoplasty, with partial excision of distal urethral segment (Richardson type procedure)

53502 Urethrorrhaphy, suture of urethral wound or injury, female

53505 Urethrorrhaphy, suture of urethral wound or injury; penile

53510   perineal

53515   prostatomembranous

Surgery: Urinary System

53520   Closure of urethrostomy or urethrocutaneous fistula, male (separate procedure)

(For closure of urethrovaginal fistula, use 57310)

(For closure of urethrorectal fistula, see 45820, 45825)

Manipulation

(For radiological supervision and interpretation, use 74485)

53600*   Dilation of urethral stricture by passage of sound or urethral dilator, male; initial

53601*   subsequent

53605   Dilation of urethral stricture or vesical neck by passage of sound or urethral dilator, male, general or conduction (spinal) anesthesia

53620*   Dilation of urethral stricture by passage of filiform and follower, male; initial

53621*   subsequent

(53640 has been deleted. To report, use 53620)

53660*   Dilation of female urethra including suppository and/or instillation; initial

53661*   subsequent

53665   Dilation of female urethra, general or conduction (spinal) anesthesia

▶(53670 has been deleted. To report, see 51701, 51702)◀

▶(53675 has been deleted. To report, use 51703)◀

Other Procedures

(53800 has been deleted. To report, use 81020)

53850   Transurethral destruction of prostate tissue; by microwave thermotherapy

53852   by radiofrequency thermotherapy

53853   by water-induced thermotherapy

53899   Unlisted procedure, urinary system

Male Genital System

Penis

Incision

54000 Slitting of prepuce, dorsal or lateral (separate procedure); newborn

▶(Do not report modifier '-63' in conjunction with 54000)◀

54001   except newborn

54015 Incision and drainage of penis, deep

(For skin and subcutaneous abscess, see 10060-10160)

Destruction

54050* Destruction of lesion(s), penis (eg, condyloma, papilloma, molluscum contagiosum, herpetic vesicle), simple; chemical

54055*   electrodesiccation

54056   cryosurgery

54057   laser surgery

54060   surgical excision

54065 Destruction of lesion(s), penis (eg, condyloma, papilloma, molluscum contagiosum, herpetic vesicle), extensive (eg, laser surgery, electrosurgery, cryosurgery, chemosurgery)

(For destruction or excision of other lesions, see **Integumentary System**)

Excision

54100 Biopsy of penis; (separate procedure)

54105   deep structures

54110 Excision of penile plaque (Peyronie disease);

54111   with graft to 5 cm in length

54112   with graft greater than 5 cm in length

54115 Removal foreign body from deep penile tissue (eg, plastic implant)

54120 Amputation of penis; partial

54125   complete

54130 Amputation of penis, radical; with bilateral inguinofemoral lymphadenectomy

54135   in continuity with bilateral pelvic lymphadenectomy, including external iliac, hypogastric and obturator nodes

(For lymphadenectomy (separate procedure), see 38760-38770)

54150 Circumcision, using clamp or other device; newborn

▶(Do not report modifier '-63' in conjunction with 54150)◀

54152   except newborn

(54154 has been deleted. To report, use 54152)

54160 Circumcision, surgical excision other than clamp, device or dorsal slit; newborn

▶(Do not report modifier '-63' in conjunction with 54160)◀

54161   except newborn

54162 Lysis or excision of penile post-circumcision adhesions

54163 Repair incomplete circumcision

54164 Frenulotomy of penis

(Do not report 54164 with circumcision codes 54150-54161, 54162, 54163)

Introduction

54200* Injection procedure for Peyronie disease;

54205   with surgical exposure of plaque

54220 Irrigation of corpora cavernosa for priapism

54230 Injection procedure for corpora cavernosography

(For radiological supervision and interpretation, use 74445)

54231 Dynamic cavernosometry, including intracavernosal injection of vasoactive drugs (eg, papaverine, phentolamine)

54235 Injection of corpora cavernosa with pharmacologic agent(s) (eg, papaverine, phentolamine)

54240 Penile plethysmography

54250 Nocturnal penile tumescence and/or rigidity test

Repair

(For other urethroplasties, see 53400-53430)

(For penile revascularization, use 37788)

54300 Plastic operation of penis for straightening of chordee (eg, hypospadias), with or without mobilization of urethra

54304 Plastic operation on penis for correction of chordee or for first stage hypospadias repair with or without transplantation of prepuce and/or skin flaps

(54305 has been deleted. To report, see 54304 et seq)

54308 Urethroplasty for second stage hypospadias repair (including urinary diversion); less than 3 cm

54312   greater than 3 cm

54316 Urethroplasty for second stage hypospadias repair (including urinary diversion) with free skin graft obtained from site other than genitalia

Surgery: Male/Female Genital System

▲=Revised Code   ●=New Code   *=Service Includes Surgical Procedure Only   American Medical Association   **169**

54318 Urethroplasty for third stage hypospadias repair to release penis from scrotum (eg, third stage Cecil repair)

(54320 has been deleted. To report, see 54308 et seq)

54322 One stage distal hypospadias repair (with or without chordee or circumcision); with simple meatal advancement (eg, Magpi, V-flap)

54324   with urethroplasty by local skin flaps (eg, flip-flap, prepucial flap)

(54325 has been deleted. To report, see 54308 et seq)

54326   with urethroplasty by local skin flaps and mobilization of urethra

54328   with extensive dissection to correct chordee and urethroplasty with local skin flaps, skin graft patch, and/or island flap

(54330 has been deleted. To report, use 54308)

54332 One stage proximal penile or penoscrotal hypospadias repair requiring extensive dissection to correct chordee and urethroplasty by use of skin graft tube and/or island flap

54336 One stage perineal hypospadias repair requiring extensive dissection to correct chordee and urethroplasty by use of skin graft tube and/or island flap

54340 Repair of hypospadias complications (ie, fistula, stricture, diverticula); by closure, incision, or excision, simple

54344   requiring mobilization of skin flaps and urethroplasty with flap or patch graft

54348   requiring extensive dissection and urethroplasty with flap, patch or tubed graft (includes urinary diversion)

54352 Repair of hypospadias cripple requiring extensive dissection and excision of previously constructed structures including re-release of chordee and reconstruction of urethra and penis by use of local skin as grafts and island flaps and skin brought in as flaps or grafts

54360 Plastic operation on penis to correct angulation

54380 Plastic operation on penis for epispadias distal to external sphincter;

54385   with incontinence

54390   with exstrophy of bladder

54400 Insertion of penile prosthesis; non-inflatable (semi-rigid)

54401   inflatable (self-contained)

(54402 has been deleted. To report, see 54415, 54416)

54405 Insertion of multi-component, inflatable penile prosthesis, including placement of pump, cylinders, and reservoir

(For reduced services, report 54405 with modifier '-52')

54406 Removal of all components of a multi-component, inflatable penile prosthesis without replacement of prosthesis

(For reduced services, report 54406 with modifier '-52')

(54407 has been deleted. To report, see 54406, 54408, 54410)

54408 Repair of component(s) of a multi-component, inflatable penile prosthesis

(54409 has been deleted. To report, use 54408)

54410 Removal and replacement of all component(s) of a multi-component, inflatable penile prosthesis at the same operative session

54411 Removal and replacement of all components of a multi-component inflatable penile prosthesis through an infected field at the same operative session, including irrigation and debridement of infected tissue

(For reduced services, report 54411 with modifier '-52')

(Do not report 11040-11043 in addition to 54411)

54415 Removal of non-inflatable (semi-rigid) or inflatable (self-contained) penile prosthesis, without replacement of prosthesis

54416 Removal and replacement of non-inflatable (semi-rigid) or inflatable (self-contained) penile prosthesis at the same operative session

54417 Removal and replacement of non-inflatable (semi-rigid) or inflatable (self-contained) penile prosthesis through an infected field at the same operative session, including irrigation and debridement of infected tissue

(Do not report 11040-11043 in addition to 54417)

54420 Corpora cavernosa-saphenous vein shunt (priapism operation), unilateral or bilateral

54430 Corpora cavernosa-corpus spongiosum shunt (priapism operation), unilateral or bilateral

54435 Corpora cavernosa-glans penis fistulization (eg, biopsy needle, Winter procedure, rongeur, or punch) for priapism

54440 Plastic operation of penis for injury

Manipulation

54450 Foreskin manipulation including lysis of preputial adhesions and stretching

Testis

Excision

54500 Biopsy of testis, needle (separate procedure)

(For fine needle aspiration, see 10021, 10022)

(For evaluation of fine needle aspirate, see 88172, 88173)

54505 Biopsy of testis, incisional (separate procedure)

(When combined with vasogram, seminal vesiculogram, or epididymogram, use 55300)

(54506 has been deleted. To report, use 54505 with modifier '-50')

(54510 has been deleted. To report, use 54512)

Surgery: Male/Female Genital System

54512 Excision of extraparenchymal lesion of testis

54520 Orchiectomy, simple (including subcapsular), with or without testicular prosthesis, scrotal or inguinal approach

(54521 has been deleted. To report, use 54520 with modifier '-50')

54522 Orchiectomy, partial

54530 Orchiectomy, radical, for tumor; inguinal approach

54535 with abdominal exploration

(For orchiectomy with repair of hernia, see 49505 or 49507 and 54520)

(For radical retroperitoneal lymphadenectomy, use 38780)

54550 Exploration for undescended testis (inguinal or scrotal area)

(54555 has been deleted. To report, use 54550 with modifier '-50')

54560 Exploration for undescended testis with abdominal exploration

(54565 has been deleted. To report, use 54560 with modifier '-50')

Repair

54600 Reduction of torsion of testis, surgical, with or without fixation of contralateral testis

54620 Fixation of contralateral testis (separate procedure)

54640 Orchiopexy, inguinal approach, with or without hernia repair

(For inguinal hernia repair performed in conjunction with inguinal orchiopexy, see 49495-49525)

(54641 has been deleted. To report, use 54640 with modifier '-50')

(54645 has been deleted)

54650 Orchiopexy, abdominal approach, for intra-abdominal testis (eg, Fowler-Stephens)

(For laparoscopic approach, use 54692)

54660 Insertion of testicular prosthesis (separate procedure)

(54661 has been deleted. To report, use 54660 with modifier '-50')

54670 Suture or repair of testicular injury

54680 Transplantation of testis(es) to thigh (because of scrotal destruction)

Laparoscopy

Surgical laparoscopy always includes diagnostic laparoscopy. To report a diagnostic laparoscopy (peritoneoscopy) (separate procedure), use 49320.

54690 Laparoscopy, surgical; orchiectomy

54692 orchiopexy for intra-abdominal testis

54699 Unlisted laparoscopy procedure, testis

Epididymis

Incision

54700 Incision and drainage of epididymis, testis and/or scrotal space (eg, abscess or hematoma)

Excision

54800 Biopsy of epididymis, needle

(For fine needle aspiration, see 10021, 10022)

(For evaluation of fine needle aspirate, see 88172, 88173)

54820 Exploration of epididymis, with or without biopsy

54830 Excision of local lesion of epididymis

54840 Excision of spermatocele, with or without epididymectomy

54860 Epididymectomy; unilateral

54861 bilateral

Repair

54900 Epididymovasostomy, anastomosis of epididymis to vas deferens; unilateral

54901 bilateral

(For operating microscope, use 69990)

Tunica Vaginalis

Incision

55000* Puncture aspiration of hydrocele, tunica vaginalis, with or without injection of medication

Excision

55040 Excision of hydrocele; unilateral

55041 bilateral

(With hernia repair, see 49495-49501)

Repair

55060 Repair of tunica vaginalis hydrocele (Bottle type)

Scrotum

Incision

55100*   Drainage of scrotal wall abscess

     (See also 54700)

55110   Scrotal exploration

55120   Removal of foreign body in scrotum

Excision

     (For excision of local lesion of skin of scrotum, see **Integumentary System**)

55150   Resection of scrotum

Repair

     (55170 has been deleted. To report, see 55175, 55180)

55175   Scrotoplasty; simple

55180   complicated

Vas Deferens

Incision

55200   Vasotomy, cannulization with or without incision of vas, unilateral or bilateral (separate procedure)

Excision

55250   Vasectomy, unilateral or bilateral (separate procedure), including postoperative semen examination(s)

Introduction

55300   Vasotomy for vasograms, seminal vesiculograms, or epididymograms, unilateral or bilateral

     (For radiological supervision and interpretation, use 74440)

     (When combined with biopsy of testis, see 54505 and use modifier '-51')

Repair

55400   Vasovasostomy, vasovasorrhaphy

     (For operating microscope, use 69990)

     (55401 has been deleted. To report, use 55400 with modifier '-50')

Suture

55450   Ligation (percutaneous) of vas deferens, unilateral or bilateral (separate procedure)

Spermatic Cord

Excision

55500   Excision of hydrocele of spermatic cord, unilateral (separate procedure)

55520   Excision of lesion of spermatic cord (separate procedure)

55530   Excision of varicocele or ligation of spermatic veins for varicocele; (separate procedure)

55535   abdominal approach

55540   with hernia repair

Laparoscopy

Surgical laparoscopy always includes diagnostic laparoscopy. To report a diagnostic laparoscopy (peritoneoscopy) (separate procedure), use 49320.

55550   Laparoscopy, surgical, with ligation of spermatic veins for varicocele

55559   Unlisted laparoscopy procedure, spermatic cord

Seminal Vesicles

Incision

55600   Vesiculotomy;

     (55601 has been deleted. To report, use 55600 with modifier '-50')

55605   complicated

Excision

55650   Vesiculectomy, any approach

     (55651 has been deleted. To report, use 55650 with modifier '-50')

55680   Excision of Mullerian duct cyst

     (For injection procedure, see 52010, 55300)

Prostate

Incision

55700   Biopsy, prostate; needle or punch, single or multiple, any approach

     (If imaging guidance is performed, use 76942)

     (For fine needle aspiration, see 10021, 10022)

     (For evaluation of fine needle aspirate, see 88172, 88173)

55705   incisional, any approach

Surgery: Male/Female Genital System

55720 Prostatotomy, external drainage of prostatic abscess, any approach; simple

55725 complicated

(For transurethral drainage, use 52700)

(55740 has been deleted. To report, use 55899)

Excision

(For transurethral removal of prostate, see 52601-52640)

(For transurethral destruction of prostate, see 53850-53852)

(For limited pelvic lymphadenectomy for staging (separate procedure), use 38562)

(For independent node dissection, see 38770-38780)

55801 Prostatectomy, perineal, subtotal (including control of postoperative bleeding, vasectomy, meatotomy, urethral calibration and/or dilation, and internal urethrotomy)

55810 Prostatectomy, perineal radical;

55812 with lymph node biopsy(s) (limited pelvic lymphadenectomy)

55815 with bilateral pelvic lymphadenectomy, including external iliac, hypogastric and obturator nodes

(If 55815 is carried out on separate days, use 38770 with modifier '-50' and 55810)

55821 Prostatectomy (including control of postoperative bleeding, vasectomy, meatotomy, urethral calibration and/or dilation, and internal urethrotomy); suprapubic, subtotal, one or two stages

55831 retropubic, subtotal

55840 Prostatectomy, retropubic radical, with or without nerve sparing;

55842 with lymph node biopsy(s) (limited pelvic lymphadenectomy)

55845 with bilateral pelvic lymphadenectomy, including external iliac, hypogastric, and obturator nodes

(If 55845 is carried out on separate days, use 38770 with modifier '-50' and 55840)

▶(For laparoscopic retropubic radical prostatectomy, use 55866)◀

55859 Transperineal placement of needles or catheters into prostate for interstitial radioelement application, with or without cystoscopy

(For interstitial radioelement application, see 77776-77778)

(For ultrasonic guidance for interstitial radioelement application, use 76965)

55860 Exposure of prostate, any approach, for insertion of radioactive substance;

(For application of interstitial radioelement, see 77776-77778)

55862 with lymph node biopsy(s) (limited pelvic lymphadenectomy)

55865 with bilateral pelvic lymphadenectomy, including external iliac, hypogastric and obturator nodes

▶Laparoscopy◀

▶Surgical laparoscopy always includes diagnostic laparoscopy. To report a diagnostic laparoscopy (peritoneoscopy) (separate procedure), use 49320.◀

● **55866** Laparoscopy, surgical prostatectomy, retropubic radical, including nerve sparing

▶(For open procedure, use 55840)◀

Other Procedures

(For artificial insemination, see 58321, 58322)

55870 Electroejaculation

55873 Cryosurgical ablation of the prostate (includes ultrasonic guidance for interstitial cryosurgical probe placement)

55899 Unlisted procedure, male genital system

Intersex Surgery

55970 Intersex surgery; male to female

55980 female to male

(56300 has been deleted. To report, use 49320)

(56301 has been deleted. To report, use 58670)

(56302 has been deleted. To report, use 58671)

(56303 has been deleted. To report, use 58662)

(56304 has been deleted. To report, use 58660)

(56305 has been deleted. To report, use 49321)

(56306 has been deleted. To report, use 49322)

(56307 has been deleted. To report, use 58661)

(56308 has been deleted. To report, use 58550)

(56309 has been deleted. To report, use 58551)

(56310 has been deleted. To report, use 44200)

(56311 has been deleted. To report, use 38570)

(56312 has been deleted. To report, use 38571)

Surgery: Male/Female Genital System

(56313 has been deleted. To report, use 38572)

(56314 has been deleted. To report, use 49323)

(56315 has been deleted. To report, use 44970)

(56316 has been deleted. To report, use 49650)

(56317 has been deleted. To report, use 49651)

(56318 has been deleted. To report, use 54690)

(56320 has been deleted. To report, use 55550)

(56321 has been deleted. To report, use 60650)

(56322 has been deleted. To report, use 43651)

(56323 has been deleted. To report, use 43652)

(56324 has been deleted. To report, use 47570)

(56340 has been deleted. To report, use 47562)

(56341 has been deleted. To report, use 47563)

(56342 has been deleted. To report, use 47564)

(56343 has been deleted. To report, use 58673)

(56344 has been deleted. To report, use 58672)

(56345 has been deleted. To report, use 38120)

(56346 has been deleted. To report, use 43653)

(56347 has been deleted. To report, use 44201)

(56348 has been deleted. To report, use 44202)

(56349 has been deleted. To report, use 43280)

(56350 has been deleted. To report, use 58555)

(56351 has been deleted. To report, use 58558)

(56352 has been deleted. To report, use 58559)

(56353 has been deleted. To report, use 58560)

(56354 has been deleted. To report, use 58561)

(56355 has been deleted. To report, use 58562)

(56356 has been deleted. To report, use 58563)

(56360 has been deleted. To report, use 49320)

(56361 has been deleted. To report, use 49321)

(56362 has been deleted. To report, use 47560)

(56363 has been deleted. To report, use 47561)

(56399 has been deleted. To report, see site-specific unlisted laparoscopy/hysteroscopy procedure codes)

Surgery: Male/Female Genital System

Female Genital System

(For pelvic laparotomy, use 49000)

(For excision or destruction of endometriomas, open method, see 49200, 49201)

(For paracentesis, see 49080, 49081)

(For secondary closure of abdominal wall evisceration or disruption, use 49900)

(For fulguration or excision of lesions, laparoscopic approach, use 58662)

(For chemotherapy, see 96400-96549)

(56000 has been deleted. To report, use 56405)

(56100 has been deleted. To report, use 56605)

(56200 has been deleted. To report, use 56810)

Vulva, Perineum and Introitus

Definitions

The following definitions apply to the vulvectomy codes (56620-56640).

A *simple* procedure is the removal of skin and superficial subcutaneous tissues.

A *radical* procedure is the removal of skin and deep subcutaneous tissue.

A *partial* procedure is the removal of less than 80% of the vulvar area.

A *complete* procedure is the removal of greater than 80% of the vulvar area.

Incision

(For incision and drainage of sebaceous cyst, furuncle, or abscess, see 10040, 10060, 10061)

(56400 has been deleted. To report, use 56405)

56405*   Incision and drainage of vulva or perineal abscess

56420*   Incision and drainage of Bartholin's gland abscess

(For incision and drainage of Skene's gland abscess or cyst, use 53060)

56440   Marsupialization of Bartholin's gland cyst

56441   Lysis of labial adhesions

Destruction

(56500 has been deleted. To report, use 56501)

56501   Destruction of lesion(s), vulva; simple (eg, laser surgery, electrosurgery, cryosurgery, chemosurgery)

(56505-56507, 56510 have been deleted. To report, use 56501)

56515   extensive (eg, laser surgery, electrosurgery, cryosurgery, chemosurgery)

(56520, 56521 have been deleted. To report, use 56501 or 56515)

(For destruction of Skene's gland cyst or abscess, use 53270)

(For cautery destruction of urethral caruncle, use 53265)

Excision

(56600 has been deleted. To report, use 56605)

56605*   Biopsy of vulva or perineum (separate procedure); one lesion

+ 56606*   each separate additional lesion (List separately in addition to code for primary procedure)

(Use 56606 in conjunction with code 56605)

(For excision of local lesion, see 11420-11426, 11620-11626)

56620   Vulvectomy simple; partial

56625   complete

(For skin graft, see 15000 et seq)

56630   Vulvectomy, radical, partial;

(For skin graft, if used, see 15000, 15120, 15121, 15240, 15241)

56631   with unilateral inguinofemoral lymphadenectomy

56632   with bilateral inguinofemoral lymphadenectomy

56633   Vulvectomy, radical, complete;

56634   with unilateral inguinofemoral lymphadenectomy

(56635 has been deleted. To report, see 56634, 56637)

(56636 has been deleted. To report, see 56634, 56637)

56637   with bilateral inguinofemoral lymphadenectomy

56640   Vulvectomy, radical, complete, with inguinofemoral, iliac, and pelvic lymphadenectomy

(56641 has been deleted. To report, use 56640 with modifier '-50')

(For lymphadenectomy, see 38760-38780)

(56680, 56685 have been deleted)

56700   Partial hymenectomy or revision of hymenal ring

(56710 has been deleted. To report, use 56700)

56720*   Hymenotomy, simple incision

56740   Excision of Bartholin's gland or cyst

(For excision of Skene's gland, use 53270)

(For excision of urethral caruncle, use 53265)

(For excision or fulguration of urethral carcinoma, use 53220)

(For excision or marsupialization of urethral diverticulum, see 53230, 53240)

Surgery: Male/Female Genital System

▲=Revised Code   ●=New Code   ✱=Service Includes Surgical Procedure Only   American Medical Association   **175**

Repair

(For repair of urethra for mucosal prolapse, use 53275)

56800   Plastic repair of introitus

56805   Clitoroplasty for intersex state

56810   Perineoplasty, repair of perineum, nonobstetrical (separate procedure)

(See also 56800)

(For repair of wounds to genitalia, see 12001-12007, 12041-12047, 13131-13133)

(For repair of recent injury of vagina and perineum, nonobstetrical, use 57210)

(For anal sphincteroplasty, see 46750, 46751)

(For episiorrhaphy, episioperineorrhaphy for recent injury of vulva and/or perineum, nonobstetrical, use 57210)

►Endoscopy◄

● **56820**   Colposcopy of the vulva;

● **56821**   with biopsy (s)

►(For colposcopic examinations/procedures involving the vagina, see 57420, 57421; cervix, see 57452-57461)◄

Vagina

Incision

57000   Colpotomy; with exploration

57010   with drainage of pelvic abscess

57020*   Colpocentesis (separate procedure)

57022   Incision and drainage of vaginal hematoma; obstetrical/postpartum

57023   non-obstetrical (eg, post-trauma, spontaneous bleeding)

Destruction

(57050, 57057, 57060 have been deleted. To report, use 57061 or 57065)

57061   Destruction of vaginal lesion(s); simple (eg, laser surgery, electrosurgery, cryosurgery, chemosurgery)

(57063 has been deleted. To report, use 57061 or 57065)

57065   extensive (eg, laser surgery, electrosurgery, cryosurgery, chemosurgery)

Excision

57100*   Biopsy of vaginal mucosa; simple (separate procedure)

57105   extensive, requiring suture (including cysts)

57106   Vaginectomy, partial removal of vaginal wall;

57107   with removal of paravaginal tissue (radical vaginectomy)

(57108 has been deleted. To report, use 57106)

57109   with removal of paravaginal tissue (radical vaginectomy) with bilateral total pelvic lymphadenectomy and para-aortic lymph node sampling (biopsy)

57110   Vaginectomy, complete removal of vaginal wall;

57111   with removal of paravaginal tissue (radical vaginectomy)

57112   with removal of paravaginal tissue (radical vaginectomy) with bilateral total pelvic lymphadenectomy and para-aortic lymph node sampling (biopsy)

57120   Colpocleisis (Le Fort type)

57130   Excision of vaginal septum

57135   Excision of vaginal cyst or tumor

Introduction

57150*   Irrigation of vagina and/or application of medicament for treatment of bacterial, parasitic, or fungoid disease

57155   Insertion of uterine tandems and/or vaginal ovoids for clinical brachytherapy

(For insertion of radioelement sources or ribbons, see 77761-77763, 77781-77784)

57160*   Fitting and insertion of pessary or other intravaginal support device

57170   Diaphragm or cervical cap fitting with instructions

57180   Introduction of any hemostatic agent or pack for spontaneous or traumatic nonobstetrical vaginal hemorrhage (separate procedure)

Repair

(For urethral suspension, Marshall-Marchetti-Krantz type, abdominal approach, see 51840, 51841)

(For laparoscopic suspension, use 51990)

57200   Colporrhaphy, suture of injury of vagina (nonobstetrical)

57210   Colpoperineorrhaphy, suture of injury of vagina and/or perineum (nonobstetrical)

57220   Plastic operation on urethral sphincter, vaginal approach (eg, Kelly urethral plication)

57230   Plastic repair of urethrocele

57240   Anterior colporrhaphy, repair of cystocele with or without repair of urethrocele

57250   Posterior colporrhaphy, repair of rectocele with or without perineorrhaphy

(For repair of rectocele (separate procedure) without posterior colporrhaphy, use 45560)

57260   Combined anteroposterior colporrhaphy;

57265   with enterocele repair

57268   Repair of enterocele, vaginal approach (separate procedure)

57270   Repair of enterocele, abdominal approach (separate procedure)

57280   Colpopexy, abdominal approach

57282   Sacrospinous ligament fixation for prolapse of vagina

57284   Paravaginal defect repair (including repair of cystocele, stress urinary incontinence, and/or incomplete vaginal prolapse)

57287   Removal or revision of sling for stress incontinence (eg, fascia or synthetic)

57288   Sling operation for stress incontinence (eg, fascia or synthetic)

(For laparoscopic approach, use 51992)

57289   Pereyra procedure, including anterior colporrhaphy

(57290 has been deleted. To report, use 57291 or 57292)

57291   Construction of artificial vagina; without graft

57292   with graft

57300   Closure of rectovaginal fistula; vaginal or transanal approach

57305   abdominal approach

57307   abdominal approach, with concomitant colostomy

57308   transperineal approach, with perineal body reconstruction, with or without levator plication

57310   Closure of urethrovaginal fistula;

57311   with bulbocavernosus transplant

57320   Closure of vesicovaginal fistula; vaginal approach

(For concomitant cystostomy, see 51005-51040)

57330   transvesical and vaginal approach

(For abdominal approach, use 51900)

57335   Vaginoplasty for intersex state

Manipulation

57400*   Dilation of vagina under anesthesia

57410*   Pelvic examination under anesthesia

57415   Removal of impacted vaginal foreign body (separate procedure) under anesthesia

(For removal without anesthesia of an impacted vaginal foreign body, use the appropriate E/M code)

Endoscopy

▶(For speculoscopy, see Category III codes 0030T, 0031T)◀

● **57420**   Colposcopy of the entire vagina, with cervix if present;

● **57421**   with biopsy(s)

▶(For colposcopic visualization of cervix and adjacent upper vagina, use 57452)◀

▶(When reporting colposcopies of multiple sites, use modifier '-51' as appropriate. For colposcopic examinations/procedures involving the vulva, see 56820, 56821; cervix, see 57452-57461)◀

(57450, 57451 have been deleted)

Cervix Uteri

▶(For cervicography, see Category III code 0003T)◀

▶Endoscopy◀

▶For colposcopic examinations/procedures involving the vulva, see 56820, 56821; vagina, see 57420, 57421◀

▲ **57452***   Colposcopy of the cervix including upper/adjacent vagina;

▶(Do not report 57452 in addition to 57454-57461)◀

▲ **57454***   with biopsy(s) of the cervix and endocervical curettage

● **57455**   with biopsy(s) of the cervix

● **57456**   with endocervical curettage

▲ **57460**   with loop electrode biopsy(s) of the cervix

● **57461**   with loop electrode conization of the cervix

▶(Do not report 57456 in addition to 57461)◀

Excision

(For radical surgical procedures, see 58200-58240)

57500*   Biopsy, single or multiple, or local excision of lesion, with or without fulguration (separate procedure)

57505   Endocervical curettage (not done as part of a dilation and curettage)

57510   Cautery of cervix; electro or thermal

57511*   cryocautery, initial or repeat

57513   laser ablation

57520   Conization of cervix, with or without fulguration, with or without dilation and curettage, with or without repair; cold knife or laser

(See also 58120)

57522   loop electrode excision

57530   Trachelectomy (cervicectomy), amputation of cervix (separate procedure)

Surgery: Male/Female Genital System

57531   Radical trachelectomy, with bilateral total pelvic lymphadenectomy and para-aortic lymph node sampling biopsy, with or without removal of tube(s), with or without removal of ovary(s)

(For radical abdominal hysterectomy, use 58210)

57540   Excision of cervical stump, abdominal approach;

57545   with pelvic floor repair

57550   Excision of cervical stump, vaginal approach;

57555   with anterior and/or posterior repair

57556   with repair of enterocele

(For insertion of intrauterine device, use 58300)

(57600-57620 have been deleted. For insertion of any hemostatic agent or pack for control of spontaneous non-obstetrical hemorrhage, use 57180)

Repair

57700   Cerclage of uterine cervix, nonobstetrical

57720   Trachelorrhaphy, plastic repair of uterine cervix, vaginal approach

Manipulation

57800*   Dilation of cervical canal, instrumental (separate procedure)

57820   Dilation and curettage of cervical stump

Corpus Uteri

Excision

58100*   Endometrial sampling (biopsy) with or without endocervical sampling (biopsy), without cervical dilation, any method (separate procedure)

(For endocervical curettage only, use 57505)

(58101, 58102, 58103 have been deleted)

58120   Dilation and curettage, diagnostic and/or therapeutic (nonobstetrical)

(For postpartum hemorrhage, use 59160)

▲**58140**   Myomectomy, excision of fibroid tumor(s) of uterus, 1 to 4 intramural myoma(s) with total weight of 250 grams or less and/or removal of surface myomas; abdominal approach

58145   vaginal approach

●**58146**   Myomectomy, excision of fibroid tumor(s) of uterus, 5 or more intramural myomas and/or intramural myomas with total weight greater than 250 grams, abdominal approach

▶(Do not report 58146 in addition to 58140-58145, 58150-58240)◀

58150   Total abdominal hysterectomy (corpus and cervix), with or without removal of tube(s), with or without removal of ovary(s);

58152   with colpo-urethrocystopexy (eg, Marshall-Marchetti-Krantz, Burch)

(For urethrocystopexy without hysterectomy, see 51840, 51841)

58180   Supracervical abdominal hysterectomy (subtotal hysterectomy), with or without removal of tube(s), with or without removal of ovary(s)

58200   Total abdominal hysterectomy, including partial vaginectomy, with para-aortic and pelvic lymph node sampling, with or without removal of tube(s), with or without removal of ovary(s)

(58205 has been deleted. For hysterectomy with pelvic lymphadenectomy, use 58210)

58210   Radical abdominal hysterectomy, with bilateral total pelvic lymphadenectomy and para-aortic lymph node sampling (biopsy), with or without removal of tube(s), with or without removal of ovary(s)

(For radical hysterectomy with ovarian transposition, use also 58825)

58240   Pelvic exenteration for gynecologic malignancy, with total abdominal hysterectomy or cervicectomy, with or without removal of tube(s), with or without removal of ovary(s), with removal of bladder and ureteral transplantations, and/or abdominoperineal resection of rectum and colon and colostomy, or any combination thereof

(For pelvic exenteration for lower urinary tract or male genital malignancy, use 51597)

▲**58260**   Vaginal hysterectomy, for uterus 250 grams or less;

58262   with removal of tube(s), and/or ovary(s)

58263   with removal of tube(s), and/or ovary(s), with repair of enterocele

(58265 has been deleted. To report, see 57240, 57250, 57260, 57265)

58267   with colpo-urethrocystopexy (Marshall-Marchetti-Krantz type, Pereyra type) with or without endoscopic control

58270   with repair of enterocele

(For repair of enterocele with removal of tubes and/or ovaries, use 58263)

58275   Vaginal hysterectomy, with total or partial vaginectomy;

58280   with repair of enterocele

58285   Vaginal hysterectomy, radical (Schauta type operation)

●**58290**   Vaginal hysterectomy, for uterus greater than 250 grams;

●**58291**   with removal of tube(s) and/or ovary(s)

●**58292**   with removal of tube(s) and/or ovary(s), with repair of enterocele

● 58293   with colpo-urethrocystopexy (Marshall-Marchetti-Krantz type, Pereyra type) with or without endoscopic control

● 58294   with repair of enterocele

Introduction

(For insertion/removal of implantable contraceptive capsules, see 11975, 11976, 11977)

58300*   Insertion of intrauterine device (IUD)

58301   Removal of intrauterine device (IUD)

(58310 has been deleted. To report, see 58321, 58322)

(58311 has been deleted. To report, use 58323)

(58320 has been deleted)

58321   Artificial insemination; intra-cervical

58322   intra-uterine

58323   Sperm washing for artificial insemination

58340*   Catheterization and introduction of saline or contrast material for hysterosonography or hysterosalpingography

(For radiological supervision and interpretation of hysterosonography, use 76831)

(For radiological supervision and interpretation of hysterosalpingography, use 74740)

(For endometrial cryoablation with ultrasonic guidance, use Category III code 0009T)

58345   Transcervical introduction of fallopian tube catheter for diagnosis and/or re-establishing patency (any method), with or without hysterosalpingography

(For radiological supervision and interpretation, use 74742)

58346   Insertion of Heyman capsules for clinical brachytherapy

(For insertion of radioelement sources or ribbons, see 77761-77763, 77781-77784)

58350*   Chromotubation of oviduct, including materials

(For materials supplied by physician, use 99070)

58353   Endometrial ablation, thermal, without hysteroscopic guidance

(For hysteroscopic procedure, use 58563)

Repair

58400   Uterine suspension, with or without shortening of round ligaments, with or without shortening of sacrouterine ligaments; (separate procedure)

58410   with presacral sympathectomy

(58430 has been deleted. To report, use 58999)

(58500 has been deleted. To report, use 58752)

58520   Hysterorrhaphy, repair of ruptured uterus (nonobstetrical)

58540   Hysteroplasty, repair of uterine anomaly (Strassman type)

(For closure of vesicouterine fistula, use 51920)

Laparoscopy/Hysteroscopy

Surgical laparoscopy always includes diagnostic laparoscopy. To report a diagnostic laparoscopy (peritoneoscopy) (separate procedure), use 49320. To report a diagnostic hysteroscopy (separate procedure), use 58555.

● 58545   Laparoscopy, surgical, myomectomy, excision; 1 to 4 intramural myomas with total weight of 250 grams or less and/or removal of surface myomas

● 58546   5 or more intramural myomas and/or intramural myomas with total weight greater than 250 grams

▲ 58550   Laparoscopy surgical, with vaginal hysterectomy, for uterus 250 grams or less;

    ▶(58551 has been deleted. To report see 58545, 58546)◀

● 58552   with removal of tube(s) and/or ovary(s)

● 58553   Laparoscopy, surgical, with vaginal hysterectomy, for uterus greater than 250 grams;

● 58554   with removal of tube(s) and/or ovary(s)

58555   Hysteroscopy, diagnostic (separate procedure)

58558   Hysteroscopy, surgical; with sampling (biopsy) of endometrium and/or polypectomy, with or without D & C

58559   with lysis of intrauterine adhesions (any method)

58560   with division or resection of intrauterine septum (any method)

58561   with removal of leiomyomata

58562   with removal of impacted foreign body

58563   with endometrial ablation (eg, endometrial resection, electrosurgical ablation, thermoablation)

58578   Unlisted laparoscopy procedure, uterus

58579   Unlisted hysteroscopy procedure, uterus

Oviduct/Ovary

Incision

58600   Ligation or transection of fallopian tube(s), abdominal or vaginal approach, unilateral or bilateral

58605   Ligation or transection of fallopian tube(s), abdominal or vaginal approach, postpartum, unilateral or bilateral, during same hospitalization (separate procedure)

(For laparoscopic procedures, use 58670, 58671)

(58610 has been deleted. To report, see 58600-58611)

Surgery: Male/Female Genital System

+ 58611 Ligation or transection of fallopian tube(s) when done at the time of cesarean delivery or intra-abdominal surgery (not a separate procedure) (List separately in addition to code for primary procedure)

58615 Occlusion of fallopian tube(s) by device (eg, band, clip, Falope ring) vaginal or suprapubic approach

(For laparoscopic approach, use 58671)

(58618 has been deleted. To report, use 58740)

Laparoscopy

Surgical laparoscopy always includes diagnostic laparoscopy. To report a diagnostic laparoscopy (peritoneoscopy) (separate procedure), use 49320.

(For laparoscopic biopsy of the ovary or fallopian tube, use 49321)

58660 Laparoscopy, surgical; with lysis of adhesions (salpingolysis, ovariolysis) (separate procedure)

58661 with removal of adnexal structures (partial or total oophorectomy and/or salpingectomy)

58662 with fulguration or excision of lesions of the ovary, pelvic viscera, or peritoneal surface by any method

58670 with fulguration of oviducts (with or without transection)

58671 with occlusion of oviducts by device (eg, band, clip, or Falope ring)

58672 with fimbrioplasty

58673 with salpingostomy (salpingoneostomy)

(Codes 58672 and 58673 are used to report unilateral procedures. For bilateral procedure, use modifier '-50')

58679 Unlisted laparoscopy procedure, oviduct, ovary

Excision

58700 Salpingectomy, complete or partial, unilateral or bilateral (separate procedure)

58720 Salpingo-oophorectomy, complete or partial, unilateral or bilateral (separate procedure)

Repair

58740 Lysis of adhesions (salpingolysis, ovariolysis)

(For laparoscopic approach, use 58660)

(For excision or destruction of endometriomas, open method, see 49200, 49201)

(For fulguration or excision of lesions, laparoscopic approach, use 58662)

58750 Tubotubal anastomosis

58752 Tubouterine implantation

58760 Fimbrioplasty

(For laparoscopic approach, use 58672)

58770 Salpingostomy (salpingoneostomy)

(For laparoscopic approach, use 58673)

Ovary

Incision

58800 Drainage of ovarian cyst(s), unilateral or bilateral, (separate procedure); vaginal approach

58805 abdominal approach

58820 Drainage of ovarian abscess; vaginal approach, open

58822 abdominal approach

58823 Drainage of pelvic abscess, transvaginal or transrectal approach, percutaneous (eg, ovarian, pericolic)

(For radiological supervision and interpretation, use 75989)

58825 Transposition, ovary(s)

Excision

58900 Biopsy of ovary, unilateral or bilateral (separate procedure)

(For laparoscopic biopsy of the ovary or fallopian tube, use 49321)

58920 Wedge resection or bisection of ovary, unilateral or bilateral

58925 Ovarian cystectomy, unilateral or bilateral

58940 Oophorectomy, partial or total, unilateral or bilateral;

(58942 has been deleted. To report, use 58952)

58943 for ovarian, tubal or primary peritoneal malignancy, with para-aortic and pelvic lymph node biopsies, peritoneal washings, peritoneal biopsies, diaphragmatic assessments, with or without salpingectomy(s), with or without omentectomy

(58945 has been deleted. To report, use 58950)

58950 Resection of ovarian, tubal or primary peritoneal malignancy with bilateral salpingo-oophorectomy and omentectomy;

58951 with total abdominal hysterectomy, pelvic and limited para-aortic lymphadenectomy

58952 with radical dissection for debulking (ie, radical excision or destruction, intra-abdominal or retroperitoneal tumors)

58953 Bilateral salpingo-oophorectomy with omentectomy, total abdominal hysterectomy and radical dissection for debulking;

58954 with pelvic lymphadenectomy and limited para-aortic lymphadenectomy

58960   Laparotomy, for staging or restaging of ovarian, tubal or primary peritoneal malignancy (second look), with or without omentectomy, peritoneal washing, biopsy of abdominal and pelvic peritoneum, diaphragmatic assessment with pelvic and limited para-aortic lymphadenectomy

In Vitro Fertilization

58970   Follicle puncture for oocyte retrieval, any method

(For radiological supervision and interpretation, use 76948)

(58972 has been deleted. To report, use 89250)

58974   Embryo transfer, intrauterine

58976   Gamete, zygote, or embryo intrafallopian transfer, any method

(58980 has been deleted. To report, use 49320)

(58982 has been deleted. To report, use 58670)

(58983 has been deleted. To report, use 58671)

(58984 has been deleted. To report, use 58662)

(58985 has been deleted. To report, use 58660)

(58986 has been deleted. To report, use 49321)

(58987 has been deleted. To report, use 49322)

(58988 has been deleted. To report, use 58661)

(58990 has been deleted. To report, use 58555)

(58992 has been deleted. To report, see 58559, 58560)

(58994 has been deleted. To report, use 58561)

(58995 has been deleted. To report, see 58559, 58561, 58563)

(58996 has been deleted. To report, use 58563)

Other Procedures

58999   Unlisted procedure, female genital system (nonobstetrical)

Maternity Care and Delivery

The services normally provided in uncomplicated maternity cases include antepartum care, delivery, and postpartum care.

Antepartum care includes the initial and subsequent history, physical examinations, recording of weight, blood pressures, fetal heart tones, routine chemical urinalysis, and monthly visits up to 28 weeks gestation, biweekly visits to 36 weeks gestation, and weekly visits until delivery. Any other visits or services within this time period should be coded separately.

Delivery services include admission to the hospital, the admission history and physical examination, management of uncomplicated labor, vaginal delivery (with or without episiotomy, with or without forceps), or cesarean delivery. Medical problems complicating labor and delivery management may require additional resources and should be identified by utilizing the codes in the **Medicine** and **Evaluation and Management Services** section in addition to codes for maternity care.

Postpartum care includes hospital and office visits following vaginal or cesarean section delivery.

For medical complications of pregnancy (eg, cardiac problems, neurological problems, diabetes, hypertension, toxemia, hyperemesis, pre-term labor, premature rupture of membranes), see services in the **Medicine** and **Evaluation and Management Services** section.

For surgical complications of pregnancy (eg, appendectomy, hernia, ovarian cyst, Bartholin cyst), see services in the **Surgery** section.

If a physician provides all or part of the antepartum and/or postpartum patient care but does not perform delivery due to termination of pregnancy by abortion or referral to another physician for delivery, see the antepartum and postpartum care codes 59425-59426 and 59430.

(For circumcision of newborn, see 54150, 54160)

Antepartum Services

(For insertion of transcervical or transvaginal fetal oximetry sensor, use Category III code 0021T)

59000*   Amniocentesis; diagnostic

(For radiological supervision and interpretation, use 76946)

59001   therapeutic amniotic fluid reduction (includes ultrasound guidance)

(59010, 59011 have been deleted)

59012   Cordocentesis (intrauterine), any method

(For radiological supervision and interpretation, use 76941)

59015   Chorionic villus sampling, any method

(For radiological supervision and interpretation, use 76945)

59020*   Fetal contraction stress test

59025   Fetal non-stress test

59030*   Fetal scalp blood sampling

(59031 has been deleted. To report, use 59030 and see modifiers '-76' and '-77')

59050   Fetal monitoring during labor by consulting physician (ie, non-attending physician) with written report; supervision and interpretation

59051   interpretation only

Excision

59100 Hysterotomy, abdominal (eg, for hydatidiform mole, abortion)

(When tubal ligation is performed at the same time as hysterotomy, use 58611 in addition to 59100)

(59101, 59105, 59106 have been deleted. To report, see 59100, 58611)

59120 Surgical treatment of ectopic pregnancy; tubal or ovarian, requiring salpingectomy and/or oophorectomy, abdominal or vaginal approach

59121 tubal or ovarian, without salpingectomy and/or oophorectomy

(59125, 59126 have been deleted. To report, see 59120, 59121)

59130 abdominal pregnancy

59135 interstitial, uterine pregnancy requiring total hysterectomy

59136 interstitial, uterine pregnancy with partial resection of uterus

59140 cervical, with evacuation

59150 Laparoscopic treatment of ectopic pregnancy; without salpingectomy and/or oophorectomy

59151 with salpingectomy and/or oophorectomy

59160 Curettage, postpartum

Introduction

(For intrauterine fetal transfusion, use 36460)

(For introduction of hypertonic solution and/or prostaglandins to initiate labor, see 59850-59857)

59200 Insertion of cervical dilator (eg, laminaria, prostaglandin) (separate procedure)

Repair

(For tracheloplasty, use 57700)

59300 Episiotomy or vaginal repair, by other than attending physician

(59305 has been deleted)

59320 Cerclage of cervix, during pregnancy; vaginal

59325 abdominal

59350 Hysterorrhaphy of ruptured uterus

(59351 has been deleted)

Vaginal Delivery, Antepartum and Postpartum Care

(For insertion of transcervical or transvaginal fetal oximetry sensor, use Category III code 0021T)

59400 Routine obstetric care including antepartum care, vaginal delivery (with or without episiotomy, and/or forceps) and postpartum care

59409 Vaginal delivery only (with or without episiotomy and/or forceps);

59410 including postpartum care

59412 External cephalic version, with or without tocolysis

(Use 59412 in addition to code(s) for delivery)

59414 Delivery of placenta (separate procedure)

(59420 has been deleted. To report, see 59425, 59426 or appropriate E/M code(s))

(For 1-3 antepartum care visits, see appropriate E/M code(s))

59425 Antepartum care only; 4-6 visits

59426 7 or more visits

59430 Postpartum care only (separate procedure)

Cesarean Delivery

(For standby attendance for infant, use 99360)

(For insertion of transcervical or transvaginal fetal oximetry sensor, use Category III code 0021T)

(59500, 59501 have been deleted. To report, see 59510, 59515, 59525)

59510 Routine obstetric care including antepartum care, cesarean delivery, and postpartum care

59514 Cesarean delivery only;

59515 including postpartum care

(59520, 59521 have been deleted. To report, see 59510, 59515, 59525)

+ 59525 Subtotal or total hysterectomy after cesarean delivery (List separately in addition to code for primary procedure)

(Use 59525 in conjunction with codes 59510, 59514, 59515, 59618, 59620, 59622)

(59540, 59541, 59560, 59561, 59580, 59581 have been deleted. To report, see 59510, 59515, 59525)

Delivery After Previous Cesarean Delivery

Patients who have had a previous cesarean delivery and now present with the expectation of a vaginal delivery are coded using codes 59610-59622. If the patient has a successful vaginal delivery after a previous cesarean delivery (VBAC), use codes 59610-59614. If the attempt is unsuccessful and another cesarean delivery is carried out, use codes 59618-59622. To report elective cesarean deliveries use code 59510, 59514 or 59515.

(For insertion of transcervical or transvaginal fetal oximetry sensor, use Category III code 0021T)

59610   Routine obstetric care including antepartum care, vaginal delivery (with or without episiotomy, and/or forceps) and postpartum care, after previous cesarean delivery

59612   Vaginal delivery only, after previous cesarean delivery (with or without episiotomy and/or forceps);

59614   including postpartum care

59618   Routine obstetric care including antepartum care, cesarean delivery, and postpartum care, following attempted vaginal delivery after previous cesarean delivery

59620   Cesarean delivery only, following attempted vaginal delivery after previous cesarean delivery;

59622   including postpartum care

Abortion

(For medical treatment of spontaneous complete abortion, any trimester, use E/M codes 99201-99233)

(59800, 59810 have been deleted. To report, see 99201-99233)

(59801, 59811 have been deleted. To report, use 59812)

59812   Treatment of incomplete abortion, any trimester, completed surgically

59820   Treatment of missed abortion, completed surgically; first trimester

59821   second trimester

59830   Treatment of septic abortion, completed surgically

59840   Induced abortion, by dilation and curettage

59841   Induced abortion, by dilation and evacuation

59850   Induced abortion, by one or more intra-amniotic injections (amniocentesis-injections), including hospital admission and visits, delivery of fetus and secundines;

59851   with dilation and curettage and/or evacuation

59852   with hysterotomy (failed intra-amniotic injection)

(For insertion of cervical dilator, use 59200)

59855   Induced abortion, by one or more vaginal suppositories (eg, prostaglandin) with or without cervical dilation (eg, laminaria), including hospital admission and visits, delivery of fetus and secundines;

59856   with dilation and curettage and/or evacuation

59857   with hysterotomy (failed medical evacuation)

Other Procedures

59866   Multifetal pregnancy reduction(s) (MPR)

59870   Uterine evacuation and curettage for hydatidiform mole

59871   Removal of cerclage suture under anesthesia (other than local)

59898   Unlisted laparoscopy procedure, maternity care and delivery

59899   Unlisted procedure, maternity care and delivery

Surgery: Male/Female Genital System

Notes

Endocrine System

(For pituitary and pineal surgery, see **Nervous System**)

Thyroid Gland

Incision

60000* Incision and drainage of thyroglossal duct cyst, infected

Excision

60001 Aspiration and/or injection, thyroid cyst

(For fine needle aspiration, see 10021, 10022)

(If imaging guidance is performed, see 76360, 76942)

60100* Biopsy thyroid, percutaneous core needle

(If imaging guidance is performed, see 76003, 76360, 76393, 76942)

(For fine needle aspiration, use 10021 or 10022)

(For evaluation of fine needle aspirate, see 88172, 88173)

60200 Excision of cyst or adenoma of thyroid, or transection of isthmus

60210 Partial thyroid lobectomy, unilateral; with or without isthmusectomy

60212 with contralateral subtotal lobectomy, including isthmusectomy

60220 Total thyroid lobectomy, unilateral; with or without isthmusectomy

60225 with contralateral subtotal lobectomy, including isthmusectomy

60240 Thyroidectomy, total or complete

(60242 has been deleted. To report, see 60210-60225)

(60245 has been deleted. To report, see 60210-60225)

(60246 has been deleted. To report, use 60271)

60252 Thyroidectomy, total or subtotal for malignancy; with limited neck dissection

60254 with radical neck dissection

60260 Thyroidectomy, removal of all remaining thyroid tissue following previous removal of a portion of thyroid

(60261 has been deleted. To report, use 60260 with modifier '-50')

60270 Thyroidectomy, including substernal thyroid; sternal split or transthoracic approach

60271 cervical approach

60280 Excision of thyroglossal duct cyst or sinus;

60281 recurrent

(For thyroid ultrasonography, use 76536)

Parathyroid, Thymus, Adrenal Glands, and Carotid Body

Excision

(For pituitary and pineal surgery, see **Nervous System**)

60500 Parathyroidectomy or exploration of parathyroid(s);

60502 re-exploration

60505 with mediastinal exploration, sternal split or transthoracic approach

(60510 has been deleted)

+ 60512 Parathyroid autotransplantation (List separately in addition to code for primary procedure)

(Use 60512 in conjunction with codes 60500, 60502, 60505, 60212, 60225, 60240, 60252, 60254, 60260, 60270, 60271)

60520 Thymectomy, partial or total; transcervical approach (separate procedure)

60521 sternal split or transthoracic approach, without radical mediastinal dissection (separate procedure)

60522 sternal split or transthoracic approach, with radical mediastinal dissection (separate procedure)

60540 Adrenalectomy, partial or complete, or exploration of adrenal gland with or without biopsy, transabdominal, lumbar or dorsal (separate procedure);

60545 with excision of adjacent retroperitoneal tumor

(For excision of remote or disseminated pheochromocytoma, see 49200, 49201)

(For laparoscopic approach, use 56321)

(60550, 60555 have been deleted. To report, use 60540 with modifier '-50')

60600 Excision of carotid body tumor; without excision of carotid artery

60605 with excision of carotid artery

Laparoscopy

Surgical laparoscopy always includes diagnostic laparoscopy. To report a diagnostic laparoscopy (peritoneoscopy) (separate procedure), use 49320.

60650 Laparoscopy, surgical, with adrenalectomy, partial or complete, or exploration of adrenal gland with or without biopsy, transabdominal, lumbar or dorsal

60659 Unlisted laparoscopy procedure, endocrine system

Other Procedures

60699 Unlisted procedure, endocrine system

Notes

Nervous System

Skull, Meninges, and Brain

(For injection procedure for cerebral angiography, see 36100-36218)

(For injection procedure for ventriculography, see 61026, 61120, 61130)

(For injection procedure for pneumoencephalography, use 61055)

Injection, Drainage, or Aspiration

61000* Subdural tap through fontanelle, or suture, infant, unilateral or bilateral; initial

61001*   subsequent taps

61020* Ventricular puncture through previous burr hole, fontanelle, suture, or implanted ventricular catheter/reservoir; without injection

(61025 has been deleted. To report, use 61026)

61026*   with injection of medication or other substance for diagnosis or treatment

(61030, 61045 have been deleted. To report, use 61026)

61050* Cisternal or lateral cervical (C1-C2) puncture; without injection (separate procedure)

(61051, 61052, 61053 have been deleted. To report, use 61055)

61055*   with injection of medication or other substance for diagnosis or treatment (eg, C1-C2)

(For radiological supervision and interpretation, see **Radiology**)

61070* Puncture of shunt tubing or reservoir for aspiration or injection procedure

(For radiological supervision and interpretation, use 75809)

Twist Drill, Burr Hole(s), or Trephine

61105* Twist drill hole for subdural or ventricular puncture;

(61106 has been deleted)

⊘ **61107***   for implanting ventricular catheter or pressure recording device

▶(For intracranial neuroendoscopic ventricular catheter placement, use 62160)◀

61108   for evacuation and/or drainage of subdural hematoma

61120 Burr hole(s) for ventricular puncture (including injection of gas, contrast media, dye, or radioactive material)

(61130 has been deleted)

61140 Burr hole(s) or trephine; with biopsy of brain or intracranial lesion

61150   with drainage of brain abscess or cyst

61151   with subsequent tapping (aspiration) of intracranial abscess or cyst

61154 Burr hole(s) with evacuation and/or drainage of hematoma, extradural or subdural

(61155 has been deleted. To report, use 61154 with modifier '-50')

61156 Burr hole(s); with aspiration of hematoma or cyst, intracerebral

⊘ **61210***   for implanting ventricular catheter, reservoir, EEG electrode(s) or pressure recording device (separate procedure)

▶(For intracranial neuroendoscopic ventricular catheter placement, use 62160)◀

61215 Insertion of subcutaneous reservoir, pump or continuous infusion system for connection to ventricular catheter

▶(For refilling and maintenance of an implantable infusion pump for spinal or brain drug therapy, use 95990)◀

(For chemotherapy, use 96450)

61250 Burr hole(s) or trephine, supratentorial, exploratory, not followed by other surgery

(61251 has been deleted. To report, use 61250 with modifier '-50')

61253 Burr hole(s) or trephine, infratentorial, unilateral or bilateral

(If burr hole(s) or trephine are followed by craniotomy at same operative session, use 61304-61321; do not use 61250 or 61253)

Craniectomy or Craniotomy

61304 Craniectomy or craniotomy, exploratory; supratentorial

61305   infratentorial (posterior fossa)

(61310, 61311 have been deleted. To report, see 61312-61315)

61312 Craniectomy or craniotomy for evacuation of hematoma, supratentorial; extradural or subdural

61313   intracerebral

61314 Craniectomy or craniotomy for evacuation of hematoma, infratentorial; extradural or subdural

61315   intracerebellar

+ ● **61316** Incision and subcutaneous placement of cranial bone graft (List separately in addition to code for primary procedure)

▶(Use 61316 in conjunction with codes 61304, 61312, 61313, 61322, 61323, 61340, 61570, 61571, 61680-61705)◀

Surgery: Nervous System

61320 Craniectomy or craniotomy, drainage of intracranial abscess; supratentorial

61321   infratentorial

● **61322** Craniectomy or craniotomy, decompressive, with or without duraplasty, for treatment of intracranial hypertension, without evacuation of associated intraparenchymal hematoma; without lobectomy

▶(Do not report 61313 in addition to 61322)◀

▶(For subtemporal decompression, use 61340)◀

● **61323**   with lobectomy

▶(Do not report 61313 in addition to 61323)◀

▶(For subtemporal decompression, use 61340)◀

61330 Decompression of orbit only, transcranial approach

(61331 has been deleted. To report, use 61330 with modifier '-50')

61332 Exploration of orbit (transcranial approach); with biopsy

61333   with removal of lesion

61334   with removal of foreign body

▲ **61340** Subtemporal cranial decompression (pseudotumor cerebri, slit ventricle syndrome)

▶(For decompressive craniotomy or craniectomy for intracranial hypertension, without hematoma evacuation, see 61322, 61323)◀

(61341 has been deleted. To report, use 61340 with modifier '-50')

61343 Craniectomy, suboccipital with cervical laminectomy for decompression of medulla and spinal cord, with or without dural graft (eg, Arnold-Chiari malformation)

61345 Other cranial decompression, posterior fossa

(For orbital decompression by lateral wall approach, Kroenlein type, use 67445)

61440 Craniotomy for section of tentorium cerebelli (separate procedure)

61450 Craniectomy, subtemporal, for section, compression, or decompression of sensory root of gasserian ganglion

61458 Craniectomy, suboccipital; for exploration or decompression of cranial nerves

61460   for section of one or more cranial nerves

61470   for medullary tractotomy

61480   for mesencephalic tractotomy or pedunculotomy

61490 Craniotomy for lobotomy, including cingulotomy

(61491 has been deleted. To report, use 61490 with modifier '-50')

61500 Craniectomy; with excision of tumor or other bone lesion of skull

61501   for osteomyelitis

61510 Craniectomy, trephination, bone flap craniotomy; for excision of brain tumor, supratentorial, except meningioma

61512   for excision of meningioma, supratentorial

61514   for excision of brain abscess, supratentorial

61516   for excision or fenestration of cyst, supratentorial

(For excision of pituitary tumor or craniopharyngioma, see 61545, 61546, 61548)

✦ ● **61517** Implantation of brain intracavitary chemotherapy agent (List separately in addition to code for primary procedure)

▶(Use 61517 only in conjunction with codes 61510 or 61518)◀

▶(Do not report 61517 for brachytherapy insertion. For intracavitary insertion of radioelement sources or ribbons, see 77781-77784)◀

61518 Craniectomy for excision of brain tumor, infratentorial or posterior fossa; except meningioma, cerebellopontine angle tumor, or midline tumor at base of skull

61519   meningioma

61520   cerebellopontine angle tumor

61521   midline tumor at base of skull

61522 Craniectomy, infratentorial or posterior fossa; for excision of brain abscess

61524   for excision or fenestration of cyst

61526 Craniectomy, bone flap craniotomy, transtemporal (mastoid) for excision of cerebellopontine angle tumor;

61530   combined with middle/posterior fossa craniotomy/craniectomy

61531 Subdural implantation of strip electrodes through one or more burr or trephine hole(s) for long term seizure monitoring

(For stereotactic implantation of electrodes, use 61760)

(61532 has been deleted. To report, see 61680-61692)

61533 Craniotomy with elevation of bone flap; for subdural implantation of an electrode array, for long term seizure monitoring

(For continuous EEG monitoring, see 95950-95954)

61534   for excision of epileptogenic focus without electrocorticography during surgery

61535   for removal of epidural or subdural electrode array, without excision of cerebral tissue (separate procedure)

61536   for excision of cerebral epileptogenic focus, with electrocorticography during surgery (includes removal of electrode array)

61538   for lobectomy with electrocorticography during surgery, temporal lobe

Surgery: Nervous System

61539   for lobectomy with electrocorticography during surgery, other than temporal lobe, partial or total

61541   for transection of corpus callosum

61542   for total hemispherectomy

61543   for partial or subtotal hemispherectomy

61544   for excision or coagulation of choroid plexus

61545   for excision of craniopharyngioma

61546   Craniotomy for hypophysectomy or excision of pituitary tumor, intracranial approach

61548   Hypophysectomy or excision of pituitary tumor, transnasal or transseptal approach, nonstereotactic

(Do not report code 69990 in addition to code 61548)

61550   Craniectomy for craniosynostosis; single cranial suture

61552   multiple cranial sutures

(61553 has been deleted. To report, see 61552, 61558, 61559)

(61555 has been deleted. To report, see 21172-21180, 61552, 61558, 61559)

(For cranial reconstruction for orbital hypertelorism, see 21260-21263)

61556   Craniotomy for craniosynostosis; frontal or parietal bone flap

61557   bifrontal bone flap

61558   Extensive craniectomy for multiple cranial suture craniosynostosis (eg, cloverleaf skull); not requiring bone grafts

61559   recontouring with multiple osteotomies and bone autografts (eg, barrel-stave procedure) (includes obtaining grafts)

(61561 has been deleted. To report, see 21172-21180)

61563   Excision, intra and extracranial, benign tumor of cranial bone (eg, fibrous dysplasia); without optic nerve decompression

61564   with optic nerve decompression

(For reconstruction, see 21181-21183)

61570   Craniectomy or craniotomy; with excision of foreign body from brain

61571   with treatment of penetrating wound of brain

(For sequestrectomy for osteomyelitis, use 61501)

61575   Transoral approach to skull base, brain stem or upper spinal cord for biopsy, decompression or excision of lesion;

61576   requiring splitting of tongue and/or mandible (including tracheostomy)

(For arthrodesis, use 22548)

Surgery of Skull Base

The surgical management of lesions involving the skull base (base of anterior, middle, and posterior cranial fossae) often requires the skills of several surgeons of different surgical specialties working together or in tandem during the operative session. These operations are usually not staged because of the need for definitive closure of dura, subcutaneous tissues, and skin to avoid serious infections such as osteomyelitis and/or meningitis.

The procedures are categorized according to: 1) *approach procedure* necessary to obtain adequate exposure to the lesion (pathologic entity), 2) *definitive procedure(s)* necessary to biopsy, excise or otherwise treat the lesion, and 3) *repair/reconstruction* of the defect present following the definitive procedure(s).

The *approach procedure* is described according to anatomical area involved, ie, anterior cranial fossa, middle cranial fossa, posterior cranial fossa, and brain stem or upper spinal cord.

The *definitive procedure(s)* describes the repair, biopsy, resection, or excision of various lesions of the skull base and, when appropriate, primary closure of the dura, mucous membranes, and skin.

The *repair/reconstruction procedure(s)* is reported separately if extensive dural grafting, cranioplasty, local or regional myocutaneous pedicle flaps, or extensive skin grafts are required.

For primary closure, see the appropriate codes, ie, 15732, 15755.

When one surgeon performs the approach procedure, another surgeon performs the definitive procedure, and another surgeon performs the repair/reconstruction procedure, each surgeon reports only the code for the specific procedure performed.

If one surgeon performs more than one procedure (ie, approach procedure and definitive procedure), then both codes are reported, adding modifier '-51' to the secondary, additional procedure(s).

Approach Procedures

Anterior Cranial Fossa

61580   Craniofacial approach to anterior cranial fossa; extradural, including lateral rhinotomy, ethmoidectomy, sphenoidectomy, without maxillectomy or orbital exenteration

61581   extradural, including lateral rhinotomy, orbital exenteration, ethmoidectomy, sphenoidectomy and/or maxillectomy

61582   extradural, including unilateral or bifrontal craniotomy, elevation of frontal lobe(s), osteotomy of base of anterior cranial fossa

61583   intradural, including unilateral or bifrontal craniotomy, elevation or resection of frontal lobe, osteotomy of base of anterior cranial fossa

61584   Orbitocranial approach to anterior cranial fossa, extradural, including supraorbital ridge osteotomy and elevation of frontal and/or temporal lobe(s); without orbital exenteration

61585   with orbital exenteration

61586   Bicoronal, transzygomatic and/or LeFort I osteotomy approach to anterior cranial fossa with or without internal fixation, without bone graft

Middle Cranial Fossa

61590   Infratemporal pre-auricular approach to middle cranial fossa (parapharyngeal space, infratemporal and midline skull base, nasopharynx), with or without disarticulation of the mandible, including parotidectomy, craniotomy, decompression and/or mobilization of the facial nerve and/or petrous carotid artery

61591   Infratemporal post-auricular approach to middle cranial fossa (internal auditory meatus, petrous apex, tentorium, cavernous sinus, parasellar area, infratemporal fossa) including mastoidectomy, resection of sigmoid sinus, with or without decompression and/or mobilization of contents of auditory canal or petrous carotid artery

61592   Orbitocranial zygomatic approach to middle cranial fossa (cavernous sinus and carotid artery, clivus, basilar artery or petrous apex) including osteotomy of zygoma, craniotomy, extra- or intradural elevation of temporal lobe

Posterior Cranial Fossa

61595   Transtemporal approach to posterior cranial fossa, jugular foramen or midline skull base, including mastoidectomy, decompression of sigmoid sinus and/or facial nerve, with or without mobilization

61596   Transcochlear approach to posterior cranial fossa, jugular foramen or midline skull base, including labyrinthectomy, decompression, with or without mobilization of facial nerve and/or petrous carotid artery

61597   Transcondylar (far lateral) approach to posterior cranial fossa, jugular foramen or midline skull base, including occipital condylectomy, mastoidectomy, resection of C1-C3 vertebral body(s), decompression of vertebral artery, with or without mobilization

61598   Transpetrosal approach to posterior cranial fossa, clivus or foramen magnum, including ligation of superior petrosal sinus and/or sigmoid sinus

Definitive Procedures

Base of Anterior Cranial Fossa

61600   Resection or excision of neoplastic, vascular or infectious lesion of base of anterior cranial fossa; extradural

61601   intradural, including dural repair, with or without graft

Base of Middle Cranial Fossa

61605   Resection or excision of neoplastic, vascular or infectious lesion of infratemporal fossa, parapharyngeal space, petrous apex; extradural

61606   intradural, including dural repair, with or without graft

61607   Resection or excision of neoplastic, vascular or infectious lesion of parasellar area, cavernous sinus, clivus or midline skull base; extradural

61608   intradural, including dural repair, with or without graft

Codes 61609-61612 are reported in addition to code(s) for primary procedure(s) 61605-61608. Report only one transection or ligation of carotid artery code per operative session.

+ 61609   Transection or ligation, carotid artery in cavernous sinus; without repair (List separately in addition to code for primary procedure)

+ 61610   with repair by anastomosis or graft (List separately in addition to code for primary procedure)

+ 61611   Transection or ligation, carotid artery in petrous canal; without repair (List separately in addition to code for primary procedure)

+ 61612   with repair by anastomosis or graft (List separately in addition to code for primary procedure)

61613   Obliteration of carotid aneurysm, arteriovenous malformation, or carotid-cavernous fistula by dissection within cavernous sinus

Base of Posterior Cranial Fossa

61615   Resection or excision of neoplastic, vascular or infectious lesion of base of posterior cranial fossa, jugular foramen, foramen magnum, or C1-C3 vertebral bodies; extradural

61616   intradural, including dural repair, with or without graft

Repair and/or Reconstruction of Surgical Defects of Skull Base

61618   Secondary repair of dura for cerebrospinal fluid leak, anterior, middle or posterior cranial fossa following surgery of the skull base; by free tissue graft (eg, pericranium, fascia, tensor fascia lata, adipose tissue, homologous or synthetic grafts)

61619   by local or regionalized vascularized pedicle flap or myocutaneous flap (including galea, temporalis, frontalis or occipitalis muscle)

Endovascular Therapy

● **61623** Endovascular temporary balloon arterial occlusion, head or neck (extracranial/intracranial) including selective catheterization of vessel to be occluded, positioning and inflation of occlusion balloon, concomitant neurological monitoring, and radiologic supervision and interpretation of all angiography required for balloon occlusion and to exclude vascular injury post occlusion

▶(If selective catheterization and angiography of arteries other than artery to be occluded is performed, use appropriate catheterization and radiologic supervision and interpretation codes)◀

▶(If complete diagnostic angiography of the artery to be occluded is performed immediately prior to temporary occlusion, use appropriate radiologic supervision and interpretation codes only)◀

▲**61624** Transcatheter permanent occlusion or embolization (eg, for tumor destruction, to achieve hemostasis, to occlude a vascular malformation), percutaneous, any method; central nervous system (intracranial, spinal cord)

(See also 37204)

(For radiological supervision and interpretation, use 75894)

61626 non-central nervous system, head or neck (extracranial, brachiocephalic branch)

(See also 37204)

(For radiological supervision and interpretation, use 75894)

Surgery for Aneurysm, Arteriovenous Malformation or Vascular Disease

Includes craniotomy when appropriate for procedure.

61680 Surgery of intracranial arteriovenous malformation; supratentorial, simple

61682 supratentorial, complex

61684 infratentorial, simple

61686 infratentorial, complex

61690 dural, simple

61692 dural, complex

61697 Surgery of complex intracranial aneurysm, intracranial approach; carotid circulation

61698 vertebrobasilar circulation

(61697, 61698 involve aneurysms that are larger than 15 mm or with calcification of the aneurysm neck, or with incorporation of normal vessels into the aneurysm neck, or a procedure requiring temporary vessel occlusion, trapping or cardiopulmonary bypass to successfully treat the aneurysm)

61700 Surgery of simple intracranial aneurysm, intracranial approach; carotid circulation

61702 vertebrobasilar circulation

61703 Surgery of intracranial aneurysm, cervical approach by application of occluding clamp to cervical carotid artery (Selverstone-Crutchfield type)

(For cervical approach for direct ligation of carotid artery, see 37600-37606)

61705 Surgery of aneurysm, vascular malformation or carotid-cavernous fistula; by intracranial and cervical occlusion of carotid artery

61708 by intracranial electrothrombosis

(For ligation or gradual occlusion of internal/common carotid artery, see 37605, 37606)

61710 by intra-arterial embolization, injection procedure, or balloon catheter

61711 Anastomosis, arterial, extracranial-intracranial (eg, middle cerebral/cortical) arteries

(For carotid or vertebral thromboendarterectomy, use 35301)

(61712 has been deleted. Use 69990 when the surgical microscope is employed for the microsurgical procedure. Do not use 69990 for visualization with magnifying loupes or corrected vision.)

Stereotaxis

61720 Creation of lesion by stereotactic method, including burr hole(s) and localizing and recording techniques, single or multiple stages; globus pallidus or thalamus

61735 subcortical structure(s) other than globus pallidus or thalamus

61750 Stereotactic biopsy, aspiration, or excision, including burr hole(s), for intracranial lesion;

▲**61751** with computed tomography and/or magnetic resonance guidance

(For radiological supervision and interpretation of computerized tomography, see 70450, 70460, or 70470 as appropriate)

(For radiological supervision and interpretation of magnetic resonance imaging, see 70551, 70552, or 70553 as appropriate)

61760 Stereotactic implantation of depth electrodes into the cerebrum for long term seizure monitoring

61770 Stereotactic localization, including burr hole(s), with insertion of catheter(s) or probe(s) for placement of radiation source

(61780 has been deleted. To report, use 61760)

Surgery: Nervous System

61790   Creation of lesion by stereotactic method, percutaneous, by neurolytic agent (eg, alcohol, thermal, electrical, radiofrequency); gasserian ganglion

61791   trigeminal medullary tract

61793   Stereotactic radiosurgery (particle beam, gamma ray or linear accelerator), one or more sessions

        (For intensity modulated beam delivery plan and treatment, see 77301, 77418)

+ 61795   Stereotactic computer assisted volumetric (navigational) procedure, intracranial, extracranial, or spinal (List separately in addition to code for primary procedure)

Neurostimulators (Intracranial)

Codes 61850-61888 apply to both simple and complex neurostimulators. For initial or subsequent electronic analysis and programming of neurostimulator pulse generators, see codes 95970-95975.

61850   Twist drill or burr hole(s) for implantation of neurostimulator electrodes, cortical

        (61855 has been deleted. To report, use 61862)

61860   Craniectomy or craniotomy for implantation of neurostimulator electrodes, cerebral, cortical

61862   Twist drill, burr hole, craniotomy, or craniectomy for stereotactic implantation of one neurostimulator array in subcortical site (eg, thalamus, globus pallidus, subthalamic nucleus, periventricular, periaqueductal gray)

        ▶(For intraoperative neurophysiologic recording, see 95961-95962)◀

        (61865 has been deleted. To report, use 61862)

61870   Craniectomy for implantation of neurostimulator electrodes, cerebellar; cortical

61875   subcortical

61880   Revision or removal of intracranial neurostimulator electrodes

61885   Incision and subcutaneous placement of cranial neurostimulator pulse generator or receiver, direct or inductive coupling; with connection to a single electrode array

61886   with connection to two or more electrode arrays

        (For open placement of cranial nerve (eg, vagal, trigeminal) neurostimulator electrode(s), use 64573)

        (For percutaneous placement of cranial nerve (eg, vagal, trigeminal) neurostimulator electrode(s), use 64553)

        (For revision or removal of cranial nerve (eg, vagal, trigeminal) neurostimulator electrode(s), use 64585)

61888   Revision or removal of cranial neurostimulator pulse generator or receiver

Repair

62000   Elevation of depressed skull fracture; simple, extradural

62005   compound or comminuted, extradural

62010   with repair of dura and/or debridement of brain

62100   Craniotomy for repair of dural/cerebrospinal fluid leak, including surgery for rhinorrhea/otorrhea

        (For repair of spinal dural/CSF leak, see 63707, 63709)

62115   Reduction of craniomegalic skull (eg, treated hydrocephalus); not requiring bone grafts or cranioplasty

62116   with simple cranioplasty

62117   requiring craniotomy and reconstruction with or without bone graft (includes obtaining grafts)

62120   Repair of encephalocele, skull vault, including cranioplasty

62121   Craniotomy for repair of encephalocele, skull base

62140   Cranioplasty for skull defect; up to 5 cm diameter

62141   larger than 5 cm diameter

62142   Removal of bone flap or prosthetic plate of skull

62143   Replacement of bone flap or prosthetic plate of skull

62145   Cranioplasty for skull defect with reparative brain surgery

62146   Cranioplasty with autograft (includes obtaining bone grafts); up to 5 cm diameter

62147   larger than 5 cm diameter

+ ● 62148   Incision and retrieval of subcutaneous cranial bone graft for cranioplasty (List separately in addition to code for primary procedure)

        ▶(Use 62148 in conjunction with codes 62140-62147)◀

▶Neuroendoscopy◀

▶Surgical endoscopy always includes diagnostic endoscopy.◀

+ ● 62160   Neuroendoscopy, intracranial, for placement or replacement of ventricular catheter and attachment to shunt system or external drainage (List separately in addition to code for primary procedure)

        ▶(Use 62160 only in conjunction with codes 61107, 61210, 62220, 62223, 62225, or 62230)◀

● 62161   Neuroendoscopy, intracranial; with dissection of adhesions, fenestration of septum pellucidum or intraventricular cysts (including placement, replacement, or removal of ventricular catheter)

● 62162   with fenestration or excision of colloid cyst, including placement of external ventricular catheter for drainage

● **62163**   with retrieval of foreign body

● **62164**   with excision of brain tumor, including placement of external ventricular catheter for drainage

● **62165**   with excision of pituitary tumor, transnasal or trans-sphenoidal approach

Cerebrospinal Fluid (CSF) Shunt

62180   Ventriculocisternostomy (Torkildsen type operation)

62190   Creation of shunt; subarachnoid/subdural-atrial, -jugular, -auricular

62192   subarachnoid/subdural-peritoneal, -pleural, other terminus

62194   Replacement or irrigation, subarachnoid/subdural catheter

62200   Ventriculocisternostomy, third ventricle;

▲ **62201**   stereotactic, neuroendoscopic method

▶(For intracranial neuroendoscopic procedures, see 62161-62165)◀

62220   Creation of shunt; ventriculo-atrial, -jugular, -auricular

▶(For intracranial neuroendoscopic ventricular catheter placement, use 62160)◀

62223   ventriculo-peritoneal, -pleural, other terminus

▶(For intracranial neuroendoscopic ventricular catheter placement, use 62160)◀

62225   Replacement or irrigation, ventricular catheter

▶(For intracranial neuroendoscopic ventricular catheter placement, use 62160)◀

62230   Replacement or revision of cerebrospinal fluid shunt, obstructed valve, or distal catheter in shunt system

▶(For intracranial neuroendoscopic ventricular catheter placement, use 62160)◀

62252   Reprogramming of programmable cerebrospinal shunt

62256   Removal of complete cerebrospinal fluid shunt system; without replacement

62258   with replacement by similar or other shunt at same operation

(For percutaneous irrigation or aspiration of shunt reservoir, use 61070)

(For reprogramming of programmable CSF shunt, use 62252)

Spine and Spinal Cord

(For application of caliper or tongs, use 20660)

(For treatment of fracture or dislocation of spine, see 22305-22327)

Injection, Drainage, or Aspiration

Injection of contrast during fluoroscopic guidance and localization is an inclusive component of codes ▶62263,◀ 62270-62273, 62280-62282, 62310-62319, ▶0027T◀. Fluoroscopic guidance and localization is reported by code 76005, unless a formal contrast study (myelography, epidurography, or arthrography) is performed, in which case the use of fluoroscopy is included in the supervision and interpretation codes.

For radiologic supervision and interpretation of epidurography, use 72275. Code 72275 is only to be used when an epidurogram is performed, recorded, and a formal radiologic report is issued.

▶Code 62263 describes a catheter-based treatment involving targeted injection of various substances (eg, hypertonic saline, steroid, anesthetic) via an indwelling epidural catheter. Code 62263 includes percutaneous insertion and removal of an epidural catheter (remaining in place over a several-day period), for the administration of multiple injections of a neurolytic agent(s) performed during serial treatment sessions (ie, spanning two or more treatment days). If required, adhesions or scarring may also be lysed by mechanical means. Code 62263 is NOT reported for each adhesiolysis treatment, but should be reported ONCE to describe the entire series of injections/infusions spanning two or more treatment days. For endoscopic lysis of adhesions, use 0027T.

Code 62264 describes multiple adhesiolysis treatment sessions performed on the same day. Adhesions or scarring may be lysed by injections of neurolytic agent(s). If required, adhesions or scarring may also be lysed mechanically using a percutaneously-deployed catheter.

Codes 62263 and 62264 include the procedure of injections of contrast for epidurography (72275) and fluoroscopic guidance and localization (76005) during initial or subsequent sessions.◀

▶(For daily hospital management of continuous epidural or subarachnoid drug administration performed in conjunction with codes 62318-62319, **see Evaluation and Management** services)◀

▶(For endoscopic lysis of epidural adhesions, use Category III code 0027T)◀

Surgery: Nervous System

▲ **62263**   Percutaneous lysis of epidural adhesions using solution injection (eg, hypertonic saline, enzyme) or mechanical means (eg, catheter) including radiologic localization (includes contrast when administered), multiple adhesiolysis sessions; 2 or more days

►(62263 includes codes 76005 and 72275)◄

● **62264**   1 day

►(Do not report 62264 with 62263)◄

►(62264 includes codes 76005 and 72275)◄

62268*   Percutaneous aspiration, spinal cord cyst or syrinx

(For radiological supervision and interpretation, see 76003, 76360, 76942)

62269*   Biopsy of spinal cord, percutaneous needle

(For radiological supervision and interpretation, see 76003, 76360, 76942)

►(For fine needle aspiration, see 10021, 10022)◄

►(For evaluation of fine needle aspirate, see 88172, 88173)◄

62270*   Spinal puncture, lumbar, diagnostic

62272*   Spinal puncture, therapeutic, for drainage of cerebrospinal fluid (by needle or catheter)

62273*   Injection, epidural, of blood or clot patch

(62274 has been deleted. To report, see 62310, 62311)

(62275 has been deleted. To report, use 62310)

(62276 has been deleted. To report, see 62318, 62319)

(62277 has been deleted. To report, see 62318, 62319)

(62278 has been deleted. To report, use 62311)

(62279 has been deleted. To report, use 62319)

62280*   Injection/infusion of neurolytic substance (eg, alcohol, phenol, iced saline solutions), with or without other therapeutic substance; subarachnoid

62281*   epidural, cervical or thoracic

62282*   epidural, lumbar, sacral (caudal)

⊘ ▲ **62284***   Injection procedure for myelography and/or computed tomography, spinal (other than C1-C2 and posterior fossa)

(For injection procedure at C1-C2, use 61055)

(For radiological supervision and interpretation, see **Radiology**)

(62286 has been deleted. To report, use 64999)

62287   Aspiration or decompression procedure, percutaneous, of nucleus pulposus of intervertebral disk, any method, single or multiple levels, lumbar (eg, manual or automated percutaneous diskectomy, percutaneous laser diskectomy)

(For fluoroscopic guidance, use 76003)

(62288 has been deleted. To report, see 62310, 62311)

(62289 has been deleted. To report, use 62311)

62290*   Injection procedure for diskography, each level; lumbar

62291*   cervical or thoracic

(For radiological supervision and interpretation, see 72285, 72295)

62292   Injection procedure for chemonucleolysis, including diskography, intervertebral disk, single or multiple levels, lumbar

(62293 has been deleted)

62294   Injection procedure, arterial, for occlusion of arteriovenous malformation, spinal

(62295-62297 have been deleted. To report, see 63001-63017)

(62298 has been deleted. To report, use 62310)

62310   Injection, single (not via indwelling catheter), not including neurolytic substances, with or without contrast (for either localization or epidurography), of diagnostic or therapeutic substance(s) (including anesthetic, antispasmodic, opioid, steroid, other solution), epidural or subarachnoid; cervical or thoracic

62311   lumbar, sacral (caudal)

62318   Injection, including catheter placement, continuous infusion or intermittent bolus, not including neurolytic substances, with or without contrast (for either localization or epidurography), of diagnostic or therapeutic substance(s) (including anesthetic, antispasmodic, opioid, steroid, other solution), epidural or subarachnoid; cervical or thoracic

62319   lumbar, sacral (caudal)

(For transforaminal epidural injection, see 64479-64484)

►(For daily hospital management of continuous epidural or subarachnoid drug administration performed in conjunction with codes 62318-62319, **see Evaluation and Management** services)◄

Catheter Implantation

(For percutaneous placement of intrathecal or epidural catheter, see codes 62270-62273, 62280-62284, 62310-62319)

(62301-62303 have been deleted. To report, see 63001-63017)

62350   Implantation, revision or repositioning of tunneled intrathecal or epidural catheter, for long-term medication administration via an external pump or implantable reservoir/infusion pump; without laminectomy

62351   with laminectomy

(For refilling and maintenance of an implantable infusion pump ►for spinal or brain drug therapy, use 95990)◄

62355   Removal of previously implanted intrathecal or epidural catheter

⊘ = Modifier '-51' Exempt   ► ◄ or ► ◄ = New or Revised Text   ✚ = Add-on Code

Reservoir/Pump Implantation

62360   Implantation or replacement of device for intrathecal or epidural drug infusion; subcutaneous reservoir

62361   non-programmable pump

62362   programmable pump, including preparation of pump, with or without programming

62365   Removal of subcutaneous reservoir or pump, previously implanted for intrathecal or epidural infusion

62367   Electronic analysis of programmable, implanted pump for intrathecal or epidural drug infusion (includes evaluation of reservoir status, alarm status, drug prescription status); without reprogramming

62368   with reprogramming

▶(For refilling and maintenance of an implantable infusion pump for spinal or brain drug therapy, use 95990)◀

Posterior Extradural Laminotomy or Laminectomy for Exploration/ Decompression of Neural Elements or Excision of Herniated Intervertebral Disks

(When 63001-63048 are followed by arthrodesis, see 22590-22614)

63001   Laminectomy with exploration and/or decompression of spinal cord and/or cauda equina, without facetectomy, foraminotomy or diskectomy, (eg, spinal stenosis), one or two vertebral segments; cervical

63003   thoracic

63005   lumbar, except for spondylolisthesis

(63010 has been deleted. To report, use 63012)

63011   sacral

63012   Laminectomy with removal of abnormal facets and/or pars inter-articularis with decompression of cauda equina and nerve roots for spondylolisthesis, lumbar (Gill type procedure)

63015   Laminectomy with exploration and/or decompression of spinal cord and/or cauda equina, without facetectomy, foraminotomy or diskectomy, (eg, spinal stenosis), more than 2 vertebral segments; cervical

63016   thoracic

63017   lumbar

63020   Laminotomy (hemilaminectomy), with decompression of nerve root(s), including partial facetectomy, foraminotomy and/or excision of herniated intervertebral disk; one interspace, cervical

(63021 has been deleted. To report, use 63020 with modifier '-50')

63030   one interspace, lumbar (including open or endoscopically-assisted approach)

(63031 has been deleted. To report, use 63030 with modifier '-50')

+ 63035   each additional interspace, cervical or lumbar (List separately in addition to code for primary procedure)

(Use 63035 in conjunction with codes 63020-63030)

63040   Laminotomy (hemilaminectomy), with decompression of nerve root(s), including partial facetectomy, foraminotomy and/or excision of herniated intervertebral disk, reexploration, single interspace; cervical

(63041 has been deleted)

63042   lumbar

(Codes 63040-63044 are unilateral procedures. For bilateral procedures, use modifier '-50')

+ 63043   each additional cervical interspace (List separately in addition to code for primary procedure)

(Use 63043 in conjunction with code 63040)

+ 63044   each additional lumbar interspace (List separately in addition to code for primary procedure)

(Use 63044 in conjunction with code 63042)

63045   Laminectomy, facetectomy and foraminotomy (unilateral or bilateral with decompression of spinal cord, cauda equina and/or nerve root(s), (eg, spinal or lateral recess stenosis)), single vertebral segment; cervical

63046   thoracic

63047   lumbar

+ 63048   each additional segment, cervical, thoracic, or lumbar (List separately in addition to code for primary procedure)

(Use 63048 in conjunction with codes 63045-63047)

Transpedicular or Costovertebral Approach for Posterolateral Extradural Exploration/Decompression

63055   Transpedicular approach with decompression of spinal cord, equina and/or nerve root(s) (eg, herniated intervertebral disk), single segment; thoracic

63056   lumbar (including transfacet, or lateral extraforaminal approach) (eg, far lateral herniated intervertebral disk)

+ 63057   each additional segment, thoracic or lumbar (List separately in addition to code for primary procedure)

(Use 63057 in conjunction with codes 63055, 63056)

(63060 has been deleted)

Surgery: Nervous System

63064 Costovertebral approach with decompression of spinal cord or nerve root(s), (eg, herniated intervertebral disk), thoracic; single segment

(63065 has been deleted)

+ 63066 each additional segment (List separately in addition to code for primary procedure)

(Use 63066 in conjunction with code 63064)

(For excision of thoracic intraspinal lesions by laminectomy, see 63266, 63271, 63276, 63281, 63286)

Anterior or Anterolateral Approach for Extradural Exploration/Decompression

For the following codes, when two surgeons work together as primary surgeons performing distinct part(s) of spinal cord exploration/decompression operation, each surgeon should report his/her distinct operative work by appending the modifier '-62' to the procedure code (and any associated add-on codes for that procedure code as long as both surgeons continue to work together as primary surgeons). In this situation, the modifier '-62' may be appended to the definitive procedure code(s) 63075, 63077, 63081, 63085, 63087, 63090 and, as appropriate, to associated additional interspace add-on code(s) 63076, 63078 or additional segment add-on code(s) 63082, 63086, 63088, 63091 as long as both surgeons continue to work together as primary surgeons.

63075 Diskectomy, anterior, with decompression of spinal cord and/or nerve root(s), including osteophytectomy; cervical, single interspace

+ 63076 cervical, each additional interspace (List separately in addition to code for primary procedure)

(Use 63076 in conjunction with code 63075)

63077 thoracic, single interspace

+ 63078 thoracic, each additional interspace (List separately in addition to code for primary procedure)

(Use 63078 in conjunction with code 63077)

(Do not report code 69990 in addition to codes 63075-63078)

63081 Vertebral corpectomy (vertebral body resection), partial or complete, anterior approach with decompression of spinal cord and/or nerve root(s); cervical, single segment

+ 63082 cervical, each additional segment (List separately in addition to code for primary procedure)

(Use 63082 in conjunction with code 63081)

(For transoral approach, see 61575, 61576)

63085 Vertebral corpectomy (vertebral body resection), partial or complete, transthoracic approach with decompression of spinal cord and/or nerve root(s); thoracic, single segment

+ 63086 thoracic, each additional segment (List separately in addition to code for primary procedure)

(Use 63086 in conjunction with code 63085)

63087 Vertebral corpectomy (vertebral body resection), partial or complete, combined thoracolumbar approach with decompression of spinal cord, cauda equina or nerve root(s), lower thoracic or lumbar; single segment

+ 63088 each additional segment (List separately in addition to code for primary procedure)

(Use 63088 in conjunction with code 63087)

63090 Vertebral corpectomy (vertebral body resection), partial or complete, transperitoneal or retroperitoneal approach with decompression of spinal cord, cauda equina or nerve root(s), lower thoracic, lumbar, or sacral; single segment

+ 63091 each additional segment (List separately in addition to code for primary procedure)

(Use 63091 in conjunction with code 63090)

(Procedures 63081-63091 include diskectomy above and/or below vertebral segment)

(If followed by arthrodesis, see 22548-22812)

(For reconstruction of spine, use appropriate vertebral corpectomy codes 63081-63091, bone graft codes 20930-20938, arthrodesis codes 22548-22812, and spinal instrumentation codes 22840-22855)

Incision

63170 Laminectomy with myelotomy (eg, Bischof or DREZ type), cervical, thoracic, or thoracolumbar

63172 Laminectomy with drainage of intramedullary cyst/syrinx; to subarachnoid space

63173 to peritoneal space

63180 Laminectomy and section of dentate ligaments, with or without dural graft, cervical; one or two segments

63182 more than two segments

63185 Laminectomy with rhizotomy; one or two segments

63190 more than two segments

63191 Laminectomy with section of spinal accessory nerve

(63192 has been deleted. To report, use 63191 with modifier '-50')

(For resection of sternocleidomastoid muscle, use 21720)

63194 Laminectomy with cordotomy, with section of one spinothalamic tract, one stage; cervical

63195 thoracic

63196 Laminectomy with cordotomy, with section of both spinothalamic tracts, one stage; cervical

63197 thoracic

63198 Laminectomy with cordotomy with section of both spinothalamic tracts, two stages within 14 days; cervical

63199 thoracic

63200 Laminectomy, with release of tethered spinal cord, lumbar

Excision by Laminectomy of Lesion Other Than Herniated Disk

(63210-63242 have been deleted. To report, see 63265-63290)

63250   Laminectomy for excision or occlusion of arteriovenous malformation of spinal cord; cervical

63251   thoracic

63252   thoracolumbar

63265   Laminectomy for excision or evacuation of intraspinal lesion other than neoplasm, extradural; cervical

63266   thoracic

63267   lumbar

63268   sacral

63270   Laminectomy for excision of intraspinal lesion other than neoplasm, intradural; cervical

63271   thoracic

63272   lumbar

63273   sacral

63275   Laminectomy for biopsy/excision of intraspinal neoplasm; extradural, cervical

63276   extradural, thoracic

63277   extradural, lumbar

63278   extradural, sacral

63280   intradural, extramedullary, cervical

63281   intradural, extramedullary, thoracic

63282   intradural, extramedullary, lumbar

63283   intradural, sacral

63285   intradural, intramedullary, cervical

63286   intradural, intramedullary, thoracic

63287   intradural, intramedullary, thoracolumbar

63290   combined extradural-intradural lesion, any level

(For drainage of intramedullary cyst/syrinx, use 63172, 63173)

Excision, Anterior or Anterolateral Approach, Intraspinal Lesion

For the following codes, when two surgeons work together as primary surgeons performing distinct part(s) of an anterior approach for an intraspinal excision, each surgeon should report his/her distinct operative work by appending the modifier '-62' to the single definitive procedure code. In this situation, the modifier '-62' may be appended to the definitive procedure code(s) 63300-63307 and, as appropriate, to the associated additional segment add-on code 63308 as long as both surgeons continue to work together as primary surgeons.

(For arthrodesis, see 22548-22585)

(For reconstruction of spine, see 20930-20938)

63300   Vertebral corpectomy (vertebral body resection), partial or complete, for excision of intraspinal lesion, single segment; extradural, cervical

63301   extradural, thoracic by transthoracic approach

63302   extradural, thoracic by thoracolumbar approach

63303   extradural, lumbar or sacral by transperitoneal or retroperitoneal approach

63304   intradural, cervical

63305   intradural, thoracic by transthoracic approach

63306   intradural, thoracic by thoracolumbar approach

63307   intradural, lumbar or sacral by transperitoneal or retroperitoneal approach

+ 63308   each additional segment (List separately in addition to codes for single segment)

(Use 63308 in conjunction with codes 63300-63307)

Stereotaxis

63600   Creation of lesion of spinal cord by stereotactic method, percutaneous, any modality (including stimulation and/or recording)

63610   Stereotactic stimulation of spinal cord, percutaneous, separate procedure not followed by other surgery

63615   Stereotactic biopsy, aspiration, or excision of lesion, spinal cord

Neurostimulators (Spinal)

Codes 63650-63688 apply to both simple and complex neurostimulators. For initial or subsequent electronic analysis and programming of neurostimulator pulse generators, see codes 95970-95975.

Codes 63650, 63655, and 63660 describe the operative placement, revision, or removal of the spinal neurostimulator system components to provide spinal electrical stimulation. A neurostimulator system includes an implanted neurostimulator, external controller, extension, and collection of contacts. Multiple contacts or electrodes (4 or more) provide the actual electrical stimulation in the epidural space.

For percutaneously placed neurostimulator systems (63650, 63660), the contacts are on a catheter-like lead. An array defines the collection of contacts that are on one catheter.

For systems placed via an open surgical exposure (63655, 63660), the contacts are on a plate or paddle-shaped surface.

Surgery: Nervous System

63650 Percutaneous implantation of neurostimulator electrode array, epidural

(63652 has been deleted)

63655 Laminectomy for implantation of neurostimulator electrodes, plate/paddle, epidural

(63656 has been deleted)

(63657 and 63658 have been deleted)

63660 Revision or removal of spinal neurostimulator electrode percutaneous array(s) or plate/paddle(s)

63685 Incision and subcutaneous placement of spinal neurostimulator pulse generator or receiver, direct or inductive coupling

63688 Revision or removal of implanted spinal neurostimulator pulse generator or receiver

(63690, 63691 have been deleted. To report, see 95970-95975)

Repair

63700 Repair of meningocele; less than 5 cm diameter

63702 larger than 5 cm diameter

▶(Do not use modifier '-63' in conjunction with 63700, 63702)◀

63704 Repair of myelomeningocele; less than 5 cm diameter

63706 larger than 5 cm diameter

▶(Do not use modifier '-63' in conjunction with 63704, 63706)◀

(For complex skin closure, see **Integumentary System**)

63707 Repair of dural/cerebrospinal fluid leak, not requiring laminectomy

(63708 has been deleted. To report, see 63707, 63709)

63709 Repair of dural/cerebrospinal fluid leak or pseudomeningocele, with laminectomy

63710 Dural graft, spinal

(For laminectomy and section of dentate ligaments, with or without dural graft, cervical, see 63180, 63182)

Shunt, Spinal CSF

63740 Creation of shunt, lumbar, subarachnoid-peritoneal, -pleural, or other; including laminectomy

63741 percutaneous, not requiring laminectomy

63744 Replacement, irrigation or revision of lumbosubarachnoid shunt

63746 Removal of entire lumbosubarachnoid shunt system without replacement

(63750 has been deleted. To report, see 62351 and 62360, 62361 or 62362)

(63780 has been deleted. To report, see 62350 and 62360, 62361 or 62362)

Extracranial Nerves, Peripheral Nerves, and Autonomic Nervous System

(For intracranial surgery on cranial nerves, see 61450, 61460, 61790)

Introduction/Injection of Anesthetic Agent (Nerve Block), Diagnostic or Therapeutic

Somatic Nerves

64400* Injection, anesthetic agent; trigeminal nerve, any division or branch

64402* facial nerve

64405* greater occipital nerve

64408* vagus nerve

64410* phrenic nerve

64412* spinal accessory nerve

64413* cervical plexus

▲ **64415*** brachial plexus, single

● **64416** brachial plexus, continuous infusion by catheter (including catheter placement) including daily management for anesthetic agent administration

▶(Do not report 01996 in addition to 64416)◀

64417* axillary nerve

64418* suprascapular nerve

64420* intercostal nerve, single

64421* intercostal nerves, multiple, regional block

64425* ilioinguinal, iliohypogastric nerves

64430* pudendal nerve

64435* paracervical (uterine) nerve

(64440 has been deleted. To report, see 64479, 64483)

(64441 has been deleted. To report, see 64480, 64484)

(64442 has been deleted. To report, use 64475)

(64443 has been deleted. To report, use 64476)

▲ **64445*** sciatic nerve, single

● **64446** sciatic nerve, continuous infusion by catheter, (including catheter placement) including daily management for anesthetic agent administration

▶(Do not report 01996 in addition to 64446)◀

● **64447** femoral nerve, single

▶(Do not report 01996 in addition to 64447)◀

Surgery: Nervous System

● **64448**   femoral nerve, continuous infusion by catheter (including catheter placement) including daily management for anesthetic agent administration

▶(Do not report 01996 in addition to 64448)◀

64450*   other peripheral nerve or branch

(For phenol destruction, see 64622-64627)

(For subarachnoid or subdural injection, see 62280, 62310-62319)

(For epidural or caudal injection, see 62273, 62281-62282, 62310-62319)

(Codes 64470-64484 are unilateral procedures. For bilateral procedures, use modifier '-50')

(For fluoroscopic guidance and localization for needle placement and injection in conjunction with codes 64470-64484, use code 76005)

64470   Injection, anesthetic agent and/or steroid, paravertebral facet joint or facet joint nerve; cervical or thoracic, single level

+ 64472   cervical or thoracic, each additional level (List separately in addition to code for primary procedure)

(Use code 64472 in conjunction with code 64470)

64475   lumbar or sacral, single level

+ 64476   lumbar or sacral, each additional level (List separately in addition to code for primary procedure)

(Use code 64476 in conjunction with code 64475)

64479   Injection, anesthetic agent and/or steroid, transforaminal epidural; cervical or thoracic, single level

+ 64480   cervical or thoracic, each additional level (List separately in addition to code for primary procedure)

(Use code 64480 in conjunction with code 64479)

64483   lumbar or sacral, single level

+ 64484   lumbar or sacral, each additional level (List separately in addition to code for primary procedure)

(Use code 64484 in conjunction with code 64483)

Sympathetic Nerves

64505*   Injection, anesthetic agent; sphenopalatine ganglion

64508*   carotid sinus (separate procedure)

64510*   stellate ganglion (cervical sympathetic)

64520*   lumbar or thoracic (paravertebral sympathetic)

64530*   celiac plexus, with or without radiologic monitoring

Neurostimulators (Peripheral Nerve)

Codes 64553-64595 apply to both simple and complex neurostimulators. For initial or subsequent electronic analysis and programming of neurostimulator pulse generators, see codes 95970-95975.

64550   Application of surface (transcutaneous) neurostimulator

64553   Percutaneous implantation of neurostimulator electrodes; cranial nerve

(For open placement of cranial nerve (eg, vagal, trigeminal) neurostimulator pulse generator or receiver, see 61885, 61886, as appropriate)

64555   peripheral nerve (excludes sacral nerve)

64560   autonomic nerve

64561   sacral nerve (transforaminal placement)

64565   neuromuscular

64573   Incision for implantation of neurostimulator electrodes; cranial nerve

(For open placement of cranial nerve (eg, vagal, trigeminal) neurostimulator pulse generator or receiver, see 61885, 61886, as appropriate)

(For revision or removal of cranial nerve (eg, vagal, trigeminal) neurostimulator pulse generator or receiver, use 61888)

64575   peripheral nerve (excludes sacral nerve)

64577   autonomic nerve

64580   neuromuscular

64581   sacral nerve (transforaminal placement)

64585   Revision or removal of peripheral neurostimulator electrodes

64590   Incision and subcutaneous placement of peripheral neurostimulator pulse generator or receiver, direct or inductive coupling

64595   Revision or removal of peripheral neurostimulator pulse generator or receiver

Destruction by Neurolytic Agent (eg, Chemical, Thermal, Electrical, Radiofrequency or Chemodenervation)

Somatic Nerves

64600   Destruction by neurolytic agent, trigeminal nerve; supraorbital, infraorbital, mental, or inferior alveolar branch

64605   second and third division branches at foramen ovale

64610   second and third division branches at foramen ovale under radiologic monitoring

Surgery: Nervous System

64612   Chemodenervation of muscle(s); muscle(s) innervated by facial nerve (eg, for blepharospasm, hemifacial spasm)

64613   cervical spinal muscle(s) (eg, for spasmodic torticollis)

64614   extremity(s) and/or trunk muscle(s) (eg, for dystonia, cerebral palsy, multiple sclerosis)

(For chemodenervation for strabismus involving the extraocular muscles, use 67345)

64620   Destruction by neurolytic agent, intercostal nerve

(Codes 64622-64627 are unilateral procedures. For bilateral procedures, use modifier '-50')

(For fluoroscopic guidance and localization for needle placement and neurolysis in conjunction with codes 64622-64627, use 76005)

64622   Destruction by neurolytic agent, paravertebral facet joint nerve; lumbar or sacral, single level

+ 64623   lumbar or sacral, each additional level (List separately in addition to code for primary procedure)

(Use 64623 in conjunction with code 64622)

64626   cervical or thoracic, single level

+ 64627   cervical or thoracic, each additional level (List separately in addition to code for primary procedure)

(Use 64627 in conjunction with code 64626)

64630   Destruction by neurolytic agent; pudendal nerve

64640   other peripheral nerve or branch

Sympathetic Nerves

64680   Destruction by neurolytic agent, celiac plexus, with or without radiologic monitoring

Neuroplasty (Exploration, Neurolysis or Nerve Decompression)

Neuroplasty is the decompression or freeing of intact nerve from scar tissue, including external neurolysis and/or transposition.

(For internal neurolysis requiring use of operating microscope, use 64727)

(For facial nerve decompression, use 69720)

64702   Neuroplasty; digital, one or both, same digit

64704   nerve of hand or foot

64708   Neuroplasty, major peripheral nerve, arm or leg; other than specified

64712   sciatic nerve

64713   brachial plexus

64714   lumbar plexus

64716   Neuroplasty and/or transposition; cranial nerve (specify)

64718   ulnar nerve at elbow

64719   ulnar nerve at wrist

64721   median nerve at carpal tunnel

(For arthroscopic procedure, use 29848)

64722   Decompression; unspecified nerve(s) (specify)

64726   plantar digital nerve

+ 64727   Internal neurolysis, requiring use of operating microscope (List separately in addition to code for neuroplasty) (Neuroplasty includes external neurolysis)

(Do not report code 69990 in addition to code 64727)

Transection or Avulsion

(For stereotactic lesion of gasserian ganglion, use 61790)

64732   Transection or avulsion of; supraorbital nerve

64734   infraorbital nerve

64736   mental nerve

64738   inferior alveolar nerve by osteotomy

64740   lingual nerve

64742   facial nerve, differential or complete

64744   greater occipital nerve

64746   phrenic nerve

(For section of recurrent laryngeal nerve, use 31595)

64752   vagus nerve (vagotomy), transthoracic

64755   vagus nerves limited to proximal stomach (selective proximal vagotomy, proximal gastric vagotomy, parietal cell vagotomy, supra- or highly selective vagotomy)

(For laparoscopic approach, use 43652)

64760   vagus nerve (vagotomy), abdominal

(For laparoscopic approach, use 43651)

64761   pudendal nerve

(64762 has been deleted. To report, use 64761 with modifier '-50')

64763   Transection or avulsion of obturator nerve, extrapelvic, with or without adductor tenotomy

(64764 has been deleted. To report, use 64763 with modifier '-50')

64766   Transection or avulsion of obturator nerve, intrapelvic, with or without adductor tenotomy

(64768 has been deleted. To report, use 64766 with modifier '-50')

64771   Transection or avulsion of other cranial nerve, extradural

64772   Transection or avulsion of other spinal nerve, extradural

(For excision of tender scar, skin and subcutaneous tissue, with or without tiny neuroma, see 11400-11446, 13100-13153)

Surgery: Nervous System

Excision

Somatic Nerves

(For Morton neurectomy, use 28080)

64774   Excision of neuroma; cutaneous nerve, surgically identifiable

64776   digital nerve, one or both, same digit

+ 64778   digital nerve, each additional digit (List separately in addition to code for primary procedure)

(Use 64778 in conjunction with code 64776)

64782   hand or foot, except digital nerve

+ 64783   hand or foot, each additional nerve, except same digit (List separately in addition to code for primary procedure)

(Use 64783 in conjunction with code 64782)

64784   major peripheral nerve, except sciatic

64786   sciatic nerve

+ 64787   Implantation of nerve end into bone or muscle (List separately in addition to neuroma excision)

(Use 64787 in conjunction with codes 64774-64786)

64788   Excision of neurofibroma or neurolemmoma; cutaneous nerve

64790   major peripheral nerve

64792   extensive (including malignant type)

64795   Biopsy of nerve

Sympathetic Nerves

64802   Sympathectomy, cervical

(64803 has been deleted. To report, use 64802 with modifier '-50')

64804   Sympathectomy, cervicothoracic

(64806 has been deleted. To report, use 64804 with modifier '-50')

64809   Sympathectomy, thoracolumbar

(64811 has been deleted. To report, use 64809 with modifier '-50')

(64814 has been deleted. To report, use 64999)

64818   Sympathectomy, lumbar

(64819 has been deleted. To report, use 64818 with modifier '-50')

64820   Sympathectomy; digital arteries, each digit

(Do not report 69990 in addition to code 64820)

(64824 has been deleted. To report, use 64999)

64821   radial artery

(Do not report 69990 in addition to code 64821)

64822   ulnar artery

(Do not report 69990 in addition to code 64822)

64823   superficial palmar arch

(Do not report 69990 in addition to code 64823)

Neurorrhaphy

(64830 has been deleted. Use 69990 when the surgical microscope is employed for the microsurgical procedure. Do not use 69990 for visualization with magnifying loupes or corrected vision)

64831   Suture of digital nerve, hand or foot; one nerve

+ 64832   each additional digital nerve (List separately in addition to code for primary procedure)

(Use 64832 in conjunction with code 64831)

64834   Suture of one nerve, hand or foot; common sensory nerve

64835   median motor thenar

64836   ulnar motor

+ 64837   Suture of each additional nerve, hand or foot (List separately in addition to code for primary procedure)

(Use 64837 in conjunction with codes 64834-64836)

64840   Suture of posterior tibial nerve

64856   Suture of major peripheral nerve, arm or leg, except sciatic; including transposition

64857   without transposition

64858   Suture of sciatic nerve

+ 64859   Suture of each additional major peripheral nerve (List separately in addition to code for primary procedure)

(Use 64859 in conjunction with codes 64856, 64857)

64861   Suture of; brachial plexus

64862   lumbar plexus

64864   Suture of facial nerve; extracranial

64865   infratemporal, with or without grafting

64866   Anastomosis; facial-spinal accessory

64868   facial-hypoglossal

64870   facial-phrenic

+ 64872   Suture of nerve; requiring secondary or delayed suture (List separately in addition to code for primary neurorrhaphy)

(Use 64872 in conjunction with codes 64831-64865)

+ 64874   requiring extensive mobilization, or transposition of nerve (List separately in addition to code for nerve suture)

(Use 64874 in conjunction with codes 64831-64865)

+ 64876   requiring shortening of bone of extremity (List separately in addition to code for nerve suture)

(Use 64876 in conjunction with codes 64831-64865)

Surgery: Nervous System

Neurorrhaphy With Nerve Graft

64885   Nerve graft (includes obtaining graft), head or neck; up to 4 cm in length

64886   more than 4 cm length

64890   Nerve graft (includes obtaining graft), single strand, hand or foot; up to 4 cm length

64891   more than 4 cm length

64892   Nerve graft (includes obtaining graft), single strand, arm or leg; up to 4 cm length

64893   more than 4 cm length

64895   Nerve graft (includes obtaining graft), multiple strands (cable), hand or foot; up to 4 cm length

64896   more than 4 cm length

64897   Nerve graft (includes obtaining graft), multiple strands (cable), arm or leg; up to 4 cm length

64898   more than 4 cm length

+ 64901   Nerve graft, each additional nerve; single strand (List separately in addition to code for primary procedure)

(Use 64901 in conjunction with codes 64885-64893)

+ 64902   multiple strands (cable) (List separately in addition to code for primary procedure)

(Use 64902 in conjunction with codes 64885, 64886, 64895-64898)

64905   Nerve pedicle transfer; first stage

64907   second stage

Other Procedures

64999   Unlisted procedure, nervous system

Eye and Ocular Adnexa

(For diagnostic and treatment ophthalmological services, see **Medicine, Ophthalmology,** and 92002 et seq)

(Do not report code 69990 in addition to codes 65091-68850)

Eyeball

Removal of Eye

65091   Evisceration of ocular contents; without implant

65093   with implant

65101   Enucleation of eye; without implant

65103   with implant, muscles not attached to implant

65105   with implant, muscles attached to implant

(For conjunctivoplasty after enucleation, see 68320 et seq)

65110   Exenteration of orbit (does not include skin graft), removal of orbital contents; only

65112   with therapeutic removal of bone

65114   with muscle or myocutaneous flap

(For skin graft to orbit (split skin), see 15120, 15121; free, full thickness, see 15260, 15261)

(For eyelid repair involving more than skin, see 67930 et seq)

Secondary Implant(s) Procedures

An ocular implant is an implant inside muscular cone; an orbital implant is an implant outside muscular cone.

65125   Modification of ocular implant with placement or replacement of pegs (eg, drilling receptacle for prosthesis appendage) (separate procedure)

65130   Insertion of ocular implant secondary; after evisceration, in scleral shell

65135   after enucleation, muscles not attached to implant

65140   after enucleation, muscles attached to implant

65150   Reinsertion of ocular implant; with or without conjunctival graft

65155   with use of foreign material for reinforcement and/or attachment of muscles to implant

65175   Removal of ocular implant

(For orbital implant (implant outside muscle cone) insertion, use 67550; removal, use 67560)

Removal of Foreign Body

(For removal of implanted material: ocular implant, use 65175; anterior segment implant, use 65920; posterior segment implant, use 67120; orbital implant, use 67560)

(For diagnostic x-ray for foreign body, use 70030)

(For diagnostic echography for foreign body, use 76529)

(For removal of foreign body from orbit: frontal approach, use 67413; lateral approach, use 67430; transcranial approach, use 61334)

(For removal of foreign body from eyelid, embedded, use 67938)

(For removal of foreign body from lacrimal system, use 68530)

65205*   Removal of foreign body, external eye; conjunctival superficial

65210*   conjunctival embedded (includes concretions), subconjunctival, or scleral nonperforating

65220*   corneal, without slit lamp

65222*   corneal, with slit lamp

(For repair of corneal laceration with foreign body, use 65275)

(65230 has been deleted. To report, use 65235)

65235   Removal of foreign body, intraocular; from anterior chamber of eye or lens

(65240, 65245 have been deleted. To report, use 65235)

(For removal of implanted material from anterior segment, use 65920)

65260   from posterior segment, magnetic extraction, anterior or posterior route

65265   from posterior segment, nonmagnetic extraction

(For removal of implanted material from posterior segment, use 67120)

Repair of Laceration

(For fracture of orbit, see 21385 et seq)

(For repair of wound of eyelid, skin, linear, simple, see 12011-12018; intermediate, layered closure, see 12051-12057; linear, complex, see 13150-13160; other, see 67930, 67935)

(For repair of wound of lacrimal system, use 68700)

(For repair of operative wound, use 66250)

65270*   Repair of laceration; conjunctiva, with or without nonperforating laceration sclera, direct closure

65272   conjunctiva, by mobilization and rearrangement, without hospitalization

65273   conjunctiva, by mobilization and rearrangement, with hospitalization

Surgery: Ocular/Auditory System

▲=Revised Code   ●=New Code   ✱=Service Includes Surgical Procedure Only

65275 cornea, nonperforating, with or without removal foreign body

65280 cornea and/or sclera, perforating, not involving uveal tissue

65285 cornea and/or sclera, perforating, with reposition or resection of uveal tissue

65286 application of tissue glue, wounds of cornea and/or sclera

(Repair of laceration includes use of conjunctival flap and restoration of anterior chamber, by air or saline injection when indicated)

(For repair of iris or ciliary body, use 66680)

65290 Repair of wound, extraocular muscle, tendon and/or Tenon's capsule

Anterior Segment

Cornea

Excision

(65300 has been deleted)

65400 Excision of lesion, cornea (keratectomy, lamellar, partial), except pterygium

65410* Biopsy of cornea

65420 Excision or transposition of pterygium; without graft

65426 with graft

Removal or Destruction

65430* Scraping of cornea, diagnostic, for smear and/or culture

65435* Removal of corneal epithelium; with or without chemocauterization (abrasion, curettage)

65436 with application of chelating agent (eg, EDTA)

(65445 has been deleted. To report, use 65450)

65450 Destruction of lesion of cornea by cryotherapy, photocoagulation or thermocauterization

(65455 has been deleted. To report, use 65450)

65600 Multiple punctures of anterior cornea (eg, for corneal erosion, tattoo)

Keratoplasty

Corneal transplant includes use of fresh or preserved grafts, and preparation of donor material.

(Keratoplasty excludes refractive keratoplasty procedures, 65760, 65765, and 65767)

65710 Keratoplasty (corneal transplant); lamellar

(65720, 65725 have been deleted. To report, use 65710)

65730 penetrating (except in aphakia)

(65740, 65745 have been deleted. To report, use 65730)

65750 penetrating (in aphakia)

65755 penetrating (in pseudophakia)

Other Procedures

65760 Keratomileusis

65765 Keratophakia

65767 Epikeratoplasty

65770 Keratoprosthesis

65771 Radial keratotomy

65772 Corneal relaxing incision for correction of surgically induced astigmatism

65775 Corneal wedge resection for correction of surgically induced astigmatism

(For fitting of contact lens for treatment of disease, use 92070)

(For unlisted procedures on cornea, use 66999)

Anterior Chamber

Incision

65800* Paracentesis of anterior chamber of eye (separate procedure); with diagnostic aspiration of aqueous

65805* with therapeutic release of aqueous

65810 with removal of vitreous and/or discission of anterior hyaloid membrane, with or without air injection

65815 with removal of blood, with or without irrigation and/or air injection

(For injection, see 66020-66030)

(For removal of blood clot, use 65930)

65820 Goniotomy

▶(Do not report modifier '-63' in conjunction with 65820)◀

(65825, 65830 have been deleted)

65850 Trabeculotomy ab externo

65855 Trabeculoplasty by laser surgery, one or more sessions (defined treatment series)

(If re-treatment is necessary after several months because of disease progression, a new treatment or treatment series should be reported with a modifier, if necessary, to indicate lesser or greater complexity)

(For trabeculectomy, use 66170)

65860 Severing adhesions of anterior segment, laser technique (separate procedure)

Other Procedures

65865   Severing adhesions of anterior segment of eye, incisional technique (with or without injection of air or liquid) (separate procedure); goniosynechiae

(For trabeculoplasty by laser surgery, use 65855)

65870   anterior synechiae, except goniosynechiae

65875   posterior synechiae

65880   corneovitreal adhesions

(For laser surgery, use 66821)

65900   Removal of epithelial downgrowth, anterior chamber of eye

65920   Removal of implanted material, anterior segment of eye

65930   Removal of blood clot, anterior segment of eye

66020   Injection, anterior chamber of eye (separate procedure); air or liquid

66030*   medication

(For unlisted procedures on anterior segment, use 66999)

Anterior Sclera

Excision

(For removal of intraocular foreign body, use 65235)

(For operations on posterior sclera, use 67250, 67255)

66130   Excision of lesion, sclera

66150   Fistulization of sclera for glaucoma; trephination with iridectomy

66155   thermocauterization with iridectomy

66160   sclerectomy with punch or scissors, with iridectomy

66165   iridencleisis or iridotasis

66170   trabeculectomy ab externo in absence of previous surgery

(For trabeculotomy ab externo, use 65850)

(For repair of operative wound, use 66250)

66172   trabeculectomy ab externo with scarring from previous ocular surgery or trauma (includes injection of antifibrotic agents)

66180   Aqueous shunt to extraocular reservoir (eg, Molteno, Schocket, Denver-Krupin)

66185   Revision of aqueous shunt to extraocular reservoir

(For removal of implanted shunt, use 67120)

Repair or Revision

(For scleral procedures in retinal surgery, see 67101 et seq)

66220   Repair of scleral staphyloma; without graft

66225   with graft

(For scleral reinforcement, see 67250, 67255)

66250   Revision or repair of operative wound of anterior segment, any type, early or late, major or minor procedure

(For unlisted procedures on anterior sclera, use 66999)

Iris, Ciliary Body

Incision

66500   Iridotomy by stab incision (separate procedure); except transfixion

66505   with transfixion as for iris bombe

(For iridotomy by photocoagulation, use 66761)

Excision

66600   Iridectomy, with corneoscleral or corneal section; for removal of lesion

66605   with cyclectomy

66625   peripheral for glaucoma (separate procedure)

66630   sector for glaucoma (separate procedure)

66635   optical (separate procedure)

(For coreoplasty by photocoagulation, use 66762)

Repair

66680   Repair of iris, ciliary body (as for iridodialysis)

(For reposition or resection of uveal tissue with perforating wound of cornea or sclera, use 65285)

66682   Suture of iris, ciliary body (separate procedure) with retrieval of suture through small incision (eg, McCannel suture)

Destruction

66700   Ciliary body destruction; diathermy

(66701, 66702 have been deleted. To report, see 66700, 66710, 66720, 66740)

66710   cyclophotocoagulation

66720   cryotherapy

(66721 has been deleted. To report, see 66700, 66710, 66720, 66740)

Surgery: Ocular/Auditory System

66740   cyclodialysis

(66741 has been deleted. To report, see 66700, 66710, 66720, 66740)

66761   Iridotomy/iridectomy by laser surgery (eg, for glaucoma) (one or more sessions)

66762   Iridoplasty by photocoagulation (one or more sessions) (eg, for improvement of vision, for widening of anterior chamber angle)

66770   Destruction of cyst or lesion iris or ciliary body (nonexcisional procedure)

(For excision lesion iris, ciliary body, see 66600, 66605; for removal of epithelial downgrowth, use 65900)

(For unlisted procedures on iris, ciliary body, use 66999)

Lens

Incision

(66800, 66801 have been deleted. To report, use 66999)

(66802 has been deleted)

66820   Discission of secondary membranous cataract (opacified posterior lens capsule and/or anterior hyaloid); stab incision technique (Ziegler or Wheeler knife)

66821   laser surgery (eg, YAG laser) (one or more stages)

66825   Repositioning of intraocular lens prosthesis, requiring an incision (separate procedure)

Removal Cataract

Lateral canthotomy, iridectomy, iridotomy, anterior capsulotomy, posterior capsulotomy, the use of viscoelastic agents, enzymatic zonulysis, use of other pharmacologic agents, and subconjunctival or sub-tenon injections are included as part of the code for the extraction of lens.

66830   Removal of secondary membranous cataract (opacified posterior lens capsule and/or anterior hyaloid) with corneo-scleral section, with or without iridectomy (iridocapsulotomy, iridocapsulectomy)

66840   Removal of lens material; aspiration technique, one or more stages

66850   phacofragmentation technique (mechanical or ultrasonic) (eg, phacoemulsification), with aspiration

66852   pars plana approach, with or without vitrectomy

(66915 has been deleted)

66920   intracapsular

66930   intracapsular, for dislocated lens

66940   extracapsular (other than 66840, 66850, 66852)

(66945 has been deleted. To report, see 66920-66940)

(For removal of intralenticular foreign body without lens extraction, use 65235)

(For repair of operative wound, use 66250)

(66980 has been deleted. To report, see 66983, 66984)

66982   Extracapsular cataract removal with insertion of intraocular lens prosthesis (one stage procedure), manual or mechanical technique (eg, irrigation and aspiration or phacoemulsification), complex, requiring devices or techniques not generally used in routine cataract surgery (eg, iris expansion device, suture support for intraocular lens, or primary posterior capsulorrhexis) or performed on patients in the amblyogenic developmental stage

66983   Intracapsular cataract extraction with insertion of intraocular lens prosthesis (one stage procedure)

66984   Extracapsular cataract removal with insertion of intraocular lens prosthesis (one stage procedure), manual or mechanical technique (eg, irrigation and aspiration or phacoemulsification)

(For complex extracapsular cataract removal, use 66982)

66985   Insertion of intraocular lens prosthesis (secondary implant), not associated with concurrent cataract removal

(To code implant at time of concurrent cataract surgery, see 66982, 66983, 66984)

(For intraocular lens prosthesis supplied by physician, use 99070)

(For ultrasonic determination of intraocular lens power, use 76519)

(For removal of implanted material from anterior segment, use 65920)

(For secondary fixation (separate procedure), use 66682)

66986   Exchange of intraocular lens

+ ● 66990   Use of ophthalmic endoscope (List separately in addition to code for primary procedure)

▶(66990 may be used only with codes 65820, 65875, 65920, 66985, 66986, 67038, 67039, 67040)◀

Other Procedures

66999   Unlisted procedure, anterior segment of eye

Posterior Segment

Vitreous

67005   Removal of vitreous, anterior approach (open sky technique or limbal incision); partial removal

67010   subtotal removal with mechanical vitrectomy

(For removal of vitreous by paracentesis of anterior chamber, use 65810)

(For removal of corneovitreal adhesions, use 65880)

67015 Aspiration or release of vitreous, subretinal or choroidal fluid, pars plana approach (posterior sclerotomy)

67025 Injection of vitreous substitute, pars plana or limbal approach, (fluid-gas exchange), with or without aspiration (separate procedure)

67027 Implantation of intravitreal drug delivery system (eg, ganciclovir implant), includes concomitant removal of vitreous

(For removal, use 67121)

67028 Intravitreal injection of a pharmacologic agent (separate procedure)

67030 Discission of vitreous strands (without removal), pars plana approach

67031 Severing of vitreous strands, vitreous face adhesions, sheets, membranes or opacities, laser surgery (one or more stages)

(67035 has been deleted. To report, use 67036)

67036 Vitrectomy, mechanical, pars plana approach;

67038   with epiretinal membrane stripping

67039   with focal endolaser photocoagulation

67040   with endolaser panretinal photocoagulation

►(For use of ophthalmic endoscope with 67038, 67039, 67040, use 66990)◄

(For associated lensectomy, use 66850)

(For use of vitrectomy in retinal detachment surgery, use 67108)

(For associated removal of foreign body, see 65260, 65265)

(For unlisted procedures on vitreous, use 67299)

Retina or Choroid

Repair

(If diathermy, cryotherapy and/or photocoagulation are combined, report under principal modality used)

67101 Repair of retinal detachment, one or more sessions; cryotherapy or diathermy, with or without drainage of subretinal fluid

(67102, 67103 have been deleted. To report, use 67101)

(67104 has been deleted. To report, use 67105)

67105   photocoagulation, with or without drainage of subretinal fluid

(67106 has been deleted. To report, use 67105)

67107 Repair of retinal detachment; scleral buckling (such as lamellar scleral dissection, imbrication or encircling procedure), with or without implant, with or without cryotherapy, photocoagulation, and drainage of subretinal fluid

67108   with vitrectomy, any method, with or without air or gas tamponade, focal endolaser photocoagulation, cryotherapy, drainage of subretinal fluid, scleral buckling, and/or removal of lens by same technique

(67109 has been deleted. To report, use 67299)

67110   by injection of air or other gas (eg, pneumatic retinopexy)

67112   by scleral buckling or vitrectomy, on patient having previous ipsilateral retinal detachment repair(s) using scleral buckling or vitrectomy techniques

(For aspiration or drainage of subretinal or subchoroidal fluid, use 67015)

67115 Release of encircling material (posterior segment)

67120 Removal of implanted material, posterior segment; extraocular

67121   intraocular

(For removal from anterior segment, use 65920)

(For removal of foreign body, see 65260, 65265)

Prophylaxis

Repetitive services. The services listed below are often performed in multiple sessions or groups of sessions. The methods of reporting vary.

The following descriptors are intended to include all sessions in a defined treatment period.

67141 Prophylaxis of retinal detachment (eg, retinal break, lattice degeneration) without drainage, one or more sessions; cryotherapy, diathermy

(67142, 67143 have been deleted. To report, use 67141)

(67144 has been deleted. To report, use 67145)

67145   photocoagulation (laser or xenon arc)

(67146 has been deleted. To report, use 67145)

Destruction

67208 Destruction of localized lesion of retina (eg, macular edema, tumors), one or more sessions; cryotherapy, diathermy

67210   photocoagulation

(67212, 67213 have been deleted. To report, use 67208)

(67214, 67216 have been deleted. To report, use 67210)

67218   radiation by implantation of source (includes removal of source)

Surgery: Ocular/Auditory System

67220 Destruction of localized lesion of choroid (eg, choroidal neovascularization); photocoagulation (eg, laser), one or more sessions

(For destruction of macular drusen, photocoagulation, use Category III code 0017T)

(For destruction of localized lesion of choroid by transpupillary thermotherapy, use Category III code 0016T)

67221 photodynamic therapy (includes intravenous infusion)

(67222, 67223 have been deleted. To report, use 67227)

(67224 has been deleted. To report, use 67228)

+ 67225 photodynamic therapy, second eye, at single session (List separately in addition to code for primary eye treatment)

(Use 67225 in conjunction with code 67221)

(67226 has been deleted. To report, use 67228)

67227 Destruction of extensive or progressive retinopathy (eg, diabetic retinopathy), one or more sessions; cryotherapy, diathermy

67228 photocoagulation (laser or xenon arc)

(For unlisted procedures on retina, use 67299)

Sclera

Repair

(For excision lesion sclera, use 66130)

67250 Scleral reinforcement (separate procedure); without graft

67255 with graft

(For repair scleral staphyloma, see 66220, 66225)

Other Procedures

67299 Unlisted procedure, posterior segment

Ocular Adnexa

Extraocular Muscles

67311 Strabismus surgery, recession or resection procedure; one horizontal muscle

67312 two horizontal muscles

(67313 has been deleted)

67314 one vertical muscle (excluding superior oblique)

67316 two or more vertical muscles (excluding superior oblique)

(For adjustable sutures, use 67335 in addition to codes 67311-67334 for primary procedure reflecting number of muscles operated on)

67318 Strabismus surgery, any procedure, superior oblique muscle

+ 67320 Transposition procedure (eg, for paretic extraocular muscle), any extraocular muscle (specify) (List separately in addition to code for primary procedure)

(Use 67320 in conjunction with codes 67311-67318)

+ 67331 Strabismus surgery on patient with previous eye surgery or injury that did not involve the extraocular muscles (List separately in addition to code for primary procedure)

(Use 67331 in conjunction with codes 67311-67318)

+ 67332 Strabismus surgery on patient with scarring of extraocular muscles (eg, prior ocular injury, strabismus or retinal detachment surgery) or restrictive myopathy (eg, dysthyroid ophthalmopathy) (List separately in addition to code for primary procedure)

(Use 67332 in conjunction with codes 67311-67318)

+ 67334 Strabismus surgery by posterior fixation suture technique, with or without muscle recession (List separately in addition to code for primary procedure)

(Use 67334 in conjunction with codes 67311-67318)

+ 67335 Placement of adjustable suture(s) during strabismus surgery, including postoperative adjustment(s) of suture(s) (List separately in addition to code for specific strabismus surgery)

(Use 67335 in conjunction with codes 67311-67334)

+ 67340 Strabismus surgery involving exploration and/or repair of detached extraocular muscle(s) (List separately in addition to code for primary procedure)

(Use 67340 in conjunction with codes 67311-67334)

67343 Release of extensive scar tissue without detaching extraocular muscle (separate procedure)

(Use 67343 in conjunction with codes 67311-67340, when such procedures are performed other than on the affected muscle)

67345 Chemodenervation of extraocular muscle

(For chemodenervation for blepharospasm and other neurological disorders, see 64612 and 64613)

Other Procedures

67350 Biopsy of extraocular muscle

(For repair of wound, extraocular muscle, tendon or Tenon's capsule, use 65290)

67399 Unlisted procedure, ocular muscle

Orbit

Exploration, Excision, Decompression

67400 Orbitotomy without bone flap (frontal or transconjunctival approach); for exploration, with or without biopsy

67405 with drainage only

67412 with removal of lesion

67413 with removal of foreign body

67414 with removal of bone for decompression

67415 Fine needle aspiration of orbital contents

(For exenteration, enucleation, and repair, see 65101 et seq; for optic nerve decompression, use 67570)

67420 Orbitotomy with bone flap or window, lateral approach (eg, Kroenlein); with removal of lesion

67430 with removal of foreign body

67440 with drainage

67445 with removal of bone for decompression

(For optic nerve sheath decompression, use 67570)

67450 for exploration, with or without biopsy

(For orbitotomy, transcranial approach, see 61330-61334)

(For orbital implant, see 67550, 67560)

(For removal of eyeball or for repair after removal, see 65091-65175)

Other Procedures

67500* Retrobulbar injection; medication (separate procedure, does not include supply of medication)

67505 alcohol

(67510 has been deleted. To report, use 67599)

67515* Injection of medication or other substance into Tenon's capsule

(For subconjunctival injection, use 68200)

67550 Orbital implant (implant outside muscle cone); insertion

67560 removal or revision

(For ocular implant (implant inside muscle cone), see 65093-65105, 65130-65175)

(For treatment of fractures of malar area, orbit, see 21355 et seq)

67570 Optic nerve decompression (eg, incision or fenestration of optic nerve sheath)

67599 Unlisted procedure, orbit

Eyelids

Incision

67700* Blepharotomy, drainage of abscess, eyelid

67710* Severing of tarsorrhaphy

67715* Canthotomy (separate procedure)

(For canthoplasty, use 67950)

(For division of symblepharon, use 68340)

Excision

Codes for removal of lesion include more than skin (ie, involving lid margin, tarsus, and/or palpebral conjunctiva).

(For removal of lesion, involving mainly skin of eyelid, see 11310-11313; 11440-11446; 11640-11646; 17000-17004)

(For repair of wounds, blepharoplasty, grafts, reconstructive surgery, see 67930-67975)

67800 Excision of chalazion; single

67801 multiple, same lid

67805 multiple, different lids

67808 under general anesthesia and/or requiring hospitalization, single or multiple

67810* Biopsy of eyelid

67820* Correction of trichiasis; epilation, by forceps only

67825* epilation by other than forceps (eg, by electrosurgery, cryotherapy, laser surgery)

67830 incision of lid margin

67835 incision of lid margin, with free mucous membrane graft

67840* Excision of lesion of eyelid (except chalazion) without closure or with simple direct closure

(For excision and repair of eyelid by reconstructive surgery, see 67961, 67966)

67850* Destruction of lesion of lid margin (up to 1 cm)

(For Mohs micrographic surgery, see 17304-17310)

(For initiation or follow-up care of topical chemotherapy (eg, 5-FU or similar agents), see appropriate office visits)

Surgery: Ocular/Auditory System

Tarsorrhaphy

67875 Temporary closure of eyelids by suture (eg, Frost suture)

67880 Construction of intermarginal adhesions, median tarsorrhaphy, or canthorrhaphy;

67882   with transposition of tarsal plate

(For severing of tarsorrhaphy, use 67710)

(For canthoplasty, reconstruction canthus, use 67950)

(For canthotomy, use 67715)

Repair (Brow Ptosis, Blepharoptosis, Lid Retraction, Ectropion, Entropion)

67900 Repair of brow ptosis (supraciliary, mid-forehead or coronal approach)

(For forehead rhytidectomy, use 15824)

67901 Repair of blepharoptosis; frontalis muscle technique with suture or other material

67902   frontalis muscle technique with fascial sling (includes obtaining fascia)

67903   (tarso) levator resection or advancement, internal approach

67904   (tarso) levator resection or advancement, external approach

67906   superior rectus technique with fascial sling (includes obtaining fascia)

(67907 has been deleted. To report, use 67999)

67908   conjunctivo-tarso-Muller's muscle-levator resection (eg, Fasanella-Servat type)

67909 Reduction of overcorrection of ptosis

67911 Correction of lid retraction

(For obtaining autogenous graft materials, see 20920, 20922 or 20926)

(For correction of trichiasis by mucous membrane graft, use 67835)

67914 Repair of ectropion; suture

67915   thermocauterization

67916   blepharoplasty, excision tarsal wedge

67917   blepharoplasty, extensive (eg, Kuhnt-Szymanowski or tarsal strip operations)

(For correction of everted punctum, use 68705)

67921 Repair of entropion; suture

67922   thermocauterization

67923   blepharoplasty, excision tarsal wedge

67924   blepharoplasty, extensive (eg, Wheeler operation)

(For repair of cicatricial ectropion or entropion requiring scar excision or skin graft, see also 67961 et seq)

Reconstruction

Codes for blepharoplasty involve more than skin (ie, involving lid margin, tarsus, and/or palpebral conjunctiva).

67930 Suture of recent wound, eyelid, involving lid margin, tarsus, and/or palpebral conjunctiva direct closure; partial thickness

67935   full thickness

67938 Removal of embedded foreign body, eyelid

(For repair of skin of eyelid, see 12011-12018; 12051-12057; 13150-13153)

(For tarsorrhaphy, canthorrhaphy, see 67880, 67882)

(For repair of blepharoptosis and lid retraction, see 67901-67911)

(For blepharoplasty for entropion, ectropion, see 67916, 67917, 67923, 67924)

(For correction of blepharochalasis (blepharorhytidectomy), see 15820-15823)

(For repair of skin of eyelid, adjacent tissue transfer, see 14060, 14061; preparation for graft, use 15000; free graft, see 15120, 15121, 15260, 15261)

(For excision of lesion of eyelid, use 67800 et seq)

(For repair of lacrimal canaliculi, use 68700)

67950 Canthoplasty (reconstruction of canthus)

67961 Excision and repair of eyelid, involving lid margin, tarsus, conjunctiva, canthus, or full thickness, may include preparation for skin graft or pedicle flap with adjacent tissue transfer or rearrangement; up to one-fourth of lid margin

67966   over one-fourth of lid margin

(For canthoplasty, use 67950)

(For free skin grafts, see 15120, 15121, 15260, 15261)

(For tubed pedicle flap preparation, use 15576; for delay, use 15630; for attachment, use 15650)

67971 Reconstruction of eyelid, full thickness by transfer of tarsoconjunctival flap from opposing eyelid; up to two-thirds of eyelid, one stage or first stage

67973   total eyelid, lower, one stage or first stage

67974   total eyelid, upper, one stage or first stage

67975   second stage

Other Procedures

67999 Unlisted procedure, eyelids

Surgery: Ocular/Auditory System

Conjunctiva

(For removal of foreign body, see 65205 et seq)

Incision and Drainage

68020 Incision of conjunctiva, drainage of cyst

68040 Expression of conjunctival follicles (eg, for trachoma)

Excision and/or Destruction

68100 Biopsy of conjunctiva

68110 Excision of lesion, conjunctiva; up to 1 cm

68115   over 1 cm

68130   with adjacent sclera

68135* Destruction of lesion, conjunctiva

Injection

(For injection into Tenon's capsule or retrobulbar injection, see 67500-67515)

68200* Subconjunctival injection

Conjunctivoplasty

(For wound repair, see 65270-65273)

68320 Conjunctivoplasty; with conjunctival graft or extensive rearrangement

68325   with buccal mucous membrane graft (includes obtaining graft)

68326 Conjunctivoplasty, reconstruction cul-de-sac; with conjunctival graft or extensive rearrangement

68328   with buccal mucous membrane graft (includes obtaining graft)

68330 Repair of symblepharon; conjunctivoplasty, without graft

68335   with free graft conjunctiva or buccal mucous membrane (includes obtaining graft)

68340   division of symblepharon, with or without insertion of conformer or contact lens

Other Procedures

68360 Conjunctival flap; bridge or partial (separate procedure)

68362   total (such as Gunderson thin flap or purse string flap)

(For conjunctival flap for perforating injury, see 65280, 65285)

(For repair of operative wound, use 66250)

(For removal of conjunctival foreign body, see 65205, 65210)

68399 Unlisted procedure, conjunctiva

Lacrimal System

Incision

68400 Incision, drainage of lacrimal gland

68420 Incision, drainage of lacrimal sac (dacryocystotomy or dacryocystostomy)

68440* Snip incision of lacrimal punctum

Excision

68500 Excision of lacrimal gland (dacryoadenectomy), except for tumor; total

68505   partial

68510 Biopsy of lacrimal gland

68520 Excision of lacrimal sac (dacryocystectomy)

68525 Biopsy of lacrimal sac

68530 Removal of foreign body or dacryolith, lacrimal passages

68540 Excision of lacrimal gland tumor; frontal approach

68550   involving osteotomy

Repair

68700 Plastic repair of canaliculi

68705 Correction of everted punctum, cautery

68720 Dacryocystorhinostomy (fistulization of lacrimal sac to nasal cavity)

68745 Conjunctivorhinostomy (fistulization of conjunctiva to nasal cavity); without tube

68750   with insertion of tube or stent

68760 Closure of the lacrimal punctum; by thermocauterization, ligation, or laser surgery

68761   by plug, each

68770 Closure of lacrimal fistula (separate procedure)

Probing and/or Related Procedures

(68800 has been deleted. To report, use 68801)

68801* Dilation of lacrimal punctum, with or without irrigation

(To report a bilateral procedure, use 68801 with modifier '-50')

Surgery: Ocular/Auditory System

68810* Probing of nasolacrimal duct, with or without irrigation;

68811 requiring general anesthesia

68815 with insertion of tube or stent

(See also 92018)

(To report a bilateral procedure, use 68810, 68811, or 68815 with modifier '-50')

(68820, 68825, 68830 have been deleted. To report, see 68810, 68811, or 68815)

68840* Probing of lacrimal canaliculi, with or without irrigation

68850* Injection of contrast medium for dacryocystography

(For radiological supervision and interpretation, see 70170, 78660)

Other Procedures

68899 Unlisted procedure, lacrimal system

Surgery: Ocular/Auditory System

Auditory System

(For diagnostic services (eg, audiometry, vestibular tests), see 92502 et seq)

External Ear

Incision

69000* Drainage external ear, abscess or hematoma; simple

69005 complicated

69020* Drainage external auditory canal, abscess

69090 Ear piercing

Excision

69100 Biopsy external ear

69105 Biopsy external auditory canal

69110 Excision external ear; partial, simple repair

69120 complete amputation

(For reconstruction of ear, see 15120 et seq)

69140 Excision exostosis(es), external auditory canal

69145 Excision soft tissue lesion, external auditory canal

69150 Radical excision external auditory canal lesion; without neck dissection

69155 with neck dissection

(For resection of temporal bone, use 69535)

(For skin grafting, see 15000-15261)

Removal of Foreign Body

69200 Removal foreign body from external auditory canal; without general anesthesia

69205 with general anesthesia

69210 Removal impacted cerumen (separate procedure), one or both ears

69220 Debridement, mastoidectomy cavity, simple (eg, routine cleaning)

(69221 has been deleted. To report, use 69220 with modifier '-50')

69222 Debridement, mastoidectomy cavity, complex (eg, with anesthesia or more than routine cleaning)

(69223 has been deleted. To report, use 69222 with modifier '-50')

Repair

(For suture of wound or injury of external ear, see 12011-14300)

69300 Otoplasty, protruding ear, with or without size reduction

(69301 has been deleted. To report, use 69300 with modifier '-50')

69310 Reconstruction of external auditory canal (meatoplasty) (eg, for stenosis due to injury, infection) (separate procedure)

69320 Reconstruction external auditory canal for congenital atresia, single stage

(For combination with middle ear reconstruction, see 69631, 69641)

(For other reconstructive procedures with grafts (eg, skin, cartilage, bone), see 13150-15760, 21230-21235)

Other Procedures

(For otoscopy under general anesthesia, use 92502)

69399 Unlisted procedure, external ear

Middle Ear

Introduction

69400 Eustachian tube inflation, transnasal; with catheterization

69401 without catheterization

69405 Eustachian tube catheterization, transtympanic

69410 Focal application of phase control substance, middle ear (baffle technique)

Incision

69420* Myringotomy including aspiration and/or eustachian tube inflation

69421* Myringotomy including aspiration and/or eustachian tube inflation requiring general anesthesia

▲ **69424** Ventilating tube removal requiring general anesthesia

▶(69424 is a unilateral procedure. To report a bilateral procedure, use 69424 with modifier '-50')◀

▶(Do not report code 69424 in conjunction with codes 69205, 69210, 69420, 69421, 69433-69676, 69710-69745, 69801-69930)◀

(69425 has been deleted. To report, use 69424 with modifier '-50')

(Tympanostomy 69431-69435 has been revised as 69433, 69436)

Surgery: Ocular/Auditory System

69433* Tympanostomy (requiring insertion of ventilating tube), local or topical anesthesia

(69434 has been deleted. To report, use 69433 with modifier '-50')

69436 Tympanostomy (requiring insertion of ventilating tube), general anesthesia

(69437 has been deleted. To report, use 69436 with modifier '-50')

69440 Middle ear exploration through postauricular or ear canal incision

(For atticotomy, see 69601 et seq)

69450 Tympanolysis, transcanal

Excision

69501 Transmastoid antrotomy (simple mastoidectomy)

69502 Mastoidectomy; complete

69505 modified radical

69511 radical

(For skin graft, see 15000 et seq)

(For mastoidectomy cavity debridement, see 69220, 69222)

69530 Petrous apicectomy including radical mastoidectomy

69535 Resection temporal bone, external approach

(For middle fossa approach, see 69950-69970)

69540 Excision aural polyp

69550 Excision aural glomus tumor; transcanal

69552 transmastoid

69554 extended (extratemporal)

Repair

69601 Revision mastoidectomy; resulting in complete mastoidectomy

69602 resulting in modified radical mastoidectomy

69603 resulting in radical mastoidectomy

69604 resulting in tympanoplasty

(For planned secondary tympanoplasty after mastoidectomy, see 69631, 69632)

69605 with apicectomy

(For skin graft, see 15120, 15121, 15260, 15261)

69610 Tympanic membrane repair, with or without site preparation or perforation for closure, with or without patch

(69611 has been deleted. To report, use 69610)

69620 Myringoplasty (surgery confined to drumhead and donor area)

69631 Tympanoplasty without mastoidectomy (including canalplasty, atticotomy and/or middle ear surgery), initial or revision; without ossicular chain reconstruction

69632 with ossicular chain reconstruction (eg, postfenestration)

69633 with ossicular chain reconstruction and synthetic prosthesis (eg, partial ossicular replacement prosthesis (PORP), total ossicular replacement prosthesis (TORP))

69635 Tympanoplasty with antrotomy or mastoidotomy (including canalplasty, atticotomy, middle ear surgery, and/or tympanic membrane repair); without ossicular chain reconstruction

69636 with ossicular chain reconstruction

69637 with ossicular chain reconstruction and synthetic prosthesis (eg, partial ossicular replacement prosthesis (PORP), total ossicular replacement prosthesis (TORP))

69641 Tympanoplasty with mastoidectomy (including canalplasty, middle ear surgery, tympanic membrane repair); without ossicular chain reconstruction

69642 with ossicular chain reconstruction

69643 with intact or reconstructed wall, without ossicular chain reconstruction

69644 with intact or reconstructed canal wall, with ossicular chain reconstruction

69645 radical or complete, without ossicular chain reconstruction

69646 radical or complete, with ossicular chain reconstruction

69650 Stapes mobilization

69660 Stapedectomy or stapedotomy with reestablishment of ossicular continuity, with or without use of foreign material;

69661 with footplate drill out

69662 Revision of stapedectomy or stapedotomy

69666 Repair oval window fistula

69667 Repair round window fistula

69670 Mastoid obliteration (separate procedure)

(69675 Tympanic neurectomy has been revised as 69676)

69676 Tympanic neurectomy

(69677 has been deleted. To report, use 69676 with modifier '-50')

Other Procedures

69700   Closure postauricular fistula, mastoid (separate procedure)

69710   Implantation or replacement of electromagnetic bone conduction hearing device in temporal bone

(Replacement procedure includes removal of old device)

69711   Removal or repair of electromagnetic bone conduction hearing device in temporal bone

69714   Implantation, osseointegrated implant, temporal bone, with percutaneous attachment to external speech processor/cochlear stimulator; without mastoidectomy

69715   with mastoidectomy

69717   Replacement (including removal of existing device), osseointegrated implant, temporal bone, with percutaneous attachment to external speech processor/cochlear stimulator; without mastoidectomy

69718   with mastoidectomy

69720   Decompression facial nerve, intratemporal; lateral to geniculate ganglion

69725   including medial to geniculate ganglion

69740   Suture facial nerve, intratemporal, with or without graft or decompression; lateral to geniculate ganglion

69745   including medial to geniculate ganglion

(For extracranial suture of facial nerve, use 64864)

69799   Unlisted procedure, middle ear

Inner Ear

Incision and/or Destruction

69801   Labyrinthotomy, with or without cryosurgery including other nonexcisional destructive procedures or perfusion of vestibuloactive drugs (single or multiple perfusions); transcanal

(69801 includes all required infusions performed on initial and subsequent days of treatment)

69802   with mastoidectomy

69805   Endolymphatic sac operation; without shunt

69806   with shunt

69820   Fenestration semicircular canal

69840   Revision fenestration operation

Excision

69905   Labyrinthectomy; transcanal

69910   with mastoidectomy

69915   Vestibular nerve section, translabyrinthine approach

(For transcranial approach, use 69950)

Introduction

69930   Cochlear device implantation, with or without mastoidectomy

Other Procedures

69949   Unlisted procedure, inner ear

Temporal Bone, Middle Fossa Approach

(For external approach, use 69535)

69950   Vestibular nerve section, transcranial approach

69955   Total facial nerve decompression and/or repair (may include graft)

69960   Decompression internal auditory canal

(69965 has been deleted. To report, use 69979)

69970   Removal of tumor, temporal bone

Other Procedures

69979   Unlisted procedure, temporal bone, middle fossa approach

Operating Microscope

The surgical microscope is employed when the surgical services are performed using the techniques of microsurgery. Code 69990 should be reported (without the modifier '-51' appended) in addition to the code for the primary procedure performed. Do not use 69990 for visualization with magnifying loupes or corrected vision. Do not report code 69990 in addition to procedures where use of the operating microscope is an inclusive component (15756-15758, 15842, 19364, 19368, 20955-20962, 20969-20973, 26551-26554, 26556, 31526, 31531, 31536, 31541, 31561, 31571, 43116, 43496, 49906, 61548, 63075-63078, 64727, 64820–64823, 65091-68850).

+ **69990**   Microsurgical techniques, requiring use of operating microscope (List separately in addition to code for primary procedure)

Surgery: Ocular/Auditory System

Notes

Radiology Guidelines (Including Nuclear Medicine and Diagnostic Ultrasound)

Items used by all physicians in reporting their services are presented in the **Introduction.** Some of the commonalities are repeated here for the convenience of those physicians referring to this section on **Radiology (Including Nuclear Medicine and Diagnostic Ultrasound).** Other definitions and items unique to Radiology are also listed.

Subject Listings

Subject listings apply when radiological services are performed by or under the responsible supervision of a physician.

Multiple Procedures

It is appropriate to designate multiple procedures that are rendered on the same date by separate entries. This can be reported by using the multiple procedure modifier '-51'. See Appendix A for modifier definitions.

Separate Procedures

Some of the procedures or services listed in *CPT* that are commonly carried out as an integral component of a total service or procedure have been identified by the inclusion of the term "separate procedure." The codes designated as "separate procedure" should not be reported in addition to the code for the total procedure or service of which it is considered an integral component.

However, when a procedure or service that is designated as a "separate procedure" is carried out independently or considered to be unrelated or distinct from other procedures/services provided at that time, it may be reported by itself, or in addition to other procedures/services by appending the modifier '-59' to the specific "separate procedure" code to indicate that the procedure is not considered to be a component of another procedure, but is a distinct, independent procedure. This may represent a different session or patient encounter, different procedure or surgery, different site or organ system, separate incision/excision, separate lesion, or separate injury (or area of injury in extensive injuries).

Subsection Information

Several of the subheadings or subsections have special needs or instructions unique to that section. Where these are indicated (eg, "Radiation Oncology") special **"Notes"** will be presented preceding those procedural terminology listings, referring to that subsection specifically. If there is an "Unlisted Procedure" code number (see section below) for the individual subsection, it will be shown. Those subsections with **"Notes"** are as follows:

Diagnostic Radiology (Diagnostic Imaging) 70010-76499
Aorta and Arteries 75600-75790
Diagnostic Ultrasound 76506-76999
Radiation Oncology 77261-77799
Clinical Treatment Planning 77261-77299
Radiation Treatment Management 77427-77499
Proton Beam Treatment Delivery 77520-77523
Hyperthermia 77600-77620
Clinical Brachytherapy 77750-77799
Nuclear Medicine 78000-78299
Musculoskeletal System 78300-78399
Cardiovascular System 78414-78499

Unlisted Service or Procedure

A service or procedure may be provided that is not listed in this edition of *CPT.* When reporting such a service, the appropriate "Unlisted Procedure" code may be used to indicate the service, identifying it by "Special Report" as discussed below. The "Unlisted Procedures" and accompanying codes for **Radiology (Including Nuclear Medicine and Diagnostic Ultrasound)** are as follows:

▶ 76496   Unlisted fluoroscopic procedure (eg, diagnostic, interventional)◀

▶ 76497   Unlisted computed tomography procedure (eg, diagnostic, interventional)◀

▶ 76498   Unlisted magnetic resonance procedure (eg, diagnostic, interventional)◀

76499   Unlisted diagnostic ▶radiographic◀ procedure

76999   Unlisted ultrasound procedure ▶(eg, diagnostic, interventional)◀

77299	Unlisted procedure, therapeutic radiology clinical treatment planning
77399	Unlisted procedure, medical radiation physics, dosimetry and treatment devices, and special services
77499	Unlisted procedure, therapeutic radiology treatment management
77799	Unlisted procedure, clinical brachytherapy
78099	Unlisted endocrine procedure, diagnostic nuclear medicine
78199	Unlisted hematopoietic, reticuloendothelial and lymphatic procedure, diagnostic nuclear medicine
78299	Unlisted gastrointestinal procedure, diagnostic nuclear medicine
78399	Unlisted musculoskeletal procedure, diagnostic nuclear medicine
78499	Unlisted cardiovascular procedure, diagnostic nuclear medicine
78599	Unlisted respiratory procedure, diagnostic nuclear medicine
78699	Unlisted nervous system procedure, diagnostic nuclear medicine
78799	Unlisted genitourinary procedure, diagnostic nuclear medicine
78999	Unlisted miscellaneous procedure, diagnostic nuclear medicine
79999	Unlisted radiopharmaceutical therapeutic procedure

Special Report

A service that is rarely provided, unusual, variable, or new may require a special report in determining medical appropriateness of the service. Pertinent information should include an adequate definition or description of the nature, extent, and need for the procedure; and the time, effort, and equipment necessary to provide the service. Additional items which may be included are:

- complexity of symptoms;
- final diagnosis;
- pertinent physical findings;
- diagnostic and therapeutic procedures;
- concurrent problems;
- follow-up care.

Supervision and Interpretation

When a procedure is performed by two physicians, the radiologic portion of the procedure is designated as "radiological supervision and interpretation." When a physician performs both the procedure and provides imaging supervision and interpretation, a combination of procedure codes outside the 70000 series and imaging supervision and interpretation codes are to be used.

(The Radiological Supervision and Interpretation codes are not applicable to the Radiation Oncology subsection.)

Administration of Contrast Material(s)

The phrase "with contrast" ►used in the codes for procedures performed using contrast for imaging enhancement◄ represents contrast material administered intravascularly, intra-articularly ►or intrathecally.◄

►For intra-articular injection, use the appropriate joint injection code. If radiographic arthrography is performed, also use the arthrography supervision and interpretation code for the appropriate joint (which includes fluoroscopy). If CT or MR arthrography are performed without radiographic arthrography, use the appropriate joint injection code, the appropriate CT or MR code ("with contrast" or "without followed by contrast"), and the appropriate imaging guidance code for needle placement for contrast injection.◄

For spine examinations using computerized tomography, magnetic resonance imaging, magnetic resonance angiography, "with contrast" includes intrathecal or intravascular injection. For intrathecal injection, use also 61055 or 62284.

Injection of ►intravascular◄ contrast material is part of the "with contrast" CT, ►CTA,◄ MRI, MRA procedure.

Oral and/or rectal contrast administration alone does not qualify as a study "with contrast."

Written Report(s)

A written report, signed by the interpreting physician, should be considered an integral part of a radiologic procedure or interpretation.

Radiology

Diagnostic Radiology (Diagnostic Imaging)

Head and Neck

(70002, 70003 have been deleted. To report, use 76499)

70010 Myelography, posterior fossa, radiological supervision and interpretation

(70011 (complete procedure) has been deleted, see 61055, 62284, 70010)

70015 Cisternography, positive contrast, radiological supervision and interpretation

(70016 (complete procedure) has been deleted, see 61055, 62284, 70015)

(70020, 70021 have been deleted. To report, use 76499)

(70022 has been deleted. To report CT guidance for stereotactic localization, use 76355)

70030 Radiologic examination, eye, for detection of foreign body

(70040, 70050 have been deleted)

70100 Radiologic examination, mandible; partial, less than four views

70110 complete, minimum of four views

70120 Radiologic examination, mastoids; less than three views per side

70130 complete, minimum of three views per side

70134 Radiologic examination, internal auditory meati, complete

70140 Radiologic examination, facial bones; less than three views

70150 complete, minimum of three views

70160 Radiologic examination, nasal bones, complete, minimum of three views

70170 Dacryocystography, nasolacrimal duct, radiological supervision and interpretation

(70171 (complete procedure) has been deleted, see 68850, 70170)

70190 Radiologic examination; optic foramina

70200 orbits, complete, minimum of four views

70210 Radiologic examination, sinuses, paranasal, less than three views

70220 Radiologic examination, sinuses, paranasal, complete, minimum of three views

(70230, 70231 have been deleted. To report, use 76499)

70240 Radiologic examination, sella turcica

70250 Radiologic examination, skull; less than four views, with or without stereo

70260 complete, minimum of four views, with or without stereo

70300 Radiologic examination, teeth; single view

70310 partial examination, less than full mouth

70320 complete, full mouth

70328 Radiologic examination, temporomandibular joint, open and closed mouth; unilateral

70330 bilateral

70332 Temporomandibular joint arthrography, radiological supervision and interpretation

(Do not report 76003 in addition to 70332)

(70333 (complete procedure) has been deleted, see 21116, 70332)

70336 Magnetic resonance (eg, proton) imaging, temporomandibular joint(s)

70350 Cephalogram, orthodontic

70355 Orthopantogram

70360 Radiologic examination; neck, soft tissue

70370 pharynx or larynx, including fluoroscopy and/or magnification technique

70371 Complex dynamic pharyngeal and speech evaluation by cine or video recording

70373 Laryngography, contrast, radiological supervision and interpretation

(70374 (complete procedure) has been deleted, see 31708, 70373)

70380 Radiologic examination, salivary gland for calculus

70390 Sialography, radiological supervision and interpretation

(70391 (complete procedure) has been deleted, see 42550, 70390)

(70400, 70401 have been deleted. To report, use 76499)

▲**70450** Computed tomography, head or brain; without contrast material

70460 with contrast material(s)

70470 without contrast material, followed by contrast material(s) and further sections

(For coronal, sagittal, and/or oblique sections, use 76375)

Radiology

▲ **70480** Computed tomography, orbit, sella, or posterior fossa or outer, middle, or inner ear; without contrast material

70481   with contrast material(s)

70482   without contrast material, followed by contrast material(s) and further sections

(For coronal, sagittal, and/or oblique sections, use 76375)

▲ **70486** Computed tomography, maxillofacial area; without contrast material

70487   with contrast material(s)

70488   without contrast material, followed by contrast material(s) and further sections

(For coronal, sagittal, and/or oblique sections, use 76375)

▲ **70490** Computed tomography, soft tissue neck; without contrast material

70491   with contrast material(s)

70492   without contrast material followed by contrast material(s) and further sections

(For coronal, sagittal, and/or oblique sections, use 76375)

(For cervical spine, see 72125, 72126)

70496 Computed tomographic angiography, head, without contrast material(s), followed by contrast material(s) and further sections, including image post-processing

70498 Computed tomographic angiography, neck, without contrast material(s), followed by contrast material(s) and further sections, including image post-processing

70540 Magnetic resonance (eg, proton) imaging, orbit, face, and neck; without contrast material(s)

(70541 has been deleted. To report head or neck magnetic resonance angiography studies, see 70544-70546, 70547-70549)

70542   with contrast material(s)

70543   without contrast material(s), followed by contrast material(s) and further sequences

70544 Magnetic resonance angiography, head; without contrast material(s)

70545   with contrast material(s)

70546   without contrast material(s), followed by contrast material(s) and further sequences

70547 Magnetic resonance angiography, neck; without contrast material(s)

70548   with contrast material(s)

70549   without contrast material(s), followed by contrast material(s) and further sequences

(70550 has been deleted. To report, use 70551)

70551 Magnetic resonance (eg, proton) imaging, brain (including brain stem); without contrast material

70552   with contrast material(s)

70553 without contrast material, followed by contrast material(s) and further sequences

(For magnetic spectroscopy, use 76390)

Chest

(71000 has been deleted)

71010 Radiologic examination, chest; single view, frontal

71015   stereo, frontal

71020 Radiologic examination, chest, two views, frontal and lateral;

71021   with apical lordotic procedure

71022   with oblique projections

71023   with fluoroscopy

71030 Radiologic examination, chest, complete, minimum of four views;

71034   with fluoroscopy

(For separate chest fluoroscopy, use 76000)

71035 Radiologic examination, chest, special views (eg, lateral decubitus, Bucky studies)

(71036 has been deleted. To report, use 76003)

(71037 (complete procedure) has been deleted, see 32400, 32405, 76003)

(71038 has been deleted. To report, use 31628)

71040 Bronchography, unilateral, radiological supervision and interpretation

(71041 (complete procedure) has been deleted, see 31656, 31708, 31710, 31715, 71040)

71060 Bronchography, bilateral, radiological supervision and interpretation

(71061 (complete procedure) has been deleted, see 31656, 31708, 31710, 31715, 71060)

71090 Insertion pacemaker, fluoroscopy and radiography, radiological supervision and interpretation

(For procedure, see appropriate organ or site)

71100 Radiologic examination, ribs, unilateral; two views

71101   including posteroanterior chest, minimum of three views

71110 Radiologic examination, ribs, bilateral; three views

71111   including posteroanterior chest, minimum of four views

71120 Radiologic examination; sternum, minimum of two views

71130   sternoclavicular joint or joints, minimum of three views

Radiology

▲ **71250**   Computed tomography, thorax; without contrast material

71260   with contrast material(s)

71270   without contrast material, followed by contrast material(s) and further sections

     (For coronal, sagittal, and/or oblique sections, use 76375)

71275   Computed tomographic angiography, chest, without contrast material(s), followed by contrast material(s) and further sections, including image post-processing

71550   Magnetic resonance (eg, proton) imaging, chest (eg, for evaluation of hilar and mediastinal lymphadenopathy); without contrast material(s)

71551   with contrast material(s)

71552   without contrast material(s), followed by contrast material(s) and further sequences

     (For breast MRI, see 76093 and 76094)

71555   Magnetic resonance angiography, chest (excluding myocardium), with or without contrast material(s)

Spine and Pelvis

72010   Radiologic examination, spine, entire, survey study, anteroposterior and lateral

72020   Radiologic examination, spine, single view, specify level

72040   Radiologic examination, spine, cervical; two or three views

72050   minimum of four views

72052   complete, including oblique and flexion and/or extension studies

72069   Radiologic examination, spine, thoracolumbar, standing (scoliosis)

72070   Radiologic examination, spine; thoracic, two views

72072   thoracic, three views

72074   thoracic, minimum of four views

72080   thoracolumbar, two views

72090   scoliosis study, including supine and erect studies

72100   Radiologic examination, spine, lumbosacral; two or three views

72110   minimum of four views

72114   complete, including bending views

72120   Radiologic examination, spine, lumbosacral, bending views only, minimum of four views

     (Contrast material in CT of spine is either by intrathecal or intravenous injection. For intrathecal injection, use also 61055 or 62284. IV injection of contrast material is part of the CT procedure)

▲ **72125**   Computed tomography, cervical spine; without contrast material

72126   with contrast material

72127   without contrast material, followed by contrast material(s) and further sections

     (For intrathecal injection procedure, see 61055, 62284)

▲ **72128**   Computed tomography, thoracic spine; without contrast material

72129   with contrast material

     (For intrathecal injection procedure, see 61055, 62284)

72130   without contrast material, followed by contrast material(s) and further sections

     (For intrathecal injection procedure, see 61055, 62284)

▲ **72131**   Computed tomography, lumbar spine; without contrast material

72132   with contrast material

72133   without contrast material, followed by contrast material(s) and further sections

     (For intrathecal injection procedure, see 61055, 62284)

     (For coronal, sagittal, and/or oblique sections, use 76375)

     (72140 has been deleted. To report, see 72141-72149)

72141   Magnetic resonance (eg, proton) imaging, spinal canal and contents, cervical; without contrast material

72142   with contrast material(s)

     (For cervical spinal canal imaging without contrast material followed by contrast material, use 72156)

     (72143 has been deleted. To report, see 72146, 72147)

     (72144 has been deleted. To report, see 72148, 72149)

     (72145 has been deleted. To report, see 72125-72133)

72146   Magnetic resonance (eg, proton) imaging, spinal canal and contents, thoracic; without contrast material

72147   with contrast material(s)

     (For thoracic spinal canal imaging without contrast material followed by contrast material, use 72157)

72148   Magnetic resonance (eg, proton) imaging, spinal canal and contents, lumbar; without contrast material

72149   with contrast material(s)

     (For lumbar spinal canal imaging without contrast material followed by contrast material, use 72158)

72156   Magnetic resonance (eg, proton) imaging, spinal canal and contents, without contrast material, followed by contrast material(s) and further sequences; cervical

72157   thoracic

72158   lumbar

Radiology

72159 Magnetic resonance angiography, spinal canal and contents, with or without contrast material(s)

72170 Radiologic examination, pelvis; one or two views

(72180 has been deleted. To report, use 72170)

72190 complete, minimum of three views

(For pelvimetry, use 74710)

72191 Computed tomographic angiography, pelvis, without contrast material(s), followed by contrast material(s) and further sections, including image post-processing

(For CTA aorto-iliofemoral runoff, use 75635)

▲**72192** Computed tomography, pelvis; without contrast material

72193 with contrast material(s)

72194 without contrast material, followed by contrast material(s) and further sections

(For coronal, sagittal, and/or oblique sections, use 76375)

72195 Magnetic resonance (eg, proton) imaging, pelvis; without contrast material(s)

72196 with contrast material(s)

72197 without contrast material(s), followed by contrast material(s) and further sequences

72198 Magnetic resonance angiography, pelvis, with or without contrast material(s)

72200 Radiologic examination, sacroiliac joints; less than three views

72202 three or more views

72220 Radiologic examination, sacrum and coccyx, minimum of two views

72240 Myelography, cervical, radiological supervision and interpretation

(72241 (complete procedure) has been deleted, see 61055, 62284, 72240)

72255 Myelography, thoracic, radiological supervision and interpretation

(72256 (complete procedure) has been deleted, see 61055, 62284, 72255)

72265 Myelography, lumbosacral, radiological supervision and interpretation

(72266 (complete procedure) has been deleted, see 61055, 62284, 72265)

72270 Myelography, entire spinal canal, radiological supervision and interpretation

(72271 (complete procedure) has been deleted, see 61055, 62284, 72270)

72275 Epidurography, radiological supervision and interpretation

►(72275 includes 76005)◄

(For injection procedure, see 62280-62282, 62310-62319, 64479-64484)

72285 Diskography, cervical or thoracic, radiological supervision and interpretation

(72286 (complete procedure) has been deleted, see 62291, 72285)

72295 Diskography, lumbar, radiological supervision and interpretation

(72296 (complete procedure) has been deleted, see 62290, 72295)

Upper Extremities

(For stress views, any joint, use 76006)

73000 Radiologic examination; clavicle, complete

73010 scapula, complete

73020 Radiologic examination, shoulder; one view

73030 complete, minimum of two views

73040 Radiologic examination, shoulder, arthrography, radiological supervision and interpretation

(Do not report 76003 in addition to 73040)

(73041 (complete procedure) has been deleted, see 23350, 73040)

73050 Radiologic examination; acromioclavicular joints, bilateral, with or without weighted distraction

73060 humerus, minimum of two views

73070 Radiologic examination, elbow; two views

73080 complete, minimum of three views

73085 Radiologic examination, elbow, arthrography, radiological supervision and interpretation

(Do not report 76003 in addition to 73085)

(73086 (complete procedure) has been deleted, see 24220, 73085)

73090 Radiologic examination; forearm, two views

73092 upper extremity, infant, minimum of two views

73100 Radiologic examination, wrist; two views

73110 complete, minimum of three views

73115 Radiologic examination, wrist, arthrography, radiological supervision and interpretation

(Do not report 76003 in addition to 73115)

(73116 (complete procedure) has been deleted, see 25246, 73115)

73120 Radiologic examination, hand; two views

73130 minimum of three views

73140 Radiologic examination, finger(s), minimum of two views

▲**73200** Computed tomography, upper extremity; without contrast material

73201 with contrast material(s)

Radiology

73202   without contrast material, followed by contrast material(s) and further sections

(For coronal, sagittal, and/or oblique sections, use 76375)

73206   Computed tomographic angiography, upper extremity, without contrast material(s), followed by contrast material(s) and further sections, including image post-processing

73218   Magnetic resonance (eg, proton) imaging, upper extremity, other than joint; without contrast material(s)

73219   with contrast material(s)

73220   without contrast material(s), followed by contrast material(s) and further sequences

73221   Magnetic resonance (eg, proton) imaging, any joint of upper extremity; without contrast material(s)

73222   with contrast material(s)

73223   without contrast material(s), followed by contrast material(s) and further sequences

73225   Magnetic resonance angiography, upper extremity, with or without contrast material(s)

Lower Extremities

(For stress views, any joint, use 76006)

73500   Radiologic examination, hip, unilateral; one view

73510   complete, minimum of two views

73520   Radiologic examination, hips, bilateral, minimum of two views of each hip, including anteroposterior view of pelvis

73525   Radiologic examination, hip, arthrography, radiological supervision and interpretation

(Do not report 76003 in addition to 73525)

(73526 (complete procedure) has been deleted, see 27093, 27095, 73525)

73530   Radiologic examination, hip, during operative procedure

(73531 has been deleted. To report, use 73530)

73540   Radiologic examination, pelvis and hips, infant or child, minimum of two views

73542   Radiological examination, sacroiliac joint arthrography, radiological supervision and interpretation

(Do not report 76003 in addition to 73542)

(For procedure, use 27096. If formal arthrography is not performed, recorded, and a formal radiologic report is not issued, use 76005 for fluoroscopic guidance for sacroiliac joint injections)

73550   Radiologic examination, femur, two views

73560   Radiologic examination, knee; one or two views

73562   three views

73564   complete, four or more views

73565   both knees, standing, anteroposterior

(73570 has been deleted. To report, see 73562, 73564)

73580   Radiologic examination, knee, arthrography, radiological supervision and interpretation

(Do not report 76003 in addition to 73580)

(73581 (complete procedure) has been deleted, see 27370, 73580)

73590   Radiologic examination; tibia and fibula, two views

73592   lower extremity, infant, minimum of two views

73600   Radiologic examination, ankle; two views

73610   complete, minimum of three views

73615   Radiologic examination, ankle, arthrography, radiological supervision and interpretation

(Do not report 76003 in addition to 73615)

(73616 (complete procedure) has been deleted, see 27648, 73615)

73620   Radiologic examination, foot; two views

73630   complete, minimum of three views

73650   Radiologic examination; calcaneus, minimum of two views

73660   toe(s), minimum of two views

▲ **73700**   Computed tomography, lower extremity; without contrast material

73701   with contrast material(s)

73702   without contrast material, followed by contrast material(s) and further sections

(For coronal, sagittal, and/or oblique sections, use 76375)

73706   Computed tomographic angiography, lower extremity, without contrast material(s), followed by contrast material(s) and further sections, including image post-processing

(For CTA aorto-iliofemoral runoff, use 75635)

73718   Magnetic resonance (eg, proton) imaging, lower extremity other than joint; without contrast material(s)

73719   with contrast material(s)

73720   without contrast material(s), followed by contrast material(s) and further sequences

73721   Magnetic resonance (eg, proton) imaging, any joint of lower extremity; without contrast material

73722   with contrast material(s)

73723   without contrast material(s), followed by contrast material(s) and further sequences

73725   Magnetic resonance angiography, lower extremity, with or without contrast material(s)

Radiology

Abdomen

74000   Radiologic examination, abdomen; single anteroposterior view

74010   anteroposterior and additional oblique and cone views

74020   complete, including decubitus and/or erect views

▲ **74022**   complete acute abdomen series, including supine, erect, and/or decubitus views, single view chest

▲ **74150**   Computed tomography, abdomen; without contrast material

74160   with contrast material(s)

74170   without contrast material, followed by contrast material(s) and further sections

(For coronal, sagittal, and/or oblique sections, use 76375)

74175   Computed tomographic angiography, abdomen, without contrast material(s), followed by contrast material(s) and further sections, including image post-processing

(For CTA aorto-iliofemoral runoff, use 75635)

74181   Magnetic resonance (eg, proton) imaging, abdomen; without contrast material(s)

74182   with contrast material(s)

74183   without contrast material(s), followed by with contrast material(s) and further sequences

74185   Magnetic resonance angiography, abdomen, with or without contrast material(s)

74190   Peritoneogram (eg, after injection of air or contrast), radiological supervision and interpretation

(For procedure, use 49400)

(For computerized axial tomography, see 72192 or 74150)

Gastrointestinal Tract

(For percutaneous placement of gastrostomy tube, use 43750)

74210   Radiologic examination; pharynx and/or cervical esophagus

74220   esophagus

74230   Swallowing function, with cineradiography/videoradiography

74235   Removal of foreign body(s), esophageal, with use of balloon catheter, radiological supervision and interpretation

(For procedure, see 43215, 43247)

74240   Radiologic examination, gastrointestinal tract, upper; with or without delayed films, without KUB

74241   with or without delayed films, with KUB

74245   with small intestine, includes multiple serial films

74246   Radiological examination, gastrointestinal tract, upper, air contrast, with specific high density barium, effervescent agent, with or without glucagon; with or without delayed films, without KUB

74247   with or without delayed films, with KUB

74249   with small intestine follow-through

74250   Radiologic examination, small intestine, includes multiple serial films;

74251   via enteroclysis tube

74260   Duodenography, hypotonic

74270   Radiologic examination, colon; barium enema, with or without KUB

(74275 has been deleted. To report, use 76499)

74280   air contrast with specific high density barium, with or without glucagon

74283   Therapeutic enema, contrast or air, for reduction of intussusception or other intraluminal obstruction (eg, meconium ileus)

(74285 has been deleted. To report, see 74270, 74280)

74290   Cholecystography, oral contrast;

74291   additional or repeat examination or multiple day examination

74300   Cholangiography and/or pancreatography; intraoperative, radiological supervision and interpretation

➕ **74301**   additional set intraoperative, radiological supervision and interpretation (List separately in addition to code for primary procedure)

(Use 74301 in conjunction with code 74300)

74305   through existing catheter, radiological supervision and interpretation

(For procedure, see 47505, 48400, 47560-47561, 47563)

(For biliary duct stone extraction, percutaneous, see 47630, 74327)

(74310, 74315 have been deleted. To report, use 76499)

74320   Cholangiography, percutaneous, transhepatic, radiological supervision and interpretation

(74321 (complete procedure) has been deleted, see 47500, 74320)

(74325, 74326 have been deleted. To report, use 76499)

74327   Postoperative biliary duct calculus removal, percutaneous via T-tube tract, basket, or snare (eg, Burhenne technique), radiological supervision and interpretation

(For procedure, use 47630)

74328   Endoscopic catheterization of the biliary ductal system, radiological supervision and interpretation

(For procedure, see 43260-43272 as appropriate)

74329   Endoscopic catheterization of the pancreatic ductal system, radiological supervision and interpretation

(For procedure, see 43260-43272 as appropriate)

74330   Combined endoscopic catheterization of the biliary and pancreatic ductal systems, radiological supervision and interpretation

(For procedure, see 43260-43272 as appropriate)

(74331 has been deleted. To report, use 43262)

74340   Introduction of long gastrointestinal tube (eg, Miller-Abbott), including multiple fluoroscopies and films, radiological supervision and interpretation

(For tube placement, use 44500)

74350   Percutaneous placement of gastrostomy tube, radiological supervision and interpretation

74355   Percutaneous placement of enteroclysis tube, radiological supervision and interpretation

(74356 (complete procedure) has been deleted, see 44015, 74355)

74360   Intraluminal dilation of strictures and/or obstructions (eg, esophagus), radiological supervision and interpretation

(74361 (complete procedure) has been deleted, see 43220, 43458, 74360)

74363   Percutaneous transhepatic dilation of biliary duct stricture with or without placement of stent, radiological supervision and interpretation

(For procedure, see 47510, 47511, 47555, 47556)

Urinary Tract

74400   Urography (pyelography), intravenous, with or without KUB, with or without tomography

(74405 has been deleted. To report, see 74400, 74410 or 74415)

74410   Urography, infusion, drip technique and/or bolus technique;

74415   with nephrotomography

74420   Urography, retrograde, with or without KUB

74425   Urography, antegrade, (pyelostogram, nephrostogram, loopogram), radiological supervision and interpretation

(74426 (complete procedure) has been deleted, see 50394, 50684, 50690, 74425)

74430   Cystography, minimum of three views, radiological supervision and interpretation

(74431 (complete procedure) has been deleted, see 51600, 51605, 74430)

74440   Vasography, vesiculography, or epididymography, radiological supervision and interpretation

(74441 (complete procedure) has been deleted, see 52010, 55300, 74440)

74445   Corpora cavernosography, radiological supervision and interpretation

(74446 (complete procedure) has been deleted, see 54230, 74445)

74450   Urethrocystography, retrograde, radiological supervision and interpretation

(74451 (complete procedure) has been deleted, see 51610, 74450)

74455   Urethrocystography, voiding, radiological supervision and interpretation

(74456 (complete procedure) has been deleted, see 51600, 74455)

(74460, 74461 have been deleted. To report, use 76499)

74470   Radiologic examination, renal cyst study, translumbar, contrast visualization, radiological supervision and interpretation

(74471 (complete procedure) has been deleted, see 50390, 74470)

74475   Introduction of intracatheter or catheter into renal pelvis for drainage and/or injection, percutaneous, radiological supervision and interpretation

(74476 (complete procedure) has been deleted, see 50392-50398, 74475)

74480   Introduction of ureteral catheter or stent into ureter through renal pelvis for drainage and/or injection, percutaneous, radiological supervision and interpretation

(74481 (complete procedure) has been deleted, see 50392-50398, 74480)

(For transurethral surgery (ureter and pelvis), see 52320-52355)

74485   Dilation of nephrostomy, ureters, or urethra, radiological supervision and interpretation

(74486 (complete procedure) has been deleted, see 50395, 53600-53621, 74485)

(For dilation of ureter without radiologic guidance, use 52341, 52344)

(For change of nephrostomy or pyelostomy tube, use 50398)

Gynecological and Obstetrical

(For abdomen and pelvis, see 72170-72190, 74000-74170)

74710   Pelvimetry, with or without placental localization

(74720, 74725 have been deleted. To report, use 74000)

(74730, 74731 have been deleted. To report, use 76499)

74740   Hysterosalpingography, radiological supervision and interpretation

(For introduction of saline or contrast for hysterosalpingography, see 58340)

(74741 (complete procedure) has been deleted, see 58340, 74740)

Radiology

74742 Transcervical catheterization of fallopian tube, radiological supervision and interpretation

(For procedure, use 58345)

(74760, 74761, 74770, 74771 have been deleted. To report, use 76499)

74775 Perineogram (eg, vaginogram, for sex determination or extent of anomalies)

Heart

(For separate injection procedures for vascular radiology, see **Surgery** section, 36000-36299)

(For cardiac catheterization procedures, see 93501-93556)

(75500 has been deleted. To report, use 93555)

(75501 (complete procedure) has been deleted, see 93501-93533, 93542, 93543, 93555)

(75505 has been deleted. To report, use 93555)

(75506 (complete procedure) has been deleted, see 36400-36425 for intravenous procedure, 36100-36248 for intra-arterial procedure and 93501-93533, 93542, 93543, 93555)

(75507 has been deleted. To report, use 93555)

(75509 (complete procedure) has been deleted. To report, see 36400-36425 for intravenous procedure, 36100-36248 for intra-arterial procedure and 93501-93533, 93542, 93543)

(75510, 75511 have been deleted. To report, use 76499)

(75519 has been deleted. To report, use 93555)

(75520 (complete procedure) has been deleted, see 36400-36425 for intravenous procedure, 36100-36248 for intra-arterial procedure, and 93501, 93542)

(75523 has been deleted. To report, use 93555)

(75524 has been deleted, see 36400-36425 for intravenous procedure, 36100-36248 for intra-arterial procedure, and 93510-93514, 93524, 93543)

(75527 has been deleted. To report, use 93555)

(75528 has been deleted, see 36400-36425 for intravenous procedure, 36100-36248 for intra-arterial procedure, and 93526-93529, 93543, and 93555)

75552 Cardiac magnetic resonance imaging for morphology; without contrast material

75553   with contrast material

75554 Cardiac magnetic resonance imaging for function, with or without morphology; complete study

75555   limited study

75556 Cardiac magnetic resonance imaging for velocity flow mapping

Aorta and Arteries

Selective vascular catheterizations should be coded to include introduction and all lesser order selective catheterizations used in the approach (eg, the description for a selective right middle cerebral artery catheterization includes the introduction and placement catheterization of the right common and internal carotid arteries).

Additional second and/or third order arterial catheterizations within the same family of arteries supplied by a single first order artery should be expressed by 36218 or 36248. Additional first order or higher catheterizations in vascular families supplied by a first order vessel different from a previously selected and coded family should be separately coded using the conventions described above.

(For intravenous procedure, see 36000-36013, 36400-36425 and 36100-36248 for intra-arterial procedure)

(For radiological supervision and interpretation, see 75600-75978)

75600 Aortography, thoracic, without serialography, radiological supervision and interpretation

(For injection procedure, use 93544)

(75601 (complete procedure) has been deleted, see 36000-36013, 36400-36425 for intravenous procedure, and 36100-36200 for intra-arterial procedure and 75600)

75605 Aortography, thoracic, by serialography, radiological supervision and interpretation

(For injection procedure, use 93544)

(75606 (complete procedure) has been deleted, see 36000-36013, 36400-36425 for intravenous procedure, and 36100-36200 for intra-arterial procedure and 75605)

(75620, 75621, 75622, 75623 have been deleted. To report, use 76499)

75625 Aortography, abdominal, by serialography, radiological supervision and interpretation

(For injection procedure, use 93544)

(75626, 75627 and 75628 have been deleted, see 36000-36013, 36400-36425 for intravenous procedure, and 36100-36200 for intra-arterial procedure and 75625)

75630 Aortography, abdominal plus bilateral iliofemoral lower extremity, catheter, by serialography, radiological supervision and interpretation

(75631 (complete procedure) has been deleted, see 36000-36013, 36400-36425 for intravenous procedure, and 36100-36200 and 36245-36248 for intra-arterial procedure and 75630)

75635 Computed tomographic angiography, abdominal aorta and bilateral iliofemoral lower extremity runoff, radiological supervision and interpretation, without contrast material(s), followed by contrast material(s) and further sections, including image post-processing

75650   Angiography, cervicocerebral, catheter, including vessel origin, radiological supervision and interpretation

(75651-75657 (complete procedure) have been deleted, see 36000-36013, 36400-36425 for intravenous procedure, and 36100-36218 for intra-arterial procedure and 75650, 75660-75685 as appropriate)

75658   Angiography, brachial, retrograde, radiological supervision and interpretation

(75659 (complete procedure) has been deleted, see 36000-36013, 36400-36425 for intravenous procedure, and 36100-36218 for intra-arterial procedure and 75658)

75660   Angiography, external carotid, unilateral, selective, radiological supervision and interpretation

(75661 (complete procedure) has been deleted, see 36000-36013, 36400-36425 for intravenous procedure, and 36100-36218 and 75660)

75662   Angiography, external carotid, bilateral, selective, radiological supervision and interpretation

(75663 (complete procedure) has been deleted, see 36000-36013, 36400-36425 for intravenous procedure, and 36100-36218 for intra-arterial procedure and 75662)

75665   Angiography, carotid, cerebral, unilateral, radiological supervision and interpretation

(75667, 75669 (complete procedure) have been deleted, see 36000-36013, 36400-36425 for intravenous procedure, and 36100-36218 for intra-arterial procedure and 75665)

75671   Angiography, carotid, cerebral, bilateral, radiological supervision and interpretation

(75672, 75673 (complete procedure) have been deleted, see 36000-36013, 36400-36425 for intravenous procedure, and 36100-36218 for intra-arterial procedure and 75671)

75676   Angiography, carotid, cervical, unilateral, radiological supervision and interpretation

(75677, 75678 (complete procedure) have been deleted, see 36000-36013, 36400-36425 for intravenous procedure, and 36100-36218 for intra-arterial procedure and 75676)

75680   Angiography, carotid, cervical, bilateral, radiological supervision and interpretation

(75681, 75682 (complete procedure) have been deleted, see 36000-36013, 36400-36425 for intravenous procedure, and 36100-36218 for intra-arterial procedure and 75680)

75685   Angiography, vertebral, cervical, and/or intracranial, radiological supervision and interpretation

(75686 has been deleted)

(75687 (complete procedure) has been deleted, see 36000-36013, 36400-36425 for intravenous procedure, and 36100-36218 for intra-arterial procedure and 75685)

(75690 (complete procedure) has been deleted, see 36000-36013, 36400-36425 for intravenous procedure, and 36100-36218 for intra-arterial procedure and 75685)

(75691 has been deleted)

(75692 (complete procedure) has been deleted, see 36000-36013, 36400-36425 for intravenous procedure, and 36100-36218 for intra-arterial procedure and 75685)

(75695 (complete procedure) has been deleted, see 36000-36013, 36400-36425 for intravenous procedure, and 36100-36218 for intra-arterial procedure and 75685)

(75696 has been deleted)

(75697 (complete procedure) has been deleted, see 36000-36013, 36400-36425 for intravenous procedure, and 36100-36218 for intra-arterial procedure and 75685)

75705   Angiography, spinal, selective, radiological supervision and interpretation

(75706 (complete procedure) has been deleted, see 36000-36013, 36400-36425 for intravenous procedure, and 36100-36248 for intra-arterial procedure and 75705)

75710   Angiography, extremity, unilateral, radiological supervision and interpretation

(75711, 75712 (complete procedure) have been deleted, see 36000-36013, 36400-36425 for intravenous procedure, and 36100-36248 for intra-arterial procedure and 75710)

75716   Angiography, extremity, bilateral, radiological supervision and interpretation

(75717, 75718 (complete procedure) have been deleted, see 36000-36013, 36400-36425 for intravenous procedure, and 36100-36248 for intra-arterial procedure and 75716)

75722   Angiography, renal, unilateral, selective (including flush aortogram), radiological supervision and interpretation

(75723 (complete procedure) has been deleted, see 36000-36013, 36400-36425 for intravenous procedure, and 36100-36200 and 36245-36248 for intra-arterial procedure and 75722)

75724   Angiography, renal, bilateral, selective (including flush aortogram), radiological supervision and interpretation

(75725 (complete procedure) has been deleted, see 36000-36013, 36400-36425 for intravenous procedure, and 36100-36200 and 36245-36248 for intra-arterial procedure and 75724)

75726   Angiography, visceral, selective or supraselective, (with or without flush aortogram), radiological supervision and interpretation

(For selective angiography, each additional visceral vessel studied after basic examination, use 75774)

(75727, 75728 (complete procedure) have been deleted, see 36000-36013, 36400-36425 for intravenous procedure, and 36100-36248 for intra-arterial procedure and 75726)

Radiology

75731 Angiography, adrenal, unilateral, selective, radiological supervision and interpretation

(75732 (complete procedure) has been deleted, see 36000-36013, 36400-36425 for intravenous procedure, and 36100-36200 and 36245-36248 for intra-arterial procedure and 75731)

75733 Angiography, adrenal, bilateral, selective, radiological supervision and interpretation

(75734 (complete procedure) has been deleted, see 36000-36013, 36400-36425 for intravenous procedure, and 36100-36200 and 36245-36248 for intra-arterial procedure and 75733)

75736 Angiography, pelvic, selective or supraselective, radiological supervision and interpretation

(75737, 75738 (complete procedure) have been deleted, see 36000-36013, 36400-36425 for intravenous procedure, and 36100-36200 and 36245-36248 for intra-arterial procedure and 75736)

75741 Angiography, pulmonary, unilateral, selective, radiological supervision and interpretation

(For injection procedure, use 93541)

(75742 (complete procedure) has been deleted, see 36000-36015, 36400-36425 for intravenous procedure and 75741)

75743 Angiography, pulmonary, bilateral, selective, radiological supervision and interpretation

(For injection procedure, use 93541)

(75744 (complete procedure) has been deleted, see 36000-36015, 36400-36425 for intravenous procedure and 75743)

75746 Angiography, pulmonary, by nonselective catheter or venous injection, radiological supervision and interpretation

(75747, 75748 (complete procedure) have been deleted, see 36000-36013, 36400-36425 for intravenous procedure, and 36100-36200 for intra-arterial procedure and 75746)

(For injection procedure, use 93541)

(75750 has been deleted. To report, use 93556)

(75751 (complete procedure) has been deleted, see 36000-36013, 36400-36425 for intravenous procedure, and 36100-36200 for intra-arterial procedure and 93556)

(For introduction of catheter, injection procedure, see 93501-93533, 93539, 93540, 93545, 93556)

(75752 has been deleted. To report, use 93556)

(75753 (complete procedure) has been deleted, see 36100-36218 for intra-arterial procedure and 93556)

(For introduction of catheter, injection procedure, see 93501-93533, 93545, 93556)

(75754 has been deleted. To report, use 93556)

(75755 (complete procedure) has been deleted, see 36100-36218 for intra-arterial procedure and 93556)

(For introduction of catheter, injection procedure, see 93501-93533, 93539, 93540, 93545, 93556)

75756 Angiography, internal mammary, radiological supervision and interpretation

(For introduction of catheter, injection procedure, see 93501-93533, 93545, 93556)

(75757 (complete procedure) has been deleted, see 36000-36013, 36400-36425 for intravenous procedure, and 36100-36218 for intra-arterial procedure and 93556)

(75762 has been deleted. To report, use 93556)

(75764 (complete procedure) has been deleted, see 36000-36013, 36400-36425 for intravenous procedure, and 36100-36218 for intra-arterial procedure and 93556)

(75766 has been deleted. To report, use 93556)

(75767 has been deleted. To report, see 36000-36013, 36400-36425 for intravenous procedure, and 36100-36218 for intra-arterial procedure and 93556)

(75772, 75773 have been deleted. To report, use 75774)

+ 75774 Angiography, selective, each additional vessel studied after basic examination, radiological supervision and interpretation (List separately in addition to code for primary procedure)

(Use 75774 in addition to code for specific initial vessel studied)

(For angiography, see codes 75600-75790)

(For catheterizations, see codes 36215-36248)

(For introduction of catheter, injection procedure, see 93501-93533, 93545, 93555, 93556)

(75775 (complete procedure) has been deleted, see 36000-36015, 36400-36425 for intravenous procedure, and 36100-36248 for intra-arterial procedure and 75774)

75790 Angiography, arteriovenous shunt (eg, dialysis patient), radiological supervision and interpretation

(For introduction of catheter, use 36140, 36145, 36215-36217, 36245-36247)

Veins and Lymphatics

(For injection procedure for venous system, see 36000-36015, 36400-36510)

(For injection procedure for lymphatic system, use 38790)

75801 Lymphangiography, extremity only, unilateral, radiological supervision and interpretation

(75802 (complete procedure) has been deleted, see 38790, 75801)

75803 Lymphangiography, extremity only, bilateral, radiological supervision and interpretation

(75804 (complete procedure) has been deleted, see 38790, 75803)

75805   Lymphangiography, pelvic/abdominal, unilateral, radiological supervision and interpretation

(75806 (complete procedure) has been deleted, see 38790, 75805)

75807   Lymphangiography, pelvic/abdominal, bilateral, radiological supervision and interpretation

(75808 (complete procedure) has been deleted, see 38790, 75807)

75809   Shuntogram for investigation of previously placed indwelling nonvascular shunt (eg, LeVeen shunt, ventriculoperitoneal shunt, indwelling infusion pump), radiological supervision and interpretation

(For procedure, see 49427 or 61070)

75810   Splenoportography, radiological supervision and interpretation

(75811 (complete procedure) has been deleted, see 38200, 75810)

75820   Venography, extremity, unilateral, radiological supervision and interpretation

(75821 (complete procedure) has been deleted, see 36000, 36005, 36406, 36410, 36420, 36425, 75820)

75822   Venography, extremity, bilateral, radiological supervision and interpretation

(75823 (complete procedure) has been deleted, see 36000, 36005, 36406, 36410, 36420, 36425, 75822)

75825   Venography, caval, inferior, with serialography, radiological supervision and interpretation

(75826 (complete procedure) has been deleted, see 36010, 75825)

75827   Venography, caval, superior, with serialography, radiological supervision and interpretation

(75828 (complete procedure) has been deleted, see 36010, 75827)

75831   Venography, renal, unilateral, selective, radiological supervision and interpretation

(75832 (complete procedure) has been deleted, see 36000-36012, 75831)

75833   Venography, renal, bilateral, selective, radiological supervision and interpretation

(75834 (complete procedure) has been deleted, see 36000-36012, 75833)

75840   Venography, adrenal, unilateral, selective, radiological supervision and interpretation

(75841 (complete procedure) has been deleted, see 36000-36012, 75840)

75842   Venography, adrenal, bilateral, selective, radiological supervision and interpretation

(75843 (complete procedure) has been deleted, see 36000-36012, 75842)

(75845, 75846, 75847, 75850, 75851 have been deleted)

75860   Venography, sinus or jugular, catheter, radiological supervision and interpretation

(75861 (complete procedure) has been deleted, see 36000-36012 for intravenous procedure and 36100-36218 for intra-arterial procedure, 75860)

75870   Venography, superior sagittal sinus, radiological supervision and interpretation

(75871 (complete procedure) has been deleted, see 36000-36012 for intravenous procedure and 36100-36218 for intra-arterial procedure, 75870)

75872   Venography, epidural, radiological supervision and interpretation

(75873 (complete procedure) has been deleted, see 36000-36012 for intravenous procedure and 36100-36218 for intra-arterial procedure, 75872)

75880   Venography, orbital, radiological supervision and interpretation

(75881 (complete procedure) has been deleted, see 36000-36012 for intravenous procedure and 36100-36218 for intra-arterial procedure, 75880)

75885   Percutaneous transhepatic portography with hemodynamic evaluation, radiological supervision and interpretation

(75886 (complete procedure) has been deleted, see 36011, 36012, 36481, 75885)

75887   Percutaneous transhepatic portography without hemodynamic evaluation, radiological supervision and interpretation

(75888 (complete procedure) has been deleted, see 36011, 36012, 36481, 75887)

75889   Hepatic venography, wedged or free, with hemodynamic evaluation, radiological supervision and interpretation

(75890 (complete procedure) has been deleted, see 36000-36012, 75889)

75891   Hepatic venography, wedged or free, without hemodynamic evaluation, radiological supervision and interpretation

(75892 (complete procedure) has been deleted, see 36000-36012, 75891)

75893   Venous sampling through catheter, with or without angiography (eg, for parathyroid hormone, renin), radiological supervision and interpretation

(For procedure, use 36500)

Radiology

Transcatheter Procedures

75894   Transcatheter therapy, embolization, any method, radiological supervision and interpretation

(75895 (complete procedure) has been deleted, see 37204, 61624, 61626, 75894)

75896   Transcatheter therapy, infusion, any method (eg, thrombolysis other than coronary), radiological supervision and interpretation

(75897 (complete procedure) has been deleted, see 37201, 37202, 75896)

(For infusion for coronary disease, see 92975, 92977)

75898   Angiography through existing catheter for follow-up study for transcatheter therapy, embolization or infusion

75900   Exchange of a previously placed arterial catheter during thrombolytic therapy with contrast monitoring, radiological supervision and interpretation

(For procedure, use 37209)

● **75901**   Mechanical removal of pericatheter obstructive material (eg, fibrin sheath) from central venous device via separate venous access, radiologic supervision and interpretation

▶(For procedure, use 36536)◀

▶(For venous catheterization, see 36010-36012)◀

● **75902**   Mechanical removal of intraluminal (intracatheter) obstructive material from central venous device through device lumen, radiologic supervision and interpretation

▶(For procedure, use 36537)◀

▶(For venous catheterization, see 36010-36012)◀

75940   Percutaneous placement of IVC filter, radiological supervision and interpretation

(75941 (complete procedure) has been deleted, see 37620, 75940)

75945   Intravascular ultrasound (non-coronary vessel), radiological supervision and interpretation; initial vessel

+ **75946**   each additional non-coronary vessel (List separately in addition to code for primary procedure)

(Use 75946 in conjunction with code 75945)

(For catheterizations, see codes 36215-36248)

(For transcatheter therapies, see codes 37200-37208, 61624, 61626)

(For procedure, see 37250, 37251)

(75950, 75951, 75955, 75956 (complete procedure) have been deleted, see 37204, 61624, 61626, 75894)

75952   Endovascular repair of infrarenal abdominal aortic aneurysm or dissection, radiological supervision and interpretation

(For implantation of endovascular grafts, see 34800-34808)

▲ **75953**   Placement of proximal or distal extension prosthesis for endovascular repair of infrarenal aortic or iliac artery aneurysm, pseudoaneurysm, or dissection, radiological supervision and interpretation

(For implantation of endovascular extension prostheses, see 34825, 34826)

● **75954**   Endovascular repair of iliac artery aneurysm, pseudoaneurysm, arteriovenous malformation, or trauma, radiological supervision and interpretation

▶(For implantation of endovascular graft, see 34900)◀

75960   Transcatheter introduction of intravascular stent(s), (non-coronary vessel), percutaneous and/or open, radiological supervision and interpretation, each vessel

(For procedure, see 37205-37208)

(For radiologic supervision and interpretation for transcatheter placement of extracranial cerebrovascular artery stent(s), use Category III code 0007T)

75961   Transcatheter retrieval, percutaneous, of intravascular foreign body (eg, fractured venous or arterial catheter), radiological supervision and interpretation

(For procedure, use 37203)

75962   Transluminal balloon angioplasty, peripheral artery, radiological supervision and interpretation

(75963 (complete procedure) has been deleted, see 35450-35460 or 35470-35476 and 75962)

+ **75964**   Transluminal balloon angioplasty, each additional peripheral artery, radiological supervision and interpretation (List separately in addition to code for primary procedure)

(Use 75964 in conjunction with code 75962)

(75965 (complete procedure) has been deleted, see 35450-35460 or 35470-35476 and 75964)

75966   Transluminal balloon angioplasty, renal or other visceral artery, radiological supervision and interpretation

(75967 (complete procedure) has been deleted, see 35450-35460 or 35470-35476 and 75966)

+ **75968**   Transluminal balloon angioplasty, each additional visceral artery, radiological supervision and interpretation (List separately in addition to code for primary procedure)

(Use 75968 in conjunction with code 75966)

(75969 (complete procedure) has been deleted, see 35450-35460 or 35470-35476 and 75968)

(For percutaneous transluminal coronary angioplasty, see 92982-92984)

75970   Transcatheter biopsy, radiological supervision and interpretation

(For injection procedure only for transcatheter therapy or biopsy, see 36100-36299)

(For transcatheter renal and ureteral biopsy, use 52007)

(For percutaneous needle biopsy of pancreas, use 48102; of retroperitoneal lymph node or mass, use 49180)

Radiology

(75971 (complete procedure) has been deleted, see 37200, 75970)

(75972-75977 have been deleted. To report, see 75962-75968)

75978 Transluminal balloon angioplasty, venous (eg, subclavian stenosis), radiological supervision and interpretation

(75979 (complete procedure) has been deleted, see 35460, 35476, 75978)

75980 Percutaneous transhepatic biliary drainage with contrast monitoring, radiological supervision and interpretation

(75981 (complete procedure) has been deleted, see 47510, 75980)

75982 Percutaneous placement of drainage catheter for combined internal and external biliary drainage or of a drainage stent for internal biliary drainage in patients with an inoperable mechanical biliary obstruction, radiological supervision and interpretation

(75983 (complete procedure) has been deleted, see 47511, 47556, 75982)

75984 Change of percutaneous tube or drainage catheter with contrast monitoring (eg, gastrointestinal system, genitourinary system, abscess), radiological supervision and interpretation

(75985 (complete procedure) has been deleted, see 43760, 47525, 47530, 50398, 50688, 51705, 51710, 75984)

(For change of nephrostomy or pyelostomy tube only, use 50398)

(For introduction procedure only for percutaneous biliary drainage, see 47510, 47511)

(For percutaneous cholecystostomy, use 47490)

(For change of percutaneous biliary drainage catheter only, use 47525)

(For percutaneous nephrostolithotomy or pyelostolithotomy, see 50080, 50081)

▲ 75989 Radiological guidance (ie, fluoroscopy, ultrasound, or computed tomography), for percutaneous drainage (eg, abscess, specimen collection), with placement of catheter, radiological supervision and interpretation

(75990 (complete procedure) has been deleted, see appropriate organ or site and 75989)

Transluminal Atherectomy

75992 Transluminal atherectomy, peripheral artery, radiological supervision and interpretation

(For procedure, see 35481-35485, 35491-35495)

+ 75993 Transluminal atherectomy, each additional peripheral artery, radiological supervision and interpretation (List separately in addition to code for primary procedure)

(Use 75993 in conjunction with code 75992)

(For procedure, see 35481-35485, 35491-35495)

75994 Transluminal atherectomy, renal, radiological supervision and interpretation

(For procedure, see 35480, 35490)

75995 Transluminal atherectomy, visceral, radiological supervision and interpretation

(For procedure, see 35480, 35490)

+ 75996 Transluminal atherectomy, each additional visceral artery, radiological supervision and interpretation (List separately in addition to code for primary procedure)

(Use 75996 in conjunction with code 75995)

(For procedure, see 35480, 35490)

Other Procedures

▶(For computed tomography cerebral perfusion analysis, see Category III code 0042T)◀

(For arthrography of shoulder, use 73040; elbow, use 73085; wrist, use 73115; hip, use 73525; knee, use 73580; ankle, use 73615)

76000 Fluoroscopy (separate procedure), up to one hour physician time, other than 71023 or 71034 (eg, cardiac fluoroscopy)

76001 Fluoroscopy, physician time more than one hour, assisting a non-radiologic physician (eg, nephrostolithotomy, ERCP, bronchoscopy, transbronchial biopsy)

76003 Fluoroscopic guidance for needle placement (eg, biopsy, aspiration, injection, localization device)

(See appropriate surgical code for procedure and anatomic location)

(Fluoroscopy 76003 is considered inclusive of all radiographic arthrography with the exception of supervision and interpretation for CT and MR arthrography)

Do not report 76003 in addition to 70332, 73040, 73085, 73115, 73525, 73580, 73615)

(Fluoroscopy 76003 is considered inclusive of organ/anatomic specific radiological supervision and interpretation procedures 74320, 74350, 74355, 74445, 74470, 74475, 75809, 75810, 75885, 75887, 75980, 75982, 75989)

76005 Fluoroscopic guidance and localization of needle or catheter tip for spine or paraspinous diagnostic or therapeutic injection procedures (epidural, transforaminal epidural, subarachnoid, paravertebral facet joint, paravertebral facet joint nerve or sacroiliac joint), including neurolytic agent destruction

(Injection of contrast during fluoroscopic guidance and localization is an inclusive component of codes ▶62263, 62264,◀ 62270-62273, 62280-62282, 62310-62319, ▶0027T)◀

Radiology

(Fluoroscopic guidance for subarachnoid puncture for diagnostic radiographic myelography is included in supervision and interpretation codes 72240, 72255, 72265, 72270)

(For epidural or subarachnoid needle or catheter placement and injection, see codes 62270-62273, 62280-62282, 62310-62319)

(For sacroiliac joint arthrography, see 27096, 73542. If formal arthrography is not performed, recorded, and a formal radiographic report is not issued, use 76005 for fluoroscopic guidance for sacroiliac joint injections)

(For paravertebral facet joint injection, see 64470-64476. For transforaminal epidural needle placement and injection, see 64479-64484)

(For destruction by neurolytic agent, see 64600-64680)

▶(For percutaneous or endoscopic lysis of epidural adhesions, codes 62263, 62264, 0027T include fluoroscopic guidance and localization)◀

+ ▲ 76006 Manual application of stress performed by physician for joint radiography, including contralateral joint if indicated

▶(For radiographic interpretation of stressed images, see appropriate anatomic site and number of views)◀

76010 Radiologic examination from nose to rectum for foreign body, single view, child

76012 Radiological supervision and interpretation, percutaneous vertebroplasty, per vertebral body; under fluoroscopic guidance

76013 under CT guidance

(For procedure, see 22520-22522)

76020 Bone age studies

76040 Bone length studies (orthoroentgenogram, scanogram)

(76060 has been deleted. See 76061, 76062)

76061 Radiologic examination, osseous survey; limited (eg, for metastases)

76062 complete (axial and appendicular skeleton)

76065 Radiologic examination, osseous survey, infant

76066 Joint survey, single view, two or more joints (specify)

▲ 76070 Computed tomography, bone mineral density study, one or more sites; axial skeleton (eg, hips, pelvis, spine)

● 76071 appendicular skeleton (peripheral) (eg, radius, wrist, heel)

76075 Dual energy x-ray absorptiometry (DEXA), bone density study, one or more sites; axial skeleton (eg, hips, pelvis, spine)

76076 appendicular skeleton (peripheral) (eg, radius, wrist, heel)

▶(To report dual energy x-ray absorptiometry (DEXA) body composition study, one or more sites, use Category III code 0028T)◀

76078 Radiographic absorptiometry (eg, photodensitometry, radiogrammetry), one or more sites

76080 Radiologic examination, abscess, fistula or sinus tract study, radiological supervision and interpretation

(76081 (complete procedure) has been deleted, see 20501, 49424, 76080)

+ ▲ 76085 Digitization of film radiographic images with computer analysis for lesion detection and further physician review for interpretation, mammography (List separately in addition to code for primary procedure)

(Use 76085 in conjunction with ▶76091,◀76092)

76086 Mammary ductogram or galactogram, single duct, radiological supervision and interpretation

(76087 (complete procedure) has been deleted, see 19030, 76086)

76088 Mammary ductogram or galactogram, multiple ducts, radiological supervision and interpretation

(76089 (complete procedure) has been deleted, see 19030, 76088)

76090 Mammography; unilateral

76091 bilateral

▶(For computer aided detection applied to a bilateral diagnostic mammogram, use 76085 in conjunction with 76091)◀

76092 Screening mammography, bilateral (two view film study of each breast)

(For computer aided detection applied to a screening mammogram, use 76085 ▶in conjunction with 76092)◀

76093 Magnetic resonance imaging, breast, without and/or with contrast material(s); unilateral

76094 bilateral

76095 Stereotactic localization guidance for breast biopsy or needle placement (eg, for wire localization or for injection), each lesion, radiological supervision and interpretation

(For procedure, see 10022, 19000, 19001, 19102, 19103, 19290, 19291)

(For injection for sentinel node localization without lymphoscintigraphy, use 38792)

76096 Mammographic guidance for needle placement, breast (eg, for wire localization or for injection), each lesion, radiological supervision and interpretation

(For procedure, see 10022, 19000, 19102, 19103, 19290, 19291)

(For injection for sentinel node localization without lymphoscintigraphy, use 38792)

(76097 has been deleted. To report, see 19291, 76096)

76098 Radiological examination, surgical specimen

76100 Radiologic examination, single plane body section (eg, tomography), other than with urography

76101   Radiologic examination, complex motion (ie, hypercycloidal) body section (eg, mastoid polytomography), other than with urography; unilateral

76102   bilateral

(For nephrotomography, use 74415)

76120   Cineradiography/videoradiography, except where specifically included

+ 76125   Cineradiography/videoradiography to complement routine examination (List separately in addition to code for primary procedure)

(76127 has been deleted. The use of photographic media is not reported separately but is considered to be a component of the basic procedure)

(76130-76137 have been deleted. To report, use code for specific radiologic examination)

76140   Consultation on x-ray examination made elsewhere, written report

76150   Xeroradiography

(76150 is to be used for non-mammographic studies only)

(76300 has been deleted. To report, use 76499)

76350   Subtraction in conjunction with contrast studies

▲ 76355   Computed tomography guidance for stereotactic localization

▲ 76360   Computed tomography guidance for needle placement (eg, biopsy, aspiration, injection, localization device), radiological supervision and interpretation

(76361 (complete procedure) has been deleted, see appropriate organ or site and 76360)

76362   Computerized axial tomographic guidance for, and monitoring of, tissue ablation

(For percutaneous radiofrequency ablation, use 47382)

(76365 has been deleted. For computed tomographic guidance for cyst aspiration, see appropriate organ or site and 76360)

(76366 (complete procedure) has been deleted, see appropriate organ or site and 76360)

▲ 76370   Computed tomography guidance for placement of radiation therapy fields

76375   Coronal, sagittal, multiplanar, oblique, 3-dimensional and/or holographic reconstruction of computerized axial tomography, magnetic resonance imaging, or other tomographic modality

(Use 76375 in addition to code for imaging procedure)

▲ 76380   Computed tomography, limited or localized follow-up study

76390   Magnetic resonance spectroscopy

(For magnetic resonance imaging, use appropriate MRI body site code)

76393   Magnetic resonance guidance for needle placement (eg, for biopsy, needle aspiration, injection, or placement of localization device) radiological supervision and interpretation

(For procedure see appropriate organ or site)

76394   Magnetic resonance guidance for, and monitoring of, tissue ablation

(For percutaneous radiofrequency ablation, use 47382)

76400   Magnetic resonance (eg, proton) imaging, bone marrow blood supply

76490   Ultrasound guidance for, and monitoring of, tissue ablation

(Do not report 76490 in addition to 76986)

(For ablation, see codes 47370-47382)

● 76496   Unlisted fluoroscopic procedure (eg, diagnostic, interventional)

● 76497   Unlisted computed tomography procedure (eg, diagnostic, interventional)

● 76498   Unlisted magnetic resonance procedure (eg, diagnostic, interventional)

▲ 76499   Unlisted diagnostic radiographic procedure

Diagnostic Ultrasound

Definitions

A-mode implies a one-dimensional ultrasonic measurement procedure.

M-mode implies a one-dimensional ultrasonic measurement procedure with movement of the trace to record amplitude and velocity of moving echo-producing structures.

B-scan implies a two-dimensional ultrasonic scanning procedure with a two-dimensional display.

Real-time scan implies a two-dimensional ultrasonic scanning procedure with display of both two-dimensional structure and motion with time.

Head and Neck

(For determination of corneal thickness (eg, pachymetry) with interpretation and report, bilateral, use Category III code 0025T)

(76500, 76505 have been deleted. To report, use 76999)

76506   Echoencephalography, B-scan and/or real time with image documentation (gray scale) (for determination of ventricular size, delineation of cerebral contents and detection of fluid masses or other intracranial abnormalities), including A-mode encephalography as secondary component where indicated

Radiology

76511 Ophthalmic ultrasound, echography, diagnostic; A-scan only, with amplitude quantification

76512 contact B-scan (with or without simultaneous A-scan)

76513 anterior segment ultrasound, immersion (water bath) B-scan or high resolution biomicroscopy

(76515 has been deleted. To report, use 76999)

76516 Ophthalmic biometry by ultrasound echography, A-scan;

(76517 has been deleted. To report, use 76999)

76519 with intraocular lens power calculation

(For partial coherence interferometry, use 92136)

76529 Ophthalmic ultrasonic foreign body localization

(76530 has been deleted. To report, use 76999)

(76535 has been deleted. To report, use 76536)

76536 Ultrasound, soft tissues of head and neck (eg, thyroid, parathyroid, parotid), B-scan and/or real time with image documentation

(76550 has been deleted. To report, see 93880-93888)

Chest

(76601 has been deleted. To report, use 76999)

76604 Ultrasound, chest, B-scan (includes mediastinum) and/or real time with image documentation

(76620, 76625 have been deleted)

(76627, 76628 have been deleted. To report, see 93307, 93308)

(76629 has been deleted)

(76632 has been deleted. To report, see 93320, 93321)

(76640 has been deleted. To report, use 76999)

76645 Ultrasound, breast(s) (unilateral or bilateral), B-scan and/or real time with image documentation

Abdomen and Retroperitoneum

76700 Ultrasound, abdominal, B-scan and/or real time with image documentation; complete

76705 limited (eg, single organ, quadrant, follow-up)

76770 Ultrasound, retroperitoneal (eg, renal, aorta, nodes), B-scan and/or real time with image documentation; complete

76775 limited

76778 Ultrasound, transplanted kidney, B-scan and/or real time with image documentation, with or without duplex Doppler study

Spinal Canal

76800 Ultrasound, spinal canal and contents

Pelvis

►Obstetrical◄

►Codes 76801 and 76802 include determination of the number of gestational sacs and fetuses, gestational sac/fetal measurements appropriate for gestation (<14 weeks 0 days), survey of visible fetal and placental anatomic structure, qualitative assessment of amniotic fluid volume/gestational sac shape and examination of the maternal uterus and adnexa.

Codes 76805 and 76810 include determination of number of fetuses and amniotic/chorionic sacs, measurements appropriate for gestational age (> or = 14 weeks 0 days), survey of intracranial/spinal/abdominal anatomy, 4 chambered heart, umbilical cord insertion site, placenta location and amniotic fluid assessment and, when visible, examination of maternal adnexa.

Codes 76811 and 76812 include all elements of codes 76805 and 76810 plus detailed anatomic evaluation of the fetal brain/ventricles, face, heart/outflow tracts and chest anatomy, abdominal organ specific anatomy, number/length/architecture of limbs and detailed evaluation of the umbilical cord and placenta and other fetal anatomy as clinically indicated.

Report should document the results of the evaluation of each element described above or the reason for non-visualization.

Code 76815 represents a focused "quick look" exam limited to the assessment of one or more of the elements listed in code 76815.

Code 76816 describes an examination designed to reassess fetal size and interval growth or reevaluate one or more anatomic abnormalities of a fetus previously demonstrated on ultrasound, and should be coded once for each fetus requiring reevaluation using modifier '-59' for each fetus after the first.

Code 76817 describes a transvaginal obstetric ultrasound performed separately or in addition to one of the transabdominal examinations described above. For transvaginal examinations performed for non-obstetrical purposes, use code 76830.◄

● **76801** Ultrasound, pregnant uterus, real time with image documentation, fetal and maternal evaluation, first trimester (<14 weeks 0 days), transabdominal approach; single or first gestation

+ ● **76802** each additional gestation (List separately in addition to code for primary procedure)

►(Use 76802 in conjunction with code 76801)◄

▲ **76805** Ultrasound, pregnant uterus, real time with image documentation, fetal and maternal evaluation, after first trimester (> or = 14 weeks 0 days), transabdominal approach; single or first gestation

+ ▲ **76810** each additional gestation (List separately in addition to code for primary procedure)

►(Use 76810 in conjunction with code 76805)◄

● **76811** Ultrasound, pregnant uterus, real time with image documentation, fetal and maternal evaluation plus detailed fetal anatomic examination, transabdominal approach; single or first gestation

+ ● **76812** each additional gestation (List separately in addition to code for primary procedure)

►(Use 76812 in conjunction with code 76811)◄

▲ **76815** Ultrasound, pregnant uterus, real time with image documentation, limited (eg, fetal heart beat, placental location, fetal position and/or qualitative amniotic fluid volume), one or more fetuses

►(Use 76815 only once per exam and not per element)◄

▲ **76816** Ultrasound, pregnant uterus, real time with image documentation, follow-up (eg, re-evaluation of fetal size by measuring standard growth parameters and amniotic fluid volume, re-evaluation of organ system(s) suspected or confirmed to be abnormal on a previous scan), transabdominal approach, per fetus

►(Report 76816 with modifier '-59' for each additional fetus examined in a multiple pregnancy)◄

● **76817** Ultrasound, pregnant uterus, real time with image documentation, transvaginal

►(For non-obstetrical transvaginal ultrasound, use 76830)◄

►(If transvaginal examination is done in addition to transabdominal obstetrical ultrasound exam, use 76817 in addition to appropriate transabdominal exam code)◄

76818 Fetal biophysical profile; with non-stress testing

76819 without non-stress testing

(Fetal biophysical profile assessments for the second and any additional fetuses, should be reported separately by code 76818 or 76819 with the modifier ►'-59'◄ appended)

(For amniotic fluid index without non-stress test, use 76815)

76825 Echocardiography, fetal, cardiovascular system, real time with image documentation (2D), with or without M-mode recording;

76826 follow-up or repeat study

76827 Doppler echocardiography, fetal, cardiovascular system, pulsed wave and/or continuous wave with spectral display; complete

76828 follow-up or repeat study

(To report the use of color mapping, use 93325)

►Non-Obstetrical◄

76830 Ultrasound, transvaginal

►(For obstetrical transvaginal ultrasound, use 76817)◄

►(If transvaginal examination is done in addition to transabdominal non-obstetrical ultrasound exam, use 76830 in addition to appropriate transabdominal exam code)◄

76831 Hysterosonography, with or without color flow Doppler

(For introduction of saline or contrast for hysterosonography, use 58340)

(76855 has been deleted. To report, see 93975-93979)

76856 Ultrasound, pelvic (nonobstetric), B-scan and/or real time with image documentation; complete

76857 limited or follow-up (eg, for follicles)

Genitalia

76870 Ultrasound, scrotum and contents

76872 Echography, transrectal;

76873 prostate volume study for brachytherapy treatment planning (separate procedure)

Extremities

76880 Ultrasound, extremity, non-vascular, B-scan and/or real time with image documentation

76885 Ultrasound, infant hips, real time with imaging documentation; dynamic (requiring physician manipulation)

76886 limited, static (not requiring physician manipulation)

Vascular Studies

(76900-76920 have been deleted. To report, see 93922-93971; for cerebrovascular studies, see 93875-93888)

(76925 has been deleted. To report, see 93922-93931 or 93965-93971)

(76926 has been deleted. To report, see 93875-93888 or 93975-93979)

Ultrasonic Guidance Procedures

76930 Ultrasonic guidance for pericardiocentesis, imaging supervision and interpretation

(76931 (complete procedure) has been deleted, see 33010, 33011, 76930)

76932 Ultrasonic guidance for endomyocardial biopsy, imaging supervision and interpretation

(76933 (complete procedure) has been deleted, see 93505, 76932)

Radiology

▲=Revised Code   ●=New Code

(76934 has been deleted. For ultrasound guidance for thoracentesis or abdominal paracentesis, see 32000 and 76942)

(76935 (complete procedure) has been deleted, see 32000, 76942)

76936 Ultrasound guided compression repair of arterial pseudoaneurysm or arteriovenous fistulae (includes diagnostic ultrasound evaluation, compression of lesion and imaging)

(76938 has been deleted. For ultrasound guidance for cyst or renal pelvis aspiration, see appropriate organ or site and 76942)

(76939 (complete procedure) has been deleted, see appropriate organ or site and 76942)

76941 Ultrasonic guidance for intrauterine fetal transfusion or cordocentesis, imaging supervision and interpretation

(For procedure, see 36460, 59012)

76942 Ultrasonic guidance for needle placement (eg, biopsy, aspiration, injection, localization device), imaging supervision and interpretation

(76943 (complete procedure) has been deleted, see appropriate organ or site and 76942)

(76944 has been deleted. To report, use 75989)

76945 Ultrasonic guidance for chorionic villus sampling, imaging supervision and interpretation

(For procedure, use 59015)

76946 Ultrasonic guidance for amniocentesis, imaging supervision and interpretation

(76947 (complete procedure) has been deleted, see 59000, 76946)

76948 Ultrasonic guidance for aspiration of ova, imaging supervision and interpretation

(76949 (complete procedure) has been deleted, see 58970, 76948)

76950 Ultrasonic guidance for placement of radiation therapy fields

(76960 has been deleted. To report, use 76950)

76965 Ultrasonic guidance for interstitial radioelement application

Other Procedures

76970 Ultrasound study follow-up (specify)

76975 Gastrointestinal endoscopic ultrasound, supervision and interpretation

(For procedure, use 43259)

(Do not report 76975 in conjunction with 43231, 43232, 43242, 45341, 45342)

76977 Ultrasound bone density measurement and interpretation, peripheral site(s), any method

(76980 has been deleted. To report, use code for specific ultrasound examination)

(76985 has been deleted. To report, use 76986)

76986 Ultrasonic guidance, intraoperative

(Do not report 76986 in addition to 47370-47382)

(For ultrasound guidance for open and laparoscopic radiofrequency tissue ablation, use 76490)

(76990 has been deleted. To report, use 76999)

(76991 has been deleted. To report, see 76830, 76872)

▲ **76999** Unlisted ultrasound procedure (eg, diagnostic, interventional)

Radiation Oncology

Listings for Radiation Oncology provide for teletherapy and brachytherapy to include initial consultation, clinical treatment planning, simulation, medical radiation physics, dosimetry, treatment devices, special services, and clinical treatment management procedures. They include normal follow-up care during course of treatment and for three months following its completion.

When a service or procedure is provided that is not listed in this edition of *CPT* it should be identified by a Special Report (see page 218) and one of the unlisted procedure codes listed below:

77299 Unlisted procedure, therapeutic radiology clinical treatment planning
77399 Unlisted procedure, medical radiation physics, dosimetry and treatment devices, and special services
77499 Unlisted procedure, therapeutic radiology treatment management
77799 Unlisted procedure, clinical brachytherapy

For treatment by injectable or ingestible isotopes, see subsection **Nuclear Medicine.**

Consultation: Clinical Management

Preliminary consultation, evaluation of patient prior to decision to treat, or full medical care (in addition to treatment management) when provided by the therapeutic radiologist may be identified by the appropriate procedure codes from **Evaluation and Management, Medicine,** or **Surgery** sections.

Radiology

Clinical Treatment Planning (External and Internal Sources)

The clinical treatment planning process is a complex service including interpretation of special testing, tumor localization, treatment volume determination, treatment time/dosage determination, choice of treatment modality, determination of number and size of treatment ports, selection of appropriate treatment devices, and other procedures.

Definitions

Simple planning requires a single treatment area of interest encompassed in a single port or simple parallel opposed ports with simple or no blocking.

Intermediate planning requires three or more converging ports, two separate treatment areas, multiple blocks, or special time dose constraints.

Complex planning requires highly complex blocking, custom shielding blocks, tangential ports, special wedges or compensators, three or more separate treatment areas, rotational or special beam considerations, combination of therapeutic modalities.

> (77260, 77265, 77270, 77275 have been deleted. To report, see 77261-77263)

77261   Therapeutic radiology treatment planning; simple

77262   intermediate

77263   complex

Definitions

Simple simulation of a single treatment area with either a single port or parallel opposed ports. Simple or no blocking.

Intermediate simulation of three or more converging ports, two separate treatment areas, multiple blocks.

Complex simulation of tangential portals, three or more treatment areas, rotation or arc therapy, complex blocking, custom shielding blocks, brachytherapy source verification, hyperthermia probe verification, any use of contrast materials.

Three-dimensional computer-generated three dimensional reconstruction of tumor volume and surrounding critical normal tissue structures from direct CT scans and/or MRI data in preparation for non-coplanar or coplanar therapy. The simulation utilizes documented three-dimensional beam's eye view volume-dose displays of multiple or moving beams. Documentation with three-dimensional volume reconstruction and dose distribution is required.

Simulation may be carried out on a dedicated simulator, a radiation therapy treatment unit, or diagnostic x-ray machine.

77280   Therapeutic radiology simulation-aided field setting; simple

77285   intermediate

77290   complex

77295   three-dimensional

77299   Unlisted procedure, therapeutic radiology clinical treatment planning

Medical Radiation Physics, Dosimetry, Treatment Devices, and Special Services

77300   Basic radiation dosimetry calculation, central axis depth dose calculation, TDF, NSD, gap calculation, off axis factor, tissue inhomogeneity factors, calculation of non-ionizing radiation surface and depth dose, as required during course of treatment, only when prescribed by the treating physician

77301   Intensity modulated radiotherapy plan, including dose-volume histograms for target and critical structure partial tolerance specifications

> (Dose plan is optimized using inverse or forward planning technique for modulated beam delivery (eg, binary, dynamic MLC) to create highly conformal dose distribution. Computer plan distribution must be verified for positional accuracy based on dosimetric verification of the intensity map with verification of treatment set-up and interpretation of verification methodology)

77305   Teletherapy, isodose plan (whether hand or computer calculated); simple (one or two parallel opposed unmodified ports directed to a single area of interest)

77310   intermediate (three or more treatment ports directed to a single area of interest)

77315   complex (mantle or inverted Y, tangential ports, the use of wedges, compensators, complex blocking, rotational beam, or special beam considerations)

> (Only one teletherapy isodose plan may be reported for a given course of therapy to a specific treatment area)

> (77320 has been deleted. To report, see 77300-77399)

77321   Special teletherapy port plan, particles, hemibody, total body

> (77325 has been deleted. To report, see 77300-77399)

Radiology

▲·**77326** Brachytherapy isodose plan; simple (calculation made from single plane, one to four sources/ribbon application, remote afterloading brachytherapy, 1 to 8 sources)

(For definition of source/ribbon, see page 239)

77327 intermediate (multiplane dosage calculations, application involving 5 to 10 sources/ribbons, remote afterloading brachytherapy, 9 to 12 sources)

77328 complex (multiplane isodose plan, volume implant calculations, over 10 sources/ribbons used, special spatial reconstruction, remote afterloading brachytherapy, over 12 sources)

(77330 has been deleted. To report, see 77300-77399)

77331 Special dosimetry (eg, TLD, microdosimetry) (specify), only when prescribed by the treating physician

77332 Treatment devices, design and construction; simple (simple block, simple bolus)

77333 intermediate (multiple blocks, stents, bite blocks, special bolus)

77334 complex (irregular blocks, special shields, compensators, wedges, molds or casts)

(77335 has been deleted. To report, see 77300-77399)

77336 Continuing medical physics consultation, including assessment of treatment parameters, quality assurance of dose delivery, and review of patient treatment documentation in support of the radiation oncologist, reported per week of therapy

(77340 has been deleted. To report, see 77300-77399)

(77345-77360 have been deleted. To report, see 77300-77399)

77370 Special medical radiation physics consultation

(77380 has been deleted. To report, use 77520)

(77381 has been deleted. To report, use 77523)

77399 Unlisted procedure, medical radiation physics, dosimetry and treatment devices, and special services

Radiation Treatment Delivery

(Radiation treatment delivery (77401-77416) recognizes the technical component and the various energy levels.)

(77400 has been deleted)

77401 Radiation treatment delivery, superficial and/or ortho voltage

77402 Radiation treatment delivery, single treatment area, single port or parallel opposed ports, simple blocks or no blocks; up to 5 MeV

77403 6-10 MeV

77404 11-19 MeV

(77405 has been deleted)

77406 20 MeV or greater

77407 Radiation treatment delivery, two separate treatment areas, three or more ports on a single treatment area, use of multiple blocks; up to 5 MeV

77408 6-10 MeV

77409 11-19 MeV

(77410 has been deleted)

77411 20 MeV or greater

77412 Radiation treatment delivery, three or more separate treatment areas, custom blocking, tangential ports, wedges, rotational beam, compensators, special particle beam (eg, electron or neutrons); up to 5 MeV

77413 6-10 MeV

77414 11-19 MeV

(77415 has been deleted. To report, use 77417)

77416 20 MeV or greater

77417 Therapeutic radiology port film(s)

77418 Intensity modulated treatment delivery, single or multiple fields/arcs, via narrow spatially and temporally modulated beams (eg, binary, dynamic MLC), per treatment session

(For intensity modulated treatment planning, use 77301)

Radiation Treatment Management

Radiation treatment management is reported in units of five fractions or treatment sessions, regardless of the actual time period in which the services are furnished. The services need not be furnished on consecutive days. Multiple fractions representing two or more treatment sessions furnished on the same day may be counted separately as long as there has been a distinct break in therapy sessions, and the fractions are of the character usually furnished on different days. Code 77427 is also reported if there are three or four fractions beyond a multiple of five at the end of a course of treatment; one or two fractions beyond a multiple of five at the end of a course of treatment are not reported separately. The professional services furnished during treatment management typically consists of:

■ Review of port films;

■ Review of dosimetry, dose delivery, and treatment parameters;

■ Review of patient treatment set-up;

■ Examination of patient for medical evaluation and management (eg, assessment of the patient's response to treatment, coordination of care and treatment, review of imaging and/or lab test results).

(77419, 77420, 77425, and 77430 have been deleted. To report radiation treatment management, use 77427)

77427 Radiation treatment management, five treatments

77431   Radiation therapy management with complete course of therapy consisting of one or two fractions only

(77431 is not to be used to fill in the last week of a long course of therapy)

77432   Stereotactic radiation treatment management of cerebral lesion(s) (complete course of treatment consisting of one session)

(77435-77460 have been deleted. To report, see 77401-77499)

(77465 has been deleted)

77470   Special treatment procedure (eg, total body irradiation, hemibody radiation, per oral, endocavitary or intraoperative cone irradiation)

(77470 assumes that the procedure is performed one or more times during the course of therapy, in addition to daily or weekly patient management)

77499   Unlisted procedure, therapeutic radiology treatment management

Proton Beam Treatment Delivery

Definitions

Simple proton treatment delivery to a single treatment area utilizing a single non-tangential/oblique port, custom block with compensation (77522) and without compensation (77520).

Intermediate proton treatment delivery to one or more treatment areas utilizing two or more ports or one or more tangential/oblique ports, with custom blocks and compensators.

Complex proton treatment delivery to one or more treatment areas utilizing two or more ports per treatment area with matching or patching fields and/or multiple isocenters, with custom blocks and compensators.

77520   Proton treatment delivery; simple, without compensation

77522   simple, with compensation

77523   intermediate

77525   complex

Hyperthermia

Hyperthermia treatments as listed in this section include external (superficial and deep), interstitial, and intracavitary.

Radiation therapy when given concurrently is listed separately.

Hyperthermia is used only as an adjunct to radiation therapy or chemotherapy. It may be induced by a variety of sources (eg, microwave, ultrasound, low energy radio-frequency conduction, or by probes).

The listed treatments include management during the course of therapy and follow-up care for three months after completion.

Preliminary consultation is not included (see **Medicine** 99241-99263).

Physics planning and interstitial insertion of temperature sensors, and use of external or interstitial heat generating sources are included.

The following descriptors are included in the treatment schedule:

77600   Hyperthermia, externally generated; superficial (ie, heating to a depth of 4 cm or less)

77605   deep (ie, heating to depths greater than 4 cm)

77610   Hyperthermia generated by interstitial probe(s); 5 or fewer interstitial applicators

77615   more than 5 interstitial applicators

Clinical Intracavitary Hyperthermia

77620   Hyperthermia generated by intracavitary probe(s)

Clinical Brachytherapy

Clinical brachytherapy requires the use of either natural or man-made radioelements applied into or around a treatment field of interest. The supervision of radioelements and dose interpretation are performed solely by the therapeutic radiologist.

Services 77750-77799 include admission to the hospital and daily visits.

For insertion of ovoids and tandems, use 57155.

For insertion of Heyman capsules, use 58346.

Definitions

(Sources refer to intracavitary placement or permanent interstitial placement; ribbons refer to temporary interstitial placement)

A simple application has one to four sources/ribbons.

An intermediate application has five to ten sources/ribbons.

A complex application has greater than ten sources/ribbons.

(77700-77749 have been deleted. To report, see 77761-77799)

77750   Infusion or instillation of radioelement solution

(77755, 77760 have been deleted. To report, see 77761-77799)

77761   Intracavitary radiation source application; simple

77762   intermediate

77763   complex

(77765, 77770, 77775 have been deleted. To report, see 77761-77799)

Radiology

77776 Interstitial radiation source application; simple

77777 intermediate

77778 complex

(77780 has been deleted. To report, see 77761-77799)

77781 Remote afterloading high intensity brachytherapy; 1-4 source positions or catheters

77782 5-8 source positions or catheters

77783 9-12 source positions or catheters

77784 over 12 source positions or catheters

(77785 has been deleted. To report, see 77761-77799)

77789 Surface application of radiation source

77790 Supervision, handling, loading of radiation source

77799 Unlisted procedure, clinical brachytherapy

(77800 has been deleted. To report, use 77331)

(77805-77810 have been deleted. To report, see 77305-77321 or 77326-77328)

(77850 has been deleted. To report, see 77300, 77336, 77370)

(77860 has been deleted. To report, use 77336)

(77999 has been deleted. To report, use 77399)

Nuclear Medicine

Listed procedures may be performed independently or in the course of overall medical care. If the physician providing these services is also responsible for diagnostic work-up and/or follow-up care of patient, see appropriate sections also.

Radioimmunoassay tests are found in the **Clinical Pathology** section (codes 82000-84999). These codes can be appropriately used by any specialist performing such tests in a laboratory licensed and/or certified for radioimmunoassays. The reporting of these tests is not confined to clinical pathology laboratories alone.

The services listed do not include the provision of radium or other radioelements. Those materials supplied by the physician should be listed separately and identified by the code 78990 for diagnostic radiopharmaceutical and 79900 for therapeutic radiopharmaceutical.

Diagnostic

Endocrine System

78000 Thyroid uptake; single determination

78001 multiple determinations

78003 stimulation, suppression or discharge (not including initial uptake studies)

78006 Thyroid imaging, with uptake; single determination

78007 multiple determinations

78010 Thyroid imaging; only

78011 with vascular flow

78015 Thyroid carcinoma metastases imaging; limited area (eg, neck and chest only)

78016 with additional studies (eg, urinary recovery)

(78017 has been deleted. To report, use 78018)

78018 whole body

(For calcitonin, use 82308)

(For triiodothyronine (true TT-3), use 84480)

(For triiodothyronine, free (FT-3), (unbound T-3 only), use 84481)

(For TT-4 thyroxine, use 84436)

(For T-4 thyroxine, neonatal, use 84437)

(For FT-4 thyroxine, free, (unbound T-4 only), use 84439)

+ 78020 Thyroid carcinoma metastases uptake (List separately in addition to code for primary procedure)

(Use 78020 in conjunction with code 78018 only)

78070 Parathyroid imaging

(For parathormone (parathyroid hormone), use 83970)

78075 Adrenal imaging, cortex and/or medulla

(For cortisol, plasma, use 82533)

(For cortisol, urine, use 82533)

(For aldosterone, double isotope technique, use 82088)

(For aldosterone, blood, use 82088)

(For aldosterone, urine, use 82088)

(For 17-ketosteroids, use 83586)

(For 17-OH ketosteroids, use 83586)

(For 17-hydroxycorticosteroids, use 83491)

(For insulin, use 83525)

(For insulin antibodies, use 86337)

(For proinsulin, use 84206)

(For glucagon, use 82943)

(For adrenocorticotropic hormone (ACTH), use 82024)

(For human growth hormone (HGH), (somatotropin), use 83003)

(For human growth antibody, use 86277)

(For thyroglobulin antibody, use 86800)

(For thyroid microsomal antibody, use 86376)

(For thyroid stimulating hormone (TSH), use 84443)

(For thyrotropin releasing factor, see 80438, 80439)

(For plus long-acting thyroid stimulator (LATS), use 84445)

(For follicle stimulating hormone (FSH component of pituitary gonadotropin), use 83001)

(For luteinizing hormone (LH component of pituitary gonadotropin), (ICSH), use 83002)

(For luteinizing releasing factor (LRH), use 83727)

(For prolactin level (mammotropin), use 84146)

(For vasopressin level (antidiuretic hormone), use 84588)

(For estradiol, use 82670)

(For progesterone, use 84144)

(For testosterone, blood, use 84403)

(For testosterone, urine, use 84403)

(For etiocholanolone, use 82696)

78099   Unlisted endocrine procedure, diagnostic nuclear medicine

(For chemical analysis, see **Chemistry** section)

Hematopoietic, Reticuloendothelial and Lymphatic System

78102   Bone marrow imaging; limited area

78103   multiple areas

78104   whole body

78110   Plasma volume, radiopharmaceutical volume-dilution technique (separate procedure); single sampling

78111   multiple samplings

78120   Red cell volume determination (separate procedure); single sampling

78121   multiple samplings

78122   Whole blood volume determination, including separate measurement of plasma volume and red cell volume (radiopharmaceutical volume-dilution technique)

78130   Red cell survival study;

78135   differential organ/tissue kinetics, (eg, splenic and/or hepatic sequestration)

78140   Labeled red cell sequestration, differential organ/tissue, (eg, splenic and/or hepatic)

78160   Plasma radioiron disappearance (turnover) rate

78162   Radioiron oral absorption

78170   Radioiron red cell utilization

78172   Chelatable iron for estimation of total body iron

(78180 has been deleted. To report, use 78199)

(For hemosiderin, use 83071)

(For intrinsic factor antibodies, use 86340)

(For cyanocobalamin (vitamin B-12), use 82607)

(For folic acid (folate) serum, use 82746)

(For hepatitis B antigen, see 87340, 87350)

(For hepatitis A antibody (HAAb), see 86708, 86709)

(For hepatitis B core antibody (HBcAb), see 86704, 86705)

(For hepatitis B surface antigen (HBsAb), use 87340)

(For hepatitis B surface antibody (HBsAb), use 86706)

(For hepatitis Be antigen (HBeAg), use 87350)

(For hepatitis Be antibody (HBeAb), use 86707)

78185   Spleen imaging only, with or without vascular flow

(If combined with liver study, use procedures 78215 and 78216)

(78186 has been deleted)

78190   Kinetics, study of platelet survival, with or without differential organ/tissue localization

78191   Platelet survival study

(78192 has been deleted. To report, use 78805)

(78193 has been deleted. To report, use 78806)

78195   Lymphatics and lymph nodes imaging

(For sentinel node identification without scintigraphy imaging, use 38792)

(For sentinal node excision, see 38500-38542)

78199   Unlisted hematopoietic, reticuloendothelial and lymphatic procedure, diagnostic nuclear medicine

(For chemical analysis, see **Chemistry** section)

Gastrointestinal System

78201   Liver imaging; static only

78202   with vascular flow

(For spleen imaging only, use 78185)

78205   Liver imaging (SPECT);

78206   with vascular flow

78215   Liver and spleen imaging; static only

78216   with vascular flow

78220   Liver function study with hepatobiliary agents, with serial images

(78221 has been deleted. To report, use 78299)

78223   Hepatobiliary ductal system imaging, including gallbladder, with or without pharmacologic intervention, with or without quantitative measurement of gallbladder function

(78225 has been deleted)

Radiology

78230	Salivary gland imaging;
78231	with serial images
78232	Salivary gland function study
	(78240 has been deleted. To report pancreas imaging, use 78299)
78258	Esophageal motility
78261	Gastric mucosa imaging
78262	Gastroesophageal reflux study
78264	Gastric emptying study
78267	Urea breath test, C-14; acquisition for analysis
78268	analysis
78270	Vitamin B-12 absorption study (eg, Schilling test); without intrinsic factor
78271	with intrinsic factor
78272	Vitamin B-12 absorption studies combined, with and without intrinsic factor
	(78276 has been deleted)
78278	Acute gastrointestinal blood loss imaging
	(78280 has been deleted)
78282	Gastrointestinal protein loss
	(78285, 78286 have been deleted. To report, use 78299)
	(For gastrin, use 82941)
	(For intrinsic factor level, use 83528)
	(For carcinoembryonic antigen level (CEA), use 82378)
78290	Intestine imaging (eg, ectopic gastric mucosa, Meckels localization, volvulus)
78291	Peritoneal-venous shunt patency test (eg, for LeVeen, Denver shunt)
	(For injection procedure, use 49427)
78299	Unlisted gastrointestinal procedure, diagnostic nuclear medicine
	(For chemical analysis, see **Chemistry** section)

Musculoskeletal System

Bone and joint imaging can be used in the diagnosis of a variety of inflammatory processes (eg, osteomyelitis), as well as for localization of primary and/or metastatic neoplasms.

78300	Bone and/or joint imaging; limited area
78305	multiple areas
78306	whole body
	(78310 has been deleted. To report, use 78445)
78315	three phase study
78320	tomographic (SPECT)

78350	Bone density (bone mineral content) study, one or more sites; single photon absorptiometry
78351	dual photon absorptiometry, one or more sites
	(78380, 78381 have been deleted. To report, see 78300, 78305)
	(For radiographic bone density (photodensitometry), use 76078)
78399	Unlisted musculoskeletal procedure, diagnostic nuclear medicine

Cardiovascular System

Myocardial perfusion and cardiac blood pool imaging studies may be performed at rest and/or during stress. When performed during exercise and/or pharmacologic stress, the appropriate stress testing code from the 93015-93018 series should be reported in addition to code(s) 78460-78465, 78472, 78473, 78478, 78480, 78481, 78483, 78491, and 78492.

	(78401-78412 have been deleted. To report, see 78472-78483)
78414	Determination of central c-v hemodynamics (non-imaging) (eg, ejection fraction with probe technique) with or without pharmacologic intervention or exercise, single or multiple determinations
	(78415 has been deleted. To report, use 78472)
	(78418-78424 have been deleted. To report, see 78460-78469)
	(78425 has been deleted. To report, use 78472)
78428	Cardiac shunt detection
	(78435 has been deleted. To report, use 78481)
78445	Non-cardiac vascular flow imaging (ie, angiography, venography)
78455	Venous thrombosis study (eg, radioactive fibrinogen)
78456	Acute venous thrombosis imaging, peptide
78457	Venous thrombosis imaging, venogram; unilateral
78458	bilateral
78459	Myocardial imaging, positron emission tomography (PET), metabolic evaluation
	(For myocardial perfusion study, see 78491-78492)
78460	Myocardial perfusion imaging; (planar) single study, at rest or stress (exercise and/or pharmacologic), with or without quantification
78461	multiple studies, (planar) at rest and/or stress (exercise and/or pharmacologic), and redistribution and/or rest injection, with or without quantification
	(78462, 78463 have been deleted. To report, see 78460, 78461)

78464   tomographic (SPECT), single study at rest or stress (exercise and/or pharmacologic), with or without quantification

78465   tomographic (SPECT), multiple studies, at rest and/or stress (exercise and/or pharmacologic) and redistribution and/or rest injection, with or without quantification

78466   Myocardial imaging, infarct avid, planar; qualitative or quantitative

(78467 has been deleted. To report, use 78466)

78468   with ejection fraction by first pass technique

78469   tomographic SPECT with or without quantification

(78470 has been deleted. To report, see 78472, 78473, or 78481)

(78471 has been deleted. To report, use 78472)

78472   Cardiac blood pool imaging, gated equilibrium; planar, single study at rest or stress (exercise and/or pharmacologic), wall motion study plus ejection fraction, with or without additional quantitative processing

(For assessment of cardiac function by first pass technique, use 78496)

78473   multiple studies, wall motion study plus ejection fraction, at rest and stress (exercise and/or pharmacologic), with or without additional quantification

(78474 has been deleted. To report, use 78472)

(78475-78477 have been deleted. To report, use 78473)

+ 78478   Myocardial perfusion study with wall motion, qualitative or quantitative study (List separately in addition to code for primary procedure)

(Use 78478 in conjunction with codes 78460, 78461, 78464, 78465)

(78479 has been deleted)

+ 78480   Myocardial perfusion study with ejection fraction (List separately in addition to code for primary procedure)

(Use 78480 in conjunction with codes 78460, 78461, 78464, 78465)

78481   Cardiac blood pool imaging, (planar), first pass technique; single study, at rest or with stress (exercise and/or pharmacologic), wall motion study plus ejection fraction, with or without quantification

78483   multiple studies, at rest and with stress (exercise and/ or pharmacologic), wall motion study plus ejection fraction, with or without quantification

(78484 has been deleted. To report, use 78481)

(78485, 78486 have been deleted. To report, use 78483)

(78487 and 78489 have been deleted. To report, use 78483)

(78490 has been deleted. To report, use 78499)

(For digoxin, use 80162)

(For cerebral blood flow study, use 78615)

78491   Myocardial imaging, positron emission tomography (PET), perfusion; single study at rest or stress

78492   multiple studies at rest and/or stress

78494   Cardiac blood pool imaging, gated equilibrium, SPECT, at rest, wall motion study plus ejection fraction, with or without quantitative processing

+ 78496   Cardiac blood pool imaging, gated equilibrium, single study, at rest, with right ventricular ejection fraction by first pass technique (List separately in addition to code for primary procedure)

(Use 78496 in conjunction with code 78472)

78499   Unlisted cardiovascular procedure, diagnostic nuclear medicine

(For chemical analysis, see **Chemistry** section)

Respiratory System

78580   Pulmonary perfusion imaging, particulate

(78581 and 78582 have been deleted)

78584   Pulmonary perfusion imaging, particulate, with ventilation; single breath

78585   rebreathing and washout, with or without single breath

78586   Pulmonary ventilation imaging, aerosol; single projection

78587   multiple projections (eg, anterior, posterior, lateral views)

78588   Pulmonary perfusion imaging, particulate, with ventilation imaging, aerosol, one or multiple projections

78591   Pulmonary ventilation imaging, gaseous, single breath, single projection

78593   Pulmonary ventilation imaging, gaseous, with rebreathing and washout with or without single breath; single projection

78594   multiple projections (eg, anterior, posterior, lateral views)

78596   Pulmonary quantitative differential function (ventilation/perfusion) study

78599   Unlisted respiratory procedure, diagnostic nuclear medicine

Nervous System

78600   Brain imaging, limited procedure; static

78601   with vascular flow

78605   Brain imaging, complete study; static

78606   with vascular flow

78607   tomographic (SPECT)

Radiology

78608 Brain imaging, positron emission tomography (PET); metabolic evaluation

78609   perfusion evaluation

78610 Brain imaging, vascular flow only

78615 Cerebral vascular flow

78630 Cerebrospinal fluid flow, imaging (not including introduction of material); cisternography

(For injection procedure, see 61000-61070, 62270-62319)

78635   ventriculography

(For injection procedure, see 61000-61070, 62270-62294)

(78640 has been deleted. To report, use 78699)

78645   shunt evaluation

(For injection procedure, see 61000-61070, 62270-62294)

78647   tomographic (SPECT)

78650 Cerebrospinal fluid leakage detection and localization

(For injection procedure, see 61000-61070, 62270-62294)

(For myelin basic protein, CSF, use 83873)

(78652 has been deleted. To report, use 78647)

(78655 has been deleted. To report, use 78800)

78660 Radiopharmaceutical dacryocystography

78699 Unlisted nervous system procedure, diagnostic nuclear medicine

Genitourinary System

78700 Kidney imaging; static only

78701   with vascular flow

78704   with function study (ie, imaging renogram)

78707 Kidney imaging with vascular flow and function; single study without pharmacological intervention

78708   single study, with pharmacological intervention (eg, angiotensin converting enzyme inhibitor and/or diuretic)

78709   multiple studies, with and without pharmacological intervention (eg, angiotensin converting enzyme inhibitor and/or diuretic)

(For introduction of radioactive substance in association with renal endoscopy, see 50559, 50578)

78710 Kidney imaging, tomographic (SPECT)

78715 Kidney vascular flow only

(78720 has been deleted. To report, use 78704)

78725 Kidney function study, non-imaging radioisotopic study

(78726 has been deleted. To report, use 78799)

(78727 has been deleted. To report, see 78700-78707)

(For renin (angiotensin I), use 84244)

(For angiotensin II, use 82163)

(For beta-2 microglobulin, use 82232)

78730 Urinary bladder residual study

(For introduction of radioactive substance in association with cystotomy or cystostomy, use 51020; in association with cystourethroscopy, use 52250)

78740 Ureteral reflux study (radiopharmaceutical voiding cystogram)

(For catheterization, see 53670, 53675)

(For estradiol, use 82670)

(For estriol, use 82677)

(For progesterone, use 84144)

(For prostatic acid phosphatase, use 84066)

78760 Testicular imaging;

78761   with vascular flow

(For testosterone, blood or urine, use 84403)

(For introduction of radioactive substance in association with ureteral endoscopy, see 50959, 50978)

(For lactogen, human placental (HPL) chorionic somatomammotropin, use 83632)

(For chorionic gonadotropin, beta subunit, see 84702, 84703)

(For pregnanediol, use 84135)

(For pregnanetriol, use 84138)

(78770, 78775 have been deleted. To report, use 78799)

78799 Unlisted genitourinary procedure, diagnostic nuclear medicine

(For chemical analysis, see **Chemistry** section)

Other Procedures

(For specific organ, see appropriate heading)

(For radiophosphorus tumor identification, ocular, see 78800)

78800 Radiopharmaceutical localization of tumor; limited area

(For specific organ, see appropriate heading)

78801   multiple areas

78802   whole body

78803   tomographic (SPECT)

78805 Radiopharmaceutical localization of inflammatory process; limited area

78806   whole body

Radiology

78807   tomographic (SPECT)

(For imaging bone infectious or inflammatory disease with a bone imaging radiopharmaceutical, see 78300, 78305, 78306)

(For RAST, see 82785, 83518, 86003, 86005)

(For gamma-E immunoglobulin, use 82785)

(For gamma-G immunoglobulin, use 82784)

(For alpha-1 antitrypsin, see 82103, 82104)

(For alpha-1 fetoprotein, see 82105, 82106)

(For amikacin, use 80150)

(For aminophylline, use 80198)

(For amitriptyline, use 80152)

(For amphetamine, chemical quantitative, use 82145)

(For chlordiazepoxide, see code for specific method)

(For chlorpromazine, see phenothiazine, urine 84022)

(For clonazepam, use 80154)

(For cocaine, quantitative, use 82520)

(For diazepam, use 80154)

(For dihydromorphinone, quantitative, use 82649)

(For diphenylhydantoin, use 80185)

(For flucytosine, see code for specific method)

(For gentamicin, use 80170)

(For lactic dehydrogenase, use 83615)

(For lysergic acid diethylamide (LSD), see 80100-80103, 80299)

(For morphine (heroin), see 80100-80103, 83925)

(For phencyclidine (PCP), see 80100-80103, 83992)

(For phenobarbital, see barbiturates 80100-80103, 82205)

(For phenytoin (diphenylthydantoin), use 80185)

(For tobramycin, use 80200)

78810   Tumor imaging, positron emission tomography (PET), metabolic evaluation

78890   Generation of automated data: interactive process involving nuclear physician and/or allied health professional personnel; simple manipulations and interpretation, not to exceed 30 minutes

78891   complex manipulations and interpretation, exceeding 30 minutes

(Use 78890 or 78891 in addition to primary procedure)

(78895 has been deleted)

78990   Provision of diagnostic radiopharmaceutical(s)

78999   Unlisted miscellaneous procedure, diagnostic nuclear medicine

Therapeutic

79000   Radiopharmaceutical therapy, hyper-thyroidism; initial, including evaluation of patient

79001   subsequent, each therapy

(For follow-up visit, see 99211-99215)

79020   Radiopharmaceutical therapy, thyroid suppression (euthyroid cardiac disease), including evaluation of patient

79030   Radiopharmaceutical ablation of gland for thyroid carcinoma

79035   Radiopharmaceutical therapy for metastases of thyroid carcinoma

79100   Radiopharmaceutical therapy, polycythemia vera, chronic leukemia, each treatment

79200   Intracavitary radioactive colloid therapy

79300   Interstitial radioactive colloid therapy

79400   Radiopharmaceutical therapy, nonthyroid, nonhematologic

79420   Intravascular radiopharmaceutical therapy, particulate

79440   Intra-articular radiopharmaceutical therapy

79900   Provision of therapeutic radiopharmaceutical(s)

79999   Unlisted radiopharmaceutical therapeutic procedure

Radiology

Notes

$\varnothing$ =Modifier '-51' Exempt ▶◀ or ▶ ◀=New or Revised Text ✚=Add-on Code

Radiology

Pathology and Laboratory Guidelines

Items used by all physicians in reporting their services are presented in the **Introduction.** Some of the commonalities are repeated here for the convenience of those physicians referring to this section on **Pathology and Laboratory.** Other definitions and items unique to Pathology and Laboratory are also listed.

Services in Pathology and Laboratory

Services in Pathology and Laboratory are provided by a physician or by technologists under responsible supervision of a physician.

Separate or Multiple Procedures

It is appropriate to designate multiple procedures that are rendered on the same date by separate entries.

Subsection Information

Several of the subheadings or subsections have special needs or instructions unique to that section. Where these are indicated, (eg, "Panel Tests"), special **"Notes"** will be presented preceding those procedural terminology listings referring to that subsection specifically. If there is an "Unlisted Procedure" code number (see section below) for the individual subsection, it will be shown. Those subsections with **"Notes"** are as follows:

Organ or Disease Panels 80048-80090
Drug Testing .80100-80103
Therapeutic Drug Assays 80150-80299
Evocative/Suppression Testing 80400-80440
Consultations
 (Clinical Pathology) 80500-80502
Urinalysis 81000-81099
Chemistry 82000-84999
Molecular Diagnostics 83890-83912
 Infectious Agent Detection 87470-87999
Infectious Agent Antibodies 86602-86804
Microbiology 87001-87254
 Infectious Agent Detection 87260-87999
Anatomic Pathology 88000-88099
Cytopathology 88104-88199
Surgical Pathology 88300-88399

Unlisted Service or Procedure

A service or procedure may be provided that is not listed in this edition of *CPT.* When reporting such a service, the appropriate "Unlisted Procedure" code may be used to indicate the service, identifying it by "Special Report" as discussed below. The "Unlisted Procedures" and accompanying codes for **Pathology and Laboratory** are as follows:

81099   Unlisted urinalysis procedure
84999   Unlisted chemistry procedure
85999   Unlisted hematology and coagulation procedure
86586   Unlisted antigen, each
86849   Unlisted immunology procedure
86999   Unlisted transfusion medicine procedure
87999   Unlisted microbiology procedure
88099   Unlisted necropsy (autopsy) procedure
88199   Unlisted cytopathology procedure
88299   Unlisted cytogenetic study
88399   Unlisted surgical pathology procedure
89399   Unlisted miscellaneous pathology test

Special Report

A service that is rarely provided, unusual, variable, or new may require a special report in determining medical appropriateness of the service. Pertinent information should include an adequate definition or description of the nature, extent, and need for the procedure; and the time, effort, and equipment necessary to provide the service. Additional items which may be included are:

- complexity of symptoms;
- final diagnosis;
- pertinent physical findings;
- diagnostic and therapeutic procedures;
- concurrent problems;
- follow-up care.

Notes

Pathology and Laboratory

(80002-80019 have been deleted. To report, see codes under Organ or Disease Oriented Panels)

(80031-80034 have been deleted. To report, see Therapeutic Drug Assays)

(80040 has been deleted. To report, see 80150-80299)

(80042 has been deleted. For serum cidal level, see 87197)

Organ or Disease Oriented Panels

These panels were developed for coding purposes only and should not be interpreted as clinical parameters. The tests listed with each panel identify the defined components of that panel.

These panel components are not intended to limit the performance of other tests. If one performs tests in addition to those specifically indicated for a particular panel, those tests should be reported separately in addition to the panel code.

80048   Basic metabolic panel

This panel must include the following:

Calcium (82310)

Carbon dioxide (82374)

Chloride (82435)

Creatinine (82565)

Glucose (82947)

Potassium (84132)

Sodium (84295)

Urea Nitrogen (BUN) (84520)

(Do not use 80048 in addition to 80053)

(80049 has been deleted. To report, use 80048)

80050   General health panel

This panel must include the following:

Comprehensive metabolic panel (80053)

Hemogram, automated, and manual differential WBC count (CBC) (85022) OR

Hemogram and platelet count, automated, and automated complete differential WBC count (CBC) (85025)

Thyroid stimulating hormone (TSH) (84443)

80051   Electrolyte panel

This panel must include the following:

Carbon dioxide (82374)

Chloride (82435)

Potassium (84132)

Sodium (84295)

(80052 has been deleted. To report, see codes for specific tests)

80053   Comprehensive metabolic panel

This panel must include the following:

Albumin (82040)

Bilirubin, total (82247)

Calcium (82310)

Carbon dioxide (bicarbonate) (82374)

Chloride (82435)

Creatinine (82565)

Glucose (82947)

Phosphatase, alkaline (84075)

Potassium (84132)

Protein, total (84155)

Sodium (84295)

Transferase, alanine amino (ALT) (SGPT) (84460)

Transferase, aspartate amino (AST) (SGOT) (84450)

Urea Nitrogen (BUN) (84520)

(Do not use 80053 in addition to 80048, 80076)

(80054 has been deleted. To report, use 80053)

80055   Obstetric panel

This panel must include the following:

Hemogram, automated, and manual differential WBC count (CBC) (85022) OR

Hemogram and platelet count, automated, and automated complete differential WBC count (CBC) (85025)

Hepatitis B surface antigen (HBsAg) (87340)

Antibody, rubella (86762)

Syphilis test, qualitative (eg, VDRL, RPR, ART) (86592)

Antibody screen, RBC, each serum technique (86850)

Blood typing, ABO (86900) AND

Blood typing, Rh (D) (86901)

(80056 has been deleted. To report, see codes for specific tests)

(80057 has been deleted. To report, see codes for specific tests)

(80058 has been deleted. To report, use 80076)

(80059 has been deleted. To report, use 80074)

(80060 has been deleted. To report, see codes for specific tests)

80061   Lipid panel

This panel must include the following:

Cholesterol, serum, total (82465)

Lipoprotein, direct measurement, high density cholesterol (HDL cholesterol) (83718)

Triglycerides (84478)

(80062 has been deleted. To report, see 80061 and/or codes for specific tests)

(80063 has been deleted. To report, see codes for specific tests)

(80064 has been deleted. To report, see codes for specific tests)

(80065 has been deleted. To report, see codes for specific tests)

(80066 has been deleted. To report, see codes for specific tests)

(80067 has been deleted. To report, see codes for specific tests)

(80068 has been deleted. To report, see codes for specific tests)

80069   Renal function panel

This panel must include the following:

Albumin (82040)

Calcium (82310)

Carbon dioxide (bicarbonate) (82374)

Chloride (82435)

Creatinine (82565)

Glucose (82947)

Phosphorus inorganic (phosphate) (84100)

Potassium (84132)

Sodium (84295)

Urea nitrogen (BUN) (84520)

(80070 has been deleted. To report, use 80091)

(80071 has been deleted. To report, see codes for specific tests)

(80072 has been deleted. To report, see 84550, 85651, 86255, 86430)

(80073 has been deleted. To report, see codes for specific tests)

80074   Acute hepatitis panel

This panel must include the following:

Hepatitis A antibody (HAAb), IgM antibody (86709)

Hepatitis B core antibody (HbcAb), IgM antibody (86705)

Hepatitis B surface antigen (HbsAg) (87340)

Hepatitis C antibody (86803)

(80075 has been deleted. To report, see codes for specific tests)

80076   Hepatic function panel

This panel must include the following:

Albumin (82040)

Bilirubin, total (82247)

Bilirubin, direct (82248)

Phosphatase, alkaline (84075)

Protein, total (84155)

Transferase, alanine amino (ALT) (SGPT) (84460)

Transferase, aspartate amino (AST) (SGOT) (84450)

(Do not use 80076 in addition to 80053)

(80080 has been deleted. To report PSA, use 84153)

(80082 has been deleted. To report, see codes for specific tests)

(80084 has been deleted. To report, see codes for specific tests)

(80085 has been deleted. To report, see codes for specific tests)

(80086 has been deleted. To report, see codes for specific tests)

(80088 has been deleted. To report, see codes for specific tests)

(80089 has been deleted. To report, see codes for specific tests)

▶(80090 has been deleted. To report, see codes for specific tests)◀

(80091 has been deleted. To report, see codes for specific tests)

Pathology and Laboratory

(80092 has been deleted. To report, see codes for specific test)

(80099 has been deleted. To report, see codes for specific tests)

Drug Testing

The following list contains examples of drugs or classes of drugs that are commonly assayed by qualitative screen, followed by confirmation with a second method.

Alcohols

Amphetamines

Barbiturates

Benzodiazepines

Cocaine and Metabolites

Methadones

Methaqualones

Opiates

Phencyclidines

Phenothiazines

Propoxyphenes

Tetrahydrocannabinoids

Tricyclic Antidepressants

Confirmed drugs may also be quantitated.

Use 80100 for each multiple drug class chromatographic procedure. Use 80102 for each procedure necessary for confirmation. For chromatography, each combination of stationary and mobile phase is to be counted as one procedure. For example, if detection of three drugs by chromatography requires one stationary phase with three mobile phases, use 80100 three (3) times. However, if multiple drugs can be detected using a single analysis (eg, one stationary phase with one mobile phase), use 80100 only once.

For quantitation of drugs screened, use appropriate code in **Chemistry** section (82000-84999) or **Therapeutic Drug Assay** section (80150-80299).

80100	Drug screen, qualitative; multiple drug classes chromatographic method, each procedure
80101	single drug class method (eg, immunoassay, enzyme assay), each drug class
80102	Drug confirmation, each procedure
80103	Tissue preparation for drug analysis

Therapeutic Drug Assays

The material for examination may be from any source. Examination is quantitative. For nonquantitative testing, see Drug Testing (80100-80103).

80150	Amikacin
80152	Amitriptyline
80154	Benzodiazepines
80156	Carbamazepine; total
80157	free
80158	Cyclosporine
80160	Desipramine
80162	Digoxin
80164	Dipropylacetic acid (valproic acid)
80166	Doxepin
80168	Ethosuximide
80170	Gentamicin
80172	Gold
80173	Haloperidol
80174	Imipramine
80176	Lidocaine
80178	Lithium
80182	Nortriptyline
80184	Phenobarbital
80185	Phenytoin; total
80186	free
80188	Primidone
80190	Procainamide;
80192	with metabolites (eg, n-acetyl procainamide)
80194	Quinidine
80196	Salicylate
80197	Tacrolimus
80198	Theophylline
80200	Tobramycin
80201	Topiramate
80202	Vancomycin
80299	Quantitation of drug, not elsewhere specified

Pathology and Laboratory

Evocative/Suppression Testing

The following test panels involve the administration of evocative or suppressive agents, and the baseline and subsequent measurement of their effects on chemical constituents. These codes are to be used for the reporting of the laboratory component of the overall testing protocol. For the physician's administration of the evocative or suppressive agents, see 90780-90784; for the supplies and drugs, see 99070. To report physician attendance and monitoring during the testing, use the appropriate evaluation and management code, including the prolonged physician care codes if required. Prolonged physician care codes are not separately reported when evocative/suppression testing involves prolonged infusions reported with 90780 and 90781. In the code descriptors where reference is made to a particular analyte (eg, Cortisol (82533 x 2)) the "x 2" refers to the number of times the test for that particular analyte is performed.

80400 ACTH stimulation panel; for adrenal insufficiency

This panel must include the following:

Cortisol (82533 x 2)

80402 for 21 hydroxylase deficiency

This panel must include the following:

Cortisol (82533 x 2)

17 hydroxyprogesterone (83498 x 2)

80406 for 3 beta-hydroxydehydrogenase deficiency

This panel must include the following:

Cortisol (82533 x 2)

17 hydroxypregnenolone (84143 x 2)

80408 Aldosterone suppression evaluation panel (eg, saline infusion)

This panel must include the following:

Aldosterone (82088 x 2)

Renin (84244 x 2)

80410 Calcitonin stimulation panel (eg, calcium, pentagastrin)

This panel must include the following:

Calcitonin (82308 x 3)

80412 Corticotropic releasing hormone (CRH) stimulation panel

This panel must include the following:

Cortisol (82533 x 6)

Adrenocorticotropic hormone (ACTH) (82024 x 6)

80414 Chorionic gonadotropin stimulation panel; testosterone response

This panel must include the following:

Testosterone (84403 x 2 on three pooled blood samples)

80415 estradiol response

This panel must include the following:

Estradiol (82670 x 2 on three pooled blood samples)

80416 Renal vein renin stimulation panel (eg, captopril)

This panel must include the following:

Renin (84244 x 6)

80417 Peripheral vein renin stimulation panel (eg, captopril)

This panel must include the following:

Renin (84244 x 2)

80418 Combined rapid anterior pituitary evaluation panel

This panel must include the following:

Adrenocorticotropic hormone (ACTH) (82024 x 4)

Luteinizing hormone (LH) (83002 x 4)

Follicle stimulating hormone (FSH) (83001 x 4)

Prolactin (84146 x 4)

Human growth hormone (HGH) (83003 x 4)

Cortisol (82533 x 4)

Thyroid stimulating hormone (TSH) (84443 x 4)

80420 Dexamethasone suppression panel, 48 hour

This panel must include the following:

Free cortisol, urine (82530 x 2)

Cortisol (82533 x 2)

Volume measurement for timed collection (81050 x 2)

(For single dose dexamethasone, use 82533)

80422 Glucagon tolerance panel; for insulinoma

This panel must include the following:

Glucose (82947 x 3)

Insulin (83525 x 3)

80424 for pheochromocytoma

This panel must include the following:

Catecholamines, fractionated (82384 x 2)

80426 Gonadotropin releasing hormone stimulation panel

This panel must include the following:

Follicle stimulating hormone (FSH) (83001 x 4)

Luteinizing hormone (LH) (83002 x 4)

Pathology and Laboratory

80428 Growth hormone stimulation panel (eg, arginine infusion, I-dopa administration)

This panel must include the following:

Human growth hormone (HGH) (83003 x 4)

80430 Growth hormone suppression panel (glucose administration)

This panel must include the following:

Glucose (82947 x 3)

Human growth hormone (HGH) (83003 x 4)

80432 Insulin-induced C-peptide suppression panel

This panel must include the following:

Insulin (83525)

C-peptide (84681 x 5)

Glucose (82947 x 5)

80434 Insulin tolerance panel; for ACTH insufficiency

This panel must include the following:

Cortisol (82533 x 5)

Glucose (82947 x 5)

80435   for growth hormone deficiency

This panel must include the following:

Glucose (82947 x 5)

Human growth hormone (HGH) (83003 x 5)

80436 Metyrapone panel

This panel must include the following:

Cortisol (82533 x 2)

11 deoxycortisol (82634 x 2)

80438 Thyrotropin releasing hormone (TRH) stimulation panel; one hour

This panel must include the following:

Thyroid stimulating hormone (TSH) (84443 x 3)

80439   two hour

This panel must include the following:

Thyroid stimulating hormone (TSH) (84443 x 4)

80440   for hyperprolactinemia

This panel must include the following:

Prolactin (84146 x 3)

Consultations (Clinical Pathology)

A clinical pathology consultation is a service, including a written report, rendered by the pathologist in response to a request from an attending physician in relation to a test result(s) requiring additional medical interpretive judgment.

Reporting of a test result(s) without medical interpretive judgment is not considered a clinical pathology consultation.

80500 Clinical pathology consultation; limited, without review of patient's history and medical records

80502   comprehensive, for a complex diagnostic problem, with review of patient's history and medical records

(These codes may also be used for pharmacokinetic consultations)

(For consultations involving the examination and evaluation of the patient, see 99241-99275)

Urinalysis

For specific analyses, see appropriate section.

▶(For urinalysis, infectious agent detection, semi-quantitative analysis of volatile compounds, use Category III code 0041T)◄

81000 Urinalysis, by dip stick or tablet reagent for bilirubin, glucose, hemoglobin, ketones, leukocytes, nitrite, pH, protein, specific gravity, urobilinogen, any number of these constituents; non-automated, with microscopy

81001   automated, with microscopy

81002   non-automated, without microscopy

81003   automated, without microscopy

(81004 has been deleted. To report, use 81000)

81005 Urinalysis; qualitative or semiquantitative, except immunoassays

(For non-immunoassay reagent strip urinalysis, see 81000, 81002)

(For immunoassay, qualitative or semiquantitative, use 83518)

(81006 has been deleted. To report, use 81099)

(For microalbumin, see 82043, 82044)

81007   bacteriuria screen, except by culture or dipstick

(For culture, see 87086-87088)

(For dipstick, use 81000 or 81002)

(81010, 81011, and 81012 have been deleted)

81015	microscopic only
81020	two or three glass test
81025	Urine pregnancy test, by visual color comparison methods
	(81030 has been deleted)
81050	Volume measurement for timed collection, each
81099	Unlisted urinalysis procedure

Chemistry

The material for examination may be from any source unless otherwise specified in the code descriptor. When an analyte is measured in multiple specimens from different sources, or in specimens that are obtained at different times, the analyte is reported separately for each source and for each specimen. The examination is quantitative unless specified. To report an organ or disease oriented panel, see codes 80048-80090.

When a code describes a method where measurement of multiple analytes may require one or several procedures, each procedure is coded separately (eg, 82491-82492, 82541-82544). For example, if two (2) analytes are measured using column chromatography using a single stationary or mobile phase, use 82492. If the same two analytes are measured using different stationary or mobile phase conditions, 82491 would be used twice. If a total of four (4) analytes are measured where two (2) analytes are measured with a single stationary and mobile phase, and the other two (2) analytes are measured using a different stationary and mobile phase, use 82492 twice. If a total of three (3) analytes are measured where two (2) analytes are measured using a single stationary or mobile phase condition, and the third analyte is measured separately using a different stationary or mobile phase procedure, use 82492 once for the (2) analytes measured under the same condition, and use 82491 once for the third analyte measured separately.

Clinical information derived from the results of laboratory data that is mathematically calculated (eg, free thyroxine index (T7)) is considered part of the test procedure and therefore is not a separately reportable service.

82000	Acetaldehyde, blood
82003	Acetaminophen
	(82005 has been deleted)
82009	Acetone or other ketone bodies, serum; qualitative
82010	quantitative
	(82011 has been deleted. To report, use 80196)
	(82012 has been deleted)

82013	Acetylcholinesterase
	(Acid, gastric, see gastric acid, 82926, 82928)
	(Acid phosphatase, see 84060-84066)
	(82015 has been deleted)
82016	Acylcarnitines; qualitative, each specimen
82017	quantitative, each specimen
	(For carnitine, use 82379)
82024	Adrenocorticotropic hormone (ACTH)
82030	Adenosine, 5-monophosphate, cyclic (cyclic AMP)
	(82035 has been deleted)
82040	Albumin; serum
82042	urine or other source, quantitative, each specimen
82043	urine, microalbumin, quantitative
82044	urine, microalbumin, semiquantitative (eg, reagent strip assay)
	(For prealbumin, use 84134)
82055	Alcohol (ethanol); any specimen except breath
	(For other volatiles, alcohol, use 84600)
	(82060, 82065, 82070 have been deleted. To report, use 82055)
	(82072 has been deleted)
82075	breath
	(82076, 82078 have been deleted. For ethanol, use 82055; for volatiles, use 84600)
82085	Aldolase
	(82086 has been deleted. To report, use 82085)
	(82087 has been deleted. To report, use 82088)
82088	Aldosterone
	(82089 has been deleted. To report, use 82088)
	(82091 has been deleted. To report, use 80408)
	(82095 has been deleted. To report, see 80100, 80101, and 80103)
	(82096 has been deleted. To report, use code for specific drug and 80103)
	(82100 has been deleted. To report, use 80100 and 80101)
	(Alkaline phosphatase, see 84075, 84080)
82101	Alkaloids, urine, quantitative
	(Alphaketoglutarate, see 82009, 82010)
	(Alpha tocopherol (Vitamin E), use 84446)
82103	Alpha-1-antitrypsin; total
82104	phenotype
82105	Alpha-fetoprotein; serum
82106	amniotic fluid

82108   Aluminum

(82112 has been deleted. To report, use 80150)

82120   Amines, vaginal fluid, qualitative

(For combined pH and amines test for vaginitis, use 82120 and 83986)

(82126 has been deleted)

82127   Amino acids; single, qualitative, each specimen

82128   multiple, qualitative, each specimen

(82130 has been deleted. To report, see 82131, 82136, 82139)

82131   single, quantitative, each specimen

(82134 has been deleted)

82135   Aminolevulinic acid, delta (ALA)

82136   Amino acids, 2 to 5 amino acids, quantitative, each specimen

(82137 has been deleted. To report, use 80198)

(82138 has been deleted. To report, use 80152)

82139   Amino acids, 6 or more amino acids, quantitative, each specimen

82140   Ammonia

(82141 has been deleted. To report, use 82140)

(82142 has been deleted)

82143   Amniotic fluid scan (spectrophotometric)

(For L/S ratio, use 83661)

(Amobarbital, see 80100-80103 for qualitative analysis, 82205 for quantitative analysis)

82145   Amphetamine or methamphetamine

(For qualitative analysis, see 80100-80103)

82150   Amylase

82154   Androstanediol glucuronide

(82155 has been deleted)

(82156 has been deleted. To report, use 82150)

82157   Androstenedione

(82159 has been deleted. To report, use 82160)

82160   Androsterone

82163   Angiotensin II

82164   Angiotensin I - converting enzyme (ACE)

(82165 has been deleted)

(Antidiuretic hormone (ADH), use 84588)

(82168 has been deleted. For antihistamines, see code for specific method)

(82170 has been deleted. To report, see 83015, 83018)

(Antimony, use 83015)

(Antitrypsin, alpha-1-, see 82103, 82104)

82172   Apolipoprotein, each

(82173 has been deleted. To report, use 80428)

82175   Arsenic

(For heavy metal screening, use 83015)

82180   Ascorbic acid (Vitamin C), blood

(Aspirin, see acetylsalicylic acid, 80196)

(Atherogenic index, blood, ultracentrifugation, quantitative, use 83717)

82190   Atomic absorption spectroscopy, each analyte

82205   Barbiturates, not elsewhere specified

(For qualitative analysis, see 80100-80103)

▶(For B-Natriuretic peptide, use 83880)◀

(82210 has been deleted. To report, see 80100-80103, 82205)

(82225, 82230 have been deleted. To report, see 83015, 83018)

(82231 has been deleted. To report, use 82232)

82232   Beta-2 microglobulin

(82235, 82236 have been deleted)

(Bicarbonate, use 82374)

82239   Bile acids; total

82240   cholylglycine

(For bile pigments, urine, see 81000-81005)

(82245 has been deleted. To report, see 81000, 81002, 81005)

82247   Bilirubin; total

82248   direct

(82250 has been deleted. To report, see 82247, 82248 as appropriate)

(82251 has been deleted. To report, use 82247 and 82248)

82252   feces, qualitative

(82260 has been deleted. To report, see 81000-81003, 82247, 82248)

82261   Biotinidase, each specimen

(82265 has been deleted. To report spectrophotometric scan, use 82143)

(82268 has been deleted. To report, see 83015, 83018)

82270   Blood, occult, by peroxidase activity (eg, guaiac), qualitative; feces, 1-3 simultaneous determinations

82273   other sources

(Blood urea nitrogen (BUN), see 84520, 84525)

(82280, 82285 have been deleted. To report, see code for specific method)

Pathology and Laboratory

82274   Blood, occult, by fecal hemoglobin determination by immunoassay, qualitative, feces, 1-3 simultaneous determinations

82286   Bradykinin

(82290, 82291 have been deleted. To report, use 84311)

82300   Cadmium

(82305 has been deleted. To report, see 82486, 82491)

82306   Calcifediol (25-OH Vitamin D-3)

82307   Calciferol (Vitamin D)

(For 1,25-Dihydroxyvitamin D, use 82652)

82308   Calcitonin

82310   Calcium; total

(82315, 82320, 82325 have been deleted. To report, use 82310)

82330   ionized

82331   after calcium infusion test

(82335 has been deleted)

82340   urine quantitative, timed specimen

(82345 has been deleted)

82355   Calculus; qualitative analysis

82360   quantitative analysis, chemical

82365   infrared spectroscopy

82370   x-ray diffraction

(82372 has been deleted. To report, use 80156)

(Carbamates, see individual listings)

82373   Carbohydrate deficient transferrin

82374   Carbon dioxide (bicarbonate)

(See also 82803)

82375   Carbon monoxide, (carboxyhemoglobin); quantitative

82376   qualitative

▶(To report end-tidal carbon monoxide, use Category III code 0043T)◀

82378   Carcinoembryonic antigen (CEA)

82379   Carnitine (total and free), quantitative, each specimen

(For acylcarnitine, see 82016, 82017)

82380   Carotene

82382   Catecholamines; total urine

82383   blood

82384   fractionated

(For urine metabolites, see 83835, 84585)

82387   Cathepsin-D

82390   Ceruloplasmin

82397   Chemiluminescent assay

(82400 has been deleted. To report, see code for specific method)

(82405 has been deleted)

82415   Chloramphenicol

(82418, 82420, 82425 have been deleted. To report, see code for specific method)

82435   Chloride; blood

82436   urine

(82437 has been deleted)

82438   other source

(For sweat collection by iontophoresis, use 89360)

82441   Chlorinated hydrocarbons, screen

(82443 has been deleted. To report, see code for specific method)

(Chlorpromazine, use 84022)

(Cholecalciferol (Vitamin D), use 82307)

82465   Cholesterol, serum or whole blood, total

(For high density lipoprotein (HDL), use 83718)

(82470 has been deleted)

82480   Cholinesterase; serum

82482   RBC

(82484 has been deleted. To report, use 82480 and 82482)

82485   Chondroitin B sulfate, quantitative

(Chorionic gonadotropin, see gonadotropin, 84702, 84703)

82486   Chromatography, qualitative; column (eg, gas liquid or HPLC), analyte not elsewhere specified

82487   paper, 1-dimensional, analyte not elsewhere specified

82488   paper, 2-dimensional, analyte not elsewhere specified

82489   thin layer, analyte not elsewhere specified

(82490 has been deleted)

82491   Chromatography, quantitative, column (eg, gas liquid or HPLC); single analyte not elsewhere specified, single stationary and mobile phase

82492   multiple analytes, single stationary and mobile phase

82495   Chromium

(82505 has been deleted)

82507   Citrate

(82512 has been deleted. To report, use 80154)

82520   Cocaine or metabolite

(Cocaine, qualitative analysis, see 80100-80103)

(Codeine, qualitative analysis, see 80100-80103)

(Codeine, quantitative analysis, see 82101)

(Complement, see 86160-86162)

82523   Collagen cross links, any method

82525   Copper

(82526 has been deleted. To report, use 82525)

(Coproporphyrin, see 84119, 84120)

(Corticosteroids, use 83491)

82528   Corticosterone

(82529 has been deleted. To report, use 82533)

82530   Cortisol; free

(82531, 82532 have been deleted)

82533   total

(82534 has been deleted. To report, use 82533)

(82536 has been deleted. To report, see 80400-80406)

(82537 has been deleted. To report, see 80400-80406)

(82538 has been deleted. To report, use 80436)

(82539 has been deleted. To report, use 80420)

(C-peptide, use 84681)

82540   Creatine

82541   Column chromatography/mass spectrometry (eg, GC/MS, or HPLC/MS), analyte not elsewhere specified; qualitative, single stationary and mobile phase

82542   quantitative, single stationary and mobile phase

82543   stable isotope dilution, single analyte, quantitative, single stationary and mobile phase

82544   stable isotope dilution, multiple analytes, quantitative, single stationary and mobile phase

(82545 has been deleted. To report, use 82540)

(82546 has been deleted. To report, see 82540, 82565)

82550   Creatine kinase (CK), (CPK); total

82552   isoenzymes

82553   MB fraction only

82554   isoforms

(82555 has been deleted)

82565   Creatinine; blood

82570   other source

82575   clearance

82585   Cryofibrinogen

82595   Cryoglobulin, qualitative or semi-quantitative (eg, cryocrit)

(For quantitative, cryoglobulin, see 82784, 82785)

(Crystals, pyrophosphate vs. urate, use 89060)

82600   Cyanide

(82601 has been deleted. To report, see 80103, 82600)

(82606 has been deleted)

82607   Cyanocobalamin (Vitamin B-12);

82608   unsaturated binding capacity

(Cyclic AMP, use 82030)

(Cyclic GMP, use 83008)

(Cyclosporine, use 80158)

(82610, 82614 have been deleted)

82615   Cystine and homocystine, urine, qualitative

(82620 has been deleted. For cystine and homocystine, quantitative, ►see 82131, 82136, 82139)◄

(82624 has been deleted)

82626   Dehydroepiandrosterone (DHEA)

82627   Dehydroepiandrosterone-sulfate (DHEA-S)

(82628 has been deleted. To report, see 80100-80103 for qualitative analysis; see 80160 for quantitative analysis)

(Delta-aminolevulinic acid (ALA), use 82135)

82633   Desoxycorticosterone, 11-

82634   Deoxycortisol, 11-

(Dexamethasone suppression test, use 80420)

(82635 has been deleted)

(Diastase, urine, use 82150)

(82636 has been deleted. To report, see 80100-80103, 80154)

82638   Dibucaine number

(82639 has been deleted. To report, use code for specific method)

(Dichloroethane, use 84600)

(Dichloromethane, use 84600)

(Diethylether, use 84600)

(82640, 82641 have been deleted)

(82643 has been deleted. To report, use 80162)

82646   Dihydrocodeinone

(For qualitative analysis, see 80100-80103)

82649   Dihydromorphinone

(For qualitative analysis, see 80100-80103)

82651   Dihydrotestosterone (DHT)

82652 Dihydroxyvitamin D, 1,25-

82654 Dimethadione

(For qualitative analysis, see 80100-80103)

(Diphenylhydantoin, use 80185)

(Dipropylacetic acid, use 80164)

(Dopamine, see 82382-82384)

(82656 has been deleted. To report, use 80166)

(Duodenal contents, see individual enzymes; for intubation and collection, use 89100)

82657 Enzyme activity in blood cells, cultured cells, or tissue, not elsewhere specified; nonradioactive substrate, each specimen

82658   radioactive substrate, each specimen

(82660 has been deleted. To report, see 80100, 80101)

(82662 has been deleted. To report, see 80100-80103)

82664 Electrophoretic technique, not elsewhere specified

(Endocrine receptor assays, see 84233-84235)

82666 Epiandrosterone

(Epinephrine, see 82382-82384)

82668 Erythropoietin

82670 Estradiol

82671 Estrogens; fractionated

82672   total

(82673, 82674, 82676 have been deleted. To report, use 82677)

(Estrogen receptor assay, use 84233)

82677 Estriol

(82678 has been deleted. To report, use 82679)

82679 Estrone

(Ethanol, see 82055 and 82075)

82690 Ethchlorvynol

(82691 has been deleted. To report, use 82690)

(82692 has been deleted. To report, use 80168)

(Ethyl alcohol, see 82055 and 82075)

82693 Ethylene glycol

(82694 has been deleted. To report, use 82696)

82696 Etiocholanolone

(For fractionation of ketosteroids, use 83593)

82705 Fat or lipids, feces; qualitative

82710   quantitative

82715 Fat differential, feces, quantitative

(82720 has been deleted)

82725 Fatty acids, nonesterified

82726 Very long chain fatty acids

(82727 has been deleted. To report ferric chloride test, urine, use 81005)

82728 Ferritin

(Fetal hemoglobin, see hemoglobin 83030, 83033, and 85460)

(Fetoprotein, alpha-1, see 82105, 82106)

(82730 has been deleted. To report fibrinogen, see 85384, 85385)

82731 Fetal fibronectin, cervicovaginal secretions, semi-quantitative

82735 Fluoride

(82740 has been deleted. To report, use 82735)

(82741 has been deleted. To report, see code for specific method)

82742 Flurazepam

(For qualitative analysis, see 80100-80103)

(Foam stability test, use 83662)

(82745 has been deleted)

82746 Folic acid; serum

82747   RBC

(Follicle stimulating hormone (FSH), use 83001)

(82750 has been deleted. To report, see code for specific method)

(82755, 82756 have been deleted)

82757 Fructose, semen

(Fructosamine, use 82985)

(Fructose, TLC screen, use 84375)

82759 Galactokinase, RBC

82760 Galactose

(82763 has been deleted. To report, use 82760 and codes for administration)

(82765 has been deleted. To report, use 82760)

82775 Galactose-1-phosphate uridyl transferase; quantitative

82776   screen

(82780 has been deleted. To report gallium, see code for specific method)

82784 Gammaglobulin; IgA, IgD, IgG, IgM, each

82785   IgE

(For allergen specific IgE, see 86003, 86005)

(82786 has been deleted)

82787 immunoglobulin subclasses, (IgG1, 2, 3, or 4), each

(Gamma-glutamyltransferase (GGT), use 82977)

(82790, 82791 have been deleted)

(82792 has been deleted. To report, see 82805, 82810)

(82793, 82795 have been deleted)

82800 Gases, blood, pH only

(82801, 82802 have been deleted. To report, use 82803)

82803 Gases, blood, any combination of pH, pCO_2, pO_2, CO_2, HCO_3 (including calculated O_2 saturation);

(Use 82803 for two or more of the above listed analytes)

(82804 has been deleted. To report, use 82803)

82805 with O_2 saturation, by direct measurement, except pulse oximetry

82810 Gases, blood, O_2 saturation only, by direct measurement, except pulse oximetry

(For pulse oximetry, use 94760)

(82812 has been deleted. To report, use 82803)

(82817 has been deleted. To report, use 82803)

82820 Hemoglobin-oxygen affinity (pO_2 for 50% hemoglobin saturation with oxygen)

82926 Gastric acid, free and total, each specimen

(82927 has been deleted. To report, use 82926)

82928 Gastric acid, free or total; each specimen

(82929, 82931, and 82932 have been deleted. To report, use 82928)

82938 Gastrin after secretin stimulation

82941 Gastrin

(Gentamicin, use 80170)

(GGT, use 82977)

(GLC, gas liquid chromatography, use 82486)

(82942 has been deleted)

82943 Glucagon

(82944 has been deleted)

82945 Glucose, body fluid, other than blood

82946 Glucagon tolerance test

82947 Glucose; quantitative, blood (except reagent strip)

82948 blood, reagent strip

(82949 has been deleted)

82950 post glucose dose (includes glucose)

82951 tolerance test (GTT), three specimens (includes glucose)

82952 tolerance test, each additional beyond three specimens

82953 tolbutamide tolerance test

(For insulin tolerance test, see 80434, 80435)

(For leucine tolerance test, use 80428)

(For semiquantitative urine glucose, see 81000, 81002, 81005, 81099)

(82954 has been deleted. To report, use 82947)

82955 Glucose-6-phosphate dehydrogenase (G6PD); quantitative

82960 screen

(82961 has been deleted)

(For glucose tolerance test with medication, use 90784 in addition)

82962 Glucose, blood by glucose monitoring device(s) cleared by the FDA specifically for home use

82963 Glucosidase, beta

82965 Glutamate dehydrogenase

82975 Glutamine (glutamic acid amide)

82977 Glutamyltransferase, gamma (GGT)

82978 Glutathione

82979 Glutathione reductase, RBC

82980 Glutethimide

(Glycohemoglobin, use 83036)

82985 Glycated protein

(82995 has been deleted. To report, use 80172)

(82996-82998 have been deleted. To report, see 84702, 84703)

(Gonadotropin, chorionic, see 84702, 84703)

(83000 has been deleted)

83001 Gonadotropin; follicle stimulating hormone (FSH)

83002 luteinizing hormone (LH)

(For luteinizing releasing factor (LRH), use 83727)

83003 Growth hormone, human (HGH) (somatotropin)

(83004 has been deleted. To report, use 80430)

(For antibody to human growth hormone, use 86277)

(83005 has been deleted)

83008 Guanosine monophosphate (GMP), cyclic

83010 Haptoglobin; quantitative

(83011 has been deleted. To report, use 83010)

83012 phenotypes

83013 Helicobacter pylori; analysis for urease activity, non-radioactive isotope

83014 drug administration and sample collection

(For H. pylori, stool, use 87338. For H. pylori, liquid scintillation counter, see 78267, 78268. For H. pylori, enzyme immunoassay, use 87339)

Pathology and Laboratory

83015 Heavy metal (eg, arsenic, barium, beryllium, bismuth, antimony, mercury); screen

83018 quantitative, each

(83019 has been deleted. To report, see 83013, 83014)

83020 Hemoglobin fractionation and quantitation; electrophoresis (eg, A2, S, C, and/or F)

83021 chromatography (eg, A2, S, C, and/or F)

83026 Hemoglobin; by copper sulfate method, non-automated

83030 F (fetal), chemical

83033 F (fetal), qualitative

83036 glycated

(For fecal hemoglobin detection by immunoassay, use 82274)

(83040 has been deleted. To report, use 83050)

83045 methemoglobin, qualitative

83050 methemoglobin, quantitative

83051 plasma

(83052, 83053 have been deleted. To report, use 85660)

83055 sulfhemoglobin, qualitative

83060 sulfhemoglobin, quantitative

83065 thermolabile

83068 unstable, screen

83069 urine

83070 Hemosiderin; qualitative

83071 quantitative

(Heroin, see 80100-80103)

(HIAA, use 83497)

(High performance liquid chromatography (HPLC), use 82486)

83080 b-Hexosaminidase, each assay

(83086, 83087 have been deleted. To report, use 82128)

83088 Histamine

(Hollander test, use 91052)

83090 Homocystine

(83093, 83095 have been deleted. For homogentisic acid, qualitative urine screen, see 81005. For quantitative assay, see code for specific method)

83150 Homovanillic acid (HVA)

(Hormones, see individual alphabetic listings in **Chemistry** section)

(Hydrogen breath test, use 91065)

(83485, 83486 have been deleted)

83491 Hydroxycorticosteroids, 17- (17-OHCS)

(For cortisol, see 82530, 82533. For deoxycortisol, use 82634)

(83492 has been deleted. To report, use 83491)

(83493 has been deleted)

(83494-83496 have been deleted. To report, use 83491)

83497 Hydroxyindolacetic acid, 5-(HIAA)

(For urine qualitative test, use 81005)

(5-Hydroxytryptamine, use 84260)

83498 Hydroxyprogesterone, 17-d

83499 Hydroxyprogesterone, 20-

83500 Hydroxyproline; free

83505 total

(83510 has been deleted. To report, use 83500 and 83505)

83516 Immunoassay for analyte other than infectious agent antibody or infectious agent antigen, qualitative or semiquantitative; multiple step method

83518 single step method (eg, reagent strip)

83519 Immunoassay, analyte, quantitative; by radiopharmaceutical technique (eg, RIA)

83520 not otherwise specified

(83523 has been deleted. To report, use 80174)

(For immunoassays for antibodies to infectious agent antigens, see analyte and method specific codes in the **Immunology** section)

(For immunoassay of tumor antigen not elsewhere specified, use 86316)

(Immunoglobulins, see 82784, 82785)

(83524 has been deleted)

83525 Insulin; total

(For proinsulin, use 84206)

(83526 has been deleted. To report, see 80434, 80435)

83527 free

83528 Intrinsic factor

(For intrinsic factor antibodies, use 86340)

(83530 has been deleted)

(83533, 83534 have been deleted. To report, use 84999)

83540 Iron

(83545, 83546 have been deleted. To report, use 83540)

83550 Iron binding capacity

(83555, 83565 have been deleted. To report, use 83550)

⊘ =Modifier '-51' Exempt ▶◀ or ▶ ◀=New or Revised Text ➕=Add-on Code

83570   Isocitric dehydrogenase (IDH)

(Isonicotinic acid hydrazide, INH, see code for specific method)

(Isopropyl alcohol, use 84600)

(83571 has been deleted. To report, use 83570)

(83576 has been deleted. To report, see code for specific method)

(83578 has been deleted)

83582   Ketogenic steroids, fractionation

(83583, 83584 have been deleted)

(Ketone bodies, for serum, see 82009, 82010; for urine, see 81000-81003)

83586   Ketosteroids, 17- (17-KS); total

(83587 has been deleted. To report, use 83593)

(83588, 83589 have been deleted. To report, use 83586)

(83590 has been deleted)

83593   fractionation

(83596 has been deleted)

(83597 has been deleted)

(83599 has been deleted. To report, use 83586)

(83600 has been deleted. To report, see code for specific method)

83605   Lactate (lactic acid)

(83610 has been deleted. To report, use 83615)

83615   Lactate dehydrogenase (LD), (LDH);

(83620 has been deleted. To report, use 83615)

(83624 has been deleted)

83625   isoenzymes, separation and quantitation

(83626 has been deleted)

(83628 has been deleted. To report, use 83625)

(83629, 83631 have been deleted. To report, use 83615)

83632   Lactogen, human placental (HPL) human chorionic somatomammotropin

83633   Lactose, urine; qualitative

83634   quantitative

(For tolerance, see 82951, 82952)

(For breath hydrogen test for lactase deficiency, use 91065)

(83645 has been deleted. To report, see quantitative code or screening for toxicity)

(83650 has been deleted)

83655   Lead

(83660 has been deleted. To report, use 83655)

83661   Fetal lung maturity assessment; lecithin sphingomyelin (L/S) ratio

83662   foam stability test

83663   fluorescence polarization

83664   lamellar body density

(For phosphatidylglycerol, use 84081)

83670   Leucine aminopeptidase (LAP)

(83675, 83680 have been deleted. To report, use 83670)

(83681 has been deleted. To report, use 80428)

(83685 has been deleted. To report, use 80176)

83690   Lipase

(83700, 83705 have been deleted. For cholesterol, see 82465, 83718-83721. For triglycerides, use 84478)

83715   Lipoprotein, blood; electrophoretic separation and quantitation

83716   high resolution fractionation and quantitation of lipoprotein cholesterols (eg, electrophoresis, nuclear magnetic resonance, ultracentrifugation)

(83717 has been deleted. To report, use 83716)

83718   Lipoprotein, direct measurement; high density cholesterol (HDL cholesterol)

83719   direct measurement, VLDL cholesterol

(83720 has been deleted)

83721   direct measurement, LDL cholesterol

(For fractionation by nuclear magnetic resonance or high resolution electrophoresis, use 83716)

(To report direct measurement, intermediate density lipoproteins (remnant lipoproteins), use Category III code 0026T)

(Luteinizing hormone (LH), use 83002)

(83725 has been deleted. To report, use 80178)

83727   Luteinizing releasing factor (LRH)

(83728 has been deleted. To report, see 80100-80103, 80299)

(83730 has been deleted)

(For qualitative analysis, see 80100-80103)

(Macroglobulins, alpha-2, use 86329)

83735   Magnesium

(83740, 83750, 83755, 83760, 83765 have been deleted. To report, use 83735)

83775   Malate dehydrogenase

(Maltose tolerance, see 82951, 82952)

(Mammotropin, use 84146)

Pathology and Laboratory

83785 Manganese

(83790 has been deleted)

(Marijuana, see 80100-80103)

(83795 has been deleted)

(83799 has been deleted. To report, use 83925)

83788 Mass spectrometry and tandem mass spectrometry (MS, MS/MS), analyte not elsewhere specified; qualitative, each specimen

83789 quantitative, each specimen

83805 Meprobamate

(For qualitative analysis, see 80100-80103)

83825 Mercury, quantitative

(83830 has been deleted. To report, use 83825)

(Mercury screen, use 83015)

83835 Metanephrines

(For catecholamines, see 82382-82384)

83840 Methadone

(For methadone qualitative analysis, see 80100-80103)

(Methamphetamine, see 80100-80103, 82145)

(Methanol, use 84600)

(83842 has been deleted. To report, see code for specific method)

(83845 has been deleted. To report, see 80101-80103)

83857 Methemalbumin

(Methemoglobin, see hemoglobin 83045, 83050)

83858 Methsuximide

(Methyl alcohol, use 84600)

(Microalbumin, see 82043 for quantitative, see 82044 for semiquantitative)

(Microglobulin, beta-2, use 82232)

(83859 has been deleted)

(83860-83862 have been deleted. To report, see 80100-80103 for qualitative analysis, 83925 for quantitative analysis)

83864 Mucopolysaccharides, acid; quantitative

(83865 has been deleted. To report, use 83864)

83866 screen

(83870 has been deleted. To report, use 84999)

83872 Mucin, synovial fluid (Ropes test)

83873 Myelin basic protein, cerebrospinal fluid

(For oligoclonal bands, use 83916)

83874 Myoglobin

(83875 has been deleted)

(83880 has been deleted. To report, use 83925)

● **83880** Natriuretic peptide

83883 Nephelometry, each analyte not elsewhere specified

83885 Nickel

83887 Nicotine

Codes 83890-83912 are intended for use with molecular diagnostic techniques for analysis of nucleic acids.

Codes 83890-83912 are coded by procedure rather than analyte.

Code separately for each procedure used in an analysis. For example, a procedure requiring isolation of DNA, restriction endonuclease digestion, electrophoresis, and nucleic acid probe amplification would be coded 83890, 83892, 83894, and 83898.

(For microbial identification, see 87797, 87798)

83890 Molecular diagnostics; molecular isolation or extraction

83891 isolation or extraction of highly purified nucleic acid

83892 enzymatic digestion

83893 dot/slot blot production

83894 separation by gel electrophoresis (eg, agarose, polyacrylamide)

(83895 has been deleted)

83896 nucleic acid probe, each

83897 nucleic acid transfer (eg, Southern, Northern)

83898 amplification of patient nucleic acid (eg, PCR, LCR), single primer pair, each primer pair

(83900 has been deleted)

83901 amplification of patient nucleic acid, multiplex, each multiplex reaction

83902 reverse transcription

83903 mutation scanning, by physical properties (eg, single strand conformational polymorphisms (SSCP), heteroduplex, denaturing gradient gel electrophoresis (DGGE), RNA'ase A), single segment, each

83904 mutation identification by sequencing, single segment, each segment

83905 mutation identification by allele specific transcription, single segment, each segment

83906 mutation identification by allele specific translation, single segment, each segment

(83910 has been deleted)

83912 interpretation and report

(83913 has been deleted. To report, use 83898)

83915 Nucleotidase 5-

83916   Oligoclonal immune (oligoclonal bands)

(83917 has been deleted)

83918   Organic acids; total, quantitative, each specimen

83919   qualitative, each specimen

(83920 has been deleted. To report, use code for specific method)

83921   Organic acid, single, quantitative

83925   Opiates, (eg, morphine, meperidine)

83930   Osmolality; blood

83935   urine

83937   Osteocalcin (bone g1a protein)

(83938 has been deleted)

83945   Oxalate

(83946 has been deleted. To report, use 80154)

(83947 has been deleted. To report, see 82009, 82010)

(83948 has been deleted. To report, see 80100-80103, 83925)

(83949 has been deleted)

(83965 has been deleted. To report, see code for specific method)

83950   Oncoprotein, HER-2/neu

(For tissue, see 88342, 88365)

83970   Parathormone (parathyroid hormone)

(83971, 83972 have been deleted. To report, see code for specific method)

(83973 has been deleted. To report, use 84375)

(83974 has been deleted)

(83975, 83985 have been deleted. To report, see code for specific method)

(Pesticide, quantitative, see code for specific method. For screen for chlorinated hydrocarbons, use 82441)

83986   pH, body fluid, except blood

(For blood pH, see 82800, 82803)

83992   Phencyclidine (PCP)

(For qualitative analysis, see 80100-80103)

(Phenobarbital, use 80184)

(83995 has been deleted. To report, see code for specific method)

(84005 has been deleted)

(84021 has been deleted. To report, see 80100, 80101, 84022)

84022   Phenothiazine

(For qualitative analysis, see 80100, 80101)

84030   Phenylalanine (PKU), blood

(Phenylalanine-tyrosine ratio, see 84030, 84510)

(84031 has been deleted)

(84033 has been deleted. To report, see code for specific method)

84035   Phenylketones, qualitative

(84037 has been deleted. To report, use 84035)

(84038 has been deleted. To report, see code for specific method)

(84039, 84040 have been deleted)

(84045 has been deleted. To report, see 80185, 80186)

84060   Phosphatase, acid; total

84061   forensic examination

(84065 has been deleted. To report, use 84066)

84066   prostatic

84075   Phosphatase, alkaline;

84078   heat stable (total not included)

84080   isoenzymes

84081   Phosphatidylglycerol

(84082 has been deleted)

(Phosphates inorganic, use 84100)

(Phosphates, organic, see code for specific method. For cholinesterase, see 82480, 82482)

(84083 has been deleted)

84085   Phosphogluconate, 6-, dehydrogenase, RBC

84087   Phosphohexose isomerase

(84090 has been deleted)

84100   Phosphorus inorganic (phosphate);

84105   urine

(Pituitary gonadotropins, see 83001-83002)

(PKU, see 84030, 84035)

84106   Porphobilinogen, urine; qualitative

84110   quantitative

(84118 has been deleted. To report, use 84120)

84119   Porphyrins, urine; qualitative

84120   quantitation and fractionation

(84121 has been deleted. To report, use 84120)

84126   Porphyrins, feces; quantitative

84127   qualitative

(84128 has been deleted)

(Porphyrin precursors, see 82135, 84106, 84110)

(For protoporphyrin, RBC, see 84202, 84203)

Pathology and Laboratory

84132	Potassium; serum
84133	urine
84134	Prealbumin

(For microalbumin, see 82043, 82044)

| 84135 | Pregnanediol |

(84136 has been deleted. To report, use 84135)

| 84138 | Pregnanetriol |

(84139 has been deleted. To report, use 84138)

| 84140 | Pregnenolone |

(84141 has been deleted. To report, use 80188)

(84142 has been deleted. To report, see 80190, 80192)

| 84143 | 17-hydroxypregnenolone |
| 84144 | Progesterone |

(Progesterone receptor assay, use 84234)

(For proinsulin, use 84206)

| 84146 | Prolactin |

(84147 has been deleted. To report, see 80100-80103)

(84149 has been deleted)

84150	Prostaglandin, each
84152	Prostate specific antigen (PSA); complexed (direct measurement)
84153	total
84154	free
84155	Protein; total, except refractometry
84160	refractometric
84165	electrophoretic fractionation and quantitation

(84170 has been deleted)

(84175 has been deleted. To report, use 84165)

(84176 has been deleted)

(84180 has been deleted. To report, use 81050 and 84155)

| 84181 | Western Blot, with interpretation and report, blood or other body fluid |
| 84182 | Western Blot, with interpretation and report, blood or other body fluid, immunological probe for band identification, each |

(For Western Blot tissue analysis, use 88371)

(84185 has been deleted)

(84190 has been deleted. To report, use 84165)

(84195 has been deleted)

(84200 has been deleted. To report, use 84165)

(84201 has been deleted. To report, see 80438, 80439)

| 84202 | Protoporphyrin, RBC; quantitative |
| 84203 | screen |

(84205 has been deleted. To report, use code for specific method)

| 84206 | Proinsulin |

(Pseudocholinesterase, use 82480)

| 84207 | Pyridoxal phosphate (Vitamin B-6) |

(84208 has been deleted. To report, use 89060)

84210	Pyruvate
84220	Pyruvate kinase
84228	Quinine

(84230 has been deleted. To report, use 80194)

(84231 has been deleted. To report radioimmunoassay not elsewhere specified, use 83519)

(84232 has been deleted)

84233	Receptor assay; estrogen
84234	progesterone
84235	endocrine, other than estrogen or progesterone (specify hormone)

(84236 has been deleted. To report, use 84233 and 84234)

| 84238 | non-endocrine (eg, acetylcholine) (specify receptor) |
| 84244 | Renin |

(84246 has been deleted)

(84250, 84251 have been deleted. To report, use 84479)

| 84252 | Riboflavin (Vitamin B-2) |

(Salicylates, use 80196)

(Secretin test, see 99070, 89100 and appropriate analyses)

| 84255 | Selenium |
| 84260 | Serotonin |

(For urine metabolites (HIAA), use 83497)

| 84270 | Sex hormone binding globulin (SHBG) |
| 84275 | Sialic acid |

(Sickle hemoglobin, use 85660)

84285	Silica
84295	Sodium; serum
84300	urine
● 84302	other source

(Somatomammotropin, use 83632)

(Somatotropin, use 83003)

| 84305 | Somatomedin |
| 84307 | Somatostatin |

(84310 has been deleted)

Pathology and Laboratory

84311	Spectrophotometry, analyte not elsewhere specified
84315	Specific gravity (except urine)

(For specific gravity, urine, see 81000-81003)

(84317 has been deleted)

(84318 has been deleted)

(Stone analysis, see 82355-82370)

(84324 has been deleted. To report, see code for specific method)

84375 Sugars, chromatographic, TLC or paper chromatography

84376 Sugars (mono-, di-, and oligosaccharides); single qualitative, each specimen

84377   multiple quantitative, each specimen

84378   single quantitative, each specimen

84379   multiple quantitative, each specimen

(84382 has been deleted)

84392 Sulfate, urine

(Sulfhemoglobin, see hemoglobin, 83055, 83060)

(84395 has been deleted)

(84397 has been deleted)

(T-3, see 84479-84481)

(T-4, see 84436-84439)

(84401 has been deleted)

84402 Testosterone; free

84403   total

(84404 has been deleted)

(84405 has been deleted. To report, use 84403)

(84406 has been deleted. For testosterone binding protein, use sex hormone binding globulin, 84270)

(84407 has been deleted. To report, see code for specific method)

(84408 has been deleted. To report, see 80100-80103, 80299)

(84409, 84410 have been deleted. To report, see code for specific method)

(84420 has been deleted. To report, use 80198)

84425 Thiamine (Vitamin B-1)

84430 Thiocyanate

84432 Thyroglobulin

(Thyroglobulin, antibody, use 86800)

(84434 has been deleted. To report, use 84022)

(Thyrotropin releasing hormone (TRH) test, see 80438, 80439)

(84435 has been deleted. To report, use 84436)

84436 Thyroxine; total

84437   requiring elution (eg, neonatal)

84439   free

(84441 has been deleted. To report, see 84436-84439)

84442 Thyroxine binding globulin (TBG)

84443 Thyroid stimulating hormone (TSH)

(84444 has been deleted. To report, see 80438, 80439)

84445 Thyroid stimulating immune globulins (TSI)

(Tobramycin, use 80200)

84446 Tocopherol alpha (Vitamin E)

(Tolbutamide tolerance, use 82953)

(84447, 84448 have been deleted. To report, see 80100-80103)

84449 Transcortin (cortisol binding globulin)

84450 Transferase; aspartate amino (AST) (SGOT)

(84455 has been deleted. To report, use 84450)

84460   alanine amino (ALT) (SGPT)

(84465 has been deleted. To report, use 84460)

84466 Transferrin

(Iron binding capacity, use 83550)

(84472 has been deleted. To report, see code for specific method)

(84474 has been deleted. To report, see code for specific method)

(84476 has been deleted. To report, use 84022)

84478 Triglycerides

84479 Thyroid hormone (T3 or T4) uptake or thyroid hormone binding ratio (THBR)

84480 Triiodothyronine T3; total (TT-3)

84481   free

84482   reverse

(84483 has been deleted. To report, see 80100-80103, 80299)

84484 Troponin, quantitative

(For Troponin, qualitative assay, use 84512)

84485 Trypsin; duodenal fluid

84488   feces, qualitative

84490   feces, quantitative, 24-hour collection

84510 Tyrosine

(Urate crystal identification, use 89060)

84512 Troponin, qualitative

(For Troponin, quantitative assay, use 84484)

84520 Urea nitrogen; quantitative

84525 semiquantitative (eg, reagent strip test)

84540 Urea nitrogen, urine

84545 Urea nitrogen, clearance

84550 Uric acid; blood

(84555 has been deleted. To report, use 84550)

84560 other source

(84565, 84570, 84575 have been deleted)

84577 Urobilinogen, feces, quantitative

84578 Urobilinogen, urine; qualitative

84580 quantitative, timed specimen

84583 semiquantitative

(84584 has been deleted)

(Uroporphyrins, use 84120)

(Valproic acid (dipropylacetic acid), use 80164)

84585 Vanillylmandelic acid (VMA), urine

84586 Vasoactive intestinal peptide (VIP)

84588 Vasopressin (antidiuretic hormone, ADH)

(84589 has been deleted. To report, use 85810)

84590 Vitamin A

(84595 has been deleted. To report, use 82380 and 84590)

(Vitamin B-1, use 84425)

(Vitamin B-2, use 84252)

(Vitamin B-6, use 84207)

(Vitamin B-12, use 82607)

(Vitamin B-12, absorption (Schilling), see 78270, 78271)

(Vitamin C, use 82180)

(Vitamin D, see 82306, 82307, 82652)

(Vitamin E, use 84446)

84591 Vitamin, not otherwise specified

84597 Vitamin K

(VMA, use 84585)

84600 Volatiles (eg, acetic anhydride, carbon tetrachloride, dichloroethane, dichloromethane, diethylether, isopropyl alcohol, methanol)

(For acetaldehyde, use 82000)

(84605 has been deleted)

(84610 has been deleted)

(Volume, blood, RISA or Cr-51, see 78110, 78111)

(84613 has been deleted)

(84615 has been deleted. To report, see code for specific method)

84620 Xylose absorption test, blood and/or urine

(For administration, use 99070)

84630 Zinc

(84635 has been deleted. To report, use 84630)

(84645 has been deleted)

(84680 has been deleted. To report, use 82677)

84681 C-peptide

(84695 has been deleted. To report, use 80170)

(84701 has been deleted. To report, see 84702-84703)

84702 Gonadotropin, chorionic (hCG); quantitative

84703 qualitative

(For urine pregnancy test by visual color comparison, use 81025)

(84800 has been deleted. To report, use 84443)

(84810 has been deleted. To report, use 80200)

84830 Ovulation tests, by visual color comparison methods for human luteinizing hormone

84999 Unlisted chemistry procedure

Hematology and Coagulation

(For blood banking procedures, see **Transfusion Medicine**)

(Agglutinins, see **Immunology**)

(Antiplasmin, use 85410)

(Antithrombin III, see 85300, 85301)

(85000 has been deleted. To report, use 85002)

85002 Bleeding time

(85003 has been deleted. To report, use 85999)

(85005 has been deleted)

● **85004** Blood count; automated differential WBC count

▲ **85007** blood smear, microscopic examination with manual differential WBC count

▲ **85008** blood smear, microscopic examination without manual differential WBC count

(See also 85585)

(For other fluids (eg, CSF), see 89050, 89051)

▲ **85009** manual differential WBC count, buffy coat

(85012 has been deleted)

(Eosinophils, nasal smear, use 89190)

85013 spun microhematocrit

▲ **85014** hematocrit (Hct)

▲ **85018**   hemoglobin (Hgb)

(For other hemoglobin determination, see 83020-83069)

(For immunoassay, hemoglobin, fecal, use 82274)

▶(85021 has been deleted)◀

▶(85022 has been deleted)◀

▶(85023 has been deleted. To report, use 85007 and 85027)◀

▶(85024 has been deleted. To report, use 85025)◀

▲ **85025**   complete (CBC), automated (Hgb, Hct, RBC, WBC and platelet count) and automated differential WBC count

▲ **85027**   complete (CBC), automated (Hgb, Hct, RBC, WBC and platelet count)

(85028 has been deleted)

(85029, 85030 have been deleted)

▶(85031 has been deleted. To report, use 85014, 85018 and 85032)◀

● **85032**   manual cell count (erythrocyte, leukocyte, or platelet) each

▲ **85041**   red blood cell (RBC), automated

▶(Do not report code 85041 in conjunction with 85025 or 85027)◀

▲ **85044**   reticulocyte, manual

▲ **85045**   reticulocyte, automated

85046   reticulocytes, hemoglobin concentration

▲ **85048**   leukocyte (WBC), automated

● **85049**   platelet, automated

85060   Blood smear, peripheral, interpretation by physician with written report

(85095 has been deleted. To report, use 38220)

(85096 has been deleted. For interpretation of smear, use 85097; for cell block interpretation, use 88305)

85097   Bone marrow, smear interpretation

(85100 has been deleted. To report, use 38220 and 85097)

(85101 has been deleted. For aspiration, use 38220)

(For special stains, see 85540, 88312, 88313)

(85102 has been deleted. To report, use 38221)

(For bone biopsy, see 20220, 20225, 20240, 20245, 20250, 20251)

(85103, 85105 have been deleted. For bone marrow biopsy interpretation, use 88305)

(85109 has been deleted)

(85120 has been deleted. To report, see 38230-38240)

85130   Chromogenic substrate assay

(85150, 85160, 85165 have been deleted)

(Circulating anti-coagulant screen (mixing studies), see 85611, 85732)

85170   Clot retraction

(85171, 85172 have been deleted)

85175   Clot lysis time, whole blood dilution

(Clotting factor I (fibrinogen), see 85384, 85385)

85210   Clotting; factor II, prothrombin, specific

(See also 85610-85613)

85220   factor V (AcG or proaccelerin), labile factor

85230   factor VII (proconvertin, stable factor)

85240   factor VIII (AHG), one stage

(85242 has been deleted)

85244   factor VIII related antigen

85245   factor VIII, VW factor, ristocetin cofactor

85246   factor VIII, VW factor antigen

85247   factor VIII, von Willebrand factor, multimetric analysis

85250   factor IX (PTC or Christmas)

85260   factor X (Stuart-Prower)

85270   factor XI (PTA)

85280   factor XII (Hageman)

85290   factor XIII (fibrin stabilizing)

85291   factor XIII (fibrin stabilizing), screen solubility

85292   prekallikrein assay (Fletcher factor assay)

85293   high molecular weight kininogen assay (Fitzgerald factor assay)

85300   Clotting inhibitors or anticoagulants; antithrombin III, activity

85301   antithrombin III, antigen assay

85302   protein C, antigen

85303   protein C, activity

85305   protein S, total

85306   protein S, free

85307   Activated Protein C (APC) resistance assay

(85310, 85311 have been deleted)

(85320 has been deleted)

(85330 has been deleted. To report, use 85335)

85335   Factor inhibitor test

85337   Thrombomodulin

(For mixing studies for inhibitors, use 85732)

(85340, 85341 have been deleted)

Pathology and Laboratory

Pathology and Laboratory

85345	Coagulation time; Lee and White
85347	activated
85348	other methods

(Differential count, see 85007 et seq)

(Duke bleeding time, use 85002)

(Eosinophils, nasal smear, use 89190)

85360	Euglobulin lysis

(Fetal hemoglobin, see 83030, 83033, 85460)

85362	Fibrin(ogen) degradation (split) products (FDP)(FSP); agglutination slide, semiquantitative

(85363, 85364 have been deleted)

(85365 has been deleted. To report, use 86320)

(Immunoelectrophoresis, use 86320)

85366	paracoagulation

(85367 has been deleted)

(85368 has been deleted. To report, use 85366)

(85369 has been deleted)

85370	quantitative

(85371 has been deleted. To report, see 85384, 85385)

(85372 has been deleted)

(85376, 85377 have been deleted. To report, see 85384, 85385)

▲ **85378**	Fibrin degradation products, D-dimer; qualitative or semiquantitative
85379	quantitative
● **85380**	ultrasensitive (eg, for evaluation for venous thromboembolism), qualitative or semiquantitative
85384	Fibrinogen; activity
85385	antigen
85390	Fibrinolysins or coagulopathy screen, interpretation and report

(85392 has been deleted)

(85395 has been deleted)

(85398 has been deleted)

85400	Fibrinolytic factors and inhibitors; plasmin
85410	alpha-2 antiplasmin
85415	plasminogen activator
85420	plasminogen, except antigenic assay
85421	plasminogen, antigenic assay

(85426 has been deleted. For von Willebrand factor assay, see 85245-85247)

(Fragility, red blood cell, see 85547, 85555-85557)

85441	Heinz bodies; direct
85445	induced, acetyl phenylhydrazine

(Hematocrit (PCV), see 85014, 85021-85031)

(Hemoglobin, see 83020-83068, 85018-85031)

85460	Hemoglobin or RBCs, fetal, for fetomaternal hemorrhage; differential lysis (Kleihauer-Betke)

(See also 83030, 83033)

(Hemolysins, see 86940, 86941)

85461	rosette
85475	Hemolysin, acid

(See also 86940, 86941)

85520	Heparin assay
85525	Heparin neutralization
85530	Heparin-protamine tolerance test

(85535 has been deleted. To report use 85536)

85536	Iron stain, peripheral blood

(For iron stains on bone marrow or other tissues with physician evaluation, use 88313)

(85538 has been deleted. For leder stain, esterase, blood or bone marrow, use 88319)

85540	Leukocyte alkaline phosphatase with count

(85544 has been deleted)

85547	Mechanical fragility, RBC

(85548 has been deleted. To report, use 85008)

85549	Muramidase

(Nitroblue tetrazolium dye test, use 86384)

85555	Osmotic fragility, RBC; unincubated

(85556 has been deleted)

85557	incubated

(Packed cell volume, use 85013)

(Partial thromboplastin time, see 85730, 85732)

(Parasites, blood (eg, malaria smears), use 87207)

(Plasmin, use 85400)

(Plasminogen, use 85420)

(Plasminogen activator, use 85415)

(85560 has been deleted. For peroxidase stain, WBC, use 88319)

(85575 has been deleted)

85576	Platelet, aggregation (in vitro), each agent

(85577 has been deleted)

(85580 has been deleted. To report, use 85590)

▶(85585 has been deleted. To report, use 85008)◀

▶(85590 has been deleted. To report, use 85032)◀

▶(85595 has been deleted. To report, use 85049)◀

85597 Platelet neutralization

85610 Prothrombin time;

85611   substitution, plasma fractions, each

85612 Russell viper venom time (includes venom); undiluted

85613   diluted

(85614 has been deleted)

(85615 has been deleted)

(85618 has been deleted)

(Red blood cell count, see ▶85025, 85027, 85041)◀

(85630 has been deleted.)

(85632 has been deleted)

85635 Reptilase test

(Reticulocyte count, see 85044, 85045)

(85650 has been deleted)

85651 Sedimentation rate, erythrocyte; non-automated

85652   automated

85660 Sickling of RBC, reduction

(Hemoglobin electrophoresis, use 83020)

(Smears (eg, for parasites, malaria), use 87207)

(85665 has been deleted. For plasminogen activator, use 85415)

(85667 has been deleted)

85670 Thrombin time; plasma

85675   titer

(85700 has been deleted)

85705 Thromboplastin inhibition; tissue

(85710, 85711 have been deleted)

(85720 has been deleted)

(For individual clotting factors, see 85245-85247)

85730 Thromboplastin time, partial (PTT); plasma or whole blood

85732   substitution, plasma fractions, each

85810 Viscosity

(85820 has been deleted. To report, use 85810)

(von Willebrand factor assay, see 85245-85247)

(WBC count, see ▶85025-85031,◀ 85048, 89050)

85999 Unlisted hematology and coagulation procedure

Immunology

(Acetylcholine receptor antibody, see 86255, 86256)

(Actinomyces, antibodies to, use 86602)

(Adrenal cortex antibodies, see 86255, 86256)

(For tuberculosis test, cell mediated immunity measurement of gamma interferon antigen response, use Category III code 0010T)

86000 Agglutinins, febrile (eg, Brucella, Francisella, Murine typhus, Q fever, Rocky Mountain spotted fever, scrub typhus), each antigen

(For antibodies to infectious agents, see 86602-86804)

86001 Allergen specific IgG quantitative or semiquantitative, each allergen

(86002 has been deleted)

(Agglutinins and autohemolysins, see 86940, 86941)

86003 Allergen specific IgE; quantitative or semiquantitative, each allergen

(For total quantitative IgE, use 82785)

(86004 has been deleted. To report, see 86940, 86941)

86005   qualitative, multiallergen screen (dipstick, paddle or disk)

(For total qualitative IgE, use 83518)

(Alpha-1 antitrypsin, see 82103, 82104)

(Alpha-1 feto-protein, see 82105, 82106)

(Anti-AChR (acetylcholine receptor) antibody titer, see 86255, 86256)

(86006 has been deleted. To report, see 83519, 86318, 86403)

(86007, 86008, 86009 have been deleted)

(86011 has been deleted. To report, use 86021)

(86012 has been deleted. To report, use 86978)

(86013 has been deleted)

(86014 has been deleted. To report, use 86022)

(86016 has been deleted. To report, use 86850)

(86017 has been deleted. To report, see 86850 and 86901)

(86018 has been deleted)

(86019 has been deleted. To report, use 86860)

(Anticardiolipin antibody, use 86147)

(Anti-DNA, use 86225)

(Anti-deoxyribonuclease titer, use 86215)

86021	Antibody identification; leukocyte antibodies
86022	platelet antibodies
86023	platelet associated immunoglobulin assay

(86024 has been deleted. For RBC antibodies, use 86870)

(86026, 86028 have been deleted)

(86031 has been deleted. To report, use 86880)

(86032 has been deleted. To report, use 86885)

(86033 has been deleted. To report, use 86886)

(86034 has been deleted. To report, see 86880-86886 and 86971)

(86035 has been deleted. To report, use 86970)

86038	Antinuclear antibodies (ANA);
86039	titer

(86045 has been deleted)

(Antistreptococcal antibody, ie, anti-DNAse, use 86215)

(Antistreptokinase titer, use 86590)

86060   Antistreptolysin O; titer

(For antibodies to infectious agents, see 86602-86804)

86063   screen

(For antibodies to infectious agents, see 86602-86804)

(86064 has been deleted. For antitrypsin, alpha-1 use 82103, for phenotyping use 82104)

(86066 has been deleted. To report, use 82104)

(86067 has been deleted. To report, use 82103)

(86068 has been deleted. For blood compatibility test, see 86920-86922)

(Blastomyces, antibodies to, use 86612)

(86069 has been deleted)

(86070 has been deleted. To report, use 86920)

(86072 has been deleted)

(86073 has been deleted. To report, see 86156, 86157, 86904)

(86074 has been deleted)

(86075, 86076 have been deleted)

86077   Blood bank physician services; difficult cross match and/or evaluation of irregular antibody(s), interpretation and written report

86078   investigation of transfusion reaction including suspicion of transmissible disease, interpretation and written report

86079   authorization for deviation from standard blood banking procedures (eg, use of outdated blood, transfusion of Rh incompatible units), with written report

(86080 has been deleted. For blood typing, see 86900-86910)

(86082 has been deleted. To report, see 86900, 86901)

(86083 has been deleted. To report, use 86850 and 86900 or 86901)

(86084 has been deleted. To report, use 86903)

(86085 has been deleted. To report, use 86904)

(86090 has been deleted)

(86095 has been deleted. To report, use 86905)

(86096 has been deleted)

(86100 has been deleted. To report, use 86901)

(86105 has been deleted. To report, use 86906)

(86115 has been deleted)

(86120 has been deleted. To report, use 86905)

(86128 has been deleted. To report, use 86890)

(86129 has been deleted)

(86130 has been deleted. To report, use 86891)

(86131, 86134, 86138 and 86139 have been deleted)

(Brucella, antibodies to, use 86622)

(Candida, antibodies to, use 86628. For skin testing, use 86485)

86140   C-reactive protein;

(Candidiasis, use 86628)

86141	high sensitivity (hsCRP)
86146	Beta 2 Glycoprotein I antibody, each
86147	Cardiolipin (phospholipid) antibody, each Ig class
86148	Anti-phosphatidylserine (phospholipid) antibody

►(To report antiprothrombin (phospholipid cofactor) antibody, use Category III code 0030T)◄

(86149 has been deleted. To report, use 82378)

(86151 has been deleted. To report, use 82378)

86155   Chemotaxis assay, specify method

(Clostridium difficile toxin, use 87230)

(Coccidioides, antibodies to, see 86635. For skin testing, use 86490)

86156	Cold agglutinin; screen
86157	titer

(86158 has been deleted)

(86159 has been deleted. To report, see 86160 and 86161)

86160 Complement; antigen, each component

86161 functional activity, each component

86162 total hemolytic (CH50)

(86163, 86164 have been deleted. To report, see 86160 and 86161)

86171 Complement fixation tests, each antigen

(Coombs test, see 86880-86886)

86185 Counterimmunoelectrophoresis, each antigen

(86201, 86202 have been deleted)

(Cryptococcus, antibodies to, use 86641)

(86209 has been deleted. To report, use 86999)

86215 Deoxyribonuclease, antibody

86225 Deoxyribonucleic acid (DNA) antibody; native or double stranded

(Echinococcus, antibodies to, see code for specific method)

(For HIV antibody tests, see 86701-86703)

86226 single stranded

(Anti D.S., DNA, IFA, eg, using C.Lucilae, see 86255 and 86256)

(86227, 86228 have been deleted. To report, use 86317)

(86229 has been deleted)

86235 Extractable nuclear antigen, antibody to, any method (eg, nRNP, SS-A, SS-B, Sm, RNP, Sc170, J01), each antibody

(86240, 86241 have been deleted)

86243 Fc receptor

(86244 has been deleted. To report fetoprotein, alpha-1, see 82105, 82106)

(86245 has been deleted)

(Filaria, antibodies to, see code for specific method)

86255 Fluorescent noninfectious agent antibody; screen, each antibody

86256 titer, each antibody

(Fluorescent technique for antigen identification in tissue, use 88346; for indirect fluorescence, use 88347)

(86265 has been deleted. To report, use 86930)

(86266 has been deleted. To report, use 86931)

(FTA, see 86781)

(86267 has been deleted. To report, use 86932)

(Gel (agar) diffusion tests, use 86331)

(86272, 86273 have been deleted)

(86274 has been deleted. To report, use 90742)

86277 Growth hormone, human (HGH), antibody

86280 Hemagglutination inhibition test (HAI)

(For rubella, use 86762)

(86281 has been deleted. To report, use 85475)

(86282 has been deleted. To report, use 86940)

(86283 has been deleted. To report, use 86941)

(86285, 86286 have been deleted)

(86287 has been deleted. To report, use 87340)

(86289 has been deleted. To report, use 86704)

(For antibodies to infectious agents, see 86602-86804)

(86290 has been deleted. To report, use 86705)

(86291 has been deleted. To report, use 86706)

(86293 has been deleted. To report, use 87350)

86294 Immunoassay for tumor antigen, qualitative or semiquantitative (eg, bladder tumor antigen)

(86295 has been deleted. To report, use 86707)

(86296 has been deleted. To report, use 86708)

(86297 has been deleted. To report, use 86708)

(86299 has been deleted. To report, use 86709)

86300 Immunoassay for tumor antigen, quantitative; CA 15-3 (27.29)

86301 CA 19-9

(86302 has been deleted. To report, use 86803)

(86303 has been deleted. To report, use 86804)

86304 CA 125

(For measurement of serum HER-2/neu oncoprotein, see 83950)

(86306 has been deleted. To report, use 87380)

(For hepatitis delta agent, antibody, use 86692)

86308 Heterophile antibodies; screening

(For antibodies to infectious agents, see 86602-86804)

86309 titer

(For antibodies to infectious agents, see 86602-86804)

86310 titers after absorption with beef cells and guinea pig kidney

(Histoplasma, antibodies to, use 86698. For skin testing, use 86510)

(For antibodies to infectious agents, see 86602-86804)

(86311 has been deleted. To report, see 87390, 87391)

(86312 has been deleted. To report, see 86701-86703)

(86313 has been deleted. To report, use 87449)

(86314 has been deleted. To report, use 86689)

(86315 has been deleted. To report, use 87450)

(Human growth hormone antibody, use 86277)

Pathology and Laboratory

86316 Immunoassay for tumor antigen; other antigen, quantitative (eg, CA 50, 72-4, 549), each

86317 Immunoassay for infectious agent antibody, quantitative, not otherwise specified

(For immunoassay techniques for antigens, see 83516, 83518, 83519, 83520, 87301-87450, 87810-87899)

(For particle agglutination procedures, use 86403)

86318 Immunoassay for infectious agent antibody, qualitative or semiquantitative, single step method (eg, reagent strip)

(86319 has been deleted. To report immunoassays for drugs, see 80100-80103)

86320 Immunoelectrophoresis; serum

86325 other fluids (eg, urine, cerebrospinal fluid) with concentration

86327 crossed (2-dimensional assay)

86329 Immunodiffusion; not elsewhere specified

86331 gel diffusion, qualitative (Ouchterlony), each antigen or antibody

86332 Immune complex assay

(86333 has been deleted. To report, use 86332)

86334 Immunofixation electrophoresis

(86335 has been deleted)

86336 Inhibin A

86337 Insulin antibodies

(86338 has been deleted. To report, use 86337)

86340 Intrinsic factor antibodies

(Leptospira, antibodies to, use 86720)

(Leukoagglutinins, use 86021)

86341 Islet cell antibody

(86342 has been deleted. To report, use 86945)

86343 Leukocyte histamine release test (LHR)

86344 Leukocyte phagocytosis

(86345, 86346, 86347 have been deleted)

(86349 has been deleted. To report, use 86950)

(86351 has been deleted)

86353 Lymphocyte transformation, mitogen (phytomitogen) or antigen induced blastogenesis

(Lymphocytes immunophenotyping, use 88180 for cytometry; see 88342, 88346 for microscopic techniques)

(86357 has been deleted. To report, see 88180, 88342, 88346)

(86358 has been deleted. To report, see 88180, 88342, 88346)

(Malaria antibodies, use 86750)

86359 T cells; total count

86360 absolute CD4 and CD8 count, including ratio

86361 absolute CD4 count

(86365 has been deleted)

86376 Microsomal antibodies (eg, thyroid or liver-kidney), each

(86377 has been deleted. To report, use 86376)

86378 Migration inhibitory factor test (MIF)

(Mitochondrial antibody, liver, see 86255, 86256)

(Mononucleosis, see 86308-86310)

86382 Neutralization test, viral

86384 Nitroblue tetrazolium dye test (NTD)

(Ouchterlony diffusion, use 86331)

(86385, 86386 have been deleted. To report, see 86910, 86911)

(86388, 86389, 86391 have been deleted)

(Platelet antibodies, see 86022, 86023)

(86392, 86393, 86398 have been deleted)

(86402 has been deleted)

86403 Particle agglutination; screen, each antibody

(86404 has been deleted. To report, use 86965)

(86405 has been deleted)

86406 titer, each antibody

(Pregnancy test, see 84702, 84703)

(86410 has been deleted. To report, use 86970)

(86411 has been deleted. To report, use 86971)

(86412 has been deleted. To report, use 86972)

(86415, 86416 have been deleted)

(86417 has been deleted. To report, use 86975)

(86418 has been deleted. To report, use 86976)

(86419 has been deleted. To report, use 86977)

(86420 has been deleted. To report, use 86978)

(86421-86423 have been deleted. To report, see 82785, 83518, 86003, 86005)

(86424, 86425, 86427 have been deleted)

(Rapid plasma reagin test (RPR), see 86592, 86593)

86430 Rheumatoid factor; qualitative

86431 quantitative

(Serologic test for syphilis, see 86592, 86593)

(86450 has been deleted)

(86455 has been deleted. To report, use 86586)

(86460, 86470, 86480 have been deleted)

Pathology and Laboratory

86485   Skin test; candida

(For antibody, candida, use 86628)

86490   coccidioidomycosis

(86495, 86500 have been deleted)

86510   histoplasmosis

(For histoplasma, antibody, use 86698)

(86520, 86530 have been deleted)

(86540 has been deleted. For mumps antibody, use 86735)

(86550, 86565, 86570 have been deleted)

86580   tuberculosis, intradermal

86585   tuberculosis, tine test

(For tuberculosis test, cell mediated immunity measurement of gamma interferon antigen response, use Category III code 0010T)

(For skin tests for allergy, see 95010-95199)

(Smooth muscle antibody, see 86255, 86256)

(Sporothrix, antibodies to, see code for specific method)

86586   unlisted antigen, each

(86587 has been deleted. To report, use 86985)

(86588 has been deleted. To report, see 86403, 87081, 87430, or 87880)

86590   Streptokinase, antibody

(For antibodies to infectious agents, see 86602-86804)

(Streptolysin O antibody, see antistreptolysin O, 86060, 86063)

86592   Syphilis test; qualitative (eg, VDRL, RPR, ART)

(For antibodies to infectious agents, see 86602-86804)

86593   quantitative

(For antibodies to infectious agents, see 86602-86804)

(Tetanus antibody, use 86774)

(Thyroglobulin antibody, use 86800)

(Thyroglobulin, use 84432)

(Thyroid microsomal antibody, use 86376)

(86594 has been deleted. To report, see 86376 and 86800)

(86595 has been deleted)

(86597 has been deleted. To report see 86812-86822)

(86600 has been deleted)

(For toxoplasma antibody, see 86777-86778)

The following codes (86602-86804) are qualitative or semiquantitative immunoassays performed by multiple step methods for the detection of antibodies to infectious agents. For immunoassays by single step method (eg, reagent strips), use code 86318. Procedures for the

identification of antibodies should be coded as precisely as possible. For example, an antibody to a virus could be coded with increasing specificity for virus, family, genus, species, or type. In some cases, further precision may be added to codes by specifying the class of immunoglobulin being detected. When multiple tests are done to detect antibodies to organisms classified more precisely than the specificity allowed by available codes, it is appropriate to code each as a separate service. For example, a test for antibody to an enterovirus is coded as 86658. Coxsackie viruses are enteroviruses, but there are no codes for the individual species of enterovirus. If assays are performed for antibodies to coxsackie A and B species, each assay should be separately coded. Similarly, if multiple assays are performed for antibodies of different immunoglobulin classes, each assay should be coded separately.

For the detection of antibodies other than those to infectious agents, see specific antibody (eg, 86021, 86022, 86023, 86376, 86800, 86850-86870) or specific method (eg, 83516, 86255, 86256).

(For infectious agent/antigen detection, see 87260-87899)

86602   Antibody; actinomyces

86603   adenovirus

86606   Aspergillus

86609   bacterium, not elsewhere specified

86611   Bartonella

86612   Blastomyces

86615   Bordetella

86617   Borrelia burgdorferi (Lyme disease) confirmatory test (eg, Western blot or immunoblot)

86618   Borrelia burgdorferi (Lyme disease)

86619   Borrelia (relapsing fever)

86622   Brucella

86625   Campylobacter

86628   Candida

(For skin test, candida, use 86485)

(86630 has been deleted)

86631   Chlamydia

86632   Chlamydia, IgM

(For chlamydia antigen, see 87270, 87320. For fluorescent antibody technique, see 86255, 86256)

86635   Coccidioides

86638   Coxiella Brunetii (Q fever)

86641   Cryptococcus

86644   cytomegalovirus (CMV)

(For TORCH panel, use 80090)

86645	cytomegalovirus (CMV), IgM		86703	HIV-1 and HIV-2, single assay
86648	Diphtheria			(For HIV-1 antigen, use 87390)
	(86650 has been deleted. To report, use 86781)			(For HIV-2 antigen, use 87391)
86651	encephalitis, California (La Crosse)			(For confirmatory test for HIV antibody (eg, Western Blot), use 86689)
86652	encephalitis, Eastern equine		86704	Hepatitis B core antibody (HBcAb); total
86653	encephalitis, St. Louis		86705	IgM antibody
86654	encephalitis, Western equine		86706	Hepatitis B surface antibody (HBsAb)
86658	enterovirus (eg, coxsackie, echo, polio)		86707	Hepatitis Be antibody (HBeAb)
	(86662 has been deleted. To report, use 86781)		86708	Hepatitis A antibody (HAAb); total
	(Trichinella, antibodies to, use 86784)		86709	IgM antibody
	(Trypanosoma, antibodies to, see code for specific method)		86710	Antibody; influenza virus
	(Tuberculosis, use 86580 for skin testing)		86713	Legionella
	(Viral antibodies, see code for specific method)		86717	Leishmania
86663	Epstein-Barr (EB) virus, early antigen (EA)		86720	Leptospira
86664	Epstein-Barr (EB) virus, nuclear antigen (EBNA)		86723	Listeria monocytogenes
86665	Epstein-Barr (EB) virus, viral capsid (VCA)		86727	lymphocytic choriomeningitis
86666	Ehrlichia		86729	Lymphogranuloma Venereum
86668	Francisella Tularensis		86732	mucormycosis
86671	fungus, not elsewhere specified		86735	mumps
86674	Giardia Lamblia		86738	Mycoplasma
86677	Helicobacter pylori		86741	Neisseria meningitidis
	(86681 has been deleted. To report, see 86255, 86256)		86744	Nocardia
86682	helminth, not elsewhere specified		86747	parvovirus
	(86683 has been deleted. To report, use 82274)		86750	Plasmodium (malaria)
86684	Hemophilus influenza		86753	protozoa, not elsewhere specified
	(86685 has been deleted. To report, see 86255, 86256)		86756	respiratory syncytial virus
86687	HTLV-I		86757	Rickettsia
86688	HTLV-II		86759	rotavirus
86689	HTLV or HIV antibody, confirmatory test (eg, Western Blot)		86762	rubella
86692	hepatitis, delta agent		86765	rubeola
	(For hepatitis delta agent, antigen, use 87380)		86768	Salmonella
86694	herpes simplex, non-specific type test		86771	Shigella
	(For TORCH panel, use 80090)		86774	tetanus
86695	herpes simplex, type 1		86777	Toxoplasma
86696	herpes simplex, type 2		86778	Toxoplasma, IgM
86698	histoplasma		86781	Treponema Pallidum, confirmatory test (eg, FTA-abs)
86701	HIV-1		86784	trichinella
86702	HIV-2		86787	varicella-zoster

Pathology and Laboratory

86790	virus, not elsewhere specified
86793	Yersinia
86800	Thyroglobulin antibody
	(For thyroglobulin, use 84432)
86803	Hepatitis C antibody;
86804	.confirmatory test (eg, immunoblot)

Tissue Typing

(For pretransplant cross-match, see appropriate code or codes)

86805	Lymphocytotoxicity assay, visual crossmatch; with titration
86806	without titration
86807	Serum screening for cytotoxic percent reactive antibody (PRA); standard method
86808	quick method
	(86810 has been deleted)
86812	HLA typing; A, B, or C (eg, A10, B7, B27), single antigen
86813	A, B, or C, multiple antigens
86816	DR/DQ, single antigen
86817	DR/DQ, multiple antigens
86821	lymphocyte culture, mixed (MLC)
86822	lymphocyte culture, primed (PLC)
86849	Unlisted immunology procedure

Transfusion Medicine

(For apheresis, use 36520)

(For therapeutic phlebotomy, use 99195)

86850	Antibody screen, RBC, each serum technique
86860	Antibody elution (RBC), each elution
86870	Antibody identification, RBC antibodies, each panel for each serum technique
86880	Antihuman globulin test (Coombs test); direct, each antiserum
86885	indirect, qualitative, each antiserum
86886	indirect, titer, each antiserum
86890	Autologous blood or component, collection processing and storage; predeposited
86891	intra- or postoperative salvage
	(For physician services to autologous donors, see 99201-99204)

86900	Blood typing; ABO
86901	Rh (D)
86903	antigen screening for compatible blood unit using reagent serum, per unit screened
86904	antigen screening for compatible unit using patient serum, per unit screened
86905	RBC antigens, other than ABO or Rh (D), each
86906	Rh phenotyping, complete
86910	Blood typing, for paternity testing, per individual; ABO, Rh and MN
86911	each additional antigen system
	▶(86915 has been deleted. To report, see 38210-38213)◀
86920	Compatibility test each unit; immediate spin technique
86921	incubation technique
86922	antiglobulin technique
86927	Fresh frozen plasma, thawing, each unit
▲ 86930	Frozen blood, each unit; freezing (includes preparation)
▲ 86931	thawing
▲ 86932	freezing (includes preparation) and thawing
86940	Hemolysins and agglutinins; auto, screen, each
86941	incubated
86945	Irradiation of blood product, each unit
86950	Leukocyte transfusion
	(For leukapheresis, use 36520)
86965	Pooling of platelets or other blood products
86970	Pretreatment of RBCs for use in RBC antibody detection, identification, and/or compatibility testing; incubation with chemical agents or drugs, each
86971	incubation with enzymes, each
86972	by density gradient separation
86975	Pretreatment of serum for use in RBC antibody identification; incubation with drugs, each
86976	by dilution
86977	incubation with inhibitors, each
86978	by differential red cell absorption using patient RBCs or RBCs of known phenotype, each absorption
86985	Splitting of blood or blood products, each unit
86999	Unlisted transfusion medicine procedure

Pathology and Laboratory

Microbiology

Includes bacteriology, mycology, parasitology, and virology.

Presumptive identification of microorganisms is defined as identification by colony morphology, growth on selective media, Gram stains, or up to three tests (eg, catalase, oxidase, indole, urease). Definitive identification of microorganisms is defined as an identification to the genus or species level that requires additional tests (eg, biochemical panels, slide cultures). If additional studies involve molecular probes, chromatography, or immunologic techniques, these should be separately coded in addition to definitive identification codes (87140-87158). For multiple specimens/sites use modifier '-59'. For repeat laboratory tests performed on the same day, use modifier '-91'.

87001	Animal inoculation, small animal; with observation
87003	with observation and dissection
87015	Concentration (any type), for infectious agents

(Do not report 87015 in conjunction with 87177)

87040	Culture, bacterial; blood, with isolation and presumptive identification of isolates (includes anaerobic culture, if appropriate)
87045	feces, with isolation and preliminary examination (eg, KIA, LIA), Salmonella and Shigella species
87046	stool, additional pathogens, isolation and preliminary examination (eg, Campylobacter, Yersinia, Vibrio, E. coli 0157), each plate

(87060 has been deleted. To report, use 87070 or 87081)

87070	any other source except urine, blood or stool, with isolation and presumptive identification of isolates

(For urine, use 87088)

87071	quantitative, aerobic with isolation and presumptive identification of isolates, any source except urine, blood or stool

(For urine, use 87088)

(87072 has been deleted. To report, use 87076 or 87077)

87073	quantitative, anaerobic with isolation and presumptive identification of isolates, any source except urine, blood or stool

(For definitive identification of isolates, use 87076 or 87077. For typing of isolates see 87140-87158)

87075	any source, anaerobic with isolation and presumptive identification of isolates
87076	anaerobic isolate, additional methods required for definitive identification, each isolate

(For gas liquid chromatography (GLC) or high pressure liquid chromatography (HPLC), use 87143)

87077	aerobic isolate, additional methods required for definitive identification, each isolate

(For gas liquid chromatography (GLC) or high pressure liquid chromatography (HPLC), use 87143)

87081	Culture, presumptive, pathogenic organisms, screening only;

(87082 and 87083 have been deleted. To report, use 87081)

87084	with colony estimation from density chart

(87085 has been deleted. To report, use 87086)

87086	Culture, bacterial; quantitative colony count, urine

(87087 has been deleted. To report, use 87088)

87088	with isolation and presumptive identification of isolates, urine
87101	Culture, fungi (mold or yeast) isolation, with presumptive identification of isolates; skin, hair, or nail
87102	other source (except blood)
87103	blood
87106	Culture, fungi, definitive identification, each organism; yeast

(Use 87106 in addition to codes 87101, 87102, or 87103 when appropriate)

87107	mold
87109	Culture, mycoplasma, any source
87110	Culture, chlamydia, any source

(For immunofluorescence staining of shell vials, use 87140)

87116	Culture, tubercle or other acid-fast bacilli (eg, TB, AFB, mycobacteria) any source, with isolation and presumptive identification of isolates

(87117 has been deleted. For concentration, use 87015)

87118	Culture, mycobacterial, definitive identification, each isolate

(For nucleic acid probe identification, use 87149)

(For GLC or HPLC identification, use 87143)

87140	Culture, typing; immunofluorescent method, each antiserum
87143	gas liquid chromatography (GLC) or high pressure liquid chromatography (HPLC) method

(87145 has been deleted)

87147	immunologic method, other than immunofluoresence (eg, agglutination grouping), per antiserum
87149	identification by nucleic acid probe

(87151 has been deleted. To report, use 87147)

87152	identification by pulse field gel typing

(87155 has been deleted. To report, use 87147)

87158   other methods

(87163 has been deleted. To report, use 87076 or 87077)

87164   Dark field examination, any source (eg, penile, vaginal, oral, skin); includes specimen collection

87166   without collection

87168   Macroscopic examination; arthropod

87169   parasite

87172   Pinworm exam (eg, cellophane tape prep)

(87173 has been deleted)

(87174 has been deleted)

(87175 has been deleted)

87176   Homogenization, tissue, for culture

87177   Ova and parasites, direct smears, concentration and identification

(Do not report 87177 in conjunction with 87015)

▶(For direct smears from a primary source, use 87207)◀

(For coccidia or microsporidia exam, use 87207)

(For trichrome, iron hemotoxylin and other special stains, use 88313)

(For nucleic acid probes in cytologic material, use 88365)

(For molecular diagnostics, see 83890-83898, 87470-87799)

(87178 has been deleted. To report, use 87797)

(87179 has been deleted. To report, use 87798)

87181   Susceptibility studies, antimicrobial agent; agar dilution method, per agent (eg, antibiotic gradient strip)

87184   disk method, per plate (12 or fewer agents)

87185   enzyme detection (eg, beta lactamase), per enzyme

87186   microdilution or agar dilution (minimum inhibitory concentration (MIC) or breakpoint), each multi-antimicrobial, per plate

+ 87187   microdilution or agar dilution, minimum lethal concentration (MLC), each plate (List separately in addition to code for primary procedure)

(Use 87187 in conjunction with 87186 or 87188)

87188   macrobroth dilution method, each agent

87190   mycobacteria, proportion method, each agent

(For other mycobacterial susceptibility studies, see 87181, 87184, 87186, or 87188)

(87192 has been deleted. For fungal susceptibility studies, see 87181, 87184, 87186, 87187, or 87188)

87197   Serum bactericidal titer (Schlicter test)

▶(87198 has been deleted. To report, use 87271)◀

▶(87199 has been deleted. To report, use 87267)◀

87205   Smear, primary source with interpretation; Gram or Giemsa stain for bacteria, fungi, or cell types

87206   fluorescent and/or acid fast stain for bacteria, fungi, parasites, viruses or cell types

▲87207   special stain for inclusion bodies or parasites (eg, malaria, coccidia, microsporidia, trypanosomes, herpes viruses)

▶(For direct smears with concentration and identification, use 87177)◀

(For thick smear preparation, use 87015)

(For complex special stains, see 88312, 88313)

(For fat, meat, fibers, nasal eosinophils, and starch, see miscellaneous section)

(87208 has been deleted)

87210   wet mount for infectious agents (eg, saline, India ink, KOH preps)

(For KOH examination of skin, hair or nails, see 87220)

(87211 has been deleted. To report, use 87177)

87220   Tissue examination by KOH slide of samples from skin, hair, or nails for fungi or ectoparasite ova or mites (eg, scabies)

87230   Toxin or antitoxin assay, tissue culture (eg, Clostridium difficile toxin)

87250   Virus isolation; inoculation of embryonated eggs, or small animal, includes observation and dissection

87252   tissue culture inoculation, observation, and presumptive identification by cytopathic effect

87253   tissue culture, additional studies or definitive identification (eg, hemabsorption, neutralization, immunofluoresence stain), each isolate

(Electron microscopy, use 88348)

(Inclusion bodies in tissue sections, see 88304-88309; in smears, see 87207-87210; in fluids, use 88106)

▲87254   centrifuge enhanced (shell vial) technique, includes identification with immunofluorescence stain, each virus

(Report 87254 in addition to 87252 as appropriate)

●87255   including identification by non-immunologic method, other than by cytopathic effect (eg, virus specific enzymatic activity)

These codes are intended for primary source only. For similar studies on culture material, refer to codes 87140-87158. Infectious agents by antigen detection, immunofluorescence microscopy, or nucleic acid probe techniques should be reported as precisely as possible. The most specific code possible should be reported. If there is no specific agent code, the general methodology code (eg, 87299, 87449, 87450, 87797, 87798, 87799, 87899) should be used. For identification of antibodies to many of the listed infectious agents, see 86602-86804.

Pathology and Laboratory

When separate assays are performed for different species or strain(s) of organisms, each assay should be reported separately.

87260   Infectious agent antigen detection by immunofluorescent technique; adenovirus

87265   Bordetella pertussis/parapertussis

● 87267   Enterovirus, direct fluorescent antibody (DFA)

87270   Chlamydia trachomatis

● 87271   Cytomegalovirus, direct fluorescent antibody (DFA)

87272   cryptosporidium/giardia

87273   Herpes simplex virus type 2

87274   Herpes simplex virus type 1

87275   Influenza B virus

87276   influenza A virus

87277   Legionella micdadei

87278   Legionella pneumophila

87279   Parainfluenza virus, each type

87280   respiratory syncytial virus

87281   Pneumocystis carinii

87283   Rubeola

87285   Treponema pallidum

87290   Varicella zoster virus

87299   not otherwise specified, each organism

87300   Infectious agent antigen detection by immunofluorescent technique, polyvalent for multiple organisms, each polyvalent antiserum

(For physician evaluation of infectious disease agents by immunofluorescence, use 88346)

87301   Infectious agent antigen detection by enzyme immunoassay technique, qualitative or semiquantitative, multiple step method; adenovirus enteric types 40/41

87320   Chlamydia trachomatis

87324   Clostridium difficile toxin(s)

87327   Cryptococcus neoformans

(For Cryptococcus latex agglutination, use 86403)

87328   cryptosporidium/giardia

87332   cytomegalovirus

87335   Escherichia coli O157

(For giardia antigen, use 87328)

87336   Entamoeba histolytica dispar group

87337   Entamoeba histolytica group

87338   Helicobacter pylori, stool

87339   Helicobacter pylori

(For H. pylori, stool, use 87338. For H. pylori, breath and blood by mass spectrometry, see 83013, 83014. For H. pylori, liquid scintillation counter, see 78267, 78268)

87340   hepatitis B surface antigen (HBsAg)

87341   hepatitis B surface antigen (HBsAg) neutralization

87350   hepatitis Be antigen (HBeAg)

87380   hepatitis, delta agent

87385   Histoplasma capsulatum

87390   HIV-1

87391   HIV-2

87400   Influenza, A or B, each

87420   respiratory syncytial virus

87425   rotavirus

87427   Shiga-like toxin

87430   Streptococcus, group A

87449   Infectious agent antigen detection by enzyme immunoassay technique qualitative or semiquantitative; multiple step method, not otherwise specified, each organism

87450   single step method, not otherwise specified, each organism

87451   multiple step method, polyvalent for multiple organisms, each polyvalent antiserum

87470   Infectious agent detection by nucleic acid (DNA or RNA); Bartonella henselae and Bartonella quintana, direct probe technique

87471   Bartonella henselae and Bartonella quintana, amplified probe technique

87472   Bartonella henselae and Bartonella quintana, quantification

87475   Borrelia burgdorferi, direct probe technique

87476   Borrelia burgdorferi, amplified probe technique

87477   Borrelia burgdorferi, quantification

87480   Candida species, direct probe technique

87481   Candida species, amplified probe technique

87482   Candida species, quantification

87485   Chlamydia pneumoniae, direct probe technique

87486   Chlamydia pneumoniae, amplified probe technique

87487   Chlamydia pneumoniae, quantification

87490   Chlamydia trachomatis, direct probe technique

87491   Chlamydia trachomatis, amplified probe technique

87492   Chlamydia trachomatis, quantification

87495   cytomegalovirus, direct probe technique

87496   cytomegalovirus, amplified probe technique

87497	cytomegalovirus, quantification
87510	Gardnerella vaginalis, direct probe technique
87511	Gardnerella vaginalis, amplified probe technique
87512	Gardnerella vaginalis, quantification
87515	hepatitis B virus, direct probe technique
87516	hepatitis B virus, amplified probe technique
87517	hepatitis B virus, quantification
87520	hepatitis C, direct probe technique
87521	hepatitis C, amplified probe technique
87522	hepatitis C, quantification
87525	hepatitis G, direct probe technique
87526	hepatitis G, amplified probe technique
87527	hepatitis G, quantification
87528	Herpes simplex virus, direct probe technique
87529	Herpes simplex virus, amplified probe technique
87530	Herpes simplex virus, quantification
87531	Herpes virus-6, direct probe technique
87532	Herpes virus-6, amplified probe technique
87533	Herpes virus-6, quantification
87534	HIV-1, direct probe technique
87535	HIV-1, amplified probe technique
87536	HIV-1, quantification
87537	HIV-2, direct probe technique
87538	HIV-2, amplified probe technique
87539	HIV-2, quantification
87540	Legionella pneumophila, direct probe technique
87541	Legionella pneumophila, amplified probe technique
87542	Legionella pneumophila, quantification
87550	Mycobacteria species, direct probe technique
87551	Mycobacteria species, amplified probe technique
87552	Mycobacteria species, quantification
87555	Mycobacteria tuberculosis, direct probe technique
87556	Mycobacteria tuberculosis, amplified probe technique
87557	Mycobacteria tuberculosis, quantification
87560	Mycobacteria avium-intracellulare, direct probe technique
87561	Mycobacteria avium-intracellulare, amplified probe technique
87562	Mycobacteria avium-intracellulare, quantification
87580	Mycoplasma pneumoniae, direct probe technique

87581	Mycoplasma pneumoniae, amplified probe technique
87582	Mycoplasma pneumoniae, quantification
87590	Neisseria gonorrhoeae, direct probe technique
87591	Neisseria gonorrhoeae, amplified probe technique
87592	Neisseria gonorrhoeae, quantification
87620	papillomavirus, human, direct probe technique
87621	papillomavirus, human, amplified probe technique
87622	papillomavirus, human, quantification
87650	Streptococcus, group A, direct probe technique
87651	Streptococcus, group A, amplified probe technique
87652	Streptococcus, group A, quantification
87797	Infectious agent detection by nucleic acid (DNA or RNA), not otherwise specified; direct probe technique, each organism
87798	amplified probe technique, each organism
87799	quantification, each organism
87800	Infectious agent detection by nucleic acid (DNA or RNA), multiple organisms; direct probe(s) technique
87801	amplified probe(s) technique
87802	Infectious agent antigen detection by immunoassay with direct optical observation; Streptococcus, group B
87803	Clostridium difficile toxin A
87804	Influenza
87810	Infectious agent detection by immunoassay with direct optical observation; Chlamydia trachomatis
87850	Neisseria gonorrhoeae
87880	Streptococcus, group A
87899	not otherwise specified
87901	Infectious agent genotype analysis by nucleic acid (DNA or RNA); HIV 1, reverse transcriptase and protease

(For infectious agent drug susceptibility phenotype prediction for HIV-1, use Category III code 0023T)

87902	Hepatitis C virus
87903	Infectious agent phenotype analysis by nucleic acid (DNA or RNA) with drug resistance tissue culture analysis, HIV 1; first through 10 drugs tested
+ 87904	each additional 1 through 5 drugs tested (List separately in addition to code for primary procedure)

(Use 87904 in conjunction with code 87903)

87999	Unlisted microbiology procedure

Pathology and Laboratory

Anatomic Pathology

Postmortem Examination

Procedures 88000 through 88099 represent physician services only. Use modifier '-90' or 09990 for outside laboratory services.

88000   Necropsy (autopsy), gross examination only; without CNS

88005   with brain

88007   with brain and spinal cord

88012   infant with brain

88014   stillborn or newborn with brain

88016   macerated stillborn

88020   Necropsy (autopsy), gross and microscopic; without CNS

88025   with brain

88027   with brain and spinal cord

88028   infant with brain

88029   stillborn or newborn with brain

88036   Necropsy (autopsy), limited, gross and/or microscopic; regional

88037   single organ

88040   Necropsy (autopsy); forensic examination

88045   coroner's call

88099   Unlisted necropsy (autopsy) procedure

Cytopathology

►(For cervicography, see Category III code 0003T)◄

88104   Cytopathology, fluids, washings or brushings, except cervical or vaginal; smears with interpretation

88106   filter method only with interpretation

88107   smears and filter preparation with interpretation

88108   Cytopathology, concentration technique, smears and interpretation (eg, Saccomanno technique)

(88109 has been deleted. For interpretation of smear, use 88104; for cell block interpretation, use 88305)

(For cervical or vaginal smears, see 88150-88155)

(For gastric intubation with lavage, see 89130-89141, 91055)

(For x-ray localization, use 74340)

88125   Cytopathology, forensic (eg, sperm)

88130   Sex chromatin identification; Barr bodies

88140   peripheral blood smear, polymorphonuclear drumsticks

(For Guard stain, use 88313)

Codes 88141-88155, 88164-88167 are used to report cervical or vaginal screening by various methods and to report physician interpretation services. Use codes 88150-88154 to report Pap smears that are examined using non-Bethesda reporting. Use codes 88164-88167 to report Pap smears that are examined using the Bethesda System of reporting. Use codes 88142-►88143◄ to report specimens collected in fluid medium with automated thin layer preparation that are examined using any system of reporting (Bethesda or non-Bethesda). Within each of these three code families choose the one code that describes the screening method(s) used. Codes 88141 and 88155 should be reported in addition to the screening code chosen when the additional services are provided.

+ 88141   Cytopathology, cervical or vaginal (any reporting system); requiring interpretation by physician (List separately in addition to code for technical service)

(Use 88141 in conjunction with codes 88142-88154, 88164-88167)

88142   Cytopathology, cervical or vaginal (any reporting system), collected in preservative fluid, automated thin layer preparation; manual screening under physician supervision

88143   with manual screening and rescreening under physician supervision

►(88144 has been deleted)◄

►(88145 has been deleted)◄

►(For automated screening of automated thin layer preparation, see 88174, 88175)◄

88147   Cytopathology smears, cervical or vaginal; screening by automated system under physician supervision

88148   screening by automated system with manual rescreening under physician supervision

88150   Cytopathology, slides, cervical or vaginal; manual screening under physician supervision

(88151 has been deleted. To report, use 88141)

88152   with manual screening and computer-assisted rescreening under physician supervision

88153   with manual screening and rescreening under physician supervision

88154   with manual screening and computer-assisted rescreening using cell selection and review under physician supervision

+ 88155 Cytopathology, slides, cervical or vaginal, definitive hormonal evaluation (eg, maturation index, karyopyknotic index, estrogenic index) (List separately in addition to code(s) for other technical and interpretation services)

(Use 88155 in conjunction with 88142-88154, 88164-88167)

(88156 has been deleted. To report, use 88164)

(88157 has been deleted. To report, use 88141)

(88158 has been deleted. To report, use 88166)

88160 Cytopathology, smears, any other source; screening and interpretation

88161 preparation, screening and interpretation

88162 extended study involving over 5 slides and/or multiple stains

(For obtaining specimen, see percutaneous needle biopsy under individual organ in **Surgery**)

(For aerosol collection of sputum, use 89350)

(For special stains, see 88312-88314)

88164 Cytopathology, slides, cervical or vaginal (the Bethesda System); manual screening under physician supervision

88165 with manual screening and rescreening under physician supervision

88166 with manual screening and computer-assisted rescreening under physician supervision

88167 with manual screening and computer-assisted rescreening using cell selection and review under physician supervision

(88170 has been deleted. To report, ►see◄ 10021, ►10022◄)

(88171 has been deleted. To report, ►see 10021,◄ 10022)

88172 Cytopathology, evaluation of fine needle aspirate; immediate cytohistologic study to determine adequacy of specimen(s)

88173 interpretation and report

● 88174 Cytopathology, cervical or vaginal (any reporting system), collected in preservative fluid, automated thin layer preparation; screening by automated system, under physician supervision

● 88175 with screening by automated system and manual rescreening, under physician supervision

►(For manual screening, see 88142, 88143)◄

88180 Flow cytometry; each cell surface, cytoplasmic or nuclear marker

88182 cell cycle or DNA analysis

(For tumor morphometry and DNA and ploidy analysis by imaging techniques, use 88358)

88199 Unlisted cytopathology procedure

(For electron microscopy, see 88348, 88349)

Cytogenetic Studies

(For acetylcholinesterase, use 82013)

(For alpha-fetoprotein, serum or amniotic fluid, see 82105, 82106)

(For laser microdissection of cells from tissue sample, see 88380)

88230 Tissue culture for non-neoplastic disorders; lymphocyte

88233 skin or other solid tissue biopsy

88235 amniotic fluid or chorionic villus cells

88237 Tissue culture for neoplastic disorders; bone marrow, blood cells

88239 solid tumor

88240 Cryopreservation, freezing and storage of cells, each cell line

►(For therapeutic cryopreservation and storage, use 38207)◄

88241 Thawing and expansion of frozen cells, each aliquot

►(For therapeutic thawing of previous harvest, use 38208)◄

88245 Chromosome analysis for breakage syndromes; baseline Sister Chromatid Exchange (SCE), 20-25 cells

88248 baseline breakage, score 50-100 cells, count 20 cells, 2 karyotypes (eg, for ataxia telangiectasia, Fanconi anemia, fragile X)

88249 score 100 cells, clastogen stress (eg, diepoxybutane, mitomycin C, ionizing radiation, UV radiation)

(88250 has been deleted. To report, use 88248)

(88260 has been deleted. To report, use 88261)

88261 Chromosome analysis; count 5 cells, 1 karyotype, with banding

88262 count 15-20 cells, 2 karyotypes, with banding

88263 count 45 cells for mosaicism, 2 karyotypes, with banding

88264 analyze 20-25 cells

(88265 has been deleted. To report, use 88262)

88267 Chromosome analysis, amniotic fluid or chorionic villus, count 15 cells, 1 karyotype, with banding

(88268 has been deleted. To report, use 88261)

88269 Chromosome analysis, in situ for amniotic fluid cells, count cells from 6-12 colonies, 1 karyotype, with banding

(88270 has been deleted. To report, use 88261)

88271 Molecular cytogenetics; DNA probe, each (eg, FISH)

88272 chromosomal in situ hybridization, analyze 3-5 cells (eg, for derivatives and markers)

Pathology and Laboratory

88273	chromosomal in situ hybridization, analyze 10-30 cells (eg, for microdeletions)
88274	interphase in situ hybridization, analyze 25-99 cells
88275	interphase in situ hybridization, analyze 100-300 cells
88280	Chromosome analysis; additional karyotypes, each study
88283	additional specialized banding technique (eg, NOR, C-banding)
88285	additional cells counted, each study
88289	additional high resolution study
88291	Cytogenetics and molecular cytogenetics, interpretation and report
88299	Unlisted cytogenetic study

Surgical Pathology

Services 88300 through 88309 include accession, examination, and reporting. They do not include the services designated in codes 88311 through 88365 and 88399, which are coded in addition when provided.

The unit of service for codes 88300 through 88309 is the specimen.

A specimen is defined as tissue or tissues that is (are) submitted for individual and separate attention, requiring individual examination and pathologic diagnosis. Two or more such specimens from the same patient (eg, separately identified endoscopic biopsies, skin lesions, etc.) are each appropriately assigned an individual code reflective of its proper level of service.

Service code 88300 is used for any specimen that in the opinion of the examining pathologist can be accurately diagnosed without microscopic examination. Service code 88302 is used when gross and microscopic examination is performed on a specimen to confirm identification and the absence of disease. Service codes 88304 through 88309 describe all other specimens requiring gross and microscopic examination, and represent additional ascending levels of physician work. Levels 88302 through 88309 are specifically defined by the assigned specimens.

Any unlisted specimen should be assigned to the code which most closely reflects the physician work involved when compared to other specimens assigned to that code.

88300	**Level I** - Surgical pathology, gross examination only
88302	**Level II** - Surgical pathology, gross and microscopic examination

Appendix, Incidental

Fallopian Tube, Sterilization

Fingers/Toes, Amputation, Traumatic

Foreskin, Newborn

Hernia Sac, Any Location

Hydrocele Sac

Nerve

Skin, Plastic Repair

Sympathetic Ganglion

Testis, Castration

Vaginal Mucosa, Incidental

Vas Deferens, Sterilization

88304	**Level III** - Surgical pathology, gross and microscopic examination

Abortion, Induced

Abscess

Aneurysm - Arterial/Ventricular

Anus, Tag

Appendix, Other than Incidental

Artery, Atheromatous Plaque

Bartholin's Gland Cyst

Bone Fragment(s), Other than Pathologic Fracture

Bursa/Synovial Cyst

Carpal Tunnel Tissue

Cartilage, Shavings

Cholesteatoma

Colon, Colostomy Stoma

Conjunctiva - Biopsy/Pterygium

Cornea

Diverticulum - Esophagus/Small Intestine

Dupuytren's Contracture Tissue

Femoral Head, Other than Fracture

Fissure/Fistula

Foreskin, Other than Newborn

Gallbladder

Ganglion Cyst

Hematoma

Hemorrhoids

Hydatid of Morgagni

Intervertebral Disc

Joint, Loose Body

Meniscus

Mucocele, Salivary

Neuroma - Morton's/Traumatic

Pilonidal Cyst/Sinus

Polyps, Inflammatory - Nasal/Sinusoidal

Skin - Cyst/Tag/Debridement

Soft Tissue, Debridement

Soft Tissue, Lipoma

Spermatocele

Tendon/Tendon Sheath

Testicular Appendage

Thrombus or Embolus

Tonsil and/or Adenoids

Varicocele

Vas Deferens, Other than Sterilization

Vein, Varicosity

88305   **Level IV** - Surgical pathology, gross and microscopic examination

Abortion - Spontaneous/Missed

Artery, Biopsy

Bone Marrow, Biopsy

Bone Exostosis

Brain/Meninges, Other than for Tumor Resection

Breast, Biopsy, Not Requiring Microscopic Evaluation of Surgical Margins

Breast, Reduction Mammoplasty

Bronchus, Biopsy

Cell Block, Any Source

Cervix, Biopsy

Colon, Biopsy

Duodenum, Biopsy

Endocervix, Curettings/Biopsy

Endometrium, Curettings/Biopsy

Esophagus, Biopsy

Extremity, Amputation, Traumatic

Fallopian Tube, Biopsy

Fallopian Tube, Ectopic Pregnancy

Femoral Head, Fracture

Fingers/Toes, Amputation, Non-traumatic

Gingiva/Oral Mucosa, Biopsy

Heart Valve

Joint, Resection

Kidney, Biopsy

Larynx, Biopsy

Leiomyoma(s), Uterine Myomectomy - without Uterus

Lip, Biopsy/Wedge Resection

Lung, Transbronchial Biopsy

Lymph Node, Biopsy

Muscle, Biopsy

Nasal Mucosa, Biopsy

Nasopharynx/Oropharynx, Biopsy

Nerve, Biopsy

Odontogenic/Dental Cyst

Omentum, Biopsy

Ovary with or without Tube, Non-neoplastic

Ovary, Biopsy/Wedge Resection

Parathyroid Gland

Peritoneum, Biopsy

Pituitary Tumor

Placenta, Other than Third Trimester

Pleura/Pericardium - Biopsy/Tissue

Polyp, Cervical/Endometrial

Polyp, Colorectal

Polyp, Stomach/Small Intestine

Prostate, Needle Biopsy

Prostate, TUR

Salivary Gland, Biopsy

Sinus, Paranasal Biopsy

Skin, Other than Cyst/Tag/Debridement/Plastic Repair

Small Intestine, Biopsy

Soft Tissue, Other than Tumor/Mass/Lipoma/Debridement

Spleen

Stomach, Biopsy

Synovium

Testis, Other than Tumor/Biopsy/Castration

Thyroglossal Duct/Brachial Cleft Cyst

Tongue, Biopsy

Tonsil, Biopsy

Trachea, Biopsy

Ureter, Biopsy

Urethra, Biopsy

Urinary Bladder, Biopsy

Uterus, with or without Tubes and Ovaries, for Prolapse

Vagina, Biopsy

Vulva/Labia, Biopsy

88307   **Level V** - Surgical pathology, gross and microscopic examination

Adrenal, Resection

Bone - Biopsy/Curettings

Pathology and Laboratory

Bone Fragment(s), Pathologic Fracture

Brain, Biopsy

Brain/Meninges, Tumor Resection

Breast, Excision of Lesion, Requiring Microscopic Evaluation of Surgical Margins

Breast, Mastectomy - Partial/Simple

Cervix, Conization

Colon, Segmental Resection, Other than for Tumor

Extremity, Amputation, Non-traumatic

Eye, Enucleation

Kidney, Partial/Total Nephrectomy

Larynx, Partial/Total Resection

Liver, Biopsy - Needle/Wedge

Liver, Partial Resection

Lung, Wedge Biopsy

Lymph Nodes, Regional Resection

Mediastinum, Mass

Myocardium, Biopsy

Odontogenic Tumor

Ovary with or without Tube, Neoplastic

Pancreas, Biopsy

Placenta, Third Trimester

Prostate, Except Radical Resection

Salivary Gland

Sentinel Lymph Node

Small Intestine, Resection, Other than for Tumor

Soft Tissue Mass (except Lipoma) - Biopsy/Simple Excision

Stomach - Subtotal/Total Resection, Other than for Tumor

Testis, Biopsy

Thymus, Tumor

Thyroid, Total/Lobe

Ureter, Resection

Urinary Bladder, TUR

Uterus, with or without Tubes and Ovaries, Other than Neoplastic/Prolapse

88309 **Level VI** - Surgical pathology, gross and microscopic examination

Bone Resection

Breast, Mastectomy - with Regional Lymph Nodes

Colon, Segmental Resection for Tumor

Colon, Total Resection

Esophagus, Partial/Total Resection

Extremity, Disarticulation

Fetus, with Dissection

Larynx, Partial/Total Resection - with Regional Lymph Nodes

Lung - Total/Lobe/Segment Resection

Pancreas, Total/Subtotal Resection

Prostate, Radical Resection

Small Intestine, Resection for Tumor

Soft Tissue Tumor, Extensive Resection

Stomach - Subtotal/Total Resection for Tumor

Testis, Tumor

Tongue/Tonsil - Resection for Tumor

Urinary Bladder, Partial/Total Resection

Uterus, with or without Tubes and Ovaries, Neoplastic

Vulva, Total/Subtotal Resection

(For fine needle aspiration, see 10021, 10022)

(For evaluation of fine needle aspirate, see 88172-88173)

+ 88311 Decalcification procedure (List separately in addition to code for surgical pathology examination)

+ 88312 Special stains (List separately in addition to code for surgical pathology examination); Group I for microorganisms (eg, Gridley, acid fast, methenamine silver), each

+ 88313 Group II, all other, (eg, iron, trichrome), except immunocytochemistry and immunoperoxidase stains, each

(For immunocytochemistry and immunoperoxidase tissue studies, use 88342)

+ 88314 histochemical staining with frozen section(s)

(88316 has been deleted. To report, use 99070)

(88317 has been deleted)

88318 Determinative histochemistry to identify chemical components (eg, copper, zinc)

88319 Determinative histochemistry or cytochemistry to identify enzyme constituents, each

88321 Consultation and report on referred slides prepared elsewhere

88323 Consultation and report on referred material requiring preparation of slides

88325 Consultation, comprehensive, with review of records and specimens, with report on referred material

88329 Pathology consultation during surgery;

88331 first tissue block, with frozen section(s), single specimen

88332 each additional tissue block with frozen section(s)

88342 Immunocytochemistry (including tissue immunoperoxidase), each antibody

(88345 has been deleted. To report, use 88346)

88346 Immunofluorescent study, each antibody; direct method

88347   indirect method

88348 Electron microscopy; diagnostic

88349   scanning

88355 Morphometric analysis; skeletal muscle

88356   nerve

88358   tumor

(When semi-thin plastic-embedded sections are performed in conjunction with morphometric analysis, only the morphometric analysis should be coded; if performed as an independent procedure, see codes 88300-88309 for surgical pathology.)

(88360 has been deleted. To report, use 88399)

88362 Nerve teasing preparations

88365 Tissue in situ hybridization, interpretation and report

(88370 has been deleted. To report, use 88342)

88371 Protein analysis of tissue by Western Blot, with interpretation and report;

88372   immunological probe for band identification, each

88380 Microdissection (eg, mechanical, laser capture)

88399 Unlisted surgical pathology procedure

Transcutaneous Procedures

88400 Bilirubin, total, transcutaneous

Other Procedures

(Basal metabolic rate has been deleted. If necessary to report, use 89399)

(89005-89007 have been deleted)

89050 Cell count, miscellaneous body fluids (eg, cerebrospinal fluid, joint fluid), except blood;

89051   with differential count

● **89055** Leukocyte count, fecal

89060 Crystal identification by light microscopy with or without polarizing lens analysis, any body fluid (except urine)

(89070, 89080 have been deleted)

89100 Duodenal intubation and aspiration; single specimen (eg, simple bile study or afferent loop culture) plus appropriate test procedure

89105   collection of multiple fractional specimens with pancreatic or gallbladder stimulation, single or double lumen tube

(For radiological localization, use 74340)

(For chemical analyses, see **Chemistry,** this section)

(Electrocardiogram, see 93000-93268)

(Esophagus acid perfusion test (Bernstein), see 91030)

89125 Fat stain, feces, urine, or respiratory secretions

89130 Gastric intubation and aspiration, diagnostic, each specimen, for chemical analyses or cytopathology;

89132   after stimulation

89135 Gastric intubation, aspiration, and fractional collections (eg, gastric secretory study); one hour

89136   two hours

89140   two hours including gastric stimulation (eg, histalog, pentagastrin)

89141   three hours, including gastric stimulation

(For gastric lavage, therapeutic, use 91105)

(For radiologic localization of gastric tube, use 74340)

(For chemical analyses, see 82926, 82928)

(Joint fluid chemistry, see **Chemistry,** this section)

89160 Meat fibers, feces

(89180 has been deleted. To report, use 89190)

89190 Nasal smear for eosinophils

(89205 has been deleted. To report, use 82273)

(Occult blood, feces, use 82270)

(Paternity tests, use 86910)

(89210 has been deleted)

89250 Culture and fertilization of oocyte(s);

89251   with co-culture of embryos

89252 Assisted oocyte fertilization, microtechnique (any method)

89253 Assisted embryo hatching, microtechniques (any method)

89254 Oocyte identification from follicular fluid

89255 Preparation of embryo for transfer (any method)

89256 Preparation of cryopreserved embryos for transfer (includes thaw)

89257 Sperm identification from aspiration (other than seminal fluid)

(For semen analysis, see 89300-89320)

(For sperm identification from testis tissue, use 89264)

89258	Cryopreservation; embryo
89259	sperm
89260	Sperm isolation; simple prep (eg, sperm wash and swim-up) for insemination or diagnosis with semen analysis
89261	complex prep (eg, Percoll gradient, albumin gradient) for insemination or diagnosis with semen analysis

(For semen analysis without sperm wash or swim-up, use 89320)

89264　Sperm identification from testis tissue, fresh or cryopreserved

(For biopsy of testis, see 54500, 54505)

(For sperm identification from aspiration, use 89257)

(For semen analysis, see 89300-89320)

89300　Semen analysis; presence and/or motility of sperm including Huhner test (post coital)

▲ **89310**　motility and count (not including Huhner test)

89320　complete (volume, count, motility, and differential)

(Skin tests, see 86485-86585 and 95010-95199)

89321　Semen analysis, presence and/or motility of sperm

(89323 has been deleted. To report, use 89325)

89325　Sperm antibodies

(For medicolegal identification of sperm, use 88125)

89329　Sperm evaluation; hamster penetration test

89330　cervical mucus penetration test, with or without spinnbarkeit test

(89345 has been deleted)

89350　Sputum, obtaining specimen, aerosol induced technique (separate procedure)

89355　Starch granules, feces

89360　Sweat collection by iontophoresis

(For chloride ▶analysis, use 82438,◀ and sodium analysis, use ▶84302)◀

89365　Water load test

89399　Unlisted miscellaneous pathology test

　⊘ = Modifier '-51' Exempt　　▶◀ or ▶ ◀ = New or Revised Text　　✚ = Add-on Code

Medicine Guidelines

In addition to the definitions and commonly used terms presented in the **Introduction**, several other items unique to this section on **Medicine** are defined or identified here.

Multiple Procedures

It is appropriate to designate multiple procedures that are rendered on the same date by separate entries. For example: If individual medical psychotherapy (90841) is rendered in addition to subsequent hospital care (eg, 99231), the psychotherapy would be reported separately from the hospital visit. In this instance, both 99231 and 90841 would be reported.

Add-on Codes

Some of the listed procedures are commonly carried out in addition to the primary procedure performed. All add-on codes found in *CPT* are exempt from the multiple procedure concept. They are exempt from the use of the modifier '-51', as these procedures are not reported as stand-alone codes. These additional or supplemental procedures are designated as "add-on" codes. Add-on codes in *CPT* can be readily identified by specific descriptor nomenclature which includes phrases such as "each additional" or "(List separately in addition to primary procedure)."

Separate Procedures

Some of the procedures or services listed in *CPT* that are commonly carried out as an integral component of a total service or procedure have been identified by the inclusion of the term "separate procedure." The codes designated as "separate procedure" should not be reported in addition to the code for the total procedure or service of which it is considered an integral component.

However, when a procedure or service that is designated as a "separate procedure" is carried out independently or considered to be unrelated or distinct from other procedures/services provided at that time, it may be reported by itself, or in addition to other procedures/services by appending the modifier '-59' to the specific "separate procedure" code to indicate that the procedure is not considered to be a component of another procedure, but is a distinct, independent procedure. This may represent a different session or patient encounter, different procedure or surgery,

different site or organ system, separate incision/excision, separate lesion, or separate injury (or area of injury in extensive injuries).

Subsection Information

Several of the subheadings or subsections have special instructions unique to that section. These special instructions will be presented preceding those procedural terminology listings, referring to that subsection specifically. If there is an "Unlisted Procedure" code number (see section below) for the individual subsection, it will also be shown. Those subsections within the **Medicine** section that have special instructions are as follows:

Immune Globulins	90281-90399
Immunization Administration for	
Vaccines/Toxoids	90471-90474
Vaccines, Toxoids	90476-90749
Therapeutic or	
Diagnostic Infusions	90780-90781
Psychiatry	90801-90899
Dialysis	90918-90999
Gastroenterology	91000-91299
Ophthalmology	92002-92499
Otorhinolaryngology	92502-92599
Echocardiography	93303-93350
Cardiac Catheterization	93501-93556
Intracardiac Electrophysiological	
Procedures/Studies	93600-93662
Peripheral Arterial Disease	
Rehabilitation	93668
Non-Invasive Vascular	
Diagnostic Studies	93875-93990
Pulmonary	94010-94799
Allergy and Clinical Immunology	95004-95199
Neurology and Neuromuscular	95805-95999
Neurostimulators,	
Analysis-Programming	95970-95975
Motion Analysis	96000-96004
Central Nervous System	
Assessments/Tests	96100-96117
Health and Behavior	
Assessment/Intervention	96150-96155
Chemotherapy Administration	96400-96549
Dermatological Procedures	96900-96999
Physical Medicine and Rehabilitation	
Modalities	97010-97028
Constant Attendance	97032-97039
Therapeutic Procedures	97110-97546
Active Wound	
Care Management	97601-97602

Osteopathic Manipulative
    Treatment 98925-98929
Chiropractic Manipulative
    Treatment 98940-98943
Special Services, Procedures and
    Reports 99000-99091
Conscious Sedation 99141-99142
Home Health
    Procedures/Services 99500-99539
Home Infusion Procedures 99551-99569

the nature, extent, and need for the procedure; and the time, effort, and equipment necessary to provide the service. Additional items which may be included are:

- complexity of symptoms;
- final diagnosis;
- pertinent physical findings;
- diagnostic and therapeutic procedures;
- concurrent problems;
- follow-up care.

Unlisted Service or Procedure

A service or procedure may be provided that is not listed in this edition of *CPT*. When reporting such a service, the appropriate "Unlisted Procedure" code may be used to indicate the service, identifying it by "Special Report" as discussed on this page. The "Unlisted Procedures" and accompanying codes for **Medicine** are as follows:

90399   Unlisted immune globulin

90749   Unlisted vaccine/toxoid

90799   Unlisted therapeutic, prophylactic or diagnostic injection

90899   Unlisted psychiatric service or procedure

90999   Unlisted dialysis procedure, inpatient or outpatient

91299   Unlisted diagnostic gastroenterology procedure

92499   Unlisted ophthalmological service or procedure

▶ **92700**   Unlisted otorhinolaryngological service or procedure◀

93799   Unlisted cardiovascular service or procedure

94799   Unlisted pulmonary service or procedure

95199   Unlisted allergy/clinical immunologic service or procedure

95999   Unlisted neurological or neuromuscular diagnostic procedure

96549   Unlisted chemotherapy procedure

96999   Unlisted special dermatological service or procedure

97039   Unlisted modality (specify type and time if constant attendance)

97139   Unlisted therapeutic procedure (specify)

97799   Unlisted physical medicine/rehabilitation service or procedure

99199   Unlisted special service, procedure or report

▶ **99600**   Unlisted home visit service or procedure◀

Materials Supplied by Physician

Supplies and materials provided by the physician (eg, sterile trays/drugs), over and above those usually included with the procedure(s) rendered are reported separately. List drugs, trays, supplies, and materials provided. Identify as 99070 or specific supply code.

Special Report

A service that is rarely provided, unusual, variable, or new may require a special report in determining medical appropriateness of the service. Pertinent information should include an adequate definition or description of

Medicine

(90000-90080 have been deleted. To report, see 99201-99215)

(90100-90170 have been deleted. To report, see 99341-99350)

(90200-90220 have been deleted. To report, see 99221-99223)

(90225 has been deleted. To report, use 99431)

(90240-90280 have been deleted. To report, see 99231-99233)

(90282 has been deleted. To report, use 99433)

(90292 has been deleted. To report, use 99238)

(90300-90370 have been deleted. To report, see 99301-99313)

(90400-90470 have been deleted. To report, see 99321-99333)

(90500-90580 have been deleted. To report, see 99281-99288)

(90590 has been deleted. To report, use 99288)

(90600-90630 have been deleted. To report, see 99241-99255)

(90640-90643 have been deleted. To report, see 99241-99245 or 99261-99263)

(90650-90654 have been deleted. To report, see 99271-99275)

(90699 has been deleted. To report, use 99499)

Immune Globulins

Codes 90281-90399 identify the immune globulin product only and must be reported in addition to the administration codes 90780-90784 as appropriate. Immune globulin products listed here include broad-spectrum and anti-infective immune globulins, antitoxins, and various isoantibodies.

⊘ **90281**   Immune globulin (Ig), human, for intramuscular use

⊘ **90283**   Immune globulin (IgIV), human, for intravenous use

⊘ **90287**   Botulinum antitoxin, equine, any route

⊘ **90288**   Botulism immune globulin, human, for intravenous use

⊘ **90291**   Cytomegalovirus immune globulin (CMV-IgIV), human, for intravenous use

⊘ **90296**   Diphtheria antitoxin, equine, any route

⊘ **90371**   Hepatitis B immune globulin (HBIg), human, for intramuscular use

⊘ **90375**   Rabies immune globulin (RIg), human, for intramuscular and/or subcutaneous use

⊘ **90376**   Rabies immune globulin, heat-treated (RIg-HT), human, for intramuscular and/or subcutaneous use

⊘ **90378**   Respiratory syncytial virus immune globulin (RSV-IgIM), for intramuscular use, 50 mg, each

⊘ **90379**   Respiratory syncytial virus immune globulin (RSV-IgIV), human, for intravenous use

⊘ **90384**   Rho(D) immune globulin (RhIg), human, full-dose, for intramuscular use

⊘ **90385**   Rho(D) immune globulin (RhIg), human, mini-dose, for intramuscular use

⊘ **90386**   Rho(D) immune globulin (RhIgIV), human, for intravenous use

⊘ **90389**   Tetanus immune globulin (TIg), human, for intramuscular use

⊘ **90393**   Vaccinia immune globulin, human, for intramuscular use

⊘ **90396**   Varicella-zoster immune globulin, human, for intramuscular use

⊘ **90399**   Unlisted immune globulin

Immunization Administration for Vaccines/Toxoids

Codes 90471-90474 must be reported in addition to the vaccine and toxoid code(s) 90476-90749.

If a significant separately identifiable Evaluation and Management service (eg, office or other outpatient services, preventive medicine services) is performed, the appropriate E/M service code should be reported in addition to the vaccine and toxoid administration codes.

(For allergy testing, see 95004 et seq)

(For skin testing of bacterial, viral, fungal extracts, see 86485-86586)

(For therapeutic or diagnostic injections, see 90782-90799)

90471   Immunization administration (includes percutaneous, intradermal, subcutaneous, intramuscular and jet injections); one vaccine (single or combination vaccine/toxoid)

+ **90472**   each additional vaccine (single or combination vaccine/toxoid) (List separately in addition to code for primary procedure)

(Use 90472 in conjunction with code 90471)

(For administration of immune globulins, use 90780-90784, and see 90281-90399)

(For intravesical administration of BCG vaccine, use 51720, and see 90586)

90473   Immunization administration by intranasal or oral route; one vaccine (single or combination vaccine/toxoid)

+ 90474   each additional vaccine (single or combination vaccine/toxoid) (List separately in addition to code for primary procedure)

(Use 90474 in conjunction with code 90473)

Vaccines, Toxoids

Codes 90476-90748 identify the vaccine product **only.** To report the administration of a vaccine/toxoid, the vaccine/toxoid product codes 90476-90749 must be used in addition to an immunization administration code(s) 90471, 90472. Do not append the modifier '-51' to the vaccine/toxoid product codes 90476-90749.

If a significantly separately identifiable Evaluation and Management service (eg, office or other outpatient services, preventive medicine services) is performed, the appropriate E/M service code should be reported in addition to the vaccine and toxoid administration codes.

To meet the reporting requirements of immunization registries, vaccine distribution programs, and reporting systems (eg, Vaccine Adverse Event Reporting System) the exact vaccine product administered needs to be reported. Multiple codes for a particular vaccine are provided in *CPT* when the schedule (number of doses or timing) differs for two or more products of the same vaccine type (eg, hepatitis A, Hib) or the vaccine product is available in more than one chemical formulation, dosage, or route of administration.

Separate codes are available for combination vaccines (eg, DTP-Hib, DtaP-Hib, HepB-Hib). It is inappropriate to code each component of a combination vaccine separately. If a specific vaccine code is not available, the unlisted procedure code should be reported, until a new code becomes available.

(For immune globulins, see codes 90281-90399, and 90780-90784 for administration of immune globulins)

⊘ **90476**   Adenovirus vaccine, type 4, live, for oral use

⊘ **90477**   Adenovirus vaccine, type 7, live, for oral use

⊘ **90581**   Anthrax vaccine, for subcutaneous use

⊘ **90585**   Bacillus Calmette-Guerin vaccine (BCG) for tuberculosis, live, for percutaneous use

⊘ **90586**   Bacillus Calmette-Guerin vaccine (BCG) for bladder cancer, live, for intravesical use

(90592 has been deleted)

⊘ **90632**   Hepatitis A vaccine, adult dosage, for intramuscular use

⊘ **90633**   Hepatitis A vaccine, pediatric/adolescent dosage-2 dose schedule, for intramuscular use

⊘ **90634**   Hepatitis A vaccine, pediatric/adolescent dosage-3 dose schedule, for intramuscular use

⊘ **90636**   Hepatitis A and hepatitis B vaccine (HepA-HepB), adult dosage, for intramuscular use

⊘ **90645**   Hemophilus influenza b vaccine (Hib), HbOC conjugate (4 dose schedule), for intramuscular use

⊘ **90646**   Hemophilus influenza b vaccine (Hib), PRP-D conjugate, for booster use only, intramuscular use

⊘ **90647**   Hemophilus influenza b vaccine (Hib), PRP-OMP conjugate (3 dose schedule), for intramuscular use

⊘ **90648**   Hemophilus influenza b vaccine (Hib), PRP-T conjugate (4 dose schedule), for intramuscular use

⊘ **90657**   Influenza virus vaccine, split virus, 6-35 months dosage, for intramuscular or jet injection use

⊘ **90658**   Influenza virus vaccine, split virus, 3 years and above dosage, for intramuscular or jet injection use

⊘ **90659**   Influenza virus vaccine, whole virus, for intramuscular or jet injection use

⊘ **90660**   Influenza virus vaccine, live, for intranasal use

⊘ **90665**   Lyme disease vaccine, adult dosage, for intramuscular use

⊘ **90669**   Pneumococcal conjugate vaccine, polyvalent, for children under five years, for intramuscular use

⊘ **90675**   Rabies vaccine, for intramuscular use

⊘ **90676**   Rabies vaccine, for intradermal use

⊘ **90680**   Rotavirus vaccine, tetravalent, live, for oral use

⊘ **90690**   Typhoid vaccine, live, oral

⊘ **90691**   Typhoid vaccine, Vi capsular polysaccharide (ViCPs), for intramuscular use

⊘ **90692**   Typhoid vaccine, heat- and phenol-inactivated (H-P), for subcutaneous or intradermal use

⊘ **90693**   Typhoid vaccine, acetone-killed, dried (AKD), for subcutaneous or jet injection use (U.S. military)

⊘ **90700**   Diphtheria, tetanus toxoids, and acellular pertussis vaccine (DTaP), for intramuscular use

⊘ **90701**   Diphtheria, tetanus toxoids, and whole cell pertussis vaccine (DTP), for intramuscular use

⊘ **90702**   Diphtheria and tetanus toxoids (DT) adsorbed for use in individuals younger than seven years, for intramuscular use

⊘ **90703**   Tetanus toxoid adsorbed, for intramuscular or jet injection use

⊘ **90704**   Mumps virus vaccine, live, for subcutaneous or jet injection use

⊘ **90705** Measles virus vaccine, live, for subcutaneous or jet injection use

⊘ **90706** Rubella virus vaccine, live, for subcutaneous or jet injection use

⊘ **90707** Measles, mumps and rubella virus vaccine (MMR), live, for subcutaneous or jet injection use

⊘ **90708** Measles and rubella virus vaccine, live, for subcutaneous or jet injection use

►(90709 has been deleted)◄

⊘ **90710** Measles, mumps, rubella, and varicella vaccine (MMRV), live, for subcutaneous use

(90711 has been deleted)

⊘ **90712** Poliovirus vaccine, (any type(s)) (OPV), live, for oral use

⊘ **90713** Poliovirus vaccine, inactivated, (IPV), for subcutaneous use

(90714 has been deleted. To report, see 90690-90693)

⊘ **90716** Varicella virus vaccine, live, for subcutaneous use

⊘ **90717** Yellow fever vaccine, live, for subcutaneous use

⊘ **90718** Tetanus and diphtheria toxoids (Td) adsorbed for use in individuals seven years or older, for intramuscular or jet injection

⊘ **90719** Diphtheria toxoid, for intramuscular use

⊘ **90720** Diphtheria, tetanus toxoids, and whole cell pertussis vaccine and Hemophilus influenza B vaccine (DTP-Hib), for intramuscular use

⊘ **90721** Diphtheria, tetanus toxoids, and acellular pertussis vaccine and Hemophilus influenza B vaccine (DtaP-Hib), for intramuscular use

(90724 has been deleted. To report, see 90657-90660)

⊘ **90723** Diphtheria, tetanus toxoids, acellular pertussis vaccine, Hepatitis B, and poliovirus vaccine, inactivated (DtaP-HepB-IPV), for intramuscular use

⊘ **90725** Cholera vaccine for injectable use

(For oral cholera, use 90592)

(90726 has been deleted. To report, see 90675, 90676)

⊘ **90727** Plague vaccine, for intramuscular or jet injection use

(90728 has been deleted. To report, see 90585, 90586)

(90730 has been deleted. To report, see 90632-90634)

(90731 has been deleted. To report, see 90744-90747)

⊘ **90732** Pneumococcal polysaccharide vaccine, 23-valent, adult or immunosuppressed patient dosage, for use in individuals 2 years or older, for subcutaneous or intramuscular use

⊘ **90733** Meningococcal polysaccharide vaccine (any group(s)), for subcutaneous or jet injection use

⊘ **90735** Japanese encephalitis virus vaccine, for subcutaneous use

(90737 has been deleted. To report, see 90645-90648)

(90741 has been deleted. To report, see 90281-90283)

(90742 has been deleted. To report, see 90287-90399)

⊘ **90740** Hepatitis B vaccine, dialysis or immunosuppressed patient dosage (3 dose schedule), for intramuscular use

⊘ **90743** Hepatitis B vaccine, adolescent (2 dose schedule), for intramuscular use

⊘ **90744** Hepatitis B vaccine, pediatric/adolescent dosage (3 dose schedule), for intramuscular use

(90745 has been deleted)

⊘ **90746** Hepatitis B vaccine, adult dosage, for intramuscular use

⊘ **90747** Hepatitis B vaccine, dialysis or immunosuppressed patient dosage (4 dose schedule), for intramuscular use

⊘ **90748** Hepatitis B and Hemophilus influenza b vaccine (HepB-Hib), for intramuscular use

⊘ **90749** Unlisted vaccine/toxoid

(90750-90754 have been deleted. To report, see 99381-99387)

(90755 has been deleted)

(90757 has been deleted. To report, use 99432)

(90760-90764 have been deleted. To report, see 99391-99397)

(90774 has been deleted. To report, use 96110)

(90778 has been deleted. To report, use 94772)

Therapeutic or Diagnostic Infusions (Excludes Chemotherapy)

These procedures encompass prolonged intravenous injections.

These codes require the presence of the physician during the infusion. These codes are not to be used for intradermal, subcutaneous or intramuscular or routine IV drug injections. For these services, see 90782-90788.

These codes may not be used in addition to prolonged services codes.

90780 Intravenous infusion for therapy/diagnosis, administered by physician or under direct supervision of physician; up to one hour

+ 90781 each additional hour, up to eight (8) hours (List separately in addition to code for primary procedure)

(Use 90781 in conjunction with code 90780)

Therapeutic, Prophylactic or Diagnostic Injections

90782   Therapeutic, prophylactic or diagnostic injection (specify material injected); subcutaneous or intramuscular

(For administration of vaccines/toxoids, see 90471-90472)

90783   intra-arterial

90784   intravenous

(90782-90784 do not include injections for allergen immunotherapy. For allergen immunotherapy injections, see 95115-95117)

90788   Intramuscular injection of antibiotic (specify)

(90790-90796 have been deleted. To report, see ▶95990◀, 96408-96414, 96420-96425, 96440, 96450, 96530, 96545, 96549)

(90798 has been deleted. To report, see 90780, 90781, 90784)

90799   Unlisted therapeutic, prophylactic or diagnostic injection

(For allergy immunizations, see 95004 et seq)

Psychiatry

(For repetitive transcranial magnetic stimulation for treatment of clinical depression, use Category III code 0018T)

Hospital care by the attending physician in treating a psychiatric inpatient or partial hospitalization may be initial or subsequent in nature (see 99221-99233) and may include exchanges with nursing and ancillary personnel. Hospital care services involve a variety of responsibilities unique to the medical management of inpatients, such as physician hospital orders, interpretation of laboratory or other medical diagnostic studies and observations.

Some patients receive hospital evaluation and management services only and others receive evaluation and management services and other procedures. If other procedures such as electroconvulsive therapy or psychotherapy are rendered in addition to hospital evaluation and management services, these should be listed separately (ie, hospital care service plus electroconvulsive therapy or when psychotherapy is done, an appropriate code defining psychotherapy with medical evaluation and management services). The modifier '-22' may be used to indicate a more extensive service. The modifier '-52' may be used to signify a service that is reduced or less extensive than the usual procedure.

Other evaluation and management services, such as office medical service or other patient encounters, may be described as listed in the section on **Evaluation and Management,** if appropriate.

The evaluation and management services should not be reported separately, when reporting codes 90805, 90807, 90809, 90811, 90813, 90815, 90817, 90819, 90822, 90824, 90827, 90829.

Consultation for psychiatric evaluation of a patient includes examination of a patient and exchange of information with the primary physician and other informants such as nurses or family members, and preparation of a report. These consultation services (99241-99263) are limited to initial or follow-up evaluation and do not involve psychiatric treatment.

Psychiatric Diagnostic or Evaluative Interview Procedures

Psychiatric diagnostic interview examination includes a history, mental status, and a disposition, and may include communication with family or other sources, ordering and medical interpretation of laboratory or other medical diagnostic studies. In certain circumstances other informants will be seen in lieu of the patient.

Interactive psychiatric diagnostic interview examination is typically furnished to children. It involves the use of physical aids and non-verbal communication to overcome barriers to therapeutic interaction between the clinician and a patient who has not yet developed, or has lost, either the expressive language communication skills to explain his/her symptoms and response to treatment, or the receptive communication skills to understand the clinician if he/she were to use ordinary adult language for communication.

90801   Psychiatric diagnostic interview examination

90802   Interactive psychiatric diagnostic interview examination using play equipment, physical devices, language interpreter, or other mechanisms of communication

Psychiatric Therapeutic Procedures

Psychotherapy is the treatment for mental illness and behavioral disturbances in which the clinician establishes a professional contract with the patient and, through definitive therapeutic communication, attempts to alleviate the emotional disturbances, reverse or change maladaptive patterns of behavior, and encourage personality growth and development. The codes for reporting psychotherapy are divided into two broad categories: Interactive Psychotherapy; and Insight Oriented, Behavior Modifying and/or Supportive Psychotherapy.

Interactive psychotherapy is typically furnished to children. It involves the use of physical aids and non-verbal communication to overcome barriers to therapeutic interaction between the clinician and a patient who has not yet developed, or has lost, either the expressive language communication skills to explain his/her symptoms and response to treatment, or the receptive communication skills to understand the clinician if he/she were to use ordinary adult language for communication.

Insight oriented, behavior modifying and/or supportive psychotherapy refers to the development of insight or affective understanding, the use of behavior modification techniques, the use of supportive interactions, the use of cognitive discussion of reality, or any combination of the above to provide therapeutic change.

Some patients receive psychotherapy only and others receive psychotherapy and medical evaluation and management services. These evaluation and management services involve a variety of responsibilities unique to the medical management of psychiatric patients, such as medical diagnostic evaluation (eg, evaluation of comorbid medical conditions, drug interactions, and physical examinations), drug management when indicated, physician orders, interpretation of laboratory or other medical diagnostic studies and observations.

In reporting psychotherapy, the appropriate code is chosen on the basis of the type of psychotherapy (interactive using non-verbal techniques versus insight oriented, behavior modifying and/or supportive using verbal techniques), the place of service (office versus inpatient), the face-to-face time spent with the patient during psychotherapy, and whether evaluation and management services are furnished on the same date of service as psychotherapy.

To report medical evaluation and management services furnished on a day when psychotherapy is not provided, select the appropriate code from the **Evaluation and Management Services Guidelines.**

Office or Other Outpatient Facility

Insight Oriented, Behavior Modifying and/or Supportive Psychotherapy

90804 Individual psychotherapy, insight oriented, behavior modifying and/or supportive, in an office or outpatient facility, approximately 20 to 30 minutes face-to-face with the patient;

90805   with medical evaluation and management services

90806 Individual psychotherapy, insight oriented, behavior modifying and/or supportive, in an office or outpatient facility, approximately 45 to 50 minutes face-to-face with the patient;

90807   with medical evaluation and management services

90808 Individual psychotherapy, insight oriented, behavior modifying and/or supportive, in an office or outpatient facility, approximately 75 to 80 minutes face-to-face with the patient;

90809   with medical evaluation and management services

Interactive Psychotherapy

90810 Individual psychotherapy, interactive, using play equipment, physical devices, language interpreter, or other mechanisms of non-verbal communication, in an office or outpatient facility, approximately 20 to 30 minutes face-to-face with the patient;

90811   with medical evaluation and management services

90812 Individual psychotherapy, interactive, using play equipment, physical devices, language interpreter, or other mechanisms of non-verbal communication, in an office or outpatient facility, approximately 45 to 50 minutes face-to-face with the patient;

90813   with medical evaluation and management services

90814 Individual psychotherapy, interactive, using play equipment, physical devices, language interpreter, or other mechanisms of non-verbal communication, in an office or outpatient facility, approximately 75 to 80 minutes face-to-face with the patient;

90815   with medical evaluation and management services

Inpatient Hospital, Partial Hospital or Residential Care Facility

Insight Oriented, Behavior Modifying and/or Supportive Psychotherapy

90816 Individual psychotherapy, insight oriented, behavior modifying and/or supportive, in an inpatient hospital, partial hospital or residential care setting, approximately 20 to 30 minutes face-to-face with the patient;

90817   with medical evaluation and management services

90818 Individual psychotherapy, insight oriented, behavior modifying and/or supportive, in an inpatient hospital, partial hospital or residential care setting, approximately 45 to 50 minutes face-to-face with the patient;

90819   with medical evaluation and management services

(90820 has been deleted. To report, use 90802)

90821 Individual psychotherapy, insight oriented, behavior modifying and/or supportive, in an inpatient hospital, partial hospital or residential care setting, approximately 75 to 80 minutes face-to-face with the patient;

90822   with medical evaluation and management services

Medicine

Interactive Psychotherapy

90823 Individual psychotherapy, interactive, using play equipment, physical devices, language interpreter, or other mechanisms of non-verbal communication, in an inpatient hospital, partial hospital or residential care setting, approximately 20 to 30 minutes face-to-face with the patient;

90824 with medical evaluation and management services

(90825 has been deleted. To report, use 90885)

90826 Individual psychotherapy, interactive, using play equipment, physical devices, language interpreter, or other mechanisms of non-verbal communication, in an inpatient hospital, partial hospital or residential care setting, approximately 45 to 50 minutes face-to-face with the patient;

90827 with medical evaluation and management services

90828 Individual psychotherapy, interactive, using play equipment, physical devices, language interpreter, or other mechanisms of non-verbal communication, in an inpatient hospital, partial hospital or residential care setting, approximately 75 to 80 minutes face-to-face with the patient;

90829 with medical evaluation and management services

(90830 has been deleted. To report, use 96100)

(90831 has been deleted. To report, see 99371-99373)

(90835 has been deleted. To report, use 90865)

(90841 has been deleted)

(90842 has been deleted. To report, see 90808, 90809, 90821, 90822)

(90843 has been deleted. To report, see 90804, 90805, 90816, 90817)

(90844 has been deleted. To report, see 90806, 90807, 90818, 90819)

Other Psychotherapy

90845 Psychoanalysis

90846 Family psychotherapy (without the patient present)

90847 Family psychotherapy (conjoint psychotherapy) (with patient present)

(90848 has been deleted. To report, use 90847)

90849 Multiple-family group psychotherapy

90853 Group psychotherapy (other than of a multiple-family group)

(90855 has been deleted. To report, see 90810-90815, and 90823-90829)

90857 Interactive group psychotherapy

Other Psychiatric Services or Procedures

90862 Pharmacologic management, including prescription, use, and review of medication with no more than minimal medical psychotherapy

90865 Narcosynthesis for psychiatric diagnostic and therapeutic purposes (eg, sodium amobarbital (Amytal) interview)

90870 Electroconvulsive therapy (includes necessary monitoring); single seizure

90871 multiple seizures, per day

(90872 has been deleted. To report, use 90899)

90875 Individual psychophysiological therapy incorporating biofeedback training by any modality (face-to-face with the patient), with psychotherapy (eg, insight oriented, behavior modifying or supportive psychotherapy); approximately 20-30 minutes

90876 approximately 45-50 minutes

90880 Hypnotherapy

90882 Environmental intervention for medical management purposes on a psychiatric patient's behalf with agencies, employers, or institutions

90885 Psychiatric evaluation of hospital records, other psychiatric reports, psychometric and/or projective tests, and other accumulated data for medical diagnostic purposes

90887 Interpretation or explanation of results of psychiatric, other medical examinations and procedures, or other accumulated data to family or other responsible persons, or advising them how to assist patient

90889 Preparation of report of patient's psychiatric status, history, treatment, or progress (other than for legal or consultative purposes) for other physicians, agencies, or insurance carriers

90899 Unlisted psychiatric service or procedure

Biofeedback

(For psychophysiological therapy incorporating biofeedback training, see 90875, 90876)

(90900 has been deleted. To report, use 90901)

90901 Biofeedback training by any modality

(90902, 90904, 90906, 90908, 90910 have been deleted. To report, use 90901)

90911 Biofeedback training, perineal muscles, anorectal or urethral sphincter, including EMG and/or manometry

▶(For incontinence treatment by pulsed magnetic neuromodulation, use Category III code 0029T)◀

(90915 has been deleted. To report, use 90901)

Dialysis

Codes 90918-90921 are reported ONCE per month to distinguish age-specific services related to the patient's end-stage renal disease (ESRD) performed in an outpatient setting. ESRD related physician services include establishment of a dialyzing cycle, outpatient evaluation and management of the dialysis visits, telephone calls, and patient management during the dialysis, provided during a full month. These codes are not used if a hospitalization occurred during the month.

Codes 90918-90921 do not include the dialysis treatment (90935, 90937, 90945, 90947) or any non-ESRD related services or other patient care services rendered outside of the dialysis setting during that month.

Evaluation and management services unrelated to ESRD services that cannot be performed during the dialysis session may be reported separately.

Codes 90922-90925 are reported when outpatient ESRD related services are not performed consecutively during an entire full month. Codes 90922-90925 are used to report ESRD related services on a per day basis for the remaining days of that month, preceding and/or following the period of hospitalization.

Example:

A four-year old receiving continuous peritoneal dialysis has sixteen days of daily outpatient care, preceding or following a period of hospitalization.

Report 90923 for each date outpatient care was performed.

For ESRD related services and dialysis procedure(s) performed during period of hospitalization: Report appropriate inpatient Evaluation and Management Service code(s) for the hospitalized period if service(s) is unrelated to ESRD services. Report 90945 or 90947 for each inpatient dialysis procedure.

End Stage Renal Disease Services

90918   End stage renal disease (ESRD) related services per full month; for patients under two years of age to include monitoring for the adequacy of nutrition, assessment of growth and development, and counseling of parents

90919   for patients between two and eleven years of age to include monitoring for the adequacy of nutrition, assessment of growth and development, and counseling of parents

90920   for patients between twelve and nineteen years of age to include monitoring for the adequacy of nutrition, assessment of growth and development, and counseling of parents

90921   for patients twenty years of age and over

90922   End stage renal disease (ESRD) related services (less than full month), per day; for patients under two years of age

90923   for patients between two and eleven years of age

90924   for patients between twelve and nineteen years of age

90925   for patients twenty years of age and over

Hemodialysis

Codes 90935, 90937 are reported to describe the hemodialysis procedure with all evaluation and management services related to the patient's renal disease on the day of the hemodialysis procedure. These codes are used for inpatient ESRD and non-ESRD procedures or for outpatient non-ESRD dialysis services. Code 90935 is reported if only one evaluation of the patient is required related to that hemodialysis procedure. Code 90937 is reported when patient re-evaluation(s) is required during a hemodialysis procedure. Utilize the modifier '-25' with Evaluation and Management codes for separately identifiable services unrelated to the dialysis procedure or renal failure which cannot be rendered during the dialysis session.

(For home visit hemodialysis services performed by a non-physician health care professional, use 99512)

(For cannula declotting, see 36831, 36833, 36860, 36861)

(For declotting of implanted vascular access device or catheter by thrombolytic agent, use 36550)

(For collection of blood specimen from a partially or completely implantable venous access device, use 36540)

(For prolonged physician attendance, see 99354-99360)

90935   Hemodialysis procedure with single physician evaluation

90937   Hemodialysis procedure requiring repeated evaluation(s) with or without substantial revision of dialysis prescription

90939   Hemodialysis access flow study to determine blood flow in grafts and arteriovenous fistulae by an indicator dilution method, hook-up; transcutaneous measurement and disconnection

90940   measurement and disconnection

(For duplex scan of hemodialysis access, use 93990)

(90941-90944 have been deleted. To report, see 90935-90937)

Miscellaneous Dialysis Procedures

Codes 90945, 90947 describe dialysis procedures other than hemodialysis (eg, peritoneal dialysis, hemofiltration or continuous renal replacement therapies), and all evaluation and management services related to the patient's renal disease on the day of the procedure. Code 90945 is reported if only one evaluation of the patient is

Medicine

required related to that procedure. Code 90947 is reported when patient re-evaluation(s) is required during a procedure. Utilize the modifier '-25' with Evaluation and Management codes for separately identifiable services unrelated to the procedure or the renal failure which cannot be rendered during the dialysis session.

(For insertion of intraperitoneal cannula or catheter, see 49420, 49421)

(For prolonged physician attendance, see 99354-99360)

90945   Dialysis procedure other than hemodialysis (eg, peritoneal dialysis, hemofiltration, or other continuous renal replacement therapies), with single physician evaluation

(For home infusion of peritoneal dialysis, use 99559)

90947   Dialysis procedure other than hemodialysis (eg, peritoneal dialysis, hemofiltration, or other continuous renal replacement therapies) requiring repeated physician evaluations, with or without substantial revision of dialysis prescription

(90951-90958 have been deleted. To report, see 90935, 90937)

(90966-90985 have been deleted. To report, see 90945, 90947)

(90988, 90991 and 90994 have been deleted. To report, see 90918-90921)

90989   Dialysis training, patient, including helper where applicable, any mode, completed course

(90990, 90992 have been deleted. To report, see 90989 and 90993)

90993   Dialysis training, patient, including helper where applicable, any mode, course not completed, per training session

(90995 has been deleted. To report, see 90918-90921)

90997   Hemoperfusion (eg, with activated charcoal or resin)

(90998 has been deleted. To report, use 90922)

90999   Unlisted dialysis procedure, inpatient or outpatient

Gastroenterology

(For duodenal intubation and aspiration, see 89100-89105)

(For gastrointestinal radiologic procedures, see 74210-74363)

(For esophagoscopy procedures, see 43200-43228; upper GI endoscopy 43234-43259; endoscopy, small intestine and stomal 44360-44393; proctosigmoidoscopy 45300-45321; sigmoidoscopy 45330-45339; colonoscopy 45355-45385; anoscopy 46600-46615)

91000   Esophageal intubation and collection of washings for cytology, including preparation of specimens (separate procedure)

91010   Esophageal motility (manometric study of the esophagus and/or gastroesophageal junction) study;

91011   with mecholyl or similar stimulant

91012   with acid perfusion studies

91020   Gastric motility (manometric) studies

91030   Esophagus, acid perfusion (Bernstein) test for esophagitis

91032   Esophagus, acid reflux test, with intraluminal pH electrode for detection of gastroesophageal reflux;

91033   prolonged recording

91052   Gastric analysis test with injection of stimulant of gastric secretion (eg, histamine, insulin, pentagastrin, calcium and secretin)

(For gastric biopsy by capsule, peroral, via tube, one or more specimens, use 43600)

(For gastric laboratory procedures, see also 89130-89141)

91055   Gastric intubation, washings, and preparing slides for cytology (separate procedure)

(For gastric lavage, therapeutic, use 91105)

91060   Gastric saline load test

(For biopsy by capsule, small intestine, per oral, via tube (one or more specimens), use 44100)

91065   Breath hydrogen test (eg, for detection of lactase deficiency)

(91090 has been deleted)

91100   Intestinal bleeding tube, passage, positioning and monitoring

91105   Gastric intubation, and aspiration or lavage for treatment (eg, for ingested poisons)

(For cholangiography, see 47500, 74320)

(For abdominal paracentesis, see 49080, 49081; with instillation of medication, see 96440, 96445)

(For peritoneoscopy, use 49320; with biopsy, use 49321)

(For peritoneoscopy and guided transhepatic cholangiography, use 47560; with biopsy, use 47561)

(For splenoportography, see 38200, 75810)

91122   Anorectal manometry

91123   Pulsed irrigation of fecal impaction

Gastric Physiology

91132   Electrogastrography, diagnostic, transcutaneous;

91133   with provocative testing

Other Procedures

91299   Unlisted diagnostic gastroenterology procedure

Ophthalmology

(For surgical procedures, see **Surgery,** Eye and Ocular Adnexa, 65091 et seq)

Definitions

Intermediate ophthalmological services describes an evaluation of a new or existing condition complicated with a new diagnostic or management problem not necessarily relating to the primary diagnosis, including history, general medical observation, external ocular and adnexal examination and other diagnostic procedures as indicated; may include the use of mydriasis for ophthalmoscopy.

For example:

a. Review of history, external examination, ophthalmoscopy, biomicroscopy for an acute complicated condition (eg, iritis) not requiring comprehensive ophthalmological services.

b. Review of interval history, external examination, ophthalmoscopy, biomicroscopy and tonometry in established patient with known cataract not requiring comprehensive ophthalmological services.

Comprehensive ophthalmological services describes a general evaluation of the complete visual system. The comprehensive services constitute a single service entity but need not be performed at one session. The service includes history, general medical observation, external and ophthalmoscopic examinations, gross visual fields and basic sensorimotor examination. It often includes, as indicated: biomicroscopy, examination with cycloplegia or mydriasis and tonometry. It always includes initiation of diagnostic and treatment programs.

Intermediate and comprehensive ophthalmological services constitute integrated services in which medical decision making cannot be separated from the examining techniques used. Itemization of service components, such as slit lamp examination, keratometry, routine ophthalmoscopy, retinoscopy, tonometry, or motor evaluation is not applicable.

For example:

The comprehensive services required for diagnosis and treatment of a patient with symptoms indicating possible disease of the visual system, such as glaucoma, cataract or retinal disease, or to rule out disease of the visual system, new or established patient.

Initiation of diagnostic and treatment program includes the prescription of medication, and arranging for special ophthalmological diagnostic or treatment services, consultations, laboratory procedures and radiological services.

Special ophthalmological services describes services in which a special evaluation of part of the visual system is made, which goes beyond the services included under general ophthalmological services, or in which special treatment is given. Special ophthalmological services may be reported in addition to the general ophthalmological services or evaluation and management services.

For example:

Fluorescein angioscopy, quantitative visual field examination, refraction or extended color vision examination (such as Nagel's anomaloscope) should be separately reported.

Prescription of lenses, when required, is included in 92015 Determination of refractive state. It includes specification of lens type (monofocal, bifocal, other), lens power, axis, prism, absorptive factor, impact resistance, and other factors.

Interpretation and report by the physician is an integral part of special ophthalmological services where indicated. Technical procedures (which may or may not be performed by the physician personally) are often part of the service, but should not be mistaken to constitute the service itself.

General Ophthalmological Services

New Patient

Solely for the purposes of distinguishing between new and established patients, **professional services** are those face-to-face services rendered by a physician and reported by a specific CPT code(s). A new patient is one who has not received any professional services from the physician or another physician of the same specialty who belongs to the same group practice within the past three years.

92002　Ophthalmological services: medical examination and evaluation with initiation of diagnostic and treatment program; intermediate, new patient

92004　　comprehensive, new patient, one or more visits

Established Patient

Solely for the purposes of distinguishing between new and established patients, **professional services** are those face-to-face services rendered by a physician and reported by a specific CPT code(s). An established patient is one who has received professional services from the physician or another physician of the same specialty who belongs to the same group practice within the past three years.

92012　Ophthalmological services: medical examination and evaluation, with initiation or continuation of diagnostic and treatment program; intermediate, established patient

92014　　comprehensive, established patient, one or more visits

(For surgical procedures, see **Surgery,** Eye and Ocular Adnexa, 65091 et seq)

Medicine

Special Ophthalmological Services

92015 Determination of refractive state

92018 Ophthalmological examination and evaluation, under general anesthesia, with or without manipulation of globe for passive range of motion or other manipulation to facilitate diagnostic examination; complete

92019   limited

92020 Gonioscopy (separate procedure)

(For gonioscopy under general anesthesia, use 92018)

92060 Sensorimotor examination with multiple measurements of ocular deviation (eg, restrictive or paretic muscle with diplopia) with interpretation and report (separate procedure)

92065 Orthoptic and/or pleoptic training, with continuing medical direction and evaluation

92070 Fitting of contact lens for treatment of disease, including supply of lens

92081 Visual field examination, unilateral or bilateral, with interpretation and report; limited examination (eg, tangent screen, Autoplot, arc perimeter, or single stimulus level automated test, such as Octopus 3 or 7 equivalent)

92082   intermediate examination (eg, at least 2 isopters on Goldmann perimeter, or semiquantitative, automated suprathreshold screening program, Humphrey suprathreshold automatic diagnostic test, Octopus program 33)

92083   extended examination (eg, Goldmann visual fields with at least 3 isopters plotted and static determination within the central 30°, or quantitative, automated threshold perimetry, Octopus program G-1, 32 or 42, Humphrey visual field analyzer full threshold programs 30-2, 24-2, or 30/60-2)

(Gross visual field testing (eg, confrontation testing) is a part of general ophthalmological services and is not reported separately)

92100 Serial tonometry (separate procedure) with multiple measurements of intraocular pressure over an extended time period with interpretation and report, same day (eg, diurnal curve or medical treatment of acute elevation of intraocular pressure)

92120 Tonography with interpretation and report, recording indentation tonometer method or perilimbal suction method

92130 Tonography with water provocation

92135 Scanning computerized ophthalmic diagnostic imaging (eg, scanning laser) with interpretation and report, unilateral

92136 Ophthalmic biometry by partial coherence interferometry with intraocular lens power calculation

92140 Provocative tests for glaucoma, with interpretation and report, without tonography

Ophthalmoscopy

Routine ophthalmoscopy is part of general and special ophthalmologic services whenever indicated. It is a non-itemized service and is not reported separately.

92225 Ophthalmoscopy, extended, with retinal drawing (eg, for retinal detachment, melanoma), with interpretation and report; initial

92226   subsequent

92230 Fluorescein angioscopy with interpretation and report

92235 Fluorescein angiography (includes multiframe imaging) with interpretation and report

92240 Indocyanine-green angiography (includes multiframe imaging) with interpretation and report

92250 Fundus photography with interpretation and report

92260 Ophthalmodynamometry

(For ophthalmoscopy under general anesthesia, use 92018)

Other Specialized Services

92265 Needle oculoelectromyography, one or more extraocular muscles, one or both eyes, with interpretation and report

92270 Electro-oculography with interpretation and report

92275 Electroretinography with interpretation and report

(92280 has been deleted. To report visual evoked potential testing of the central nervous system, use 95930)

(For electronystagmography for vestibular function studies, see 92541 et seq)

(For ophthalmic echography (diagnostic ultrasound), see 76511-76529)

92283 Color vision examination, extended, eg, anomaloscope or equivalent

(Color vision testing with pseudoisochromatic plates (such as HRR or Ishihara) is not reported separately. It is included in the appropriate general or ophthalmological service, or 99172)

92284 Dark adaptation examination with interpretation and report

92285 External ocular photography with interpretation and report for documentation of medical progress (eg, close-up photography, slit lamp photography, goniophotography, stereo-photography)

92286 Special anterior segment photography with interpretation and report; with specular endothelial microscopy and cell count

92287   with fluorescein angiography

Contact Lens Services

The prescription of contact lens includes specification of optical and physical characteristics (such as power, size, curvature, flexibility, gas-permeability). It is NOT a part of the general ophthalmological services.

The fitting of contact lens includes instruction and training of the wearer and incidental revision of the lens during the training period.

Follow-up of successfully fitted extended wear lenses is reported as part of a general ophthalmological service (92012 et seq).

The supply of contact lenses may be reported as part of the service of fitting. It may also be reported separately by using 92391 or 92396 and modifier '-26' for the service of fitting without supply.

> (For therapeutic or surgical use of contact lens, see 68340, 92070)

92310   Prescription of optical and physical characteristics of and fitting of contact lens, with medical supervision of adaptation; corneal lens, both eyes, except for aphakia

> (For prescription and fitting of one eye, add modifier '-52')

92311   corneal lens for aphakia, one eye

92312   corneal lens for aphakia, both eyes

92313   corneoscleral lens

92314   Prescription of optical and physical characteristics of contact lens, with medical supervision of adaptation and direction of fitting by independent technician; corneal lens, both eyes except for aphakia

> (For prescription and fitting of one eye, add modifier '-52')

92315   corneal lens for aphakia, one eye

92316   corneal lens for aphakia, both eyes

92317   corneoscleral lens

92325   Modification of contact lens (separate procedure), with medical supervision of adaptation

92326   Replacement of contact lens

Ocular Prosthetics, Artificial Eye

92330   Prescription, fitting, and supply of ocular prosthesis (artificial eye), with medical supervision of adaptation

> (If supply is not included, use modifier '-26'; to report supply separately, use 92393)

92335   Prescription of ocular prosthesis (artificial eye) and direction of fitting and supply by independent technician, with medical supervision of adaptation

Spectacle Services (Including Prosthesis for Aphakia)

Prescription of lenses, when required, is included in 92015 Determination of refractive state. It includes specification of lens type (monofocal, bifocal, other), lens power, axis, prism, absorptive factor, impact resistance, and other factors.

Fitting of spectacles is a separate service; when provided by the physician, it is reported as indicated by 92340-92371.

Fitting includes measurement of anatomical facial characteristics, the writing of laboratory specifications, and the final adjustment of the spectacles to the visual axes and anatomical topography. Presence of physician is not required.

Supply of materials is a separate service component; it is not part of the service of fitting spectacles.

92340   Fitting of spectacles, except for aphakia; monofocal

92341   bifocal

92342   multifocal, other than bifocal

92352   Fitting of spectacle prosthesis for aphakia; monofocal

92353   multifocal

92354   Fitting of spectacle mounted low vision aid; single element system

92355   telescopic or other compound lens system

92358   Prosthesis service for aphakia, temporary (disposable or loan, including materials)

92370   Repair and refitting spectacles; except for aphakia

92371   spectacle prosthesis for aphakia

Supply of Materials

92390   Supply of spectacles, except prosthesis for aphakia and low vision aids

92391   Supply of contact lenses, except prosthesis for aphakia

> (For supply of contact lenses reported as part of the service of fitting, see 92310-92313)

> (For replacement of contact lens, use 92326)

92392   Supply of low vision aids (A low vision aid is any lens or device used to aid or improve visual function in a person whose vision cannot be normalized by conventional spectacle correction. Includes reading additions up to 4D.)

92393   Supply of ocular prosthesis (artificial eye)

> (For supply reported as part of the service of fitting, use 92330)

Medicine

92395   Supply of permanent prosthesis for aphakia; spectacles

(For temporary spectacle correction, use 92358)

92396   contact lenses

(For supply reported as part of the service of fitting, see 92311, 92312)

(Use 99070 for the supply of other materials, drugs, trays, etc.)

Other Procedures

92499   Unlisted ophthalmological service or procedure

Special Otorhinolaryngologic Services

Diagnostic or treatment procedures usually included in a comprehensive otorhinolaryngologic evaluation or office visit, are reported as an integrated medical service, using appropriate descriptors from the 99201 series. Itemization of component procedures (eg, otoscopy, rhinoscopy, tuning fork test) does not apply.

Special otorhinolaryngologic services are those diagnostic and treatment services not usually included in a comprehensive otorhinolaryngologic evaluation or office visit. These services are reported separately, using descriptors from the 92500 series.

All services include medical diagnostic evaluation. Technical procedures (which may or may not be performed by the physician personally) are often part of the service, but should not be mistaken to constitute the service itself.

(For laryngoscopy with stroboscopy, use 31579)

92502   Otolaryngologic examination under general anesthesia

92504   Binocular microscopy (separate diagnostic procedure)

92506   Evaluation of speech, language, voice, communication, auditory processing, and/or aural rehabilitation status

92507   Treatment of speech, language, voice, communication, and/or auditory processing disorder (includes aural rehabilitation); individual

92508   group, two or more individuals

92510   Aural rehabilitation following cochlear implant (includes evaluation of aural rehabilitation status and hearing, therapeutic services) with or without speech processor programming

92511   Nasopharyngoscopy with endoscope (separate procedure)

92512   Nasal function studies (eg, rhinomanometry)

92516   Facial nerve function studies (eg, electroneuronography)

92520   Laryngeal function studies

▶(92525 has been deleted. To report, see 92610-92611 for specific evaluation)◀

92526   Treatment of swallowing dysfunction and/or oral function for feeding

Vestibular Function Tests, With Observation and Evaluation by Physician, Without Electrical Recording

92531   Spontaneous nystagmus, including gaze

92532   Positional nystagmus test

92533   Caloric vestibular test, each irrigation (binaural, bithermal stimulation constitutes four tests)

92534   Optokinetic nystagmus test

Vestibular Function Tests, With Recording (eg, ENG, PENG), and Medical Diagnostic Evaluation

92541   Spontaneous nystagmus test, including gaze and fixation nystagmus, with recording

92542   Positional nystagmus test, minimum of 4 positions, with recording

92543   Caloric vestibular test, each irrigation (binaural, bithermal stimulation constitutes four tests), with recording

92544   Optokinetic nystagmus test, bidirectional, foveal or peripheral stimulation, with recording

92545   Oscillating tracking test, with recording

92546   Sinusoidal vertical axis rotational testing

+ 92547   Use of vertical electrodes (List separately in addition to code for primary procedure)

(Use 92547 in conjunction with codes 92541-92546)

(For unlisted vestibular tests, use 92599)

92548   Computerized dynamic posturography

Audiologic Function Tests With Medical Diagnostic Evaluation

The audiometric tests listed below imply the use of calibrated electronic equipment. Other hearing tests (such as whispered voice, tuning fork) are considered part of the general otorhinolaryngologic services and are not reported separately. All descriptors refer to testing both ears. Use the modifier '-52' if a test is applied to one ear instead of to two ears. All descriptors (except 92559) apply to testing of individuals; for testing of groups, use 92559 and specify test(s) used.

(For evaluation of speech, language and/or hearing problems through observation and assessment of performance, use 92506)

| 92551 | Screening test, pure tone, air only |

92552   Pure tone audiometry (threshold); air only

92553   air and bone

92555   Speech audiometry threshold;

92556   with speech recognition

92557   Comprehensive audiometry threshold evaluation and speech recognition (92553 and 92556 combined)

(For hearing aid evaluation and selection, see 92590-92595)

92559   Audiometric testing of groups

92560   Bekesy audiometry; screening

92561   diagnostic

92562   Loudness balance test, alternate binaural or monaural

92563   Tone decay test

92564   Short increment sensitivity index (SISI)

92565   Stenger test, pure tone

(92566 has been deleted. To report, use 92567)

92567   Tympanometry (impedance testing)

92568   Acoustic reflex testing

92569   Acoustic reflex decay test

92571   Filtered speech test

92572   Staggered spondaic word test

92573   Lombard test

(92574 has been deleted)

92575   Sensorineural acuity level test

92576   Synthetic sentence identification test

92577   Stenger test, speech

(92578 has been deleted)

92579   Visual reinforcement audiometry (VRA)

(92580 has been deleted)

(92581 has been deleted. To report, use 92585)

92582   Conditioning play audiometry

92583   Select picture audiometry

92584   Electrocochleography

92585   Auditory evoked potentials for evoked response audiometry and/or testing of the central nervous system; comprehensive

92586   limited

92587   Evoked otoacoustic emissions; limited (single stimulus level, either transient or distortion products)

92588   comprehensive or diagnostic evaluation (comparison of transient and/or distortion product otoacoustic emissions at multiple levels and frequencies)

92589   Central auditory function test(s) (specify)

92590   Hearing aid examination and selection; monaural

92591   binaural

92592   Hearing aid check; monaural

92593   binaural

92594   Electroacoustic evaluation for hearing aid; monaural

92595   binaural

92596   Ear protector attenuation measurements

▲ 92597   Evaluation for use and/or fitting of voice prosthetic device to supplement oral speech

▶(To report augmentative and alternative communication device services, see 92605, 92607, 92608)◀

▶(92598 has been deleted)◀

▶(92599 has been deleted. To report use 92700)◀

▶Evaluative and Therapeutic Services◀

▶Codes 92601 and 92603 describe post-operative analysis and fitting of previously placed external devices, connection to the cochlear implant, and programming of the stimulator. Codes 92602 and 92604 describe subsequent sessions for measurements and adjustment of the external transmitter and re-programming of the internal stimulator.◀

▶(For placement of cochlear implant, use 69930)◀

● 92601   Diagnostic analysis of cochlear implant, patient under 7 years of age; with programming

● 92602   subsequent reprogramming

▶(Do not report 92602 in addition to 92601)◀

▶(For aural rehabilitation services following cochlear implant, including evaluation of rehabilitation status, use 92507)◀

● 92603   Diagnostic analysis of cochlear implant, age 7 years or older; with programming

● 92604   subsequent reprogramming

▶(Do not report 92604 in addition to 92603)◀

● 92605   Evaluation for prescription of non-speech-generating augmentative and alternative communication device

● 92606   Therapeutic service(s) for the use of non-speech-generating device, including programming and modification

● 92607   Evaluation for prescription for speech-generating augmentative and alternative communication device, face-to-face with the patient; first hour

▶(For evaluation for prescription of a non-speech-generating device, use 92605)◀

+ ● 92608   each additional 30 minutes (List separately in addition to code for primary procedure)

▶(Use 92608 in conjunction with 92607)◀

Medicine

▲=Revised Code   ●=New Code

● **92609**   Therapeutic services for the use of speech-generating device, including programming and modification

▶(For therapeutic service(s) for the use of a non-speech-generating device, use 92606)◀

● **92610**   Evaluation of oral and pharyngeal swallowing function

▶(For motion fluoroscopic evaluation of swallowing function, use 92611)◀

▶(For flexible endoscopic examination, use 92612-92617)◀

● **92611**   Motion fluoroscopic evaluation of swallowing function by cine or video recording

▶(For radiological supervision and interpretation, use 74230)◀

▶(For evaluation of oral and pharyngeal swallowing function, use 92610)◀

● **92612**   Flexible fiberoptic endoscopic evaluation of swallowing by cine or video recording;

▶(If flexible fiberoptic or endoscopic evaluation of swallowing is performed without cine or video recording, use 92700)◀

● **92613**   physician interpretation and report only

▶(To report an evaluation of oral and pharyngeal swallowing function, use 92610)◀

▶(To report motion fluoroscopic evaluation of swallowing function, use 92611)◀

● **92614**   Flexible fiberoptic endoscopic evaluation, laryngeal sensory testing by cine or video recording;

● **92615**   physician interpretation and report only

● **92616**   Flexible fiberoptic endoscopic evaluation of swallowing and laryngeal sensory testing by cine or video recording;

● **92617**   physician interpretation and report only

▶Other Procedures◀

● **92700**   Unlisted otorhinolaryngological service or procedure

Cardiovascular

Therapeutic Services

(For non-surgical septal reduction therapy (eg, alcohol ablation), use Category III code 0024T)

92950   Cardiopulmonary resuscitation (eg, in cardiac arrest)

(See also critical care services, 99291, 99292)

92953   Temporary transcutaneous pacing

(For physician direction of ambulance or rescue personnel outside the hospital, use 99288)

92960   Cardioversion, elective, electrical conversion of arrhythmia; external

92961   internal (separate procedure)

(Do not report 92961 in addition to codes 93662, 93618-93624, 93631, 93640-93642, 93650-93652, 93741-93744)

92970   Cardioassist-method of circulatory assist; internal

92971   external

(For balloon atrial-septostomy, use 92992)

(For placement of catheters for use in circulatory assist devices such as intra-aortic balloon pump, use 33970)

+ **92973**   Percutaneous transluminal coronary thrombectomy (List separately in addition to code for primary procedure)

(Use 92973 in conjunction with codes 92980, 92982)

+ **92974**   Transcatheter placement of radiation delivery device for subsequent coronary intravascular brachytherapy (List separately in addition to code for primary procedure)

(Use 92974 in conjunction with codes 92980, 92982, 93508)

(For intravascular radioelement application, see 77781-77784)

92975   Thrombolysis, coronary; by intracoronary infusion, including selective coronary angiography

92977   by intravenous infusion

(For thrombolysis of vessels other than coronary, see 37201, 75896)

(For cerebral thrombolysis, use 37195)

+ **92978**   Intravascular ultrasound (coronary vessel or graft) during diagnostic evaluation and/or therapeutic intervention including imaging supervision, interpretation and report; initial vessel (List separately in addition to code for primary procedure)

+ **92979**   each additional vessel (List separately in addition to code for primary procedure)

(Use 92979 in conjunction with code 92978)

(Intravascular ultrasound services include all transducer manipulations and repositioning within the specific vessel being examined, both before and after therapeutic intervention (eg, stent placement))

92980   Transcatheter placement of an intracoronary stent(s), percutaneous, with or without other therapeutic intervention, any method; single vessel

+ **92981**   each additional vessel (List separately in addition to code for primary procedure)

(Use 92981 in conjunction with code 92980)

(To report additional vessels treated by angioplasty or atherectomy only during the same session, see 92984, 92996)

Medicine

(To report transcatheter placement of radiation delivery device for coronary intravascular brachytherapy, use 92974)

(For intravascular radioelement application, see 77781-77784)

92982 Percutaneous transluminal coronary balloon angioplasty; single vessel

+ 92984 each additional vessel (List separately in addition to code for primary procedure)

(Use 92984 in conjunction with codes 92980, 92982, 92995)

(For stent placement following completion of angioplasty or atherectomy, see 92980, 92981)

(To report transcatheter placement of radiation delivery device for coronary intravascular brachytherapy, use 92974)

(For intravascular radioelement application, see 77781-77784)

92986 Percutaneous balloon valvuloplasty; aortic valve

92987 mitral valve

92990 pulmonary valve

92992 Atrial septectomy or septostomy; transvenous method, balloon (eg, Rashkind type) (includes cardiac catheterization)

92993 blade method (Park septostomy) (includes cardiac catheterization)

92995 Percutaneous transluminal coronary atherectomy, by mechanical or other method, with or without balloon angioplasty; single vessel

+ 92996 each additional vessel (List separately in addition to code for primary procedure)

(Use 92996 in conjunction with code(s) 92980, 92982, 92995)

(For stent placement following completion of angioplasty or atherectomy, see 92980, 92981)

(To report additional vessels treated by angioplasty only during the same session, use 92984)

92997 Percutaneous transluminal pulmonary artery balloon angioplasty; single vessel

+ 92998 each additional vessel (List separately in addition to code for primary procedure)

(Use 92998 in conjunction with code 92997)

Cardiography

(For echocardiography, see 93303-93350)

93000 Electrocardiogram, routine ECG with at least 12 leads; with interpretation and report

93005 tracing only, without interpretation and report

93010 interpretation and report only

(For ECG monitoring, see 99354-99360)

▲ 93012 Telephonic transmission of post-symptom electrocardiogram rhythm strip(s), 24-hour attended monitoring, per 30 day period of time; tracing only

93014 physician review with interpretation and report only

93015 Cardiovascular stress test using maximal or submaximal treadmill or bicycle exercise, continuous electrocardiographic monitoring, and/or pharmacological stress; with physician supervision, with interpretation and report

93016 physician supervision only, without interpretation and report

93017 tracing only, without interpretation and report

93018 interpretation and report only

93024 Ergonovine provocation test

93025 Microvolt T-wave alternans for assessment of ventricular arrhythmias

93040 Rhythm ECG, one to three leads; with interpretation and report

93041 tracing only without interpretation and report

93042 interpretation and report only

(93045 has been deleted. To report, use 93615)

(93201, 93202, 93204, 93205, 93208, 93209 and 93210 have been deleted. To report, use 93799)

(93220, 93221, 93222 have been deleted. To report, use 93799)

93224 Electrocardiographic monitoring for 24 hours by continuous original ECG waveform recording and storage, with visual superimposition scanning; includes recording, scanning analysis with report, physician review and interpretation

93225 recording (includes hook-up, recording, and disconnection)

93226 scanning analysis with report

93227 physician review and interpretation

93230 Electrocardiographic monitoring for 24 hours by continuous original ECG waveform recording and storage without superimposition scanning utilizing a device capable of producing a full miniaturized printout; includes recording, microprocessor-based analysis with report, physician review and interpretation

93231 recording (includes hook-up, recording, and disconnection)

93232 microprocessor-based analysis with report

93233 physician review and interpretation

Medicine

93235 Electrocardiographic monitoring for 24 hours by continuous computerized monitoring and non-continuous recording, and real-time data analysis utilizing a device capable of producing intermittent full-sized waveform tracings, possibly patient activated; includes monitoring and real-time data analysis with report, physician review and interpretation

93236 monitoring and real-time data analysis with report

93237 physician review and interpretation

(93255 has been deleted)

(93258, 93259, 93262, 93263, 93266 have been deleted. To report, see 93224-93237)

▲ **93268** Patient demand single or multiple event recording with presymptom memory loop, 24-hour attended monitoring, per 30 day period of time; includes transmission, physician review and interpretation

(93269 has been deleted. To report, use 93268)

93270 recording (includes hook-up, recording, and disconnection)

93271 monitoring, receipt of transmissions, and analysis

93272 physician review and interpretation only

(For postsymptom recording, see 93012, 93014)

(For implanted patient activated cardiac event recording, see 33282, 93727)

(93273-93277 have been deleted. To report, see 93224-93237)

93278 Signal-averaged electrocardiography (SAECG), with or without ECG

(For interpretation and report only, use 93278 with modifier '-26')

(For unlisted cardiographic procedure, use 93799)

(93280 has been deleted. To report, use 76000)

Echocardiography

Echocardiography includes obtaining ultrasonic signals from the heart and great arteries, with two-dimensional image and/or Doppler ultrasonic signal documentation, and interpretation and report. When interpretation is performed separately use modifier '-26'.

(For fetal echocardiography, see 76825-76828)

(93300 has been deleted)

93303 Transthoracic echocardiography for congenital cardiac anomalies; complete

93304 follow-up or limited study

(93305 has been deleted)

93307 Echocardiography, transthoracic, real-time with image documentation (2D) with or without M-mode recording; complete

93308 follow-up or limited study

(93309 has been deleted. To report, see 93307, 93308)

93312 Echocardiography, transesophageal, real time with image documentation (2D) (with or without M-mode recording); including probe placement, image acquisition, interpretation and report

93313 placement of transesophageal probe only

93314 image acquisition, interpretation and report only

93315 Transesophageal echocardiography for congenital cardiac anomalies; including probe placement, image acquisition, interpretation and report

93316 placement of transesophageal probe only

93317 image acquisition, interpretation and report only

93318 Echocardiography, transesophageal (TEE) for monitoring purposes, including probe placement, real time 2-dimensional image acquisition and interpretation leading to ongoing (continuous) assessment of (dynamically changing) cardiac pumping function and to therapeutic measures on an immediate time basis

✚ **93320** Doppler echocardiography, pulsed wave and/or continuous wave with spectral display (List separately in addition to codes for echocardiographic imaging); complete

(Use 93320 in conjunction with codes 93303, 93304, 93307, 93308, 93312, 93314, 93315, 93317, 93350)

✚ **93321** follow-up or limited study (List separately in addition to codes for echocardiographic imaging)

(Use 93321 in conjunction with codes 93303, 93304, 93307, 93308, 93312, 93314, 93315, 93317, 93950)

✚ **93325** Doppler echocardiography color flow velocity mapping (List separately in addition to codes for echocardiography)

(Use 93325 in conjunction with codes 76825, 76826, 76827, 76828, 93303, 93304, 93307, 93308, 93312, 93314, 93315, 93317, 93320, 93321, 93350)

93350 Echocardiography, transthoracic, real-time with image documentation (2D), with or without M-mode recording, during rest and cardiovascular stress test using treadmill, bicycle exercise and/or pharmacologically induced stress, with interpretation and report

(The appropriate stress testing code from the 93015-93018 series should be reported in addition to 93350 to capture the exercise stress portion of the study)

Cardiac Catheterization

Cardiac catheterization is a diagnostic medical procedure which includes introduction, positioning and repositioning of catheter(s), when necessary, recording of intracardiac and intravascular pressure, obtaining blood samples for measurement of blood gases or dilution curves and cardiac output measurements (Fick or other method, with or without rest and exercise and/or studies) with or without electrode catheter placement, final evaluation and report of procedure. When selective injection procedures are performed without a preceding cardiac catheterization, these services should be reported using codes in the Vascular Injection Procedures section, 36011-36015 and 36215-36218.

When coronary artery, arterial coronary conduit or venous bypass graft angiography is performed without concomitant left heart cardiac catheterization, use 93508. Injection procedures 93539, 93540, 93544, and 93545 represent separate identifiable services and may be coded in conjunction with one another in addition to code 93508, as appropriate. To report imaging supervision, interpretation and report in conjunction with code 93508, use code 93556.

Modifier '-51' should not be appended to codes 93501-93533, 93539-93556

⊘ **93501**   Right heart catheterization

(For bundle of His recording, use 93600)

⊘ **93503**   Insertion and placement of flow directed catheter (eg, Swan-Ganz) for monitoring purposes

(For subsequent monitoring, see 99356-99357)

⊘ **93505**   Endomyocardial biopsy

⊘ **93508**   Catheter placement in coronary artery(s), arterial coronary conduit(s), and/or venous coronary bypass graft(s) for coronary angiography without concomitant left heart catheterization

(93508 is to be used only when left heart catheterization 93510, 93511, 93524, 93526 is not performed)

(93508 is to be used only once per procedure)

(To report transcatheter placement of radiation delivery device for coronary intravascular brachytherapy, use 92974)

(For intravascular radioelement application, see 77781-77784)

⊘ **93510**   Left heart catheterization, retrograde, from the brachial artery, axillary artery or femoral artery; percutaneous

⊘ **93511**   by cutdown

⊘ **93514**   Left heart catheterization by left ventricular puncture

(93515 has been deleted. To report, use 93524)

⊘ **93524**   Combined transseptal and retrograde left heart catheterization

⊘ **93526**   Combined right heart catheterization and retrograde left heart catheterization

⊘ **93527**   Combined right heart catheterization and transseptal left heart catheterization through intact septum (with or without retrograde left heart catheterization)

⊘ **93528**   Combined right heart catheterization with left ventricular puncture (with or without retrograde left heart catheterization)

⊘ **93529**   Combined right heart catheterization and left heart catheterization through existing septal opening (with or without retrograde left heart catheterization)

⊘ **93530**   Right heart catheterization, for congenital cardiac anomalies

⊘ **93531**   Combined right heart catheterization and retrograde left heart catheterization, for congenital cardiac anomalies

⊘ **93532**   Combined right heart catheterization and transseptal left heart catheterization through intact septum with or without retrograde left heart catheterization, for congenital cardiac anomalies

⊘ **93533**   Combined right heart catheterization and transseptal left heart catheterization through existing septal opening, with or without retrograde left heart catheterization, for congenital cardiac anomalies

(93535 has been deleted. To report, see 33971)

(93536 has been deleted. To report, use 33967)

(When injection procedures are performed in conjunction with cardiac catheterization, these services do not include introduction of catheters but do include repositioning of catheters when necessary and use of automatic power injectors. Injection procedures 93539-93545 represent separate identifiable services and may be coded in conjunction with one another when appropriate. The technical details of angiography, supervision of filming and processing, interpretation and report are not included. To report imaging supervision, interpretation and report, use 93555 and/or 93556. Modifier '-51' should not be appended to 93539-93556.)

⊘ **93539**   Injection procedure during cardiac catheterization; for selective opacification of arterial conduits (eg, internal mammary), whether native or used for bypass

⊘ **93540**   for selective opacification of aortocoronary venous bypass grafts, one or more coronary arteries

⊘ **93541**   for pulmonary angiography

⊘ **93542**   for selective right ventricular or right atrial angiography

⊘ **93543**   for selective left ventricular or left atrial angiography

⊘ **93544**   for aortography

Medicine

⊘ **93545**   for selective coronary angiography (injection of radiopaque material may be by hand)

(93546 has been deleted. To report, use 93510 and 93543)

(To report imaging supervision and interpretation, use 93555)

(93547 has been deleted. To report, use 93510, 93543, and 93545)

(To report imaging supervision and interpretation, use 93555 and 93556)

(93548 has been deleted. To report, use 93510, 93543, 93544, 93545)

(To report imaging supervision and interpretation, use 93555 and 93556)

(93549 has been deleted. To report, use 93526, 93527 or 93528; 93543, 93545)

(To report imaging supervision and interpretation, use 93555 and 93556)

(93550 has been deleted. To report, use 93526 or 93527 or 93528; 93540, 93543; and 93545)

(To report imaging supervision and interpretation, use 93555 and 93556)

(93551 has been deleted. To report, use 93539 or 93540)

(93552 has been deleted. To report, use 93510; 93539 or 93540; 93543 and 93545)

(To report imaging supervision and interpretation, use 93555 and 93556)

(93553 has been deleted. To report, use 93510; 93539 or 93540; 93543, 93544, 93545)

(To report imaging supervision and interpretation, use 93555 and 93556)

⊘ **93555**   Imaging supervision, interpretation and report for injection procedure(s) during cardiac catheterization; ventricular and/or atrial angiography

⊘ **93556**   pulmonary angiography, aortography, and/or selective coronary angiography including venous bypass grafts and arterial conduits (whether native or used in bypass)

(Codes 93561 and 93562 are not to be used with cardiac catheterization codes)

93561   Indicator dilution studies such as dye or thermal dilution, including arterial and/or venous catheterization; with cardiac output measurement (separate procedure)

93562   subsequent measurement of cardiac output

(For radioisotope method of cardiac output, see 78472, 78473, or 78481)

(93570 has been deleted. To report, use 92982)

+ **93571**   Intravascular doppler velocity and/or pressure derived coronary flow reserve measurement (coronary vessel or graft) during coronary angiography including pharmacologically induced stress; initial vessel (List separately in addition to code for primary procedure)

+ **93572**   each additional vessel (List separately in addition to code for primary procedure)

(Intravascular distal coronary blood flow velocity measurements include all Doppler transducer manipulations and repositioning within the specific vessel being examined, during coronary angiography or therapeutic intervention (eg, angioplasty))

(For unlisted cardiac catheterization procedure, use 93799)

►Repair of Septal Defect◄

● **93580**   Percutaneous transcatheter closure of congenital interatrial communication (ie, fontan fenestration, atrial septal defect) with implant

►(Percutaneous transcatheter closure of atrial septal defect includes a right heart catheterization procedure. Code 93580 includes injection of contrast for atrial and ventricular angiograms. Codes 93501, 93529-93533, 93539, 93543, 93555 should not be reported separately in addition to code 93580)◄

● **93581**   Percutaneous transcatheter closure of a congenital ventricular septal defect with implant

►(Percutaneous transcatheter closure of ventricular septal defect (ie, fontan fenestration) includes a right heart catheterization procedure. Code 93581 includes injection of contrast for atrial and ventricular angiograms. Codes 93501, 93529-93533, 93539, 93543, 93555 should not be reported separately in addition to code 93581)◄

►(For echocardiographic services performed in addition to 93580, 93581, see 93303-93317 as appropriate)◄

Intracardiac Electrophysiological Procedures/Studies

Intracardiac electrophysiologic studies (EPS) are an invasive diagnostic medical procedure which include the insertion and repositioning of electrode catheters, recording of electrograms before and during pacing or programmed stimulation of multiple locations in the heart, analysis of recorded information, and report of the procedure. Electrophysiologic studies are most often performed with two or more electrode catheters. In many circumstances, patients with arrhythmias are evaluated and treated at the same encounter. In this situation, a diagnostic *electrophysiologic study* is performed, induced tachycardia(s) are *mapped*, and on the basis of the diagnostic and mapping information, the tissue is *ablated*. Electrophysiologic study(ies), mapping, and ablation represent distinctly different procedures, requiring individual reporting whether performed on the same or subsequent dates.

Definitions

Arrhythmia Induction: In most electrophysiologic studies, an attempt is made to induce arrhythmia(s) from single or multiple sites within the heart. Arrhythmia induction is achieved by performing pacing at different rates, programmed stimulation (introduction of critically timed electrical impulses), and other techniques. Because arrhythmia induction occurs via the same catheter(s) inserted for the electrophysiologic study(ies), catheter insertion and temporary pacemaker codes are not additionally reported. Codes 93600-93603, 93610-93612 and 93618 are used to describe unusual situations where there may be recording, pacing or an attempt at arrhythmia induction from only one site in the heart. Code 93619 describes only evaluation of the sinus node, atrioventricular node and His-Purkinje conduction system, without arrhythmia induction. Codes 93620-93624 and 93640-93642 all include recording, pacing and attempted arrhythmia induction from one or more site(s) in the heart.

Mapping: Mapping is a distinct procedure performed in addition to a diagnostic electrophysiologic procedure and should be separately reported using code 93609 or 93613. ▶Do not report standard mapping (93609) in addition to 3-D mapping (93613).◀ When a tachycardia is induced, the site of tachycardia origination or its electrical path through the heart is often defined by mapping. Mapping creates a multidimensional depiction of a tachycardia by recording multiple electrograms obtained sequentially or simultaneously from multiple catheter sites in the heart. Depending upon the technique, certain types of mapping catheters may be repositioned from point-to-point within the heart, allowing sequential recording from the various sites to construct maps. Other types of mapping catheters allow mapping without a point-to-point technique by allowing simultaneous recording from many electrodes on the same catheter and computer-assisted three dimensional reconstruction of the tachycardia activation sequence.

Ablation: Once the part of the heart involved in the tachycardia is localized, the tachycardia may be treated by ablation (the delivery of a radiofrequency energy to the area to selectively destroy cardiac tissue). Ablation procedures (93651-93652) may be performed: independently on a date subsequent to a diagnostic electrophysiologic study and mapping; or, at the time a diagnostic electrophysiologic study, tachycardia(s) induction and mapping is performed. When an electrophysiologic study, mapping, and ablation are performed on the same date, each procedure should be separately reported. In reporting catheter ablation, code 93651 and/or 93652 should be reported once to describe ablation of cardiac arrhythmias, regardless of the number of arrhythmias ablated.

Modifier '-51' should not be appended to 93600-93660.

⊘ **93600**   Bundle of His recording

⊘ **93602**   Intra-atrial recording

⊘ **93603**   Right ventricular recording

(93604, 93606 have been deleted. To report, see 93603, 93609, and 93622 as appropriate)

(93605 has been deleted. To report, use 93609)

(93607 has been deleted. To report, use 93622)

(93608 has been deleted. To report, use 93609)

+ **93609**   Intraventricular and/or intra-atrial mapping of tachycardia site(s) with catheter manipulation to record from multiple sites to identify origin of tachycardia (List separately in addition to code for primary procedure)

(Use 93609 in conjunction with codes 93620, 93651, 93652)

▶(Do not report 93609 in addition to 93613)◀

⊘ **93610**   Intra-atrial pacing

⊘ **93612**   Intraventricular pacing

(Do not report 93612 in conjunction with codes 93620-93622)

+ **93613**   Intracardiac electrophysiologic 3-dimensional mapping (List separately in addition to code for primary procedure)

(Use 93613 in conjunction with codes 93620, 93651, 93652)

▶(Do not report 93613 in addition to 93609)◀

(93614 has been deleted)

⊘ **93615**   Esophageal recording of atrial electrogram with or without ventricular electrogram(s);

⊘ **93616**   with pacing

⊘ **93618**   Induction of arrhythmia by electrical pacing

(For intracardiac phonocardiogram, use 93799)

⊘ **93619**   Comprehensive electrophysiologic evaluation with right atrial pacing and recording, right ventricular pacing and recording, His bundle recording, including insertion and repositioning of multiple electrode catheters, without induction or attempted induction of arrhythmia

(Do not report 93619 in conjunction with codes 93600, 93602, 93610, 93612, 93618, or 93620-93622)

⊘ ▲ **93620**   Comprehensive electrophysiologic evaluation including insertion and repositioning of multiple electrode catheters with induction or attempted induction of arrhythmia; with right atrial pacing and recording, right ventricular pacing and recording, His bundle recording

(Do not report 93620 in conjunction with codes 93600, 93602, 93610, 93612, 93618 or 93619)

+ **93621**   with left atrial pacing and recording from coronary sinus or left atrium (List separately in addition to code for primary procedure)

(Use 93621 in conjunction with code 93620)

+ **93622**   with left ventricular pacing and recording (List separately in addition to code for primary procedure)

(Use 93622 in conjunction with code 93620)

Medicine

+ 93623 Programmed stimulation and pacing after intravenous drug infusion (List separately in addition to code for primary procedure)

(Use 93623 in conjunction with codes 93619, 93620)

⊘ 93624 Electrophysiologic follow-up study with pacing and recording to test effectiveness of therapy, including induction or attempted induction of arrhythmia

(93630 has been deleted. To report, use 93631 and 33261)

⊘ 93631 Intra-operative epicardial and endocardial pacing and mapping to localize the site of tachycardia or zone of slow conduction for surgical correction

⊘ 93640 Electrophysiologic evaluation of single or dual chamber pacing cardioverter-defibrillator leads including defibrillation threshold evaluation (induction of arrhythmia, evaluation of sensing and pacing for arrhythmia termination) at time of initial implantation or replacement;

⊘ 93641 with testing of single or dual chamber pacing cardioverter-defibrillator pulse generator

(For subsequent or periodic electronic analysis and/or reprogramming of single or dual chamber pacing cardioverter-defibrillators, see 93642, 93741-93744)

⊘ 93642 Electrophysiologic evaluation of single or dual chamber pacing cardioverter-defibrillator (includes defibrillation threshold evaluation, induction of arrhythmia, evaluation of sensing and pacing for arrhythmia termination, and programming or reprogramming of sensing or therapeutic parameters)

⊘ 93650 Intracardiac catheter ablation of atrioventricular node function, atrioventricular conduction for creation of complete heart block, with or without temporary pacemaker placement

⊘ 93651 Intracardiac catheter ablation of arrhythmogenic focus; for treatment of supraventricular tachycardia by ablation of fast or slow atrioventricular pathways, accessory atrioventricular connections or other atrial foci, singly or in combination

⊘ 93652 for treatment of ventricular tachycardia

⊘ 93660 Evaluation of cardiovascular function with tilt table evaluation, with continuous ECG monitoring and intermittent blood pressure monitoring, with or without pharmacological intervention

(For testing of autonomic nervous system function, see 95921-95923)

+ 93662 Intracardiac echocardiography during therapeutic/diagnostic intervention, including imaging supervision and interpretation (List separately in addition to code for primary procedure)

(Use 93662 in conjunction with codes 93621, 93622, 93651, or 93652, as appropriate)

(Do not report 92961 in addition to 93662)

Peripheral Arterial Disease Rehabilitation

Peripheral arterial disease (PAD) rehabilitative physical exercise consists of a series of sessions, lasting 45-60 minutes per session, involving use of either a motorized treadmill or a track to permit each patient to achieve symptom-limited claudication. Each session is supervised by an exercise physiologist or nurse. The supervising provider monitors the individual patient's claudication threshold and other cardiovascular limitations for adjustment of workload. During this supervised rehabilitation program, the development of new arrhythmias, symptoms that might suggest angina or the continued inability of the patient to progress to an adequate level of exercise may require physician review and examination of the patient. These physician services would be separately reported with an appropriate level E/M service code.

93668 Peripheral arterial disease (PAD) rehabilitation, per session

Other Vascular Studies

(For arterial cannulization and recording of direct arterial pressure, use 36620)

(For radiographic injection procedures, see 36000-36299)

(For vascular cannulization for hemodialysis, see 36800-36821)

(For chemotherapy for malignant disease, see 96408-96549)

(For penile plethysmography, use 54240)

(93700 has been deleted)

93701 Bioimpedance, thoracic, electrical

(93710 has been deleted)

93720 Plethysmography, total body; with interpretation and report

93721 tracing only, without interpretation and report

93722 interpretation and report only

(For regional plethysmography, see 93875-93931)

93724 Electronic analysis of antitachycardia pacemaker system (includes electrocardiographic recording, programming of device, induction and termination of tachycardia via implanted pacemaker, and interpretation of recordings)

(93725-93730 have been deleted. To report, see 93875-93971)

93727 Electronic analysis of implantable loop recorder (ILR) system (includes retrieval of recorded and stored ECG data, physician review and interpretation of retrieved ECG data and reprogramming)

93731   Electronic analysis of dual-chamber pacemaker system (includes evaluation of programmable parameters at rest and during activity where applicable, using electrocardiographic recording and interpretation of recordings at rest and during exercise, analysis of event markers and device response); without reprogramming

93732   with reprogramming

93733   Electronic analysis of dual chamber internal pacemaker system (may include rate, pulse amplitude and duration, configuration of wave form, and/or testing of sensory function of pacemaker), telephonic analysis

93734   Electronic analysis of single chamber pacemaker system (includes evaluation of programmable parameters at rest and during activity where applicable, using electrocardiographic recording and interpretation of recordings at rest and during exercise, analysis of event markers and device response); without reprogramming

93735   with reprogramming

93736   Electronic analysis of single chamber internal pacemaker system (may include rate, pulse amplitude and duration, configuration of wave form, and/or testing of sensory function of pacemaker), telephonic analysis

(93737 has been deleted. To report, use 93741 or 93743)

(93738 has been deleted. To report, use 93742 or 93744)

93740   Temperature gradient studies

(93750 has been deleted. To report, see 93875-93971)

93741   Electronic analysis of pacing cardioverter-defibrillator (includes interrogation, evaluation of pulse generator status, evaluation of programmable parameters at rest and during activity where applicable, using electrocardiographic recording and interpretation of recordings at rest and during exercise, analysis of event markers and device response); single chamber, without reprogramming

93742   single chamber, with reprogramming

93743   dual chamber, without reprogramming

93744   dual chamber, with reprogramming

93760   Thermogram; cephalic

93762   peripheral

93770   Determination of venous pressure

(For central venous cannulization and pressure measurements, see 36488-36491, 36500)

(93780, 93781 have been deleted)

93784   Ambulatory blood pressure monitoring, utilizing a system such as magnetic tape and/or computer disk, for 24 hours or longer; including recording, scanning analysis, interpretation and report

93786   recording only

93788   scanning analysis with report

93790   physician review with interpretation and report

(93791-93796 have been deleted. To report, see 93731-93736)

Other Procedures

93797   Physician services for outpatient cardiac rehabilitation; without continuous ECG monitoring (per session)

93798   with continuous ECG monitoring (per session)

93799   Unlisted cardiovascular service or procedure

Non-Invasive Vascular Diagnostic Studies

Vascular studies include patient care required to perform the studies, supervision of the studies and interpretation of study results with copies for patient records of hard copy output with analysis of all data, including bidirectional vascular flow or imaging when provided.

The use of a simple hand-held or other Doppler device that does not produce hard copy output, or that produces a record that does not permit analysis of bidirectional vascular flow, is considered to be part of the physical examination of the vascular system and is not separately reported.

Duplex scan ▶(eg, 93880, 93882)◀ describes an ultrasonic scanning procedure ▶for characterizing the pattern and direction of blood flow in arteries or veins with the production of real time images integrating B-mode two-dimensional vascular structure with spectral and/or color flow Doppler mapping or imaging.◀

▶Non-invasive physiologic studies are performed using equipment separate and distinct from the duplex scanner. Codes 93875, 93965, 93922, 93923, and 93924 describe the evaluation of non-imaging physiologic recordings of pressures, Doppler analysis of bi-directional blood flow, plethysmography, and/or oxygen tension measurements appropriate for the anatomic area studied.◀

Cerebrovascular Arterial Studies

(93850, 93860 have been deleted. To report, see 93875-93882)

(93870 has been deleted. To report, see 93880 and 93882)

93875   Non-invasive physiologic studies of extracranial arteries, complete bilateral study (eg, periorbital flow direction with arterial compression, ocular pneumoplethysmography, Doppler ultrasound spectral analysis)

Medicine

93880 Duplex scan of extracranial arteries; complete bilateral study

93882 unilateral or limited study

93886 Transcranial Doppler study of the intracranial arteries; complete study

93888 limited study

Extremity Arterial Studies (Including Digits)

(93890, 93910 have been deleted. To report, see 93922-93931)

(93920, 93921 have been deleted. To report, see 93922-93924)

93922 Non-invasive physiologic studies of upper or lower extremity arteries, single level, bilateral (eg, ankle/brachial indices, Doppler waveform analysis, volume plethysmography, transcutaneous oxygen tension measurement)

93923 Non-invasive physiologic studies of upper or lower extremity arteries, multiple levels or with provocative functional maneuvers, complete bilateral study (eg, segmental blood pressure measurements, segmental Doppler waveform analysis, segmental volume plethysmography, segmental transcutaneous oxygen tension measurements, measurements with postural provocative tests, measurements with reactive hyperemia)

93924 Non-invasive physiologic studies of lower extremity arteries, at rest and following treadmill stress testing, complete bilateral study

93925 Duplex scan of lower extremity arteries or arterial bypass grafts; complete bilateral study

93926 unilateral or limited study

93930 Duplex scan of upper extremity arteries or arterial bypass grafts; complete bilateral study

93931 unilateral or limited study

Extremity Venous Studies (Including Digits)

(93950, 93960 have been deleted. To report, see 93965-93971)

93965 Non-invasive physiologic studies of extremity veins, complete bilateral study (eg, Doppler waveform analysis with responses to compression and other maneuvers, phleborheography, impedance plethysmography)

93970 Duplex scan of extremity veins including responses to compression and other maneuvers; complete bilateral study

93971 unilateral or limited study

Visceral and Penile Vascular Studies

93975 Duplex scan of arterial inflow and venous outflow of abdominal, pelvic, scrotal contents and/or retroperitoneal organs; complete study

93976 limited study

93978 Duplex scan of aorta, inferior vena cava, iliac vasculature, or bypass grafts; complete study

93979 unilateral or limited study

93980 Duplex scan of arterial inflow and venous outflow of penile vessels; complete study

93981 follow-up or limited study

Extremity Arterial-Venous Studies

93990 Duplex scan of hemodialysis access (including arterial inflow, body of access and venous outflow)

(For measurement of hemodialysis access flow using indicator dilution methods, use 90940)

Pulmonary

Items 94010-94799 include laboratory procedure(s) and interpretation of test results. If a separate identifiable Evaluation and Management service is performed, the appropriate E/M service code should be reported in addition to 94010-94799.

94010 Spirometry, including graphic record, total and timed vital capacity, expiratory flow rate measurement(s), with or without maximal voluntary ventilation

94014 Patient-initiated spirometric recording per 30-day period of time; includes reinforced education, transmission of spirometric tracing, data capture, analysis of transmitted data, periodic recalibration and physician review and interpretation

94015 recording (includes hook-up, reinforced education, data transmission, data capture, trend analysis, and periodic recalibration)

94016 physician review and interpretation only

94060 Bronchospasm evaluation: spirometry as in 94010, before and after bronchodilator (aerosol or parenteral)

(For prolonged exercise test for bronchospasm with pre- and post-spirometry, use 94620)

94070 Prolonged postexposure evaluation of bronchospasm with multiple spirometric determinations after antigen, cold air, methacholine or other chemical agent, with subsequent spirometrics

94150 Vital capacity, total (separate procedure)

(94160 has been deleted. For vital capacity measurement only, use 94150. For spirometry with timed expiratory volumes, use 94010)

94200 Maximum breathing capacity, maximal voluntary ventilation

94240 Functional residual capacity or residual volume: helium method, nitrogen open circuit method, or other method

94250 Expired gas collection, quantitative, single procedure (separate procedure)

94260 Thoracic gas volume

(For plethysmography, see 93720-93722)

94350 Determination of maldistribution of inspired gas: multiple breath nitrogen washout curve including alveolar nitrogen or helium equilibration time

94360 Determination of resistance to airflow, oscillatory or plethysmographic methods

94370 Determination of airway closing volume, single breath tests

94375 Respiratory flow volume loop

94400 Breathing response to CO_2 (CO_2 response curve)

94450 Breathing response to hypoxia (hypoxia response curve)

94620 Pulmonary stress testing; simple (eg, prolonged exercise test for bronchospasm with pre- and post-spirometry)

94621 complex (including measurements of CO_2 production, O_2 uptake, and electrocardiographic recordings)

▲**94640** Pressurized or nonpressurized inhalation treatment for acute airway obstruction or for sputum induction for diagnostic purposes (eg, with an aerosol generator, nebulizer, metered dose inhaler or intermittent positive pressure breathing (IPPB) device)

►(For more than one inhalation treatment performed on the same date, append modifier '-76')◄

94642 Aerosol inhalation of pentamidine for pneumocystis carinii pneumonia treatment or prophylaxis

►(94650, 94651, 94652 have been deleted)◄

94656 Ventilation assist and management, initiation of pressure or volume preset ventilators for assisted or controlled breathing; first day

94657 subsequent days

94660 Continuous positive airway pressure ventilation (CPAP), initiation and management

94662 Continuous negative pressure ventilation (CNP), initiation and management

▲**94664** Demonstration and/or evaluation of patient utilization of an aerosol generator, nebulizer, metered dose inhaler or IPPB device

►(94664 can be reported one time only per day of service)◄

►(94665 has been deleted)◄

94667 Manipulation chest wall, such as cupping, percussing, and vibration to facilitate lung function; initial demonstration and/or evaluation

94668 subsequent

94680 Oxygen uptake, expired gas analysis; rest and exercise, direct, simple

94681 including CO_2 output, percentage oxygen extracted

94690 rest, indirect (separate procedure)

(94700, 94705, 94710 have been deleted. For analysis of arterial blood gas results, see appropriate Evaluation and Management code. For test procedure, see 82800-82810)

(For single arterial puncture, use 36600)

(94715 has been deleted. To report, use 82820)

94720 Carbon monoxide diffusing capacity (eg, single breath, steady state)

94725 Membrane diffusion capacity

94750 Pulmonary compliance study (eg, plethysmography, volume and pressure measurements)

94760 Noninvasive ear or pulse oximetry for oxygen saturation; single determination

(For blood gases, see 82803-82810)

94761 multiple determinations (eg, during exercise)

94762 by continuous overnight monitoring (separate procedure)

94770 Carbon dioxide, expired gas determination by infrared analyzer

(For bronchoscopy, see 31622-31656)

(For placement of flow directed catheter, use 93503)

(For venipuncture, use 36410)

(For central venous catheter placement, see 36488-36491)

(For arterial puncture, use 36600)

(For arterial catheterization, use 36620)

(For thoracentesis, use 32000)

(For phlebotomy, therapeutic, use 99195)

(For lung biopsy, needle, use 32405)

(For intubation, orotracheal or nasotracheal, use 31500)

94772 Circadian respiratory pattern recording (pediatric pneumogram), 12 to 24 hour continuous recording, infant

(Separate procedure codes for electromyograms, EEG, ECG, and recordings of respiration are excluded when 94772 is reported)

94799 Unlisted pulmonary service or procedure

Allergy and Clinical Immunology

Definitions

Allergy sensitivity tests describe the performance and evaluation of selective cutaneous and mucous membrane tests in correlation with the history, physical examination, and other observations of the patient. The number of tests performed should be judicious and dependent upon the history, physical findings, and clinical judgment. All patients should not necessarily receive the same tests nor the same number of sensitivity tests.

Immunotherapy (desensitization, hyposensitization) is the parenteral administration of allergenic extracts as antigens at periodic intervals, usually on an increasing dosage scale to a dosage which is maintained as maintenance therapy. Indications for immunotherapy are determined by appropriate diagnostic procedures coordinated with clinical judgment and knowledge of the natural history of allergic diseases.

Other therapy: for medical conferences on the use of mechanical and electronic devices (precipitators, air conditioners, air filters, humidifiers, dehumidifiers), climatotherapy, physical therapy, occupational and recreational therapy, see **Evaluation and Management** section.

Allergy Testing

(95000-95003 have been deleted. To report, use 95004)

95004   Percutaneous tests (scratch, puncture, prick) with allergenic extracts, immediate type reaction, specify number of tests

(95005-95007 have been deleted. To report, use 95010)

95010   Percutaneous tests (scratch, puncture, prick) sequential and incremental, with drugs, biologicals or venoms, immediate type reaction, specify number of tests

(95011 has been deleted. To report, use 95010)

(95014 has been deleted. To report, use 95015)

95015   Intracutaneous (intradermal) tests, sequential and incremental, with drugs, biologicals, or venoms, immediate type reaction, specify number of tests

(95016-95018 have been deleted. To report, use 95015)

(95020-95023 have been deleted. To report, use 95024)

95024   Intracutaneous (intradermal) tests with allergenic extracts, immediate type reaction, specify number of tests

▲ 95027   Intracutaneous (intradermal) tests, sequential and incremental, with allergenic extracts for airborne allergens, immediate type reaction, specify number of tests

95028   Intracutaneous (intradermal) tests with allergenic extracts, delayed type reaction, including reading, specify number of tests

(95030-95034 have been deleted. To report, use 95028)

(95040-95043 have been deleted. To report, use 95044)

95044   Patch or application test(s) (specify number of tests)

(95050, 95051 have been deleted. To report, use 95052)

95052   Photo patch test(s) (specify number of tests)

95056   Photo tests

95060   Ophthalmic mucous membrane tests

95065   Direct nasal mucous membrane test

95070   Inhalation bronchial challenge testing (not including necessary pulmonary function tests); with histamine, methacholine, or similar compounds

95071   with antigens or gases, specify

(For pulmonary function tests, see 94060, 94070)

95075   Ingestion challenge test (sequential and incremental ingestion of test items, eg, food, drug or other substance such as metabisulfite)

(95077 has been deleted)

95078   Provocative testing (eg, Rinkel test)

(95080-95082 have been deleted)

(For allergy laboratory tests, see 86000-86999)

(For intravenous therapy for severe or intractable allergic disease, see 90780, 90781, 90784)

(95105 has been deleted. To report, see appropriate E/M code(s))

Allergen Immunotherapy

Codes 95115-95199 include the professional services necessary for allergen immunotherapy. Office visit codes may be used in addition to allergen immunotherapy if other identifiable services are provided at that time.

95115   Professional services for allergen immunotherapy not including provision of allergenic extracts; single injection

95117   two or more injections

95120   Professional services for allergen immunotherapy in prescribing physicians office or institution, including provision of allergenic extract; single injection

95125   two or more injections

95130   single stinging insect venom

95131   two stinging insect venoms

95132   three stinging insect venoms

95133   four stinging insect venoms

95134   five stinging insect venoms

(95135 has been deleted. To report, use 95144)

(95140 has been deleted. To report, use 95144)

95144   Professional services for the supervision of preparation and provision of antigens for allergen immunotherapy; single dose vial(s) (specify number of vials)

(A single dose vial contains a single dose of antigen administered in one injection)

95145   Professional services for the supervision of preparation and provision of antigens for allergen immunotherapy (specify number of doses); single stinging insect venom

95146   two single stinging insect venoms

95147   three single stinging insect venoms

95148   four single stinging insect venoms

95149   five single stinging insect venoms

(95150, 95155 have been deleted. To report, use 95165)

(95160 has been deleted. To report, see 95145-95149)

95165   Professional services for the supervision of preparation and provision of antigens for allergen immunotherapy; single or multiple antigens (specify number of doses)

95170   whole body extract of biting insect or other arthropod (specify number of doses)

(For allergy immunotherapy reporting, a dose is the amount of antigen(s) administered in a single injection from a multiple dose vial)

95180   Rapid desensitization procedure, each hour (eg, insulin, penicillin, equine serum)

95199   Unlisted allergy/clinical immunologic service or procedure

(For skin testing of bacterial, viral, fungal extracts, see 95028, 86485-86586)

(For special reports on allergy patients, use 99080)

(For testing procedures such as radioallergosorbent testing (RAST), rat mast cell technique (RMCT), mast cell degranulation test (MCDT), lymphocytic transformation test (LTT), leukocyte histamine release (LHR), migration inhibitory factor test (MIF), transfer factor test (TFT), nitroblue tetrazolium dye test (NTD), see Immunology section in **Pathology** or use 95199)

Endocrinology

95250   Glucose monitoring for up to 72 hours by continuous recording and storage of glucose values from interstitial tissue fluid via a subcutaneous sensor (includes hook-up, calibration, patient initiation and training, recording, disconnection, downloading with printout of data)

(Do not report 95250 in conjunction with 99091)

(To report physician review, interpretation and written report associated with code 95250, see **Evaluation and Management** services codes)

Neurology and Neuromuscular Procedures

Neurologic services are typically consultative, and any of the levels of consultation (99241-99263) may be appropriate.

In addition, services and skills outlined under **Evaluation and Management** levels of service appropriate to neurologic illnesses should be coded similarly.

The EEG, autonomic function, and evoked potential services (95812-95829, 95920-95930 and 95950-95962) include recording, interpretation by a physician, and report. For interpretation only, use modifier '-26'.

(For repetitive transcranial magnetic stimulation for treatment of clinical depression, use Category III code 0018T)

(Do not report codes 95860-95875 in addition to 96000-96004)

Sleep Testing

Sleep studies and polysomnography refer to the continuous and simultaneous monitoring and recording of various physiological and pathophysiological parameters of sleep for 6 or more hours with physician review, interpretation and report. The studies are performed to diagnose a variety of sleep disorders and to evaluate a patient's response to therapies such as nasal continuous positive airway pressure (NCPAP). Polysomnography is distinguished from sleep studies by the inclusion of sleep staging which is defined to include a 1-4 lead electroencephalogram (EEG), an electro-oculogram (EOG), and a submental electromyogram (EMG). Additional parameters of sleep include: 1) ECG; 2) airflow; 3) ventilation and respiratory effort; 4) gas exchange by oximetry, transcutaneous monitoring, or end tidal gas analysis; 5) extremity muscle activity, motor activity-movement; 6) extended EEG monitoring; 7) penile tumescence; 8) gastroesophageal reflux; 9) continuous blood pressure monitoring; 10) snoring; 11) body positions; etc.

The sleep services (95805-95811) include recording, interpretation and report. For interpretation only, use modifier '-26'.

For a study to be reported as polysomnography, sleep must be recorded and staged.

(Report with a '-52' modifier if less than 6 hours of recording or in other cases of reduced services as appropriate)

(For unattended sleep study, use 95806)

95805   Multiple sleep latency or maintenance of wakefulness testing, recording, analysis and interpretation of physiological measurements of sleep during multiple trials to assess sleepiness

95806 Sleep study, simultaneous recording of ventilation, respiratory effort, ECG or heart rate, and oxygen saturation, unattended by a technologist

95807 Sleep study, simultaneous recording of ventilation, respiratory effort, ECG or heart rate, and oxygen saturation, attended by a technologist

95808 Polysomnography; sleep staging with 1-3 additional parameters of sleep, attended by a technologist

95810 sleep staging with 4 or more additional parameters of sleep, attended by a technologist

95811 sleep staging with 4 or more additional parameters of sleep, with initiation of continuous positive airway pressure therapy or bilevel ventilation, attended by a technologist

▶Routine Electroencephalography (EEG)◀

▶EEG codes 95812-95822 include hyperventilation and/or photic stimulation when appropriate. Routine EEG codes 95816-95822 include 20 to 40 minutes of recording. Extended EEG codes 95812-95813 include reporting times longer than 40 minutes.◀

▲**95812** Electroencephalogram (EEG) extended monitoring; 41-60 minutes

95813 greater than one hour

▲**95816** Electroencephalogram (EEG); including recording awake and drowsy

(95817 has been deleted. To report, use 95816)

▲**95819** including recording awake and asleep

(95821 has been deleted. To report, use 95819)

▲**95822** recording in coma or sleep only

(95823 has been deleted. To report, use 95954)

95824 cerebral death evaluation only

(95826 has been deleted. To report, use 95829, 95951 or 95956)

▲**95827** all night recording

(For 24-hour EEG monitoring, ▶see 95950-95953 or 95956◀)

(For EEG during nonintracranial surgery, use 95955)

(For Wada ▶test◀, use 95958)

▶(For digital analysis of EEG, use 95957)◀

(95828 has been deleted. To report, see 95807-95810)

95829 Electrocorticogram at surgery (separate procedure)

95830 Insertion by physician of sphenoidal electrodes for electroencephalographic (EEG) recording

▶Muscle and Range of Motion Testing◀

95831 Muscle testing, manual (separate procedure) with report; extremity (excluding hand) or trunk

95832 hand, with or without comparison with normal side

95833 total evaluation of body, excluding hands

95834 total evaluation of body, including hands

(95842 has been deleted. To report, use 95999)

95851 Range of motion measurements and report (separate procedure); each extremity (excluding hand) or each trunk section (spine)

95852 hand, with or without comparison with normal side

95857 Tensilon test for myasthenia gravis;

95858 with electromyographic recording

▶Electromyography and Nerve Conduction Tests◀

95860 Needle electromyography; one extremity with or without related paraspinal areas

95861 two extremities with or without related paraspinal areas

(For dynamic electromyography performed during motion analysis studies, see 96002-96003)

95863 three extremities with or without related paraspinal areas

95864 four extremities with or without related paraspinal areas

▲**95867** cranial nerve supplied muscle(s), unilateral

95868 cranial nerve supplied muscles, bilateral

▲**95869** thoracic paraspinal muscles (excluding T1 or T12)

95870 limited study of muscles in one extremity or non-limb (axial) muscles (unilateral or bilateral), other than thoracic paraspinal, cranial nerve supplied muscles, or sphincters

(To report a complete study of the extremities, see 95860-95864)

(For anal or urethral sphincter, detrusor, urethra, perineum musculature, see 51785-51792)

(For eye muscles, use 92265)

95872 Needle electromyography using single fiber electrode, with quantitative measurement of jitter, blocking and/or fiber density, any/all sites of each muscle studied

▲**95875** Ischemic limb exercise test with serial specimen(s) acquisition for muscle(s) metabolite(s)

(95880 has been deleted. To report, use 96105)

(95881 has been deleted. To report, use 96111)

(95882 has been deleted. To report, use 96115)

(95883 has been deleted. To report, use 96117)

⊘ **95900** Nerve conduction, amplitude and latency/velocity study, each nerve; motor, without F-wave study

⊘ **95903** motor, with F-wave study

⊘ **95904** sensory

(Report 95900, 95903, and/or 95904 only once when multiple sites on the same nerve are stimulated or recorded)

▶Intraoperative Neurophysiology◄

+ **95920** Intraoperative neurophysiology testing, per hour (List separately in addition to code for primary procedure)

(Use code 95920 in conjunction with the study performed, 92585, 95822, 95860, 95861, 95867, 95868, 95900, 95904, 95925, 95926, 95927, 95930, 95933, 95934, 95936, 95937)

(Code 95920 describes ongoing electrophysiologic testing and monitoring performed during surgical procedures. Code 95920 is reported per hour of service, and includes only the ongoing electrophysiologic monitoring time distinct from performance of specific type(s) of baseline electrophysiologic study(ies) (95860, 95861, 95867, 95868, 95900, 95904, 95933, 95934, 95936, 95937) or interpretation of specific type(s) of baseline electrophysiologic study(ies) (92585, 95822, 95925, 95926, 95927, 95930). The time spent performing or interpreting the baseline electrophysiologic study(ies) should not be counted as intraoperative monitoring, but represents separately reportable procedures. Code 95920 should be used once per hour even if multiple electrophysiologic studies are performed. The baseline electrophysiologic study(ies) should be used once per operative session.)

▶(For electrocorticography, use 95829)◄

▶(For intraoperative EEG during nonintracranial surgery, use 95955)◄

▶(For intraoperative functional cortical or subcortical mapping, see 95961-95962)◄

▶(For intraoperative neurostimulator programming and analysis, see 95970-95975)◄

▶Autonomic Function Tests◄

95921 Testing of autonomic nervous system function; cardiovagal innervation (parasympathetic function), including two or more of the following: heart rate response to deep breathing with recorded R-R interval, Valsalva ratio, and 30:15 ratio

95922 vasomotor adrenergic innervation (sympathetic adrenergic function), including beat-to-beat blood pressure and R-R interval changes during Valsalva maneuver and at least five minutes of passive tilt

95923 sudomotor, including one or more of the following: quantitative sudomotor axon reflex test (QSART), silastic sweat imprint, thermoregulatory sweat test, and changes in sympathetic skin potential

▶Evoked Potentials and Reflex Tests◄

95925 Short-latency somatosensory evoked potential study, stimulation of any/all peripheral nerves or skin sites, recording from the central nervous system; in upper limbs

95926 in lower limbs

95927 in the trunk or head

(To report a unilateral study, use modifier '-52')

(For auditory evoked potentials, use 92585)

95930 Visual evoked potential (VEP) testing central nervous system, checkerboard or flash

95933 Orbicularis oculi (blink) reflex, by electrodiagnostic testing

95934 H-reflex, amplitude and latency study; record gastrocnemius/soleus muscle

(95935 has been deleted. To report, see 95903, 95934, 95936)

95936 record muscle other than gastrocnemius/soleus muscle

(To report a bilateral study, use modifier '-50')

95937 Neuromuscular junction testing (repetitive stimulation, paired stimuli), each nerve, any one method

▶Special EEG Tests◄

95950 Monitoring for identification and lateralization of cerebral seizure focus, electroencephalographic (eg, 8 channel EEG) recording and interpretation, each 24 hours

95951 Monitoring for localization of cerebral seizure focus by cable or radio, 16 or more channel telemetry, combined electroencephalographic (EEG) and video recording and interpretation (eg, for presurgical localization), each 24 hours

(95952 has been deleted. To report, use 95950)

95953 Monitoring for localization of cerebral seizure focus by computerized portable 16 or more channel EEG, electroencephalographic (EEG) recording and interpretation, each 24 hours

95954 Pharmacological or physical activation requiring physician attendance during EEG recording of activation phase (eg, thiopental activation test)

95955 Electroencephalogram (EEG) during nonintracranial surgery (eg, carotid surgery)

Medicine

95956 Monitoring for localization of cerebral seizure focus by cable or radio, 16 or more channel telemetry, electroencephalographic (EEG) recording and interpretation, each 24 hours

95957 Digital analysis of electroencephalogram (EEG) (eg, for epileptic spike analysis)

95958 Wada activation test for hemispheric function, including electroencephalographic (EEG) monitoring

95961 Functional cortical and subcortical mapping by stimulation and/or recording of electrodes on brain surface, or of depth electrodes, to provoke seizures or identify vital brain structures; initial hour of physician attendance

+ 95962 each additional hour of physician attendance (List separately in addition to code for primary procedure)

(Use 95962 in conjunction with code 95961)

95965 Magnetoencephalography (MEG), recording and analysis; for spontaneous brain magnetic activity (eg, epileptic cerebral cortex localization)

95966 for evoked magnetic fields, single modality (eg, sensory, motor, language, or visual cortex localization)

+ 95967 for evoked magnetic fields, each additional modality (eg, sensory, motor, language, or visual cortex localization) (List separately in addition to code for primary procedure)

(Use 95967 in conjunction with code 95966)

(For electroencephalography performed in addition to magnetoencephalography, see 95812-95827)

(For somatosensory evoked potentials, auditory evoked potentials, and visual evoked potentials performed in addition to magnetic evoked field responses, see 92585, 95925, 95926, and/or 95930)

(For computerized tomography performed in addition to magnetoencephalography, see 70450-70470, 70496)

(For magnetic resonance imaging performed in addition to magnetoencephalography, see 70551-70553)

Neurostimulators, Analysis-Programming

A simple neurostimulator pulse generator/transmitter (95970, 95971) is one capable of affecting 3 or fewer of the following: pulse amplitude, pulse duration, pulse frequency, 8 or more electrode contacts, cycling, stimulation train duration, train spacing, number of programs, number of channels, alternating electrode polarities, dose time (stimulation parameters changing in time periods of minutes including dose lockout times), more than 1 clinical feature (eg, rigidity, dyskinesia, tremor). A complex neurostimulator pulse generator/transmitter (95970, 95972, 95973, 95974, 95975) is one capable of affecting more than 3 of the above.

Code 95970 describes subsequent electronic analysis of a previously-implanted simple or complex brain, spinal cord, or peripheral neurostimulator pulse generator system, without reprogramming. Code 95971 describes intraoperative or subsequent electronic analysis of an implanted simple brain, spinal cord, or peripheral (ie, peripheral nerve, autonomic nerve, neuromuscular) neurostimulator pulse generator system, with programming. Codes 95972 and 95973 describe intraoperative (at initial insertion/revision) or subsequent electronic analysis of an implanted complex brain, spinal cord or peripheral (except cranial nerve) neurostimulator pulse generator system, with programming. Codes 95974 and 95975 describe intraoperative (at initial insertion/revision) or subsequent electronic analysis of an implanted complex cranial nerve neurostimulator pulse generator system, with programming.

(For insertion of neurostimulator pulse generator, see 61885, 63685, 63688, 64590)

(For revision or removal of neurostimulator pulse generator or receiver, see 61888, 63688, 64595)

(For implantation of neurostimulator electrodes, see 61850-61875, 63650-63655, 64553-64580. For revision or removal of neurostimulator electrodes, see 61880, 63660, 64585)

95970 Electronic analysis of implanted neurostimulator pulse generator system (eg, rate, pulse amplitude and duration, configuration of wave form, battery status, electrode selectability, output modulation, cycling, impedance and patient compliance measurements); simple or complex brain, spinal cord, or peripheral (ie, cranial nerve, peripheral nerve, autonomic nerve, neuromuscular) neurostimulator pulse generator/transmitter, without reprogramming

95971 simple brain, spinal cord, or peripheral (ie, peripheral nerve, autonomic nerve, neuromuscular) neurostimulator pulse generator/transmitter, with intraoperative or subsequent programming

95972 complex brain, spinal cord, or peripheral (except cranial nerve) neurostimulator pulse generator/transmitter, with intraoperative or subsequent programming, first hour

+ 95973 complex brain, spinal cord, or peripheral (except cranial nerve) neurostimulator pulse generator/transmitter, with intraoperative or subsequent programming, each additional 30 minutes after first hour (List separately in addition to code for primary procedure)

(Use 95973 in conjunction with code 95972)

95974 complex cranial nerve neurostimulator pulse generator/transmitter, with intraoperative or subsequent programming, with or without nerve interface testing, first hour

95975   complex cranial nerve neurostimulator pulse generator/transmitter, with intraoperative or subsequent programming, each additional 30 minutes after first hour (List separately in addition to code for primary procedure)

(Use 95975 in conjunction with code 95974)

Other Procedures

● 95990   Refilling and maintenance of implantable pump or reservoir for drug delivery, spinal (intrathecal, epidural) or brain (intraventricular)

▶(For analysis and/or reprogramming of implantable infusion pump, see 62367-62368)◀

▶(For refill and maintenance of implanted infusion pump or reservoir for systemic drug therapy (eg, chemotherapy or insulin, use 96530)◀

95999   Unlisted neurological or neuromuscular diagnostic procedure

Motion Analysis

Codes 96000-96004 describe services performed as part of a major therapeutic or diagnostic decision making process. Motion analysis is performed in a dedicated motion analysis laboratory (ie, a facility capable of performing videotaping from the front, back and both sides, computerized 3-D kinematics, 3-D kinetics, and dynamic electromyography). Code 96000 may include 3-D kinetics and stride characteristics. Codes 96002-96003 describe dynamic electromyography. Do not report codes 95860-95875 in addition to the motion analysis codes.

Code 96004 should only be reported once regardless of the number of study(ies) reviewed/interpreted.

(For performance of needle electromyography procedures, see 95860-95875)

(For gait training, use 97116)

96000   Comprehensive computer-based motion analysis by video-taping and 3-D kinematics;

96001   with dynamic plantar pressure measurements during walking

96002   Dynamic surface electromyography, during walking or other functional activities, 1-12 muscles

96003   Dynamic fine wire electromyography, during walking or other functional activities, 1 muscle

(Do not report codes 95860-95875 in addition to 96002, 96003)

96004   Physician review and interpretation of comprehensive computer based motion analysis, dynamic plantar pressure measurements, dynamic surface electromyography during walking or other functional activities, and dynamic fine wire electromyography, with written report

Central Nervous System Assessments/Tests (eg, Neuro-Cognitive, Mental Status, Speech Testing)

The following codes are used to report the services provided during testing of the cognitive function of the central nervous system. The testing of cognitive processes, visual motor responses, and abstractive abilities is accomplished by the combination of several types of testing procedures. It is expected that the administration of these tests will generate material that will be formulated into a report.

(For development of cognitive skills, see 97532, 97533)

96100   Psychological testing (includes psychodiagnostic assessment of personality, psychopathology, emotionality, intellectual abilities, eg, WAIS-R, Rorschach, MMPI) with interpretation and report, per hour

96105   Assessment of aphasia (includes assessment of expressive and receptive speech and language function, language comprehension, speech production ability, reading, spelling, writing, eg, by Boston Diagnostic Aphasia Examination) with interpretation and report, per hour

96110   Developmental testing; limited (eg, Developmental Screening Test II, Early Language Milestone Screen), with interpretation and report

96111   extended (includes assessment of motor, language, social, adaptive and/or cognitive functioning by standardized developmental instruments, eg, Bayley Scales of Infant Development) with interpretation and report, per hour

96115   Neurobehavioral status exam (clinical assessment of thinking, reasoning and judgment, eg, acquired knowledge, attention, memory, visual spatial abilities, language functions, planning) with interpretation and report, per hour

(For mini-mental status examination performed by a physician, see **Evaluation and Management** services codes)

96117   Neuropsychological testing battery (eg, Halstead-Reitan, Luria, WAIS-R) with interpretation and report, per hour

Medicine

Health and Behavior Assessment/Intervention

▶Health and behavior assessment procedures are used to identify the psychological, behavioral, emotional, cognitive, and social factors important to the prevention, treatment, or management of physical health problems.

The focus of the assessment is not on mental health but on the biopsychosocial factors important to physical health problems and treatments. The focus of the intervention is to improve the patient's health and well-being utilizing cognitive, behavioral, social, and/or psychophysiological procedures designed to ameliorate specific disease-related problems.◀

Codes 96150-96155 describe services ▶offered to patients who present with established illnesses or symptoms, who are not diagnosed with mental illness, and may benefit from evaluations that focus on the biopsychosocial factors related to the patient's physical health status. These services do not represent preventive medicine counseling and risk factor reduction interventions.◀

For patients that require psychiatric services (90801-90899) as well as health and behavior assessment/intervention (96150-96155), report the predominant service performed. Do not report codes 96150-96155 in addition to codes 90801-90899 on the same date.

Evaluation and Management services codes ▶(including **Preventive Medicine, Individual Counseling** codes 99401-99404, and **Preventive Medicine, Group Counseling** codes 99411-99412),◀ should not be reported on the same day.

> ▶(For health and behavior assessment and/or intervention performed by a physician, see **Evaluation and Management** or **Preventive Medicine** services codes)◀

96150   Health and behavior assessment (eg, health-focused clinical interview, behavioral observations, psychophysiological monitoring, health-oriented questionnaires), each 15 minutes face-to-face with the patient; initial assessment

96151   re-assessment

96152   Health and behavior intervention, each 15 minutes, face-to-face; individual

96153   group (2 or more patients)

96154   family (with the patient present)

96155   family (without the patient present)

Chemotherapy Administration

Procedures 96400-96549 are independent of the patient's visit.

If a significant separately identifiable Evaluation and Management service is performed, the appropriate E/M service code should be reported in addition to 96400-96549.

Either may occur independently on any date of service, or they may occur sequentially on the same day.

Preparation of chemotherapy agent(s) is included in the service for administration of the agent.

Regional (isolation) chemotherapy perfusion should be reported using the codes for arterial infusion (96420-96425). Placement of the intra-arterial catheter should be reported using the appropriate code from the **Cardiovascular Surgery** section. Placement of arterial and venous cannula(s) for extracorporeal circulation via a membrane oxygenator perfusion pump should be reported using code 36823. Code 36823 includes dose calculation and administration of the chemotherapy agent by injection into the perfusate. Do not report code(s) 96408-96425 in conjunction with code 36823.

Report separate codes for each parenteral method of administration employed when chemotherapy is administered by different techniques. Medications (eg, antibiotics, steroidal agents, antiemetics, narcotics, analgesics, biological agents) administered independently or sequentially as supportive management of chemotherapy administration, should be separately reported using 90780-90788, as appropriate.

96400   Chemotherapy administration, subcutaneous or intramuscular, with or without local anesthesia

96405   Chemotherapy administration, intralesional; up to and including 7 lesions

96406   more than 7 lesions

96408   Chemotherapy administration, intravenous; push technique

96410   infusion technique, up to one hour

✚ 96412   infusion technique, one to 8 hours, each additional hour (List separately in addition to code for primary procedure)

> (Use 96412 in conjunction with code 96410)

96414   infusion technique, initiation of prolonged infusion (more than 8 hours), requiring the use of a portable or implantable pump

> ▶(For refilling and maintenance of a portable pump or an implantable infusion pump or reservoir for drug delivery,◀ see 96520, 96530)

96420   Chemotherapy administration, intra-arterial; push technique

96422   infusion technique, up to one hour

+ 96423   infusion technique, one to 8 hours, each additional hour (List separately in addition to code for primary procedure)

(Use 96423 in conjunction with code 96422)

(For regional chemotherapy perfusion via membrane oxygenator perfusion pump to an extremity, use 36823)

96425   infusion technique, initiation of prolonged infusion (more than 8 hours), requiring the use of a portable or implantable pump

▶(For refilling and maintenance of a portable pump or an implantable infusion pump or reservoir for drug delivery,◀ see 96520, 96530)

96440   Chemotherapy administration into pleural cavity, requiring and including thoracentesis

96445   Chemotherapy administration into peritoneal cavity, requiring and including peritoneocentesis

96450   Chemotherapy administration, into CNS (eg, intrathecal), requiring and including spinal puncture

(For intravesical (bladder) chemotherapy administration, use 51720)

(For insertion of subarachnoid catheter and reservoir for infusion of drug, see 62350, 62351, 62360, 62361, 62362; for insertion of intraventricular catheter and reservoir, see 61210, 61215)

(96500-96512 have been deleted. To report, see 96408-96414)

96520   Refilling and maintenance of portable pump

(96524, 96526 have been deleted. To report, see 96420-96425)

▲**96530**   Refilling and maintenance of implantable pump or reservoir for drug delivery, systemic (eg, intravenous, intra-arterial)

▶(For refilling and maintenance of an implantable infusion pump for spinal or brain drug infusion, use 95990)◀

(For collection of blood specimen from a partially or completely implantable venous access device, use 36540)

(96535 has been deleted. To report, see 96440, 96445)

(96540 has been deleted. To report, use 96542)

96542   Chemotherapy injection, subarachnoid or intraventricular via subcutaneous reservoir, single or multiple agents

96545   Provision of chemotherapy agent

(For radioactive isotope therapy, see 79000-79999)

96549   Unlisted chemotherapy procedure

Photodynamic Therapy

96567   Photodynamic therapy by external application of light to destroy premalignant and/or malignant lesions of the skin and adjacent mucosa (eg, lip) by activation of photosensitive drug(s), each phototherapy exposure session

(96570, 96571 are to be used in addition to bronchoscopy, endoscopy codes)

(To report ocular photodynamic therapy, use 67221)

+ 96570   Photodynamic therapy by endoscopic application of light to ablate abnormal tissue via activation of photosensitive drug(s); first 30 minutes (List separately in addition to code for endoscopy or bronchoscopy procedures of lung and esophagus)

+ 96571   each additional 15 minutes (List separately in addition to code for endoscopy or bronchoscopy procedures of lung and esophagus)

(Use 96570, 96571 in conjunction with codes 31641, 43228 as appropriate)

Special Dermatological Procedures

Dermatologic services are typically consultative, and any of the five levels of consultation (99241-99263) may be appropriate.

In addition, services and skills outlined under **Evaluation and Management** levels of service appropriate to dermatologic illnesses should be coded similarly.

▶(For whole body photography, see Category III code 0044T)◀

(For intralesional injections, see 11900, 11901)

(For Tzanck smear, use 87207)

96900   Actinotherapy (ultraviolet light)

96902   Microscopic examination of hairs plucked or clipped by the examiner (excluding hair collected by the patient) to determine telogen and anagen counts, or structural hair shaft abnormality

96910   Photochemotherapy; tar and ultraviolet B (Goeckerman treatment) or petrolatum and ultraviolet B

96912   psoralens and ultraviolet A (PUVA)

Medicine

96913   Photochemotherapy (Goeckerman and/or PUVA) for severe photoresponsive dermatoses requiring at least four to eight hours of care under direct supervision of the physician (includes application of medication and dressings)

● 96920   Laser treatment for inflammatory skin disease (psoriasis); total area less than 250 sq cm

● 96921   250 sq cm to 500 sq cm

● 96922   over 500 sq cm

96999   Unlisted special dermatological service or procedure

Physical Medicine and Rehabilitation

(For muscle testing, range of joint motion, electromyography, see 95831 et seq)

(For biofeedback training by EMG, use 90901)

(For transcutaneous nerve stimulation (TNS), use 64550)

(97000 has been deleted. To report, see 97010-97039)

97001   Physical therapy evaluation

97002   Physical therapy re-evaluation

97003   Occupational therapy evaluation

97004   Occupational therapy re-evaluation

97005   Athletic training evaluation

97006   Athletic training re-evaluation

Modalities

Any physical agent applied to produce therapeutic changes to biologic tissue; includes but not limited to thermal, acoustic, light, mechanical, or electric energy.

Supervised

The application of a modality that does not require direct (one-on-one) patient contact by the provider.

97010   Application of a modality to one or more areas; hot or cold packs

97012   traction, mechanical

97014   electrical stimulation (unattended)

(For acupuncture with electrical stimulation, use 97781)

97016   vasopneumatic devices

97018   paraffin bath

97020   microwave

97022   whirlpool

97024   diathermy

97026   infrared

97028   ultraviolet

Constant Attendance

The application of a modality that requires direct (one-on-one) patient contact by the provider.

97032   Application of a modality to one or more areas; electrical stimulation (manual), each 15 minutes

97033   iontophoresis, each 15 minutes

97034   contrast baths, each 15 minutes

97035   ultrasound, each 15 minutes

97036   Hubbard tank, each 15 minutes

97039   Unlisted modality (specify type and time if constant attendance)

Therapeutic Procedures

A manner of effecting change through the application of clinical skills and/or services that attempt to improve function.

Physician or therapist required to have direct (one-on-one) patient contact.

(97100 has been deleted. To report, see 97110-97139)

(97101 has been deleted. To report, see 97110-97139)

97110   Therapeutic procedure, one or more areas, each 15 minutes; therapeutic exercises to develop strength and endurance, range of motion and flexibility

97112   neuromuscular reeducation of movement, balance, coordination, kinesthetic sense, posture, and/or proprioception for sitting and/or standing activities

97113   aquatic therapy with therapeutic exercises

(97114 has been deleted. To report, use 97530)

97116   gait training (includes stair climbing)

(Use 96000-96003 to report comprehensive gait and motion analysis procedures)

(97118 has been deleted. To report, use 97032)

(97120 has been deleted. To report, use 97033)

(97122 has been deleted. To report, use 97140)

97124   massage, including effleurage, petrissage and/or tapotement (stroking, compression, percussion)

(For myofascial release, use 97140)

(97126 has been deleted. To report, use 97034)

(97128 has been deleted. To report, use 97035)

97139   Unlisted therapeutic procedure (specify)

97140   Manual therapy techniques (eg, mobilization/manipulation, manual lymphatic drainage, manual traction), one or more regions, each 15 minutes

(97145 has been deleted. To report, see 97110-97139)

97150   Therapeutic procedure(s), group (2 or more individuals)

(Report 97150 for each member of group)

(Group therapy procedures involve constant attendance of the physician or therapist, but by definition do not require one-on-one patient contact by the physician or therapist)

(97200, 97201 have been deleted. To report, see 97010-97039, 97110-97139)

(97220, 97221 have been deleted. To report, use 97036)

(97240, 97241 have been deleted. To report, see 97036, 97113)

(97250 has been deleted. To report, use 97140)

(97260, 97261 have been deleted. To report, use 97140)

(97265 has been deleted. To report, use 97140)

(For manipulation under general anesthesia, see appropriate anatomic section in **Musculoskeletal System**)

(For osteopathic manipulative treatment (OMT), see 98925-98929)

(97500, 97501 have been deleted. To report, use 97504)

97504   Orthotic(s) fitting and training, upper extremity(ies), lower extremity(ies), and/or trunk, each 15 minutes

(Code 97504 should not be reported with 97116)

(For casting and strapping of fracture, injury or dislocation, see 29000, 29590)

97520   Prosthetic training, upper and/or lower extremities, each 15 minutes

(97521 has been deleted. To report, use 97520)

97530   Therapeutic activities, direct (one-on-one) patient contact by the provider (use of dynamic activities to improve functional performance), each 15 minutes

(97531 has been deleted. To report, use 97530)

97532   Development of cognitive skills to improve attention, memory, problem solving, (includes compensatory training), direct (one-on-one) patient contact by the provider, each 15 minutes

97533   Sensory integrative techniques to enhance sensory processing and promote adaptive responses to environmental demands, direct (one-on-one) patient contact by the provider, each 15 minutes

97535   Self-care/home management training (eg, activities of daily living (ADL) and compensatory training, meal preparation, safety procedures, and instructions in use of assistive technology devices/adaptive equipment) direct one-on-one contact by provider, each 15 minutes

97537   Community/work reintegration training (eg, shopping, transportation, money management, avocational activities and/or work environment/modification analysis, work task analysis), direct one-on-one contact by provider, each 15 minutes

(97540 has been deleted. To report, see 97535, 97537)

(97541 has been deleted. To report, see 97535, 97537)

(For wheelchair management/propulsion training, use 97542)

97542   Wheelchair management/propulsion training, each 15 minutes

97545   Work hardening/conditioning; initial 2 hours

+ 97546   each additional hour (List separately in addition to code for primary procedure)

(Use 97546 in conjunction with code 97545)

Active Wound Care Management

Active wound care procedures are performed to promote healing, and involve selective and non-selective debridement techniques.

(Do not report 97601, 97602 in addition to 11040-11044)

97601   Removal of devitalized tissue from wound(s); selective debridement, without anesthesia (eg, high pressure waterjet, sharp selective debridement with scissors, scalpel and tweezers), including topical application(s), wound assessment, and instruction(s) for ongoing care, per session

97602   non-selective debridement, without anesthesia (eg, wet-to-moist dressings, enzymatic, abrasion), including topical application(s), wound assessment, and instruction(s) for ongoing care, per session

Tests and Measurements

(For muscle testing, manual or electrical, joint range of motion, electromyography or nerve velocity determination, see 95831-95904)

(97700, 97701 have been deleted. To report, use 97703)

97703   Checkout for orthotic/prosthetic use, established patient, each 15 minutes

(97720, 97721 have been deleted. To report, use 97750)

(97740, 97741 have been deleted. To report, use 97530)

97750   Physical performance test or measurement (eg, musculoskeletal, functional capacity), with written report, each 15 minutes

(97752 has been deleted. To report, use 97750)

Medicine

Other Procedures

(For extracorporeal shock wave musculoskeletal therapy, use Category III code 0019T)

(97770 has been deleted. To report, see 97532, 97533)

97780 Acupuncture, one or more needles; without electrical stimulation

97781   with electrical stimulation

97799 Unlisted physical medicine/rehabilitation service or procedure

(98900-98902 have been deleted. To report, use appropriate category and level of **Evaluation and Management** codes)

(98910-98912 have been deleted. To report, see 99361-99362)

(98920-98922 have been deleted. To report, see 99371-99373)

Medical Nutrition Therapy

97802 Medical nutrition therapy; initial assessment and intervention, individual, face-to-face with the patient, each 15 minutes

97803   re-assessment and intervention, individual, face-to-face with the patient, each 15 minutes

97804   group (2 or more individual(s)), each 30 minutes

(For medical nutrition therapy assessment and/or intervention performed by a physician, see **Evaluation and Management** or **Preventive Medicine** service codes)

Osteopathic Manipulative Treatment

Osteopathic manipulative treatment is a form of manual treatment applied by a physician to eliminate or alleviate somatic dysfunction and related disorders. This treatment may be accomplished by a variety of techniques.

Evaluation and Management services may be reported separately if, using the modifier '-25,' the patient's condition requires a significant separately identifiable E/M service, above and beyond the usual preservice and postservice work associated with the procedure. The E/M service may be caused or prompted by the same symptoms or condition for which the OMT service was provided. As such, different diagnoses are not required for the reporting of the OMT and E/M service on the same date.

Body regions referred to are: head region; cervical region; thoracic region; lumbar region; sacral region; pelvic region; lower extremities; upper extremities; rib cage region; abdomen and viscera region.

98925 Osteopathic manipulative treatment (OMT); one to two body regions involved

98926   three to four body regions involved

98927   five to six body regions involved

98928   seven to eight body regions involved

98929   nine to ten body regions involved

Chiropractic Manipulative Treatment

Chiropractic manipulative treatment (CMT) is a form of manual treatment to influence joint and neurophysiological function. This treatment may be accomplished using a variety of techniques.

The chiropractic manipulative treatment codes include a pre-manipulation patient assessment. Additional Evaluation and Management services may be reported separately using the modifier '-25', if the patient's condition requires a significant separately identifiable E/M service, above and beyond the usual preservice and postservice work associated with the procedure. The E/M service may be caused or prompted by the same symptoms or condition for which the CMT service was provided. As such, different diagnoses are not required for the reporting of the CMT and E/M service on the same date.

For purposes of CMT, the five spinal regions referred to are: cervical region (includes atlanto-occipital joint); thoracic region (includes costovertebral and costotransverse joints); lumbar region; sacral region; and pelvic (sacro-iliac joint) region. The five extraspinal regions referred to are: head (including temporomandibular joint, excluding atlanto-occipital) region; lower extremities; upper extremities; rib cage (excluding costotransverse and costovertebral joints) and abdomen.

98940 Chiropractic manipulative treatment (CMT); spinal, one to two regions

98941   spinal, three to four regions

98942   spinal, five regions

98943   extraspinal, one or more regions

Special Services, Procedures and Reports

The procedures with code numbers 99000 through 99091 provide the reporting physician with the means of identifying the completion of special reports and services that are an adjunct to the basic services rendered. The specific number assigned indicates the special circumstances under which a basic procedure is performed.

Code 99091 should be reported no more than once in a 30 day period to include the physician or health care provider time involved with data accession, review and interpretation, modification of care plan as necessary (including communication to patient and/or caregiver), and associated documentation.

If the services described by code 99091 are provided on the same day the patient presents for an E/M service, these services should be considered part of the E/M service and not separately reported.

Do not report 99091 if it occurs within 30 days of care plan oversight services 99374-99380. Do not report 99091 if other more specific CPT codes exist (eg, 93014, 93227, 93233, 93272 for cardiographic services; 95250 for continuous glucose monitoring). Do not report 99091 for transfer and interpretation of data from hospital or clinical laboratory computers.

Miscellaneous Services

99000 Handling and/or conveyance of specimen for transfer from the physician's office to a laboratory

99001 Handling and/or conveyance of specimen for transfer from the patient in other than a physician's office to a laboratory (distance may be indicated)

99002 Handling, conveyance, and/or any other service in connection with the implementation of an order involving devices (eg, designing, fitting, packaging, handling, delivery or mailing) when devices such as orthotics, protectives, prosthetics are fabricated by an outside laboratory or shop but which items have been designed, and are to be fitted and adjusted by the attending physician

(For routine collection of venous blood, use 36415)

(99012, 99013, 99014, 99015 have been deleted. To report, see 99371-99373)

99024 Postoperative follow-up visit, included in global service

(As a component of a surgical "package," see **Surgery Guidelines**)

99025 Initial (new patient) visit when starred (*) surgical procedure constitutes major service at that visit

● **99026** Hospital mandated on call service; in-hospital, each hour

● **99027**   out-of-hospital, each hour

▶(For physician standby services requiring prolonged physician attendance, use 99360, as appropriate. Time spent performing separately reportable procedure(s) or service(s) should not be included in the time reported as mandated on call service)◀

99050 Services requested after office hours in addition to basic service

99052 Services requested between 10:00 PM and 8:00 AM in addition to basic service

99054 Services requested on Sundays and holidays in addition to basic service

99056 Services provided at request of patient in a location other than physician's office which are normally provided in the office

99058 Office services provided on an emergency basis

(99062, 99064, 99065 have been deleted. To report, see 99281-99285)

99070 Supplies and materials (except spectacles), provided by the physician over and above those usually included with the office visit or other services rendered (list drugs, trays, supplies, or materials provided)

(For spectacles, see 92390-92395)

99071 Educational supplies, such as books, tapes, and pamphlets, provided by the physician for the patient's education at cost to physician

99075 Medical testimony

99078 Physician educational services rendered to patients in a group setting (eg, prenatal, obesity, or diabetic instructions)

99080 Special reports such as insurance forms, more than the information conveyed in the usual medical communications or standard reporting form

99082 Unusual travel (eg, transportation and escort of patient)

99090 Analysis of clinical data stored in computers (eg, ECGs, blood pressures, hematologic data)

(For physician/health care professional collection and interpretation of physiologic data stored/transmitted by patient/caregiver, see 99091)

(Do not report 99090 if other more specific CPT codes exist, eg, 93014, 93227, 93233, 93272 for cardiographic services; 95250 for continuous glucose monitoring, 97750 for musculoskeletal function testing)

Medicine

99091   Collection and interpretation of physiologic data (eg, ECG, blood pressure, glucose monitoring) digitally stored and/or transmitted by the patient and/or caregiver to the physician or other qualified health care professional, requiring a minimum of 30 minutes of time

Qualifying Circumstances for Anesthesia

(For explanation of these services, see **Anesthesia Guidelines**)

+ 99100   Anesthesia for patient of extreme age, under 1 year and over 70 (List separately in addition to code for primary anesthesia procedure)

▶(For procedure performed on infants less than 1 year of age at time of surgery, see 00833, 00834)◀

+ 99116   Anesthesia complicated by utilization of total body hypothermia (List separately in addition to code for primary anesthesia procedure)

+ 99135   Anesthesia complicated by utilization of controlled hypotension (List separately in addition to code for primary anesthesia procedure)

+ 99140   Anesthesia complicated by emergency conditions (specify) (List separately in addition to code for primary anesthesia procedure)

(An emergency is defined as existing when delay in treatment of the patient would lead to a significant increase in the threat to life or body part.)

Sedation With or Without Analgesia (Conscious Sedation)

Sedation with or without analgesia (conscious sedation) is used to achieve a medically controlled state of depressed consciousness while maintaining the patient's airway, protective reflexes and ability to respond to stimulation or verbal commands. Conscious sedation includes performance and documentation of pre- and post-sedation evaluations of the patient, administration of the sedation and/or analgesic agent(s), and monitoring of cardiorespiratory function (ie, pulse oximetry, cardiorespiratory monitor, and blood pressure). The use of these codes requires the presence of an independent trained observer to assist the physician in monitoring the patient's level of consciousness and physiological status.

(If the sedation with or without analgesia (conscious sedation) is administered in support of a procedure provided by another physician, see **Anesthesia** section)

⊘ **99141**   Sedation with or without analgesia (conscious sedation); intravenous, intramuscular or inhalation

(94760-94762 may not be reported in addition to 99141)

⊘ **99142**   oral, rectal and/or intranasal

(94760-94762 may not be reported in addition to 99142)

(99150, 99151 have been deleted. To report, see 99354-99360)

Other Services and Procedures

99170   Anogenital examination with colposcopic magnification in childhood for suspected trauma

(For conscious sedation, use 99141, 99142)

99172   Visual function screening, automated or semi-automated bilateral quantitative determination of visual acuity, ocular alignment, color vision by pseudoisochromatic plates, and field of vision (may include all or some screening of the determination(s) for contrast sensitivity, vision under glare)

(This service must employ graduated visual acuity stimuli that allow a quantitative determination of visual acuity (eg, Snellen chart). This service may not be used in addition to a general ophthalmological service or an E/M service)

(Do not report 99172 in conjunction with code 99173)

99173   Screening test of visual acuity, quantitative, bilateral

(The screening test used must employ graduated visual acuity stimuli that allow a quantitative estimate of visual acuity (eg, Snellen chart). Other identifiable services unrelated to this screening test provided at the same time may be reported separately (eg, preventive medicine services). When acuity is measured as part of a general ophthalmological service or of an E/M service of the eye, it is a diagnostic examination and not a screening test.)

(Do not report 99173 in conjunction with code 99172)

99175   Ipecac or similar administration for individual emesis and continued observation until stomach adequately emptied of poison

(For diagnostic intubation, see 82926-82928, 89130-89141)

(For gastric lavage for diagnostic purposes, see 91055)

(99178 has been deleted. To report, use 96110)

(99180 has been deleted. To report, use 99183)

(99182 has been deleted. To report, use 99183)

Medicine

99183   Physician attendance and supervision of hyperbaric oxygen therapy, per session

(Evaluation and Management services and/or procedures (eg, wound debridement) provided in a hyperbaric oxygen treatment facility in conjunction with a hyperbaric oxygen therapy session should be reported separately)

99185   Hypothermia; regional

99186   total body

99190   Assembly and operation of pump with oxygenator or heat exchanger (with or without ECG and/or pressure monitoring); each hour

99191   3/4 hour

99192   1/2 hour

99195   Phlebotomy, therapeutic (separate procedure)

99199   Unlisted special service, procedure or report

Home Health Procedures/Services

These codes are used by non-physician health care professionals. Physicians should utilize the home visit codes 99341-99350, and utilize CPT codes other than 99500-▶99600◀ for any additional procedure/service provided to a patient living in a residence.

The following codes are used to report services provided in a patient's residence (including assisted living apartments, group homes, non-traditional private homes, custodial care facilities, or schools).

Health care professionals who are authorized to use Evaluation and Management Home Visit codes (99341-99350) may report codes 99500-▶99600◀ in addition to codes 99341-99350 if both services are performed. Evaluation and Management services may be reported separately, using the modifier '-25', if the patient's condition requires a significant separately identifiable E/M service, above and beyond the home health service(s)/procedure(s) codes 99500-▶99600.◀

▶Codes 99551-99600 include a home visit by a health care professional in a single 24-hour period. All solutions, equipment, supplies and drugs are excluded and should be reported separately. If more than one therapy is given in a 24-hour period, the most complex therapy should be reported first and 99600 should be reported separately for each additional therapy given in that 24-hour period. These codes do not represent self-administration of medications by the patient.◀

99500   Home visit for prenatal monitoring and assessment to include fetal heart rate, non-stress test, uterine monitoring, and gestational diabetes monitoring

99501   Home visit for postnatal assessment and follow-up care

99502   Home visit for newborn care and assessment

99503   Home visit for respiratory therapy care (eg, bronchodilator, oxygen therapy, respiratory assessment, apnea evaluation)

▲ **99504**   Home visit for mechanical ventilation care

99505   Home visit for stoma care and maintenance including colostomy and cystostomy

99506   Home visit for intramuscular injections

99507   Home visit for care and maintenance of catheter(s) (eg, urinary, drainage, and enteral)

▶(99508 has been deleted. To report see 95806-95811)◀

99509   Home visit for assistance with activities of daily living and personal care

(To report self-care/home management training, see 97535)

(To report home medical nutrition assessment and intervention services, see 97802-97804)

(To report home speech therapy services, see 92507-92508)

99510   Home visit for individual, family, or marriage counseling

99511   Home visit for fecal impaction management and enema administration

99512   Home visit for hemodialysis, per diem

(For home infusion of peritoneal dialysis, use 99559)

▶(99539 has been deleted. To report, use 99600)◀

Home Infusion Procedures▶/Services◀

▲ **99551**   Home infusion for pain management (intravenous or subcutaneous), per visit

▲ **99552**   Home infusion for pain management (epidural or intrathecal), per visit

▲ **99553**   Home infusion for tocolytic therapy, per visit

▲ **99554**   Home infusion for hematopoietic hormones (eg, erythropoietin, G-CSF, CM-CSF) or platelets, per visit

▲ **99555**   Home infusion for chemotherapy, per visit

▲ **99556**   Home infusion for antibiotics/antifungals/antivirals, per visit

▲ **99557**   Home infusion of continuous anticoagulant therapy (eg, heparin), per visit

▲ **99558**   Home infusion of immunotherapy, per visit

▲ **99559**   Home infusion of peritoneal dialysis, per visit

(For home visit for hemodialysis, use 99512)

▲ **99560**   Home infusion of enteral nutrition, per visit

▲ **99561**   Home infusion of hydration therapy, per visit

Medicine

▲ **99562**   Home infusion of total parenteral nutrition, per visit

▲ **99563**   Home administration of aerosolized pentamidine, per visit

▲ **99564**   Home infusion for anti-hemophilic agents (eg, Factor VIII), per visit

▲ **99565**   Home infusion of alpha-1-proteinase inhibitor (eg, Prolastin), per visit

▲ **99566**   Home infusion for uninterrupted, long-term intravenous treatment (eg, epoprostenol), per visit

▲ **99567**   Home infusion of sympathomimetic agents (eg, dobutamine), per visit

▲ **99568**   Home infusion of miscellaneous drugs, per visit

+ ▲ **99569**   Home infusion, each additional therapy given on same day (List separately in addition to code for primary visit), per visit

● **99600**   Unlisted home visit service or procedure

Medicine

Category III Codes

The following section contains a set of temporary codes for emerging technology, services, and procedures. Category III codes will allow data collection for these services/procedures. Use of unlisted codes does not offer the opportunity for the collection of specific data. If a Category III code is available, this code must be reported instead of a Category I unlisted code. This is an activity that is critically important in the evaluation of health care delivery and the formation of public and private policy. The use of the codes in this section will allow physicians and other qualified health care professionals, insurers, health services researchers, and health policy experts to identify emerging technology, services, and procedures for clinical efficacy, utilization and outcomes.

The inclusion of a service or procedure in this section neither implies nor endorses clinical efficacy, safety or the applicability to clinical practice. The codes in this section do not conform to the usual requirements for CPT Category I codes established by the Editorial Panel. For Category I codes, the Panel requires that the service/ procedure be performed by many health care professionals in clinical practice in multiple locations and that FDA approval, as appropriate, has already been received. The nature of emerging technology, services, and procedures is such that these requirements may not be met. For these reasons, temporary codes for emerging technology, services, and procedures have been placed in a separate section of the CPT book and the codes are differentiated from Category I CPT codes by the use of alphanumeric characters.

Services/procedures described in this section make use of alphanumeric characters. These codes have an alpha character as the 5th character in the string, preceded by four digits. The digits are not intended to reflect the placement of the code in the Category I section of CPT nomenclature. Codes in this section may or may not eventually receive a Category I CPT code. In either case, a given Category III code will be archived after five years of its inception unless it is demonstrated that a temporary code is still needed. New codes in this section are released semi-annually via the AMA/CPT internet site, to expedite dissemination for reporting. The full set of temporary codes for emerging technology, services, and procedures are published annually in the *CPT* book.

0001T   Endovascular repair of infrarenal abdominal aortic aneurysm or dissection; modular bifurcated prosthesis (two docking limbs)

0002T   aorto-uni-iliac or aorto-unifemoral prosthesis

(For radiological supervision and interpretation, use 75952 in conjunction with 0001T-0002T)

0003T   Cervicography

(0004T has been deleted. To report, use 88380)

0005T   Transcatheter placement of extracranial cerebrovascular artery stent(s), percutaneous; initial vessel

+ 0006T   each additional vessel (List separately in addition to code for primary procedure

(Use 0006T in conjunction with code 0005T)

(For radiological supervision and interpretation, use 0007T)

0007T   Transcatheter placement of extracranial cerebrovascular artery stent(s), percutaneous, radiological supervision and interpretation, each vessel

(For procedure, see 0005T, 0006T)

0008T   Upper gastrointestinal endoscopy including esophagus, stomach, and either the duodenum and/or jejunum as appropriate; with suturing of the esophagogastric junction

0009T   Endometrial cryoablation with ultrasonic guidance

0010T   Tuberculosis test, cell mediated immunity measurement of gamma interferon antigen response

0012T   Arthroscopy, knee, surgical, implantation of osteochondral graft(s) for treatment of articular surface defect; autografts

0013T   allografts

0014T   Meniscal transplantation, medial or lateral, knee (any method)

0016T   Destruction of localized lesion of choroid (eg, choroidal neovascularization), transpupillary thermotherapy

0017T   Destruction of macular drusen, photocoagulation

0018T   Delivery of high power, focal magnetic pulses for direct stimulation to cortical neurons

0019T   Extracorporeal shock wave therapy; involving musculoskeletal system

0020T   involving plantar fascia

0021T   Insertion of transcervical or transvaginal fetal oximetry sensor

0023T   Infectious agent drug susceptibility phenotype prediction using genotypic comparison to known genotypic/ phenotypic database, HIV 1

0024T   Non-surgical septal reduction therapy (eg, alcohol ablation), for hypertrophic obstructive cardiomyopathy; with coronary arteriograms, with or without temporary pacemaker

0025T   Determination of corneal thickness (eg, pachymetry) with interpretation and report, bilateral

0026T   Lipoprotein, direct measurement, intermediate density lipoproteins (IDL) (remnant lipoproteins)

Category III Codes

● **0027T** Endoscopic lysis of epidural adhesions with direct visualization using mechanical means (eg, spinal endoscopic catheter system) or solution injection (eg, normal saline) including radiologic localization and epidurography

▶(For diagnostic epidurography, use 64999)◀

● **0028T** Dual energy x-ray absorptiometry (DEXA) body composition study, one or more sites

● **0029T** Treatment(s) for incontinence, pulsed magnetic neuromodulation, per day

● **0030T** Antiprothrombin (phospholipid cofactor) antibody, each Ig class

● **0031T** Speculoscopy;

● **0032T**   with directed sampling

● **0033T** Endovascular repair of descending thoracic aortic aneurysm, pseudoaneurysm or dissection; involving coverage of left subclavian artery origin, initial endoprosthesis

▶(For radiological supervision and interpretation, use 0038T)◀

● **0034T**   not involving coverage of left subclavian artery origin, initial endoprosthesis

▶(For radiological supervision and interpretation, use 0038T)◀

● **0035T** Placement of proximal or distal extension prosthesis for endovascular repair of descending thoracic aortic aneurysm, pseudoaneurysm or dissection; initial extension

▶(For radiological supervision and interpretation, use 0040T)◀

▶(Do not report 0034T and 0035T when placement of extension converts repair to cover left subclavian origin, use only 0033T)◀

✚ ● **0036T**   each additional extension (List separately in addition to code for primary procedure)

▶(Use 0036T in conjunction with code 0035T)◀

▶(For radiological supervision and interpretation, use 0040T)◀

● **0037T** Open subclavian to carotid artery transposition performed in conjunction with endovascular thoracic aneurysm repair, by neck incision, unilateral

▶(For bilateral procedure, use modifier '-50')◀

▶(Do not report 0037T in addition to 35694)◀

● **0038T** Endovascular repair of descending thoracic aortic aneurysm, pseudoaneurysm or dissection involving coverage of left subclavian artery origin, initial endoprosthesis, radiological supervision and interpretation

▶(For implantation of endovascular graft, use 0033T)◀

● **0039T** Endovascular repair of descending thoracic aortic aneurysm, pseudoaneurysm or dissection not involving coverage of left subclavian artery origin, initial endoprosthesis, radiological supervision and interpretation

▶(For implantation of endovascular graft, use 0034T)◀

● **0040T** Placement of proximal or distal extension prosthesis for endovascular repair of descending thoracic aortic aneurysm, pseudoaneurysm or dissection, each extension, radiological supervision and interpretation

▶(For implantation of endovascular graft extensions, see 0035T, 0036T)◀

● **0041T** Urinalysis infectious agent detection, semi-quantitative analysis of volatile compounds

● **0042T** Cerebral perfusion analysis using computed tomography with contrast administration, including post-processing of parametric maps with determination of cerebral blood flow, cerebral blood volume, and mean transit time

● **0043T** Carbon monoxide, expired gas analysis (eg, $ETCO_c$/hemolysis breath test)

● **0044T** Whole body integumentary photography, at request of a physician, for monitoring of high-risk patients with dysplastic nevus syndrome or familial melanoma

Category III Codes

Appendix A

Modifiers

This list includes all of the modifiers applicable to *CPT* 2003 codes.

Note: For all *CPT* modifiers in Appendix A, references to the five digit modifier codes have been deleted.

-21 Prolonged Evaluation and Management Services: When the face-to-face or floor/unit service(s) provided is prolonged or otherwise greater than that usually required for the highest level of evaluation and management service within a given category, it may be identified by adding modifier '-21' to the evaluation and management code number. A report may also be appropriate.

-22 Unusual Procedural Services: When the service(s) provided is greater than that usually required for the listed procedure, it may be identified by adding modifier '-22' to the usual procedure number. A report may also be appropriate.

-23 Unusual Anesthesia: Occasionally, a procedure, which usually requires either no anesthesia or local anesthesia, because of unusual circumstances must be done under general anesthesia. This circumstance may be reported by adding the modifier '-23' to the procedure code of the basic service.

-24 Unrelated Evaluation and Management Service by the Same Physician During a Postoperative Period: The physician may need to indicate that an evaluation and management service was performed during a postoperative period for a reason(s) unrelated to the original procedure. This circumstance may be reported by adding the modifier '-24' to the appropriate level of E/M service.

-25 Significant, Separately Identifiable Evaluation and Management Service by the Same Physician on the Same Day of the Procedure or Other Service: The physician may need to indicate that on the day a procedure or service identified by a CPT code was performed, the patient's condition required a significant, separately identifiable E/M service above and beyond the other service provided or beyond the usual preoperative and postoperative care associated with the procedure that was performed. The E/M service may be prompted by the symptom or condition for which the procedure and/or service was provided. As such, different diagnoses are not required for reporting of the E/M services on the same date. This circumstance may be reported by adding the modifier '-25' to the appropriate level of E/M service. **Note:** This modifier is not used to report an E/M service that resulted in a decision to perform surgery. See modifier '-57.'

-26 Professional Component: Certain procedures are a combination of a physician component and a technical component. When the physician component is reported separately, the service may be identified by adding the modifier '-26' to the usual procedure number.

-32 Mandated Services: Services related to *mandated* consultation and/or related services (eg, PRO, third party payer, governmental, legislative or regulatory requirement) may be identified by adding the modifier '-32' to the basic procedure.

-47 Anesthesia by Surgeon: Regional or general anesthesia provided by the surgeon may be reported by adding the modifier '-47' to the basic service. (This does not include local anesthesia.) **Note:** Modifier '-47' would not be used as a modifier for the anesthesia procedures.

-50 Bilateral Procedure: Unless otherwise identified in the listings, bilateral procedures that are performed at the same operative session, should be identified by adding the modifier '-50' to the appropriate five digit code.

-51 Multiple Procedures: When multiple procedures, other than E/M services, are performed at the same session by the same provider, the primary procedure or service may be reported as listed. The additional procedure(s) or service(s) may be identified by appending the modifier '-51' to the additional procedure or service code(s). **Note:** This modifier should not be appended to designated "add-on" codes (see Appendix D).

-52 Reduced Services: Under certain circumstances a service or procedure is partially reduced or eliminated at the physician's discretion. Under these circumstances the service provided can be identified by its usual procedure number and the addition of the modifier '-52', signifying that the service is reduced. This provides a means of reporting reduced services without disturbing the identification of the basic service. **Note:** For hospital outpatient reporting of a previously scheduled procedure/service that is partially reduced or cancelled as a result of extenuating circumstances or those that threaten the well-being of the patient prior to or after administration of anesthesia, see modifiers '-73' and '-74' (see modifiers approved for ASC hospital outpatient use).

-53 Discontinued Procedure: Under certain circumstances, the physician may elect to terminate a surgical or diagnostic procedure. Due to extenuating circumstances or those that threaten the well being of the patient, it may be necessary to indicate that a surgical or diagnostic procedure was started but discontinued. This circumstance may be reported by adding the modifier '-53' to the code reported by the physician for the discontinued procedure. **Note:** This modifier is not used to report the elective cancellation of a procedure prior to the patient's anesthesia induction and/or surgical preparation in the operating suite. For outpatient hospital/ambulatory surgery center (ASC) reporting of a previously scheduled procedure/service that is partially reduced or cancelled as a result of extenuating circumstances or those that threaten the well being of the patient prior to or after administration of anesthesia, see modifiers '-73' and '-74' (see modifiers approved for ASC hospital outpatient use).

-54 **Surgical Care Only:** When one physician performs a surgical procedure and another provides preoperative and/or postoperative management, surgical services may be identified by adding the modifier '-54' to the usual procedure number.

-55 **Postoperative Management Only:** When one physician performed the postoperative management and another physician performed the surgical procedure, the postoperative component may be identified by adding the modifier '-55' to the usual procedure number.

-56 **Preoperative Management Only:** When one physician performed the preoperative care and evaluation and another physician performed the surgical procedure, the preoperative component may be identified by adding the modifier '-56' to the usual procedure number.

-57 **Decision for Surgery:** An evaluation and management service that resulted in the initial decision to perform the surgery may be identified by adding the modifier '-57' to the appropriate level of E/M service.

-58 **Staged or Related Procedure or Service by the Same Physician During the Postoperative Period:** The physician may need to indicate that the performance of a procedure or service during the postoperative period was: a) planned prospectively at the time of the original procedure (staged); b) more extensive than the original procedure; or c) for therapy following a diagnostic surgical procedure. This circumstance may be reported by adding the modifier '-58' to the staged or related procedure. **Note:** This modifier is not used to report the treatment of a problem that requires a return to the operating room. See modifier '-78.'

-59 **Distinct Procedural Service:** Under certain circumstances, the physician may need to indicate that a procedure or service was distinct or independent from other services performed on the same day. Modifier '-59' is used to identify procedures/services that are not normally reported together, but are appropriate under the circumstances. This may represent a different session or patient encounter, different procedure or surgery, different site or organ system, separate incision/excision, separate lesion, or separate injury (or area of injury in extensive injuries) not ordinarily encountered or performed on the same day by the same physician. However, when another already established modifier is appropriate it should be used rather than modifier '-59.' Only if no more descriptive modifier is available, and the use of modifier '-59' best explains the circumstances, should modifier '-59' be used.

-62 **Two Surgeons:** When two surgeons work together as primary surgeons performing distinct part(s) of a procedure, each surgeon should report his/her distinct operative work by adding the modifier '-62' to the procedure code and any associated add-on code(s) for that procedure as long as both surgeons continue to work

together as primary surgeons. Each surgeon should report the co-surgery once using the same procedure code. If additional procedure(s) (including add-on procedure(s) are performed during the same surgical session, separate code(s) may also be reported with the modifier '-62' added. **Note:** If a co-surgeon acts as an assistant in the performance of additional procedure(s) during the same surgical session, those services may be reported using separate procedure code(s) with the modifier '-80' or modifier '-82' added, as appropriate.

▶ -63 **Procedure Performed on Infants less than 4 kg:** Procedures performed on neonates and infants up to a present body weight of 4 kg may involve significantly increased complexity and physician work commonly associated with these patients. This circumstance may be reported by adding the modifier '-63' to the procedure number. **Note:** Unless otherwise designated, this modifier may only be appended to procedures/services listed in the 20000-69999 code series. Modifier '-63' should not be appended to any CPT codes listed in the **Evaluation and Management Services, Anesthesia, Radiology, Pathology/Laboratory, or Medicine** sections.◀

-66 **Surgical Team:** Under some circumstances, highly complex procedures (requiring the concomitant services of several physicians, often of different specialties, plus other highly skilled, specially trained personnel, various types of complex equipment) are carried out under the "surgical team" concept. Such circumstances may be identified by each participating physician with the addition of the modifier '-66' to the basic procedure number used for reporting services.

-76 **Repeat Procedure by Same Physician:** The physician may need to indicate that a procedure or service was repeated subsequent to the original procedure or service. This circumstance may be reported by adding the modifier '-76' to the repeated procedure/service.

-77 **Repeat Procedure by Another Physician:** The physician may need to indicate that a basic procedure or service performed by another physician had to be repeated. This situation may be reported by adding modifier '-77' to the repeated procedure/service.

-78 **Return to the Operating Room for a Related Procedure During the Postoperative Period:** The physician may need to indicate that another procedure was performed during the postoperative period of the initial procedure. When this subsequent procedure is related to the first, and requires the use of the operating room, it may be reported by adding the modifier '-78' to the related procedure. (For repeat procedures on the same day, see '-76'.)

-79 **Unrelated Procedure or Service by the Same Physician During the Postoperative Period:** The physician may need to indicate that the performance of a procedure or service during the postoperative period was unrelated to the original procedure. This circumstance may be reported by using the modifier '-79'. (For repeat procedures on the same day, see '-76'.)

-80 Assistant Surgeon: Surgical assistant services may be identified by adding the modifier '-80' to the usual procedure number(s).

-81 Minimum Assistant Surgeon: Minimum surgical assistant services are identified by adding the modifier '-81' to the usual procedure number.

-82 Assistant Surgeon (when qualified resident surgeon not available): The unavailability of a qualified resident surgeon is a prerequisite for use of modifier '-82' appended to the usual procedure code number(s).

-90 Reference (Outside) Laboratory: When laboratory procedures are performed by a party other than the treating or reporting physician, the procedure may be identified by adding the modifier '-90' to the usual procedure number.

-91 Repeat Clinical Diagnostic Laboratory Test: In the course of treatment of the patient, it may be necessary to repeat the same laboratory test on the same day to obtain subsequent (multiple) test results. Under these circumstances, the laboratory test performed can be identified by its usual procedure number and the addition of the modifier '-91'. **Note:** This modifier may not be used when tests are rerun to confirm initial results; due to testing problems with specimens or equipment; or for any other reason when a normal, one-time, reportable result is all that is required. This modifier may not be used when other code(s) describe a series of test results (eg, glucose tolerance tests, evocative/suppression testing). This modifier may only be used for laboratory test(s) performed more than once on the same day on the same patient.

-99 Multiple Modifiers: Under certain circumstances two or more modifiers may be necessary to completely delineate a service. In such situations modifier '-99' should be added to the basic procedure, and other applicable modifiers may be listed as part of the description of the service.

Anesthesia Physical Status Modifiers

The Physical Status modifiers are consistent with the American Society of Anesthesiologists ranking of patient physical status, and distinguish various levels of complexity of the anesthesia service provided. All anesthesia services are reported by use of the anesthesia five-digit procedure code (00100-03108) with the appropriate physical status modifier appended.

Example: 00100-P1

Under certain circumstances, when another established modifier(s) is appropriate, it should be used in addition to the physical status modifier.

Example: 00100-P4-53

Physical Status Modifier P1: A normal healthy patient

Physical Status Modifier P2: A patient with mild systemic disease

Physical Status Modifier P3: A patient with severe systemic disease

Physical Status Modifier P4: A patient with severe systemic disease that is a constant threat to life

Physical Status Modifier P5: A moribund patient who is not expected to survive without the operation

Physical Status Modifier P6: A declared brain-dead patient whose organs are being removed for donor purposes

Modifiers Approved for Ambulatory Surgery Center (ASC) Hospital Outpatient Use

CPT Level I Modifiers

-25 Significant, Separately Identifiable Evaluation and Management Service by the Same Physician on the Same Day of the Procedure or Other Service: The physician may need to indicate that on the day a procedure or service identified by a CPT code was performed, the patient's condition required a significant, separately identifiable E/M service above and beyond the other service provided or beyond the usual preoperative and postoperative care associated with the procedure that was performed. The E/M service may be prompted by the symptom or condition for which the procedure and/or service was provided. As such, different diagnoses are not required for reporting of the E/M services on the same date. This circumstance may be reported by adding the modifier '-25' to the appropriate level of E/M service. **Note:** This modifier is not used to report an E/M service that resulted in a decision to perform surgery. See modifier '-57.'

-27 Multiple Outpatient Hospital E/M Encounters on the Same Date: For hospital outpatient reporting purposes, utilization of hospital resources related to separate and distinct E/M encounters performed in multiple outpatient hospital settings on the same date may be reported by adding the modifier '-27' to each appropriate level outpatient and/or emergency department E/M code(s). This modifier provides a means of reporting circumstances involving evaluation and management services provided by physician(s) in more than one (multiple) outpatient hospital setting(s) (eg, hospital emergency department, clinic). **Note:** This modifier is not to be used for physician reporting of multiple E/M services performed by the same physician on the same date. For physician reporting of all outpatient evaluation and management services provided by the same physician on the same date and performed in multiple outpatient setting(s) (eg, hospital emergency department, clinic), see **Evaluation and Management, Emergency Department, or Preventive Medicine Services** codes.

-50 Bilateral Procedure: Unless otherwise identified in the listings, bilateral procedures that are performed at the same operative session should be identified by adding the modifier '-50' to the appropriate five digit code.

-52 Reduced Services: Under certain circumstances a service or procedure is partially reduced or eliminated at the physician's discretion. Under these circumstances the service provided can be identified by its usual procedure number and the addition of the modifier '-52', signifying that the service is reduced. This provides a means of reporting reduced services without disturbing the identification of the basic service. **Note:** For hospital outpatient reporting of a previously scheduled procedure/service that is partially reduced or cancelled as a result of extenuating circumstances or those that threaten the well-being of the patient prior to or after administration of anesthesia, see modifiers '-73' and '-74'.

-58 Staged or Related Procedure or Service by the Same Physician During the Postoperative Period: The physician may need to indicate that the performance of a procedure or service during the postoperative period was: a) planned prospectively at the time of the original procedure (staged); b) more extensive than the original procedure; or c) for therapy following a diagnostic surgical procedure. This circumstance may be reported by adding the modifier '-58' to the staged or related procedure. **Note:** This modifier is not used to report the treatment of a problem that requires a return to the operating room. See modifier '-78.'

-59 Distinct Procedural Service: Under certain circumstances, the physician may need to indicate that a procedure or service was distinct or independent from other services performed on the same day. Modifier '-59' is used to identify procedures/services that are not normally reported together, but are appropriate under the circumstances. This may represent a different session or patient encounter, different procedure or surgery, different site or organ system, separate incision/excision, separate lesion, or separate injury (or area of injury in extensive injuries) not ordinarily encountered or performed on the same day by the same physician. However, when another already established modifier is appropriate it should be used rather than modifier '-59.' Only if no more descriptive modifier is available, and the use of modifier '-59' best explains the circumstances, should modifier '-59' be used.

-73 Discontinued Out-Patient Hospital/Ambulatory Surgery Center (ASC) Procedure Prior to the Administration of Anesthesia: Due to extenuating circumstances or those that threaten the well being of the patient, the physician may cancel a surgical or diagnostic procedure subsequent to the patient's surgical preparation (including sedation when provided, and being taken to the room where the procedure is to be performed), but prior to the administration of anesthesia (local, regional block(s) or general). Under these circumstances, the intended service that is prepared for but cancelled can be reported by its usual procedure number and the addition of the modifier '-73'. **Note:** The elective cancellation of a service prior to the administration of anesthesia and/or surgical preparation of the patient should not be reported. For physician reporting of a discontinued procedure, see modifier '-53.'

-74 Discontinued Out-Patient Hospital/Ambulatory Surgery Center (ASC) Procedure After Administration of Anesthesia: Due to extenuating circumstances or those that threaten the well being of the patient, the physician may terminate a surgical or diagnostic procedure after the administration of anesthesia (local, regional block(s), general) or after the procedure was started (incision made, intubation started, scope inserted, etc). Under these circumstances, the procedure started but terminated can be reported by its usual procedure number and the addition of the modifier '-74'. **Note:** The elective cancellation of a service prior to the administration of anesthesia and/or surgical preparation of the patient should not be reported. For physician reporting of a discontinued procedure, see modifier '-53.'

-76 Repeat Procedure by Same Physician: The physician may need to indicate that a procedure or service was repeated subsequent to the original procedure or service. This circumstance may be reported by adding the modifier '-76' to the repeated procedure/service.

-77 Repeat Procedure by Another Physician: The physician may need to indicate that a basic procedure or service performed by another physician had to be repeated. This situation may be reported by adding modifier '-77' to the repeated procedure/service.

-78 Return to the Operating Room for a Related Procedure During the Postoperative Period: The physician may need to indicate that another procedure was performed during the postoperative period of the initial procedure. When this subsequent procedure is related to the first, and requires the use of the operating room, it may be reported by adding the modifier '-78' to the related procedure. (For repeat procedures on the same day, see '-76'.)

-79 Unrelated Procedure or Service by the Same Physician During the Postoperative Period: The physician may need to indicate that the performance of a procedure or service during the postoperative period was unrelated to the original procedure. This circumstance may be reported by using the modifier '-79'. (For repeat procedures on the same day, see '-76'.)

-91 Repeat Clinical Diagnostic Laboratory Test: In the course of treatment of the patient, it may be necessary to repeat the same laboratory test on the same day to obtain subsequent (multiple) test results. Under these circumstances, the laboratory test performed can be identified by its usual procedure number and the addition of the modifier '-91'. **Note:** This modifier may not be used when tests are rerun to confirm initial results; due to testing problems with specimens or equipment; or for any other reason when a normal, one-time, reportable result is all that is required. This modifier may not be used when other code(s) describe a series of test results (eg, glucose tolerance tests, evocative/suppression testing). This modifier may only be used for laboratory test(s) performed more than once on the same day on the same patient.

Level II (HCPCS/National) Modifiers

-E1   Upper left, eyelid

-E2   Lower left, eyelid

-E3   Upper right, eyelid

-E4   Lower right, eyelid

-F1   Left hand, second digit

-F2   Left hand, third digit

-F3   Left hand, fourth digit

-F4   Left hand, fifth digit

-F5   Right hand, thumb

-F6   Right hand, second digit

-F7   Right hand, third digit

-F8   Right hand, fourth digit

-F9   Right hand, fifth digit

-FA   Left hand, thumb

-LC   Left circumflex coronary artery (Hospitals use with codes 92980-92984, 92995, 92996)

-LD   Left anterior descending coronary artery (Hospitals use with codes 92980-92984, 92995, 92996)

-LT   Left side (used to identify procedures performed on the left side of the body)

-QM   Ambulance service provided under arrangement by a provider of services

-QN   Ambulance service furnished directly by a provider of services

-RC   Right coronary artery (Hospitals use with codes 92980-92984, 92995, 92996)

-RT   Right side (used to identify procedures performed on the right side of the body)

-T1   Left foot, second digit

-T2   Left foot, third digit

-T3   Left foot, fourth digit

-T4   Left foot, fifth digit

-T5   Right foot, great toe

-T6   Right foot, second digit

-T7   Right foot, third digit

-T8   Right foot, fourth digit

-T9   Right foot, fifth digit

-TA   Left foot, great toe

Appendix B

Summary of Additions, Deletions, and Revisions

For *CPT 2003* we revised the format of Appendix B. In past additions of the *CPT* book, Appendix B contained code numbers with abbreviated descriptors, and indicated whether the codes were added, revised, or deleted.

This year we updated this appendix to show the changes that occurred in the code descriptors. Deleted language appears with a ~~strikethrough~~, while new text appears underlined. This enhancement will give users a quick reference to the changes, without having to refer to the previous edition for the original code language.

New codes appear with a bullet (●) and are indicated as "Code added." Revised codes are preceded with a triangle (▲). Revisions to the notes, introductory paragraphs, and cross-references are not included in this appendix, but are identified in the main text of the book with the "► ◄" symbols and presented in green. Codes listed as "Grammatical change" contain minor revisions that do not change the original intent of the codes, and therefore are not preceded with a triangle symbol.

Evaluation and Management

▲ 99289   Critical care services delivered by a physician, face-to-face, during an interfacility transport of ~~Physician constant attention of the~~ critically ill or critically injured pediatric patient, 24 months of age or less, ~~during an interfacility transport~~; first 30-74 minutes of hands on care during transport

● 99293   Code added

● 99294   Code added

▲ 99295   **Initial neonatal ~~intensive~~ critical care,** per day, for the evaluation and management of a critically ill neonate, ~~and infant~~ 30 days of age or less

▲ 99296   **Subsequent neonatal ~~intensive~~ critical care,** per day, for the evaluation and management of a critically ill ~~and unstable~~ neonate, ~~or infant~~ 30 days of age or less

~~99297~~   ~~Subsequent neonatal intensive care, per day, for the evaluation and management of a critically ill though stable neonate or infant~~

▲ 99298   **Subsequent ~~neonatal~~ intensive care,** per day, for the evaluation and management of the recovering very low birth weight infant (present body weight less than 1500 grams)

● 99299   Code added

Anesthesia

▲ 00320   Anesthesia for all procedures on esophagus, thyroid, larynx, trachea and lymphatic system of neck; not otherwise specified, age 1 year or older

● 00326   Code added

● 00539   Code added

● 00541   Code added

● 00640   Code added

● 00834   Code added

● 00836   Code added

~~00869~~   ~~vasectomy, unilateral/bilateral~~

● 00921   Code added

▲ 01382   Anesthesia for diagnostic arthroscopic procedures of knee joint

▲ 01400   Anesthesia for open or surgical arthroscopic procedures on knee joint; not otherwise specified

▲ 01464   Anesthesia for arthroscopic procedures of ankle ~~joint~~ and/or foot

▲ 01622   Anesthesia for diagnostic arthroscopic procedures of shoulder joint

▲ 01630   Anesthesia for open or surgical arthroscopic procedures on humeral head and neck, sternoclavicular joint, acromioclavicular joint, and shoulder joint; not otherwise specified

▲ 01732   Anesthesia for diagnostic arthroscopic procedures of elbow joint

▲ 01740   Anesthesia for open or surgical arthroscopic procedures of~~a humerus and~~ the elbow; not otherwise specified

● 01829   Code added

▲ 01830   Anesthesia for open or surgical arthroscopic/endoscopic procedures on distal radius, distal ulna, wrist, or hand ~~bones~~ joints; not otherwise specified

01960   Grammatical change

▲ 01961   Anesthesia for cesarean delivery only

▲ 01962   Anesthesia for urgent hysterectomy following delivery

▲ 01963   Anesthesia for cesarean hysterectomy without any labor analgesia/anesthesia care

▲ 01964   Anesthesia for abortion procedures

+▲ 01968   Anesthesia for ~~C~~cesarean delivery following neuraxial labor analgesia/anesthesia (List separately in addition to code for primary procedure performed)

+▲ 01969   Anesthesia for ~~C~~cesarean hysterectomy following neuraxial labor analgesia/anesthesia (List separately in addition to code for primary procedure performed)

● 01991   Code added

● 01992   Code added

▲ 01996   Daily hospital management of epidural or subarachnoid continuous drug administration

Surgery

▲ 11400   Excision, benign lesion including margins, except skin tag (unless listed elsewhere), trunk, arms or legs; ~~lesion~~ excised diameter 0.5 cm or less

▲ 11401   ~~lesion~~ excised diameter 0.6 to 1.0 cm

▲ 11402   ~~lesion~~ excised diameter 1.1 to 2.0 cm

▲ 11403   ~~lesion~~ excised diameter 2.1 to 3.0 cm

▲ 11404   ~~lesion~~ excised diameter 3.1 to 4.0 cm

▲ 11406   ~~lesion~~ excised diameter over 4.0 cm

▲ 11420 Excision, benign lesion <u>including margins</u>, except skin tag (unless listed elsewhere), scalp, neck, hands, feet, genitalia; ~~lesion~~ <u>excised</u> diameter 0.5 cm or less

▲ 11421 ~~lesion~~ <u>excised</u> diameter 0.6 to 1.0 cm

▲ 11422 ~~lesion~~ <u>excised</u> diameter 1.1 to 2.0 cm

▲ 11423 ~~lesion~~ <u>excised</u> diameter 2.1 to 3.0 cm

▲ 11424 ~~lesion~~ <u>excised</u> diameter 3.1 to 4.0 cm

▲ 11426 ~~lesion~~ <u>excised</u> diameter over 4.0 cm

▲ 11440 Excision, other benign lesion <u>including margins</u> (unless listed elsewhere), face, ears, eyelids, nose, lips, mucous membrane; ~~lesion~~ <u>excised</u> diameter 0.5 cm or less

▲ 11441 ~~lesion~~ <u>excised</u> diameter 0.6 to 1.0 cm

▲ 11442 ~~lesion~~ <u>excised</u> diameter 1.1 to 2.0 cm

▲ 11443 ~~lesion~~ <u>excised</u> diameter 2.1 to 3.0 cm

▲ 11444 ~~lesion~~ <u>excised</u> diameter 3.1 to 4.0 cm

▲ 11446 ~~lesion~~ <u>excised</u> diameter over 4.0 cm

▲ 11600 Excision, malignant lesion <u>including margins</u>, trunk, arms, or legs; ~~lesion~~ <u>excised</u> diameter 0.5 cm or less

▲ 11601 ~~lesion~~ <u>excised</u> diameter 0.6 to 1.0 cm

▲ 11602 ~~lesion~~ <u>excised</u> diameter 1.1 to 2.0 cm

▲ 11603 ~~lesion~~ <u>excised</u> diameter 2.1 to 3.0 cm

▲ 11604 ~~lesion~~ <u>excised</u> diameter 3.1 to 4.0 cm

▲ 11606 ~~lesion~~ <u>excised</u> diameter over 4.0 cm

▲ 11620 Excision, malignant lesion <u>including margins</u>, scalp, neck, hands, feet, genitalia; ~~lesion~~ <u>excised</u> diameter 0.5 cm or less

▲ 11621 ~~lesion~~ <u>excised</u> diameter 0.6 to 1.0 cm

▲ 11622 ~~lesion~~ <u>excised</u> diameter 1.1 to 2.0 cm

▲ 11623 ~~lesion~~ <u>excised</u> diameter 2.1 to 3.0 cm

▲ 11624 ~~lesion~~ <u>excised</u> diameter 3.1 to 4.0 cm

▲ 11626 ~~lesion~~ <u>excised</u> diameter over 4.0 cm

▲ 11640 Excision, malignant lesion <u>including margins</u>, face, ears, eyelids, nose, lips; ~~lesion~~ <u>excised</u> diameter 0.5 cm or less

▲ 11641 ~~lesion~~ <u>excised</u> diameter 0.6 to 1.0 cm

▲ 11642 ~~lesion~~ <u>excised</u> diameter 1.1 to 2.0 cm

▲ 11643 ~~lesion~~ <u>excised</u> diameter 2.1 to 3.0 cm

▲ 11644 ~~lesion~~ <u>excised</u> diameter 3.1 to 4.0 cm

▲ 11646 ~~lesion~~ <u>excised</u> diameter over 4.0 cm

▲ 15756 Free muscle <u>or myocutaneous</u> flap ~~with or without skin~~ with microvascular anastomosis

⊘▲ 17304 Chemosurgery (Mohs micrographic technique), including removal of all gross tumor, surgical excision of tissue specimens, mapping, color coding of specimens, microscopic examination of specimens by the surgeon, and complete histopathological preparation <u>including the first routine stain (eg, hematoxylin and eosin, toluidine blue);</u> first stage, fresh tissue technique, up to 5 specimens

+▲ 17310 <u>each additional specimen,</u> ~~more than~~ <u>after the first</u> 5 specimens, fixed or fresh tissue, any stage <u>(List separately in addition to code for primary procedure)</u>

▲ 20550 Injection<u>(s)</u>; tendon sheath, ligament~~, ganglion cyst~~

▲ 20552 single or multiple trigger point(s), one or two muscle<u>(s)</u> ~~group(s)~~

▲ 20553 single or multiple trigger point(s), three or more muscle<u>(s)</u> ~~groups~~

▲ 20600* Arthrocentesis, aspiration and/or injection; small joint or bursa ~~or ganglion cyst~~ (eg, fingers, toes)

▲ 20605* intermediate joint or bursa ~~or ganglion cyst~~ (eg, temporomandibular, acromioclavicular, wrist, elbow or ankle, olecranon bursa)

● 20612 Code added

▲ 21030 Excision of benign tumor or cyst of ~~facial bone other than mandible~~ <u>maxilla or zygoma</u>, by enucleation and curettage

▲ 21034 Excision of malignant tumor of ~~facial bone other than mandible~~ <u>maxilla or zygoma</u>

▲ 21040 Excision of benign ~~cyst or tumor~~ <u>tumor or cyst</u> of mandible<u>; by enucleation and/or curettage</u> ~~simple~~

~~21041~~ ~~complex~~

● 21046 Code added

● 21047 Code added

● 21048 Code added

● 21049 Code added

▲ 21740 Reconstructive repair of pectus excavatum or carinatum<u>; open</u>

● 21742 Code added

● 21743 Code added

▲ 23410 Repair of ruptured musculotendinous cuff (eg, rotator cuff) <u>open</u>; acute

▲ 24516 ~~Open t~~<u>T</u>reatment of humeral shaft fracture, with insertion of intramedullary implant, with or without cerclage and/or locking screws

▲ 25320 Capsulorrhaphy or reconstruction, wrist, <u>open</u> ~~any method~~ (eg, capsulodesis, ligament repair, tendon transfer or graft) (includes synovectomy, capsulotomy and open reduction) for carpal instability

25430 Grammatical change

26440 Grammatical change

▲ 27235 Percutaneous skeletal fixation of femoral fracture, proximal end, neck~~, undisplaced, mildly displaced, or impacted fracture~~

▲ 27244 ~~Open t~~<u>T</u>reatment of intertrochanteric, pertrochanteric, or subtrochanteric femoral fracture; with plate/screw type implant, with or without cerclage

▲ 27425 Lateral retinacular release <u>open</u> ~~any method~~

▲ 27730 Arrest, epiphyseal (epiphysiodesis) ~~any method~~ <u>open</u>; distal tibia

▲ 27759 ~~Open t~~<u>T</u>reatment of tibial shaft fracture (with or without fibular fracture) by intramedullary implant, with or without interlocking screws and/or cerclage

▲ 27870 Arthrodesis, ankle, <u>open</u> ~~any method~~

▲ 29540 ankle <u>and/or foot</u>

● 29827 Code added

● 29873 Code added

● 29899 Code added

● 33215 Code added

▲ 33216   Insertion ~~or repositioning~~ of a transvenous electrode; single chamber (one electrode) permanent pacemaker or single chamber pacing cardioverter-defibrillator

● 33224   Code added

+● 33225   Code added

● 33226   Code added

+● 33508   Code added

▲ 34812   Open femoral artery exposure for delivery of ~~aortic~~ endovascular prosthesis, by groin incision, unilateral

▲ 34825   Placement of proximal or distal extension prosthesis for endovascular repair of infrarenal abdominal aortic <u>or iliac</u> aneurysm<u>, false aneurysm, or dissection</u>; initial vessel

● 34833   Code added

● 34834   Code added

● 34900   Code added

+● 35572   Code added

▲ 36415   ~~Routine venipuncture of finger/heel/ear stick for collection of specimen(s)~~ <u>Collection of venous blood by venipuncture</u>

● 36416   Code added

● 36511   Code added

● 36512   Code added

● 36513   Code added

● 36514   Code added

● 36515   Code added

● 36516   Code added

36520   ~~Therapeutic apheresis; plasma and/or cell exchange~~

36521   ~~with extracorporeal affinity column adsorption and plasma reinfusion~~

● 36536   Code added

● 36537   Code added

▲ 36540   Collection of blood specimen from a ~~partially or~~ completely implantable venous access device

▲ 36830   nonautogenous graft <u>(eg, biological collagen, thermoplastic graft)</u>

▲ 37140   Venous anastomosis, <u>open</u>; portocaval

● 37182   Code added

● 37183   Code added

● 37500   Code added

● 37501   Code added

▲ 37760   Ligation of perforator <u>veins</u>, subfascial, radical (Linton type), with or without skin graft<u>, open</u>

● 38204   Code added

● 38205   Code added

● 38206   Code added

● 38207   Code added

● 38208   Code added

● 38209   Code added

● 38210   Code added

● 38211   Code added

● 38212   Code added

● 38213   Code added

● 38214   Code added

● 38215   Code added

▲ 38220   Bone marrow<u>;</u> aspiration <u>only</u>

▲ 38221   ~~Bone marrow~~ biopsy, needle or trocar

38231   ~~Blood-derived peripheral stem cell harvesting for transplantation, per collection~~

● 38242   Code added

● 43201   Code added

● 43236   Code added

● 44206   Code added

● 44207   Code added

● 44208   Code added

44209   ~~Unlisted laparoscopy procedure, intestine (except rectum)~~

● 44210   Code added

● 44211   Code added

● 44212   Code added

● 44238   Code added

● 44239   Code added

+● 44701   Code added

● 45335   Code added

● 45340   Code added

● 45381   Code added

● 45386   Code added

● 46706   Code added

▲ 49200   Excision or destruction<u>, open,</u> ~~by any method of~~ intra-abdominal or retroperitoneal tumors or cysts or endometriomas;

● 49419   Code added

49491   Grammatical change

49495   Grammatical change

● 49904   Code added

+▲ 49905   Omental flap<u>, intra-abdominal</u> ~~(eg, for reconstruction of sternal and chest wall defects)~~ (List separately in addition to code for primary procedure)

● 50542   Code added

● 50543   Code added

● 50562   Code added

● 51701   Code added

● 51702   Code added

● 51703   Code added

● 51798   Code added

▲ 52001   Cystourethroscopy with irrigation and evacuation of <u>multiple obstructing</u> clots

▲ 52354 with biopsy and/or fulguration of <u>ureteral or renal pelvic</u> lesion

▲ 52355 with resection of <u>ureteral or renal pelvic</u> tumor

▲ 53440 <u>Sling o</u>~~O~~peration for correction of male urinary incontinence <u>(eg, fascia or synthetic)</u>~~, with or without introduction of prosthesis~~

▲ 53442 Removal <u>or revision of sling for male urinary</u> ~~of perineal prosthesis introduced for~~ incontinence <u>(eg, fascia or synthetic)</u>

~~53670~~ ~~Catheterization, urethra; simple~~

~~53675~~ ~~complicated (may include difficult removal of balloon catheter)~~

● 55866 Code added

● 56820 Code added

● 56821 Code added

● 57420 Code added

● 57421 Code added

▲ 57452 Colposcopy ~~(vaginoscopy)~~ <u>of the cervix including upper/adjacent vagina;</u> ~~(separate procedure)~~

▲ 57454 with biopsy(s) of the cervix and~~/or~~ endocervical curettage

● 57455 Code added

● 57456 Code added

▲ 57460 with loop electrode ~~excision procedure~~ <u>biopsy(s)</u> of the cervix

● 57461 Code added

▲ 58140 Myomectomy, excision of ~~leiomyomata~~ <u>fibroid tumor(s)</u> of uterus<u>, 1 to 4 intramural myoma(s) with total weight of 250 grams or</u> less <u>and/or removal of surface myomas</u> ~~single or multiple (separate procedure)~~; abdominal approach

● 58146 Code added

▲ 58260 Vaginal hysterectomy~~,~~<u>.</u> <u>for uterus 250 grams or less;</u>

58267 Grammatical change

● 58290 Code added

● 58291 Code added

● 58292 Code added

● 58293 Code added

● 58294 Code added

● 58545 Code added

● 58546 Code added

▲ 58550 Laparoscopy surgical~~,~~ <u>.</u>with vaginal hysterectomy<u>, for uterus 250 grams or less;</u> ~~with or without removal of tube(s), with or without removal of ovary(s) (laparoscopic assisted vaginal hysterectomy~~

~~58551~~ ~~with removal of leiomyomata (single or multiple)~~

● 58552 Code added

● 58553 Code added

● 58554 Code added

+● 61316 Code added

● 61322 Code added

● 61323 Code added

▲ 61340 ~~Other cranial decompression (eg, subtemporal), supratentorial~~ <u>Subtemporal cranial decompression (pseudotumor cerebri, slit ventricle syndrome)</u>

+● 61517 Code added

● 61623 Code added

▲ 61624 Transcatheter <u>permanent</u> occlusion or embolization (eg, for tumor destruction, to achieve hemostasis, to occlude a vascular malformation), percutaneous, any method; central nervous system (intracranial, spinal cord)

▲ 61751 Stereotactic biopsy, aspiration, or excision, including burr hole(s), for intracranial lesion; with ~~computerized axial tomography~~ <u>computed tomography</u> and/or magnetic resonance guidance

+● 62148 Code added

+● 62160 Code added

● 62161 Code added

● 62162 Code added

● 62163 Code added

● 62164 Code added

● 62165 Code added

▲ 62201 stereotactic<u>, neuroendoscopic</u> method

▲ 62263 Percutaneous lysis of epidural adhesions using solution injection (eg, hypertonic saline, enzyme) or mechanical means (eg, ~~spring-wound~~ catheter) including radiologic localization (includes contrast when administered)<u>, multiple adhesiolysis sessions; 2 or more days</u>

● 62264 Code added

▲ 62284 Injection procedure for myelography and/or ~~computerized axial tomography~~ <u>computed tomography</u>, spinal (other than C1-C2 and posterior fossa)

▲ 64415 brachial plexus<u>, single</u>

● 64416 Code added

▲ 64445 sciatic nerve<u>, single</u>

● 64446 Code added

● 64447 Code added

● 64448 Code added

+● 66990 Code added

▲ 69424 Ventilating tube removal ~~when originally inserted by another physician~~ <u>requiring general anesthesia</u>

Radiology

▲ 70450 ~~Computerized axial tomography~~ <u>Computed tomography</u>, head or brain; without contrast material

▲ 70480 ~~Computerized axial tomography~~ <u>Computed tomography</u>, orbit, sella, or posterior fossa or outer, middle, or inner ear; without contrast material

▲ 70486 ~~Computerized axial tomography~~ <u>Computed tomography</u>, maxillofacial area; without contrast material

▲ 70490 ~~Computerized axial tomography~~ <u>Computed tomography</u>, soft tissue neck; without contrast material

▲ 71250 ~~Computerized axial tomography~~ <u>Computed tomography</u>, thorax; without contrast material

▲ 72125 ~~Computerized axial tomography~~ <u>Computed tomography</u>, cervical spine; without contrast material

▲ 72128 ~~Computerized axial tomography~~ <u>Computed tomography</u>, thoracic spine; without contrast material

▲ 72131 ~~Computerized axial tomography~~ <u>Computed tomography</u>, lumbar spine; without contrast material

▲ 72192   ~~Computerized axial tomography~~ Computed tomography, pelvis; without contrast material

▲ 73200   ~~Computerized axial tomography~~ Computed tomography, upper extremity; without contrast material

▲ 73700   ~~Computerized axial tomography~~ Computed tomography, lower extremity; without contrast material

▲ 74022   complete acute abdomen series, including supine, erect, and/or decubitus views, ~~upright PA~~ single view chest

▲ 74150   ~~Computerized axial tomography~~ Computed tomography, abdomen; without contrast material

● 75901   Code added

● 75902   Code added

▲ 75953   Placement of proximal or distal extension prosthesis for endovascular repair of infrarenal aortic or iliac artery aneurysm, pseudoaneurysm, or dissection, radiological supervision and interpretation

● 75954   Code added

▲ 75989   Radiological guidance (ie, fluoroscopy, ultrasound, or computed ~~axial~~ tomography), for percutaneous drainage ~~of abscess, or specimen collection~~ (eg, abscess, specimen collection), with placement of ~~indwelling~~ catheter, radiological supervision and interpretation

▲ 76006   ~~Radiologic examination, stress view(s) any joint,~~ Manual application of stress ~~applied~~ performed by ~~a~~ physician ~~(includes comparison views)~~ for joint radiography, including contralateral joint if indicated

▲ 76070   ~~Computerized axial tomography~~ Computed tomography, bone mineral density study, one or more sites; axial skeleton (eg, hips, pelvis, spine)

● 76071   Code added

+▲ 76085   Digitization of film radiographic images with computer analysis for lesion detection and further physician review for interpretation, ~~screening~~ mammography (List separately in addition to code for primary procedure)

▲ 76355   ~~Computerized axial tomography~~ Computed tomography guidance for stereotactic localization

▲ 76360   ~~Computerized axial tomography~~ Computed tomography guidance for needle placement (eg, biopsy, aspiration, injection, localization device), radiological supervision and interpretation

▲ 76370   ~~Computerized axial tomography~~ Computed tomography guidance for placement of radiation therapy fields

▲ 76380   ~~Computerized axial tomography~~ Computed tomography, limited or localized follow-up study

● 76496   Code added

● 76497   Code added

● 76498   Code added

▲ 76499   Unlisted diagnostic ~~radiologic~~ radiographic procedure

● 76801   Code added

+● 76802   Code added

▲ 76805   Ultrasound, pregnant uterus, ~~B-scan and/or~~ real time with image documentation~~;~~, ~~complete (complete~~ fetal and maternal evaluation~~)~~, after first trimester (> or = 14 weeks 0 days), transabdominal approach; single or first gestation

+▲ 76810   ~~complete (complete fetal and maternal evaluation), multiple gestation, after the first trimester~~ each additional gestation (List separately in addition to code for primary procedure performed)

● 76811   Code added

+● 76812   Code added

▲ 76815   Ultrasound, pregnant uterus, real time with image documentation, limited (eg, fetal heart beat, placental location, fetal position and/or qualitative amniotic fluid volume ~~or emergency in the delivery room~~), one or more fetuses

▲ 76816   Ultrasound, pregnant uterus, real time with image documentation, follow-up ~~or repeat~~ (eg, re-evaluation of fetal size by measuring standard growth parameters and amniotic fluid volume, re-evaluation of organ system(s) suspected or confirmed to be abnormal on a previous scan), transabdominal approach, per fetus

● 76817   Code added

▲ 76999   Unlisted ultrasound procedure (eg, diagnostic, interventional)

▲ 77326   Brachytherapy isodose ~~calculation~~ plan; simple (calculation made from single plane, one to four sources/ribbon application, remote afterloading brachytherapy, 1 to 8 sources)

Pathology and Laboratory

~~80090~~   ~~TORCH antibody panel~~

83015   Grammatical change

● 83880   Code added

● 84302   Code added

● 85004   Code added

▲ 85007   ~~Blood count;~~ blood smear, microscopic examination with manual differential WBC count ~~(includes RBC morphology and platelet estimation)~~

▲ 85008   ~~manual blood smear examination without differential parameters~~ blood smear microscopic examination without manual differential WBC count

▲ 85009   manual differential WBC count, buffy coat

▲ 85014   ~~other than spun~~ hematocrit (Hct)

▲ 85018   hemoglobin (Hgb)

~~85021~~   ~~hemogram, automated (RBC, WBC, Hgb, Hct & indices only)~~

~~85022~~   ~~hemogram, automated, manual differential WBC count (CBC)~~

~~85023~~   ~~hemogram and platelet count, automated, manual differential WBC count (CBC)~~

~~85024~~   ~~hemogram and platelet count, automated, and automated partial differential WBC count (CBC)~~

▲ 85025   ~~hemogram and platelet count, automated, and automated complete differential WBC count (CBC)~~ complete (CBC), automated (Hgb, Hct, RBC, WBC and platelet count) and automated differential WBC count

▲ 85027   ~~hemogram & platelet count, automated~~ complete (CBC), automated (Hgb, Hct, RBC, WBC and platelet count)

~~85031~~   ~~Blood count; hemogram, manual, complete CBC (RBC, WBC, Hgb, Hct, & indices)~~

● 85032   Code added

▲ 85041   red blood cell (RBC) ~~only~~, automated

▲ 85044   reticulocyte ~~count~~, manual

▲ 85045   reticulocyte ~~count, flow cytometry~~ automated

▲ 85048   leukocyte ~~white blood cell~~ (WBC), automated

● 85049   Code added

▲ 85378   Fibrin degradation products, D-dimer; <u>qualitative or</u> semiquantitative

● 85380   Code added

85576   Grammatical change

~~85585~~   ~~estimation on smear, only~~

~~85590~~   ~~manual count~~

~~85595~~   ~~automated count~~

~~86915~~   ~~Bone marrow or peripheral stem cell harvest, modification or treatment to eliminate cell type(s) (eg, T cells, metastatic carcinoma)~~

▲ 86930   Frozen blood, ~~preparation for freezing,~~ each unit; <u>freezing (includes preparation)</u>

▲ 86931   ~~with~~ thawing

▲ 86932   ~~with~~ freezing <u>(includes preparation)</u> and thawing

▲ 87207   special stain for inclusion bodies or ~~intracellular~~ parasites (eg, malaria, coccidia, microsporidia, ~~cytomegalovirus,~~ <u>trypanosomes,</u> herpes viruses)

▲ 87254   <u>centrifuge enhanced</u> (shell vial) <u>technique</u>, includes identification with immunofluorescence stain, each virus

● 87255   Code added

● 87267   Code added

● 87271   Code added

~~88144~~   ~~with manual screening and computer-assisted rescreening under physician supervision~~

~~88145~~   ~~with manual screening and computer-assisted rescreening using cell selection and review under physician supervision~~

● 88174   Code added

● 88175   Code added

+● 89055   Code added

▲ 89310   motility and count <u>(not including Huhner test)</u>

Medicine

⊘ ~~90709~~   ~~Rubella and mumps virus vaccine, live, for subcutaneous use~~

~~92525~~   ~~Evaluation of swallowing and oral function for feeding~~

▲ 92597   Evaluation for use and/or fitting of voice prosthetic ~~or augmentative/alternative communication~~ device to supplement oral speech

~~92598~~   ~~Modification of voice prosthetic or augmentative/alternative communication device to supplement oral speech~~

~~92599~~   ~~Unlisted otorhinolaryngological service or procedure~~

● 92601   Code added

● 92602   Code added

● 92603   Code added

● 92604   Code added

● 92605   Code added

● 92606   Code added

● 92607   Code added

+● 92608   Code added

● 92609   Code added

● 92610   Code added

● 92611   Code added

● 92612   Code added

● 92613   Code added

● 92614   Code added

● 92615   Code added

● 92616   Code added

● 92617   Code added

● 92700   Code added

▲ 93012   Telephonic transmission of post-symptom electrocardiogram rhythm strip(s), <u>24 attended monitoring,</u> per 30 day period of time; tracing only

▲ 93268   Patient demand single or multiple event recording with presymptom memory loop, <u>24-hour attended monitoring,</u> per 30 day period of time; includes transmission, physician review and interpretation

● 93580   Code added

● 93581   Code added

⊘▲ 93620   Comprehensive electrophysiologic evaluation <u>including insertion and repositioning of multiple electrode catheters with induction or attempted induction of arrhythmia;</u> with right atrial pacing and recording, right ventricular pacing and recording, His bundle recording~~; including insertion and repositioning of multiple electrode catheters with induction or attempted induction of arrhythmia;~~

+▲ 94640   <u>Pressurized or</u> nonpressurized inhalation treatment for acute airways obstruction <u>or for sputum induction for diagnostic purposes eg, with an aerosol generator, nebulizer, metered dose inhaler or intermittent positive pressure breathing (IPPB) device</u>

~~94650~~   ~~Intermittent positive pressure breathing (IPPB) treatment, air or oxygen, with or without nebulized medication; initial demonstration and/or evaluation~~

~~94651~~   ~~subsequent~~

~~94652~~   ~~newborn infants~~

▲ 94664   ~~Aerosol or vapor inhalations for sputum mobilization, bronchodilation, or sputum induction for diagnostic purposes; initial demonstration or evaluation~~ <u>Demonstration and/or evaluation of patient utilization of an aerosol generator, nebulizer, metered dose inhaler or IPPB device</u>

~~94665~~   ~~subsequent~~

▲ 95027   ~~Skin end point titration~~ <u>Intracutaneous (intradermal) tests, sequential and incremental, with allergenic extracts for airborne allergens, immediate type reaction, specify number of tests allergen(s) tested</u>

▲ 95812   Electroencephalogram (EEG) extended monitoring; ~~up to one hour~~ <u>41-60 minutes</u>

▲ 95816   Electroencephalogram (EEG)<u>;</u> including recording awake and drowsy ~~(including hyperventilation and/or photic stimulation when appropriate)~~

▲ 95819   ~~Electroencephalogram (EEG)~~ including recording awake and asleep ~~(including hyperventilation and/or photic stimulation when appropriate)~~

▲ 95822   ~~Electroencephalogram (EEG);~~ <u>recording in coma or</u> sleep only

▲ 95827   all night <u>recording</u> ~~sleep only~~

95860   Grammatical change

95861	Grammatical change	
95863	Grammatical change	
95864	Grammatical change	
▲ 95867	~~Needle electromyography,~~ cranial nerve supplied muscle(s), unilateral	
95868	Grammatical change	
▲ 95869	~~Needle electromyography,~~ thoracic paraspinal muscles (excluding T1 or T12)	
▲ 95875	Ischemic limb exercise test with serial specimen(s) acquisition for muscle(s) metabolite(s)	
● 95990	Code added	
▲ 96530	Refilling and maintenance of an implantable pump or reservoir for drug delivery, systemic (eg, intravenous, intra-arterial)	
● 96920	Code added	
● 96921	Code added	
● 96922	Code added	
● 99026	Code added	
● 99027	Code added	
99100	Grammatical change	
▲ 99504	Home visit for ~~patients receiving~~ mechanical ventilation care	
~~99508~~	~~Home visit for polysomnography and sleep studies~~	
~~99539~~	~~Unlisted home visit service or procedure~~	
▲ 99551	Home infusion for pain management (intravenous or subcutaneous), ~~per diem~~ per visit	
▲ 99552	Home infusion for pain management (epidural or intrathecal), ~~per diem~~ per visit	
▲ 99553	Home infusion for tocolytic therapy, ~~per diem~~ per visit	
▲ 99554	Home infusion for hematopoietic hormones (eg, erythropoietin, G-CSF, GM-CSF) or platelets, ~~per diem~~ per visit	
▲ 99555	Home infusion for chemotherapy, ~~per diem~~ per visit	
▲ 99556	Home infusion for antibiotics/antifungals/antivirals, ~~per diem~~ per visit	
▲ 99557	Home infusion of continuous anticoagulant therapy (eg, heparin), ~~per diem~~ per visit	
▲ 99558	Home infusion of immunotherapy, ~~per diem~~ per visit	
▲ 99559	Home infusion of peritoneal dialysis, ~~per diem~~ per visit	
▲ 99560	Home infusion of enteral nutrition, ~~per diem~~ per visit	
▲ 99561	Home infusion of hydration therapy, ~~per diem~~ per visit	
▲ 99562	Home infusion of total parenteral nutrition, ~~per diem~~ per visit	
▲ 99563	Home administration of aerosolized pentamidine, ~~per diem~~ per visit	
▲ 99564	Home infusion for anti-hemophilic agents (eg, Factor VIII), ~~per diem~~ per visit	
▲ 99565	Home infusion of alpha-1-proteinase inhibitor (eg, Prolastin), ~~per diem~~ per visit	
▲ 99566	Home infusion for uninterrupted, long-term intravenous treatment (eg, epoprostenol), ~~per diem~~ per visit	
▲ 99567	Home infusion of sympathomimetic agents (eg, dobutamine), ~~per diem~~ per visit	

▲ 99568	Home infusion of miscellaneous drugs, ~~per diem~~ per visit	
+▲ 99569	Home infusion, each additional therapy given on same day (List separately in addition to code for primary visit), per visit	
● 99600	Code added	

Category III Codes

● 0027T	Code added	
● 0028T	Code added	
● 0029T	Code added	
● 0030T	Code added	
● 0031T	Code added	
● 0032T	Code added	
● 0033T	Code added	
● 0034T	Code added	
● 0035T	Code added	
+● 0036T	Code added	
● 0037T	Code added	
● 0038T	Code added	
● 0039T	Code added	
● 0040T	Code added	
● 0041T	Code added	
● 0042T	Code added	
● 0043T	Code added	
● 0044T	Code added	

Appendix C

Clinical Examples

As described in *CPT 2003*, clinical examples of the CPT codes for Evaluation and Management (E/M) services are intended to be an important element of the coding system. The clinical examples, when used with the E/M descriptors contained in the full text of *CPT*, provide a comprehensive and powerful new tool for physicians to report the services provided to their patients.

The American Medical Association is pleased to provide you with these clinical examples for *CPT 2003*. The clinical examples that are provided in this supplement are limited to Office or Other Outpatient Services, Hospital Inpatient Services, Consultations, Critical Care, Prolonged Services and Care Plan Oversight.

These clinical examples do not encompass the entire scope of medical practice. Inclusion or exclusion of any particular specialty group does not infer any judgment of importance or lack thereof; nor does it limit the applicability of the example to any particular specialty.

Of utmost importance is that these clinical examples are just that: examples. A particular patient encounter, depending on the specific circumstances, must be judged by the services provided by the physician for that particular patient. Simply because the patient's complaints, symptoms, or diagnoses match those of a particular clinical example, does not automatically assign that patient encounter to that particular level of service. The three key components (history, examination, and medical decision making) must be met and documented in the medical record to report a particular level of service.

Office or Other Outpatient Services

New Patient

99201   Initial office visit for a 50-year-old male from out-of-town who needs a prescription refill for a nonsteroidal anti-inflammatory drug. (Anesthesiology)

Initial office visit for a 40-year-old female, new patient, requesting information about local pain clinics. (Anesthesiology/Pain Medicine)

Initial office visit for a 10-year-old girl for determination of visual acuity as part of a summer camp physical (does not include determination of refractive error). (Ophthalmology)

Initial office visit for an out-of-town patient requiring topical refill. (Dermatology)

Initial office visit for a 65-year-old male for reassurance about an isolated seborrheic keratosis on upper back. (Plastic Surgery)

Initial office visit for an out-of-state visitor who needs refill of topical steroid to treat lichen planus. (Dermatology)

Initial office visit for an 86-year-old male, out-of-town visitor, who needs prescription refilled for an anal skin preparation that he forgot. (General Surgery/Colon & Rectal Surgery)

Initial office visit for a transient patient with alveolar osteitis for repacking. (Oral & Maxillofacial Surgery)

Initial office visit for a patient with a pedunculated lesion of the neck which is unsightly. (Dermatology)

Initial office visit for a 10-year-old male, for limited subungual hematoma not requiring drainage. (Internal Medicine)

Initial office visit with an out-of-town visitor who needs a prescription refilled because she forgot her hay fever medication. (Allergy & Immunology/Internal Medicine)

Initial office visit with a 9-month-old female with diaper rash. (Pediatrics)

Initial office visit with a 10-year-old male with severe rash and itching for the past 24 hours, positive history for contact with poison oak 48 hours prior to the visit. (Family Medicine)

Initial office visit with a 5-year-old female to remove sutures from simple wound placed by another physician. (Plastic Surgery)

Initial office visit for a 22-year-old male with a small area of sunburn requiring first aid. (Dermatology/Family Medicine/Internal Medicine)

Initial office visit for the evaluation and management of a contusion of a finger. (Orthopaedic Surgery)

99202   Initial office visit for a 13-year-old patient with comedopapular acne of the face unresponsive to over-the-counter medications. (Family Medicine)

Initial office visit for a patient with a clinically benign lesion or nodule of the lower leg which has been present for many years. (Dermatology)

Initial office visit for a patient with a circumscribed patch of dermatitis of the leg. (Dermatology)

Initial office visit for a patient with papulosquamous eruption of elbows. (Dermatology)

Initial office visit for a 9-year-old patient with erythematous, grouped, vesicular eruption of the lip of three days' duration. (Pediatrics)

Initial office visit for an 18-year-old male referred by an orthodontist for advice regarding removal of four wisdom teeth. (Oral & Maxillofacial Surgery)

Initial office visit for a 14-year-old male, who was referred by his orthodontist, for advice on the exposure of impacted maxillary cuspids. (Oral & Maxillofacial Surgery)

Initial office visit for a patient presenting with itching patches on the wrists and ankles. (Dermatology)

Initial office visit for a 30-year-old male for evaluation and discussion of treatment of rhinophyma. (Plastic Surgery)

Initial office visit for a 16-year-old male with severe cystic acne, new patient. (Dermatology)

Initial office evaluation for gradual hearing loss, 58-year-old male, history and physical examination, with interpretation of complete audiogram, air bone, etc. (Otolaryngology)

Initial evaluation and management of recurrent urinary infection in female. (Internal Medicine)

Initial office visit with a 10-year-old girl with history of chronic otitis media and a draining ear. (Pediatrics)

Initial office visit for a 10-year-old female with acute maxillary sinusitis. (Family Medicine)

Initial office visit for a patient with recurring episodes of herpes simplex who has developed a clustering of vesicles on the upper lip. (Internal Medicine)

Initial office visit for a 25-year-old patient with single season allergic rhinitis. (Allergy & Immunology)

Initial office visit to plan transient dialysis for a 56-year-old stable dialysis patient who has accompanying records. (Nephrology)

99203   Initial office visit for a 76-year-old male with a stasis ulcer of three months' duration. (Dermatology)

Initial office visit for a 30-year-old female with pain in the lateral aspect of the forearm. (Physical Medicine & Rehabilitation)

Initial office visit for a 15-year-old patient with a four-year history of moderate comedopapular acne of the face, chest, and back with early scarring. Discussion of use of systemic medication. (Dermatology)

Initial office visit for a patient with papulosquamous eruption of the elbow with pitting of nails and itchy scalp. (Dermatology)

Initial office visit for a 57-year-old female who complains of painful parotid swelling for one week's duration. (Oral & Maxillofacial Surgery)

Initial office visit for a patient with an ulcerated non-healing lesion or nodule on the tip of the nose. (Dermatology)

Initial office visit for a patient with dermatitis of the antecubital and popliteal fossae. (Dermatology)

Initial office visit for a 22-year-old female with irregular menses. (Family Medicine)

Initial office visit for a 50-year-old female with dyspepsia and nausea. (Family Medicine)

Initial office visit for a 53-year-old laborer with degenerative joint disease of the knee with no prior treatment. (Orthopaedic Surgery)

Initial office visit for a 60-year-old male with Dupuytren's contracture of one hand with multiple digit involvement. (Orthopaedic Surgery)

Initial office visit for a 33-year-old male with painless gross hematuria without cystoscopy. (Internal Medicine)

Initial office visit for a 55-year-old female with chronic blepharitis. There is a history of use of many medications. (Ophthalmology)

Initial office visit for an 18-year-old female with a two-day history of acute conjunctivitis. Extensive history of possible exposures, prior normal ocular history, and medication use is obtained. (Ophthalmology)

Initial office visit for a 14-year-old male with unilateral anterior knee pain. (Physical Medicine & Rehabilitation)

Initial office visit of an adult who presents with symptoms of an upper-respiratory infection that has progressed to unilateral purulent nasal discharge and discomfort in the right maxillary teeth. (Otolaryngology, Head & Neck Surgery)

Initial office visit of a 40-year-old female with symptoms of atopic allergies including eye and sinus congestion, often associated with infections. She would like to be tested for allergies. (Otolaryngology, Head & Neck Surgery)

Initial office visit of a 65-year-old with nasal stuffiness. (Otolaryngology, Head & Neck Surgery)

Initial office visit for initial evaluation of a 48-year-old man with recurrent low back pain radiating to the leg. (General Surgery)

Initial office visit for evaluation, diagnosis and management of painless gross hematuria in a new patient, without cystoscopy. (Internal Medicine)

Initial office visit with couple for counseling concerning voluntary vasectomy for sterility. Spent 30 minutes discussing procedure, risks and benefits, and answering questions. (Urology)

Initial office visit of a 49-year-old male with nasal obstruction. Detailed exam with topical anesthesia. (Plastic Surgery)

Initial office visit for evaluation of a 13-year-old female with progressive scoliosis. (Physical Medicine & Rehabilitation)

Initial office visit for a 21-year-old female desiring counseling and evaluation of initiation of contraception. (Family Practice/Internal Medicine/Obstetrics & Gynecology)

Initial office visit for a 49-year-old male presenting with painless blood per rectum associated with bowel movement. (Colon & Rectal Surgery)

Initial office visit for a 19-year-old football player with three-day-old acute knee injury; now with swelling and pain. (Orthopaedic Surgery)

99204   Initial office visit for a 13-year-old female with progressive scoliosis. (Orthopaedic Surgery)

Initial office visit for a 34-year-old female with primary infertility for evaluation and counseling. (Obstetrics & Gynecology)

Initial office visit for a 6-year-old male with multiple upper respiratory infections. (Allergy & Immunology)

Initial office visit for a patient with generalized dermatitis of 80 percent of the body surface area. (Dermatology)

Initial office visit for an adolescent who was referred by school counselor because of repeated skipping school. (Psychiatry)

Initial office visit for a 50-year-old machinist with a generalized eruption. (Dermatology)

Initial office visit for a 45-year-old female who has been abstinent from alcohol and benzodiazepines for three months but complains of headaches, insomnia, and anxiety. (Psychiatry)

Initial office visit for a 60-year-old male with recent change in bowel habits, weight loss, and abdominal pain. (Abdominal Surgery/General Surgery)

Initial office visit for a 50-year-old male with an aortic aneurysm who is considering surgery. (General Surgery)

Initial office visit for a 17-year-old female with depression. (Internal Medicine)

Initial office visit of a 40-year-old with chronic draining ear, imbalance, and probable cholesteatoma. (Otolaryngology, Head & Neck Surgery)

Initial office visit for initial evaluation of a 63-year-old male with chest pain on exertion. (Cardiology/Internal Medicine)

Initial office visit for evaluation of a 70-year-old patient with recent onset of episodic confusion. (Internal Medicine)

Initial office visit for a 7-year-old female with juvenile diabetes mellitus, new to area, past history of hospitalization times three. (Pediatrics)

Initial office visit of a 50-year-old female with progressive solid food dysphagia. (Gastroenterology)

Initial office visit for a 34-year-old patient with primary infertility, including counseling. (Obstetrics & Gynecology)

Initial office visit for evaluation of a 70-year-old female with polyarthralgia. (Rheumatology)

Initial office visit for a patient with papulosquamous eruption involving 60 percent of the cutaneous surface with joint pain. Combinations of topical and systemic treatments discussed. (Dermatology)

99205 Initial office visit for a patient with disseminated lupus erythematosus with kidney disease, edema, purpura, and scarring lesions on the extremities plus cardiac symptoms. (Dermatology/General Surgery/Internal Medicine)

Initial office visit for a 25-year-old female with systemic lupus erythematosus, fever, seizures, and profound thrombocytopenia. (Rheumatology/Allergy & Immunology)

Initial office visit for an adult with multiple cutaneous blisters, denuded secondarily infected ulcerations, oral lesions, weight loss, and increasing weakness refractory to high dose corticosteroid. Initiation of new immunosuppressive therapy. (Dermatology)

Initial office visit for a 28-year-old male with systemic vasculitis and compromised circulation to the limbs. (Rheumatology)

Initial office visit for a 41-year-old female new to the area requesting rheumatologic care, on disability due to scleroderma and recent hospitalization for malignant hypertension. (Rheumatology)

Initial office visit for a 52-year-old female with acute four extremity weakness and shortness of breath one week post-flu vaccination. (Physical Medicine & Rehabilitation)

Initial office visit for a 60-year-old male with previous back surgery; now presents with back and pelvic pain, two-month history of bilateral progressive calf and thigh tightness and weakness when walking, causing several falls. (Orthopaedic Surgery)

Initial office visit for an adolescent referred from ER after making suicide gesture. (Psychiatry)

Initial office visit for a 49-year-old female with a history of headaches and dependence on opioids. She reports weight loss, progressive headache, and depression. (Psychiatry)

Initial office visit for a 50-year-old female with symptoms of rash, swellings, recurrent arthritic complaints, and diarrhea and lymphadenopathy. Patient has had a 25 lb. weight loss and was recently camping in the Amazon. (Allergy & Immunology)

Initial office visit for a 34-year-old uremic Type I diabetic patient referred for ESRD modality assessment and planning. (Nephrology)

Initial office visit for a 75-year-old female with neck and bilateral shoulder pain, brisk deep tendon reflexes, and stress incontinence. (Physical Medicine & Rehabilitation)

Initial office visit for an 8-year-old male with cerebral palsy and spastic quadriparesis. (Physical Medicine & Rehabilitation)

Initial office visit for a 73-year-old male with known prostate malignancy, who presents with severe back pain and a recent onset of lower extremity weakness. (Physical Medicine & Rehabilitation)

Initial office visit for a 38-year-old male with paranoid delusions and a history of alcohol abuse. (Psychiatry)

Initial office visit for a 12-week-old with bilateral hip dislocations and bilateral club feet. (Orthopaedic Surgery)

Initial office visit for a 29-year-old female with acute orbital congestion, eyelid retraction, and bilateral visual loss from optic neuropathy. (Ophthalmology)

Initial office visit for a 70-year-old diabetic patient with progressive visual field loss, advanced optic disc cupping and neovascularization of retina. (Ophthalmology)

Initial office visit for a newly diagnosed Type I diabetic patient. (Endocrinology)

Initial office evaluation of a 65-year-old female with exertional chest pain, intermittent claudication, syncope and a murmur of aortic stenosis. (Cardiology)

Initial office visit for a 73-year-old male with an unexplained 20 lb. weight loss. (Hematology/Oncology)

Initial office evaluation, patient with systemic lupus erythematosus, fever, seizures and profound thrombocytopenia. (Allergy & Immunology/Internal Medicine/Rheumatology)

Initial office evaluation and management of patient with systemic vasculitis and compromised circulation to the limbs. (Rheumatology)

Initial office visit for a 24-year-old homosexual male who has a fever, a cough, and shortness of breath. (Infectious Disease)

Initial outpatient evaluation of a 69-year-old male with severe chronic obstructive pulmonary disease, congestive heart failure, and hypertension. (Family Medicine)

Initial office visit for a 17-year-old female, who is having school problems and has told a friend she is considering suicide. The patient and her family are consulted in regard to treatment options. (Psychiatry)

Initial office visit for a female with severe hirsutism, amenorrhea, weight loss and a desire to have children. (Endocrinology/Obstetrics & Gynecology)

Initial office visit for a 42-year-old male on hypertensive medication, newly arrived to the area, with diastolic blood pressure of 110, history of recurrent calculi, episodic headaches, intermittent chest pain and orthopnea. (Internal Medicine)

Established Patient

99211 Office visit for an 82-year-old female, established patient, for a monthly B12 injection with documented Vitamin B12 deficiency. (Geriatrics/Internal Medicine/Family Medicine)

Office visit for a 50-year-old male, established patient, for removal of uncomplicated facial sutures. (Plastic Surgery)

Office visit for an established patient who lost prescription for lichen planus. Returned for new copy. (Dermatology)

Office visit for an established patient undergoing orthodontics who complains of a wire which is irritating his/her cheek and asks you to check it. (Oral & Maxillofacial Surgery)

Office visit for a 50-year-old female, established patient, seen for her gold injection by the nurse. (Rheumatology)

Office visit for a 73-year-old female, established patient, with pernicious anemia for weekly B12 injection. (Gastroenterology)

Office visit for an established patient for dressing change on a skin biopsy. (Dermatology)

Office visit for a 19-year-old, established patient, for removal of sutures from a two cm. laceration of forehead, which you placed four days ago in ER. (Plastic Surgery)

Office visit of a 20-year-old female, established patient, who receives an allergy vaccine injection and is observed for a reaction by the nurse. (Otolaryngology, Head & Neck Surgery)

Office visit for a 45-year-old male, established patient, with chronic renal failure for the administration of erythropoietin. (Nephrology)

Office visit for an established patient, a Peace Corps enlistee, who requests documentation that third molars have been removed. (Oral & Maxillofacial Surgery)

Office visit for a 69-year-old female, established patient, for partial removal of antibiotic gauze from an infected wound site. (Plastic Surgery)

Office visit for a 9-year-old, established patient, successfully treated for impetigo, requiring release to return to school. (Dermatology/Pediatrics)

Office visit for an established patient requesting a return-to-work certificate for resolving contact dermatitis. (Dermatology)

Office visit for an established patient who is performing glucose monitoring and wants to check accuracy of machine with lab blood glucose by technician who checks accuracy and function of patient machine. (Endocrinology)

Follow-up office visit for a 65-year-old female with a chronic indwelling percutaneous nephrostomy catheter seen for routine pericatheter skin care and dressing change. (Interventional Radiology)

Outpatient visit with 19-year-old male, established patient, for supervised drug screen. (Addiction Medicine)

Office visit with 12-year-old male, established patient, for cursory check of hematoma one day after venipuncture. (Internal Medicine)

Office visit with 31-year-old female, established patient, for return to work certificate. (Anesthesiology)

Office visit for a 42-year-old, established patient, to read tuberculin test results. (Allergy & Immunology)

Office visit for 14-year-old, established patient, to re-dress an abrasion. (Orthopaedic Surgery)

Office visit for a 45-year-old female, established patient, for a blood pressure check. (Obstetrics & Gynecology)

Office visit for a 23-year-old, established patient, for instruction in use of peak flow meter. (Allergy & Immunology)

Office visit for prescription refill for a 35-year-old female, established patient, with schizophrenia who is stable but has run out of neuroleptic and is scheduled to be seen in a week. (Psychiatry)

99212 Office visit for an 11-year-old, established patient, seen in follow-up for mild comedonal acne of the cheeks on topical desquamating agents. (Dermatology/Family Medicine/Pediatrics)

Office visit for a 10-year-old female, established patient, who has been swimming in a lake, now presents with a one-day history of left ear pain with purulent drainage. (Family Medicine)

Office visit of a child, established patient, with chronic secretory otitis media. (Otolaryngology, Head & Neck Surgery)

Office visit for an established patient seen in follow-up of clearing patch of localized contact dermatitis. (Family Medicine/Dermatology)

Office visit for an established patient returning for evaluation of response to treatment of lichen planus on wrists and ankles. (Dermatology)

Office visit for an established patient with tinea pedis being treated with topical therapy. (Dermatology)

Office visit for an established patient with localized erythematous plaque of psoriasis with topical hydration. (Dermatology)

Office visit for a 50-year-old male, established patient, recently seen for acute neck pain, diagnosis of spondylosis, responding to physical therapy and intermittent cervical traction. Returns for evaluation for return to work. (Neurology)

Office visit for an established patient with recurring episodes of herpes simplex who has developed a clustering of vesicles on the upper lip. (Oral & Maxillofacial Surgery)

Evaluation for a 50-year-old male, established patient, who has experienced a recurrence of knee pain after he discontinued NSAID. (Anesthesiology/Pain Medicine)

Office visit for an established patient with an irritated skin tag for reassurance. (Dermatology)

Office visit for a 40-year-old, established patient, who has experienced a systemic allergic reaction following administration of immunotherapy. The dose must be readjusted. (Allergy & Immunology)

Office visit for a 33-year-old, established patient, for contusion and abrasion of lower extremity. (Orthopaedic Surgery)

Office visit for a 22-year-old male, established patient, one month after I & D of "wrestler's ear." (Plastic Surgery)

Office visit for a 21-year-old, established patient, who is seen in follow-up after antibiotic therapy for acute bacterial tonsillitis. (Otolaryngology, Head & Neck Surgery)

Office visit for a 4-year-old, established patient, with tympanostomy tubes, check-up. (Otolaryngology, Head & Neck Surgery)

Office visit for an established patient who has had needle aspiration of a peritonsillar abscess. (Otolaryngology, Head & Neck Surgery)

Follow-up office examination for evaluation and treatment of acute draining ear in a 5-year-old with tympanotomy tubes. (Otolaryngology, Head & Neck Surgery)

Office visit, established patient, 6-year-old with sore throat and headache. (Family Medicine/Pediatrics)

Office evaluation for possible purulent bacterial conjunctivitis with one- to two-day history of redness and discharge, 16-year-old female, established patient. (Pediatrics/Internal Medicine/Family Medicine)

Office visit with a 65-year-old female, established patient, returns for three-week follow-up for resolving severe ankle sprain. (Orthopaedic Surgery)

Office visit, sore throat, fever and fatigue in a 19-year-old college student, established patient. (Internal Medicine)

Office visit with a 33-year-old female, established patient, recently started on treatment for hemorrhoidal complaints, for re-evaluation. (Colon & Rectal Surgery)

Office visit with a 36-year-old male, established patient, for follow-up on effectiveness of medicine management of oral candidiasis. (Oral & Maxillofacial Surgery)

Office visit for a 27-year-old female, established patient, with complaints of vaginal itching. (Obstetrics & Gynecology)

Office visit for a 65-year-old male, established patient, with eruptions on both arms from poison oak exposure. (Allergy & Immunology/Internal Medicine)

99213   Office visit for an established patient with new lesions of lichen planus in spite of topical therapies. (Dermatology)

Office visit for the quarterly follow-up of a 45-year-old male with stable chronic asthma requiring regular drug therapy. (Allergy & Immunology)

Office visit for a 13-year-old, established patient, with comedopapular acne of the face which has shown poor response to topical medication. Discussion of use of systemic medication. (Dermatology)

Office visit for a 62-year-old female, established patient, for follow-up for stable cirrhosis of the liver. (Internal Medicine/Family Medicine)

Office visit for a 3-year-old, established patient, with atopic dermatitis and food hypersensitivity for quarterly follow-up evaluation. The patient is on topical lotions and steroid creams as well as oral antihistamines. (Allergy & Immunology)

Office visit for an 80-year-old female, established patient, to evaluate medical management of osteoarthritis of the temporomandibular joint. (Rheumatology)

Office visit for a 70-year-old female, established patient, one year post excision of basal cell carcinoma of nose with nasolabial flap. Now presents with new suspicious recurrent lesion and suspicious lesion of the back. (Plastic Surgery)

Office visit for a 68-year-old female, established patient, with polymyalgia rheumatic, maintained on chronic low-dose corticosteroid, with no new complaints. (Rheumatology)

Office visit for a 3-year-old female, established patient, for earache and dyshidrosis of feet. (Pediatrics/Family Medicine)

Office visit for an established patient for 18 months post-operative follow-up of TMJ repair. (Oral & Maxillofacial Surgery)

Office visit for a 45-year-old male, established patient, being re-evaluated for recurrent acute prostatitis. (Urology)

Office visit for a 43-year-old male, established patient, with known reflex sympathetic dystrophy. (Anesthesiology)

Office visit for an established patient with an evenly pigmented superficial nodule of leg which is symptomatic. (Dermatology)

Office visit for an established patient with psoriasis involvement of the elbows, pitting of the nails, and itchy scalp. (Dermatology)

Office visit for a 27-year-old male, established patient, with deep follicular and perifollicular inflammation unable to tolerate systemic antibiotics due to GI upset, requires change of systemic medication. (Dermatology)

Office visit for a 16-year-old male, established patient, who is on medication for exercise-induced bronchospasm. (Allergy & Immunology)

Office visit for a 60-year-old, established patient, with chronic essential hypertension on multiple drug regimen, for blood pressure check. (Family Medicine)

Office visit for a 20-year-old male, established patient, for removal of sutures in hand. (Family Medicine)

Office visit for a 58-year-old female, established patient, with unilateral painful bunion. (Orthopaedic Surgery)

Office visit for a 45-year-old female, established patient, with known osteoarthritis and painful swollen knees. (Rheumatology)

Office visit for a 25-year-old female, established patient, complaining of bleeding and heavy menses. (Obstetrics & Gynecology)

Office visit for a 55-year-old male, established patient, with hypertension managed by a beta blocker/thiazide regime; now experiencing mild fatigue. (Nephrology)

Office visit for a 65-year-old female, established patient, with primary glaucoma for interval determination of intraocular pressure and possible adjustment of medication. (Ophthalmology)

Office visit for a 56-year-old man, established patient, with stable exertional angina who complains of new onset of calf pain while walking. (Cardiology)

Office visit for a 63-year-old female, established patient, with rheumatoid arthritis on auranofin and ibuprofin, seen for routine follow-up visit. (Rheumatology)

Office visit for an established patient with Graves' disease, three months post I-131 therapy, who presents with lassitude and malaise. (Endocrinology)

Office visit for the quarterly follow-up of a 63-year-old male, established patient, with chronic myofascial pain syndrome, effectively managed by doxepin, who presents with new onset urinary hesitancy. (Pain Medicine)

Office visit for the biannual follow-up of an established patient with migraine variant having infrequent, intermittent, moderate to severe headaches with nausea and vomiting, which are sometimes effectively managed by ergotamine tartrate and an antiemetic, but occasionally requiring visits to an emergency department. (Pain Medicine)

Office visit for an established patient after discharge from a pain rehabilitation program to review and adjust medication dosage. (Pain Medicine)

Office visit with 55-year-old male, established patient, for management of hypertension, mild fatigue, on beta blocker/thiazide regimen. (Family Medicine/Internal Medicine)

Outpatient visit with 37-year-old male, established patient, who is three years post total colectomy for chronic ulcerative colitis, presents for increased irritation at his stoma. (General Surgery)

Office visit for a 70-year-old diabetic hypertensive established patient with recent change in insulin requirement. (Internal Medicine/Nephrology)

Office visit with 80-year-old female, established patient, for follow-up osteoporosis, status-post compression fractures. (Rheumatology)

Office visit for an established patient with stable cirrhosis of the liver. (Gastroenterology)

Routine, follow-up office evaluation at a three-month interval for a 77-year-old female, established patient, with nodular small cleaved-cell lymphoma. (Hematology/Oncology)

Quarterly follow-up office visit for a 45-year-old male, established patient, with stable chronic asthma, on steroid and bronchodilator therapy. (Pulmonary Medicine)

Office visit for a 50-year-old female, established patient, with insulin-dependent diabetes mellitus and stable coronary artery disease, for monitoring. (Family Medicine/Internal Medicine)

99214 Office visit for an established patient now presenting with generalized dermatitis of 80 percent of the body surface area. (Dermatology)

Office visit for a 32-year-old female, established patient, with new onset right lower quadrant pain. (Family Medicine)

Office visit for reassessment and reassurance/counseling of a 40-year-old female, established patient, who is experiencing increased symptoms while on a pain management treatment program. (Pain Medicine)

Office visit for a 30-year-old, established patient, under management for intractable low back pain, who now presents with new onset right posterior thigh pain. (Pain Medicine)

Office visit for an established patient with frequent intermittent, moderate to severe headaches requiring beta blocker or tricyclic antidepressant prophylaxis, as well as four symptomatic treatments, but who is still experiencing headaches at a frequency of several times a month that are unresponsive to treatment. (Pain Medicine)

Office visit for an established patient with psoriasis with extensive involvement of scalp, trunk, palms, and soles with joint pain. Combinations of topical and systemic treatments discussed and instituted. (Dermatology)

Office visit for a 55-year-old male, established patient, with increasing night pain, limp, and progressive varus of both knees. (Orthopaedic Surgery)

Follow-up visit for a 15-year-old withdrawn patient with four-year history of papulocystic acne of the face, chest, and back with early scarring and poor response to past treatment. Discussion of use of systemic medication. (Dermatology)

Office visit for a 28-year-old male, established patient, with regional enteritis, diarrhea, and low-grade fever. (Internal Medicine)

Office visit for a 25-year-old female, established patient, following recent arthrogram and MR imaging for TMJ pain. (Oral & Maxillofacial Surgery)

Office visit for a 32-year-old female, established patient, with large obstructing stone in left mid-ureter, to discuss management options including urethroscopy with extraction or ESWL. (Urology)

Evaluation for a 28-year-old male, established patient, with new onset of low back pain. (Anesthesiology/Pain Medicine)

Office visit for a 28-year-old female, established patient, with right lower quadrant abdominal pain, fever, and anorexia. (Internal Medicine/Family Medicine)

Office visit for a 45-year-old male, established patient, four months follow-up of L4-5 diskectomy, with persistent incapacitating low back and leg pain. (Orthopaedic Surgery)

Outpatient visit for a 77-year-old male, established patient, with hypertension, presenting with a three-month history of episodic substernal chest pain on exertion. (Cardiology)

Office visit for a 25-year-old female, established patient, for evaluation of progressive saddle nose deformity of unknown etiology. (Plastic Surgery)

Office visit for a 65-year-old male, established patient, with BPH and severe bladder outlet obstruction, to discuss management options such as TURP. (Urology)

Office visit for an adult diabetic established patient with a past history of recurrent sinusitis who presents with a one-week history of double vision. (Otolaryngology, Head & Neck Surgery)

Office visit for an established patient with lichen planus and 60 percent of the cutaneous surface involved, not responsive to systemic steroids, as well as developing symptoms of progressive heartburn and paranoid ideation. (Dermatology)

Office visit for a 52-year-old male, established patient, with a 12-year history of bipolar disorder responding to lithium carbonate and brief psychotherapy. Psychotherapy and prescription provided. (Psychiatry)

Office visit for a 63-year-old female, established patient, with a history of familial polyposis, status post-colectomy with sphincter sparing procedure, who now presents with rectal bleeding and increase in stooling frequency. (General Surgery)

Office visit for a 68-year-old male, established patient, with the sudden onset of multiple flashes and floaters in the right eye due to a posterior vitreous detachment. (Ophthalmology)

Office visit for a 55-year-old female, established patient, on cyclosporin for treatment of resistant, small vessel vasculitis. (Rheumatology)

Follow-up office visit for a 55-year-old male, two months after iliac angioplasty with new onset of contralateral extremity claudication. (Interventional Radiology)

Office visit for a 68-year-old male, established patient, with stable angina, two months post myocardial infarction, who is not tolerating one of his medications. (Cardiology)

Weekly office visit for 5FU therapy for an ambulatory established patient with metastatic colon cancer and increasing shortness of breath. (Hematology/Oncology)

Follow-up office visit for a 60-year-old male, established patient, whose post-traumatic seizures have disappeared on medication and who now raises the question of stopping the medication (Neurology)

Office evaluation on new onset RLQ pain in a 32-year-old woman, established patient. (Urology/General Surgery/Internal Medicine/Family Medicine)

Office evaluation of 28-year-old, established patient, with regional enteritis, diarrhea and low-grade fever. (Family Medicine/Internal Medicine)

Office visit with 50-year-old female, established patient, diabetic, blood sugar controlled by diet. She now complains of frequency of urination and weight loss, blood sugar of 320 and negative ketones on dipstick. (Internal Medicine)

Follow-up office visit for a 45-year-old, established patient, with rheumatoid arthritis on gold, methotrexate, or immunosuppressive therapy. (Rheumatology)

Office visit for a 60-year-old male, established patient, two years post-removal of intracranial meningioma, now with new headaches and visual disturbance. (Neurosurgery)

Office visit for a 68-year-old female, established patient, for routine review and follow-up of non-insulin dependent diabetes, obesity, hypertension and congestive heart failure. Complains of vision difficulties and admits dietary noncompliance. Patient is counseled concerning diet and current medications adjusted. (Family Medicine)

99215 Office visit for an established patient who developed persistent cough, rectal bleeding, weakness, and diarrhea plus pustular infection on skin. Patient on immunosuppressive therapy. (Dermatology)

Office visit for an established patient with disseminated lupus erythematosus, extensive edema of extremities kidney disease, and weakness requiring monitored course on azathioprene, corticosteroid and complicated by acute depression. (Dermatology/Internal Medicine/Rheumatology)

Office visit for an established patient with progressive dermatomyositis and recent onset of fever, nasal speech, and regurgitation of fluids through the nose. (Dermatology)

Office visit for a 28-year-old female, established patient, who is abstinent from previous cocaine dependence, but reports progressive panic attacks and chest pains. (Psychiatry)

Office visit for an established adolescent patient with history of bipolar disorder treated with lithium; seen on urgent basis at family's request because of severe depressive symptoms. (Psychiatry)

Office visit for an established patient having acute migraine with new onset neurological symptoms and whose headaches are unresponsive to previous attempts at management with a combination of preventive and abortive medication. (Pain Medicine)

Office visit for an established patient with exfoliative lichen planus with daily fever spikes, disorientation, and shortness of breath. (Dermatology)

Office visit for a 25-year-old, established patient, two years post-burn with bilateral ectropion, hypertrophic facial burn scars, near absence of left breast, and burn syndactyly of both hands. Discussion of treatment options following examination. (Plastic Surgery)

Office visit for a 6-year-old, established patient, to review newly diagnosed immune deficiency with recommendations for therapy including IV immunoglobulin and chronic antibiotics. (Allergy & Immunology)

Office visit for a 36-year-old, established patient, three months status post-transplant, with new onset of peripheral edema, increased blood pressure, and progressive fatigue. (Nephrology)

Office visit for an established patient with Kaposi's sarcoma who presents with fever and widespread vesicles. (Dermatology)

Office visit for a 27-year-old female, established patient, with bipolar disorder who was stable on lithium carbonate and monthly supportive psychotherapy but now has developed symptoms of hypomania. (Psychiatry)

Office visit for a 25-year-old male, established patient with a history of schizophrenia who has been seen bi-monthly but is complaining of auditory hallucinations. (Psychiatry)

Office visit for a 62-year-old male, established patient, three years post-op abdominal perineal resection, now with a rising carcinoembryonic antigen, weight loss, and pelvic pain. (Abdominal Surgery)

Office visit for a 42-year-old male, established patient, nine months post-op emergency vena cava shunt for variceal bleeding, now presents with complaints of one episode of "dark" bowel movement, weight gain, tightness in abdomen, whites of eyes seem "yellow" and occasional drowsiness after eating hamburgers. (Abdominal Surgery)

Office visit for a 68-year-old male, established patient, with biopsy-proven rectal carcinoma, for evaluation and discussion of treatment options. (General Surgery)

Office visit for a 60-year-old, established patient, with diabetic nephropathy with increasing edema and dyspnea. (Endocrinology)

Office visit with 30-year-old male, established patient for three-month history of fatigue, weight loss, intermittent fever, and presenting with diffuse adenopathy and splenomegaly. (Family Medicine)

Office visit for restaging of an established patient with new lymphadenopathy one year post-therapy for lymphoma. (Hematology/Oncology)

Office visit for evaluation of recent onset syncopal attacks in a 70-year-old woman, established patient. (Internal Medicine)

Follow-up visit, 40-year-old mother of three, established patient, with acute rheumatoid arthritis, anatomical Stage 3, ARA function Class 3 rheumatoid arthritis, and deteriorating function. (Rheumatology)

Office evaluation and discussion of treatment options for a 68-year-old male, established patient, with a biopsy-proven rectal carcinoma. (General Surgery)

Follow-up office visit for a 65-year-old male, established patient, with a fever of recent onset while on outpatient antibiotic therapy for endocarditis. (Infectious Disease)

Office visit for a 75-year-old, established patient, with ALS (amyotrophic lateral sclerosis), who is no longer able to swallow. (Neurology)

Office visit for a 70-year-old female, established patient, with diabetes mellitus and hypertension, presenting with a two-month history of increasing confusion, agitation and short-term memory loss. (Family Medicine/Internal Medicine)

Hospital Inpatient Services

Initial Hospital Care

New or Established Patient

99221 Initial hospital visit following admission for a 42-year-old male for observation following an uncomplicated mandible fracture. (Plastic Surgery/Oral & Maxillofacial Surgery)

Initial hospital visit for a 40-year-old patient with a thrombosed synthetic arteriovenous conduit. (Nephrology)

Initial hospital visit for a healthy 24-year-old male with an acute onset of low back pain following a lifting injury. (Internal Medicine/Anesthesiology/Pain Medicine)

Initial hospital visit for a 69-year-old female with controlled hypertension, scheduled for surgery. (Internal Medicine/Cardiology)

Initial hospital visit for a 24-year-old healthy female with benign tumor of palate. (Oral & Maxillofacial Surgery)

Initial hospital visit for a 14-year-old female with infectious mononucleosis and dehydration. (Internal Medicine)

Initial hospital visit for a 62-year-old female with stable rheumatoid arthritis, admitted for total joint replacement. (Rheumatology)

Initial hospital visit for a 12-year-old patient with a laceration of the upper eyelid, involving the lid margin and superior canaliculus, admitted prior to surgery for IV antibiotic therapy. (Plastic Surgery)

Initial hospital visit for a 69-year-old female with controlled hypertension, scheduled for surgery. (Cardiology)

Hospital admission, examination, and initiation of treatment program for a 67-year-old male with uncomplicated pneumonia who requires IV antibiotic therapy. (Internal Medicine)

Hospital admission for an 18-month-old with 10 percent dehydration. (Pediatrics)

Hospital admission for a 12-year-old with a laceration of the upper eyelid involving the lid margin and superior canaliculus, admitted prior to surgery for IV antibiotic therapy. (Ophthalmology)

Hospital admission for a 32-year-old female with severe flank pain, hematuria and presumed diagnosis of ureteral calculus as determined by Emergency Department physician. (Urology)

Initial hospital visit for a patient with several large venous stasis ulcers not responding to outpatient therapy. (Dermatology)

Initial hospital visit for 21-year-old pregnant patient (nine weeks gestation) with hyperemesis gravidarum. (Obstetrics & Gynecology)

Initial hospital visit for a 73-year-old female with acute pyelonephritis who is otherwise generally healthy. (Geriatrics)

Initial hospital visit for 62-year-old patient with cellulitis of the foot requiring bedrest and intravenous antibiotics. (Orthopaedic Surgery)

99222 Initial hospital visit for a 50-year-old patient with lower quadrant abdominal pain and increased temperature, but without septic picture. (General Surgery/Abdominal Surgery/Colon & Rectal Surgery)

Initial hospital visit for airway management, due to a benign laryngeal mass. (Otolaryngology, Head & Neck Surgery)

Initial hospital visit for a 66-year-old female with an L-2 vertebral compression fracture with acute onset of paralytic ileus; seen in the office two days previously. (Orthopaedic Surgery)

Initial hospital visit and evaluation of a 15-year-old male admitted with peritonsillar abscess or cellulitis requiring intravenous antibiotic therapy. (Otolaryngology, Head & Neck Surgery)

Initial hospital visit for a 42-year-old male with vertebral compression fracture following a motor vehicle accident. (Orthopaedic Surgery)

Initial hospital visit for a patient with generalized atopic dermatitis and secondary infection. (Dermatology)

Initial hospital visit for a 3-year-old patient with high temperature, limp, and painful hip motion of 18 hours' duration. (Pediatrics/Orthopaedic Surgery)

Initial hospital visit for a young adult, presenting with an acute asthma attack unresponsive to outpatient therapy. (Allergy & Immunology)

Initial hospital visit for an 18-year-old male who has suppurative sialoadenitis and dehydration. (Oral & Maxillofacial Surgery)

Initial hospital visit for a 65-year-old female for acute onset of thrombotic cerebrovascular accident with contralateral paralysis and aphasia. (Neurology)

Initial hospital visit for a 50-year-old male chronic paraplegic patient with pain and spasm below the lesion. (Anesthesiology)

Partial hospital admission for an adolescent patient from chaotic blended family, transferred from inpatient setting, for continued treatment to control symptomatic expressions of hostility and depression. (Psychiatry)

Initial hospital visit for a 15-year-old male with acute status asthmaticus, unresponsive to outpatient therapy. (Internal Medicine)

Initial hospital visit for a 61-year-old male with history of previous myocardial infarction, who now complains of chest pain. (Internal Medicine)

Initial hospital visit of a 15-year-old on medications for a sore throat over the last two weeks. The sore throat has worsened and now has dysphagia. The exam shows large necrotic tonsils with an adequate airway and small palpable nodes. The initial mono test was negative. (Otolaryngology, Head & Neck Surgery)

Initial hospital evaluation of a 23-year-old allergy patient admitted with eyelid edema and pain on fifth day of oral antibiotic therapy. (Otolaryngology, Head & Neck Surgery)

Hospital admission, young adult patient, failed previous therapy and now presents in acute asthmatic attack. (Family Medicine/Allergy & Immunology)

Hospital admission of a 62-year-old smoker, established patient, with bronchitis in acute respiratory distress. (Internal Medicine/Pulmonary Medicine)

Hospital admission, examination, and initiation of a treatment program for a 65-year-old female with new onset of right-sided paralysis and aphasia. (Neurology)

Hospital admission for a 50-year-old with left lower quadrant abdominal pain and increased temperature, but without septic picture. (General Surgery)

Hospital admission, examination, and initiation of treatment program for a 66-year-old chronic hemodialysis patient with fever and a new pulmonary infiltrate. (Nephrology)

Hospital admission for an 8-year-old febrile patient with chronic sinusitis and severe headache, unresponsive to oral antibiotics. (Allergy & Immunology)

Hospital admission for a 40-year-old male with submaxillary cellulitis and trismus from infected lower molar. (Oral & Maxillofacial Surgery)

99223 Initial hospital visit for a 45-year-old female, who has a history of rheumatic fever as a child and now has anemia, fever, and congestive heart failure. (Cardiology)

Initial hospital visit for a 50-year-old male with acute chest pain and diagnostic electrocardiographic changes of an acute anterior myocardial infarction. (Cardiology/Family Medicine/Internal Medicine)

Initial hospital visit of a 75-year-old with progressive stridor and dysphagia with history of cancer of the larynx treated by radiation therapy in the past. Exam shows a large recurrent tumor of the glottis with a mass in the neck. (Otolaryngology, Head & Neck Surgery)

Initial hospital visit for a 70-year-old male admitted with chest pain, complete heart block, and congestive heart failure. (Cardiology)

Initial hospital visit for an 82-year-old male who presents with syncope, chest pain, and ventricular arrhythmias. (Cardiology)

Initial hospital visit for a 75-year-old male with history of arteriosclerotic coronary vascular disease, who is severely dehydrated, disoriented, and experiencing auditory hallucinations. (Psychiatry)

Initial hospital visit for a 70-year-old male with alcohol and sedative-hypnotic dependence, admitted by family for severe withdrawal, hypertension, and diabetes mellitus. (Psychiatry)

Initial hospital visit for a persistently suicidal latency-aged child whose parents have requested admission to provide safety during evaluation, but are anxious about separation from her. (Psychiatry)

Initial psychiatric visit for an adolescent patient without previous psychiatric history, who was transferred from the medical ICU after a significant overdose. (Psychiatry)

Initial hospital visit for a 35-year-old female with severe systemic lupus erythematosus on corticosteroid and cyclophosphamide, with new onset of fever, chills, rash, and chest pain. (Rheumatology)

Initial hospital visit for a 52-year-old male with known rheumatic heart disease who presents with anasarca, hypertension, and history of alcohol abuse. (Cardiology)

Initial hospital visit for a 55-year-old female with a history of congenital heart disease; now presents with cyanosis. (Cardiology)

Initial hospital visit for a psychotic, hostile, violently combative adolescent, involuntarily committed, for seclusion and restraint in order to provide for safety on unit. (Psychiatry)

Initial hospital visit for a now subdued and sullen teenage male with six-month history of declining school performance, increasing self-endangerment, and resistance of parental expectations, including running away past weekend after physical fight with father. (Psychiatry)

Initial partial hospital admission for a 17-year-old female with history of borderline mental retardation who has developed auditory hallucinations. Parents are known to abuse alcohol, and Child Protective Services is investigating allegations of sexual abuse of a younger sibling. (Psychiatry)

Initial hospital visit of a 67-year old male admitted with a large neck mass, dysphagia, and history of myocardial infarction three months before. (Otolaryngology, Head & Neck Surgery)

Initial hospital visit for a patient with suspected cerebrospinal fluid rhinorrhea which developed two weeks after head injury. (Otolaryngology, Head & Neck Surgery)

Initial hospital visit for a 25-year-old female with history of poly-substance abuse and psychiatric disorder. The patient appears to be psychotic with markedly elevated vital signs. (Psychiatry)

Initial hospital visit for a 70-year-old male with cutaneous T-cell lymphoma who has developed fever and lymphadenopathy. (Internal Medicine)

Initial hospital visit for a 62-year-old female with known coronary artery disease, for evaluation of increasing edema, dyspnea on exertion, confusion, and sudden onset of fever with productive cough. (Internal Medicine)

Initial hospital visit for a 3-year-old female with 36-hour history of sore throat and high fever; now with sudden onset of lethargy, irritability, photophobia, and nuchal rigidity. (Pediatrics)

Initial hospital visit for a 26-year-old female for evaluation of severe facial fractures (LeFort's II/III). (Plastic Surgery)

Initial hospital visit for a 55-year-old female for bilateral mandibular fractures resulting in flail mandible and airway obstruction. (Plastic Surgery)

Initial hospital visit for a 71-year-old patient with a red painful eye four days following uncomplicated cataract surgery due to endophthalmitis. (Ophthalmology)

Initial hospital visit for a 45-year-old patient involved in a motor vehicle accident who suffered a perforating corneoscleral laceration with loss of vision. (Ophthalmology)

Initial hospital visit for a 58-year-old male who has Ludwig's angina and progressive airway compromise. (Oral & Maxillofacial Surgery)

Initial hospital visit for a patient with generalized systemic sclerosis, receiving immunosuppressive therapy because of recent onset of cough, fever, and inability to swallow. (Dermatology)

Initial hospital visit for an 82-year-old male who presents with syncope, chest pain, and ventricular arrhythmias. (Cardiology)

Initial hospital visit for a 62-year-old male with history of previous myocardial infarction, comes in with recurrent, sustained ventricular tachycardia. (Cardiology)

Initial hospital visit for a chronic dialysis patient with infected PTFE fistula, septicemia, and shock. (Nephrology)

Initial hospital visit for a 1-year-old male, victim of child abuse, with central nervous system depression, skull fracture, and retinal hemorrhage. (Family Medicine/Neurology)

Initial hospital visit for a 25-year-old female with recent C4-5 quadriplegia, admitted for rehabilitation. (Physical Medicine & Rehabilitation)

Initial hospital visit for an 18-year-old male, post-traumatic brain injury with multiple impairment. (Physical Medicine & Rehabilitation)

Initial partial hospital admission for 16-year-old male, sullen and subdued, with six-month history of declining school performance, increasing self-endangerment, and resistance to parental expectations. (Psychiatry)

Initial hospital visit for a 16-year-old primigravida at 32 weeks gestation with severe hypertension (200/110), thrombocytopenia, and headache. (Obstetrics & Gynecology)

Initial hospital visit for a 49-year-old male with cirrhosis of liver with hematemesis, hepatic encephalopathy, and fever. (Gastroenterology)

Initial hospital visit for a 55-year-old female in chronic pain who has attempted suicide. (Psychiatry)

Initial hospital visit for a 70-year-old male, with multiple organ system disease, admitted with history of being aneuric and septic for 24 hours prior to admission. (Urology)

Initial hospital visit for a 3-year-old female with 36-hour history of sore throat and high fever, now with sudden onset of lethargy, irritability, photophobia, and nuchal rigidity. (Internal Medicine)

Initial hospital visit for a 78-year-old male, transfers from nursing home with dysuria and pyuria, increasing confusion, and high fever. (Internal Medicine)

Initial hospital visit for a 1-day-old male with cyanosis, respiratory distress, and tachypnea. (Cardiology)

Initial hospital visit for a 3-year-old female with recurrent tachycardia and syncope. (Cardiology)

Initial hospital visit for a thyrotoxic patient who presents with fever, atrial fibrillation, and delirium. (Endocrinology)

Initial hospital visit for a 50-year-old Type I diabetic who presents with diabetic ketoacidosis with fever and obtundation. (Endocrinology)

Initial hospital visit for a 40-year-old female with anatomical stage 3, ARA functional class 3 rheumatoid arthritis on methotrexate, corticosteroid, and nonsteroidal anti-inflammatory drugs. Patient presents with severe arthritis flare, new oral ulcers, abdominal pain, and leukopenia. (Rheumatology)

Initial hospital exam of a pediatric patient with high fever and proptosis. (Otolaryngology, Head & Neck Surgery)

Initial hospital visit for a 25-year-old patient admitted for the first time to the rehab unit, with recent C-4-5 quadriplegia. (Physical Medicine & Rehabilitation)

Hospital admission, examination, and initiation of treatment program for a previously unknown 58-year-old male who presents with acute chest pain (Cardiology)

Hospital admission, examination, and initiation of induction chemotherapy for a 42-year-old patient with newly diagnosed acute myelogenous leukemia. (Hematology/Oncology)

Hospital admission following a motor vehicle accident of a 24-year-old male with fracture dislocation of C5-6; neurologically intact. (Neurosurgery)

Hospital admission for a 78-year-old female with left lower lobe pneumonia and a history of coronary artery disease, congestive heart failure, osteoarthritis and gout. (Family Medicine)

Hospital admission, examination, and initiation of treatment program for a 65-year-old immunosuppressed male with confusion, fever, and a headache. (Infectious Disease)

Hospital admission for a 9-year-old with vomiting, dehydration, fever, tachypnea and an admitting diagnosis of diabetic ketoacidosis. (Pediatrics)

Initial hospital visit for a 65-year-old male who presents with acute myocardial infarction, oliguria, hypotension, and altered state of consciousness. (Cardiology)

Initial hospital visit for a hostile/resistant adolescent patient who is severely depressed and involved in poly-substance abuse. Patient is experiencing significant conflict in his chaotic family situation and was suspended from school following an attack on a teacher with a baseball bat. (Psychiatry)

Initial hospital visit for 89-year-old female with fulminant hepatic failure and encephalopathy. (Gastroenterology)

Initial hospital visit for a 42-year-old female with rapidly progressing scleroderma, malignant hypertension, digital infarcts, and oligurea. (Rheumatology)

Subsequent Hospital Care

99231 Subsequent hospital visit for a 65-year-old female, post-open reduction and internal fixation of a fracture. (Physical Medicine & Rehabilitation)

Subsequent hospital visit for a 33-year-old patient with pelvic pain who is responding to pain medication and observation. (Obstetrics & Gynecology)

Subsequent hospital visit for a 21-year-old female with hyperemesis who has responded well to intravenous fluids. (Obstetrics & Gynecology)

Subsequent hospital visit to re-evaluate post-op pain and titrate patient-controlled analgesia for a 27-year-old female. (Anesthesiology)

Follow-up hospital visit for a 35-year-old female, status post-epidural analgesia. (Anesthesiology/Pain Medicine)

Subsequent hospital visit for a 56-year-old male, post-gastrectomy, for maintenance of analgesia using an intravenous dilaudid infusion. (Anesthesiology)

Subsequent hospital visit for a 4-year-old on day three receiving medication for uncomplicated pneumonia. (Allergy & Immunology)

Subsequent hospital visit for a 30-year-old female with urticaria which has stabilized with medication. (Allergy & Immunology)

Subsequent hospital visit for a 76-year-old male with venous stasis ulcers. (Dermatology)

Subsequent hospital visit for a 24-year-old female with otitis externa, seen two days before in consultation, now to have otic wick removal. (Otolaryngology, Head & Neck Surgery)

Subsequent hospital visit for a 27-year-old with acute labyrinthitis. (Otolaryngology, Head & Neck Surgery)

Subsequent hospital visit for a 10-year-old male admitted for lobar pneumonia with vomiting and dehydration; is becoming afebrile and tolerating oral fluids. (Family Medicine/Pediatrics)

Subsequent hospital visit for a 62-year-old patient with resolving cellulitis of the foot. (Orthopaedic Surgery)

Subsequent hospital visit for a 25-year-old male admitted for supra-ventricular tachycardia and converted on medical therapy. (Cardiology)

Subsequent hospital visit for a 27-year-old male two days after open reduction and internal fixation for malar complex fracture. (Plastic Surgery)

Subsequent hospital visit for a 76-year-old male with venous stasis ulcers. (Geriatrics)

Subsequent hospital visit for a 67-year-old female admitted three days ago with bleeding gastric ulcer; now stable. (Gastroenterology)

Subsequent hospital visit for stable 33-year-old male, status post-lower gastrointestinal bleeding. (General Surgery/Gastroenterology)

Subsequent hospital visit for a 29-year-old auto mechanic with effort thrombosis of left upper extremity. (General Surgery)

Subsequent hospital visit for a 14-year-old female in middle phase of inpatient treatment, who is now behaviorally stable and making satisfactory progress in treatment. (Psychiatry)

Subsequent hospital visit for an 18-year-old male with uncomplicated asthma who is clinically stable. (Allergy & Immunology)

Subsequent hospital visit for a 55-year-old male with rheumatoid arthritis, two days following an uncomplicated total joint replacement. (Rheumatology)

Subsequent hospital visit for a 60-year-old dialysis patient with an access infection, now afebrile on antibiotic. (Nephrology)

Subsequent hospital visit for a 36-year-old female with stable post-rhinoplasty epistaxis. (Plastic Surgery)

Subsequent hospital visit for a 66-year-old female with L-2 vertebral compression fracture with resolving ileus. (Orthopaedic Surgery)

Subsequent hospital visit for a patient with peritonsillar abscess. (Otolaryngology, Head & Neck Surgery)

Subsequent hospital visit for an 18-year-old female responding to intravenous antibiotic therapy for ear or sinus infection. (Otolaryngology, Head & Neck Surgery)

Subsequent hospital visit for a 70-year-old male admitted with congestive heart failure who has responded to therapy. (Cardiology)

Follow-up hospital visit for a 32-year-old female with left ureteral calculus; being followed in anticipation of spontaneous passage. (Urology)

Subsequent hospital visit for a 4-year-old female, admitted for acute gastroenteritis and dehydration, requiring IV hydration; now stable. (Family Medicine)

Subsequent hospital visit for a 50-year-old Type II diabetic who is clinically stable and without complications requiring regulation of a single dose of insulin daily. (Endocrinology)

Subsequent hospital visit to reassesses the status of a 65-year-old patient post-open reduction and internal fixation of hip fracture, on the rehab unit. (Physical Medicine & Rehabilitation)

Subsequent hospital visit for a 78-year-old male with cholangiocarcinoma managed by biliary drainage. (Interventional Radiology)

Subsequent hospital visit for a 50-year-old male with uncomplicated myocardial infarction who is clinically stable and without chest pain. (Family Medicine/Cardiology/Internal Medicine)

Subsequent hospital visit for a stable 72-year-old lung cancer patient undergoing a five-day course of infusion chemotherapy. (Hematology/Oncology)

Subsequent hospital visit, two days post admission for a 65-year-old male with a CVA (cerebral vascular accident) and left hemiparesis, who is clinically stable. (Neurology/Physical Medicine and Rehabilitation)

Subsequent hospital visit for now stable, 33-year-old male, status post lower gastrointestinal bleeding. (General Surgery)

Subsequent visit on third day of hospitalization for a 60-year-old female recovering from an uncomplicated pneumonia. (Infectious Disease/Internal Medicine/Pulmonary Medicine)

Subsequent hospital visit for a 3-year-old patient in traction for a congenital dislocation of the hip. (Orthopaedic Surgery)

Subsequent hospital visit for a 4-year-old female, admitted for acute gastroenteritis and dehydration, requiring IV hydration; now stable. (Family Medicine/Internal Medicine)

Subsequent hospital visit for 50-year-old female with resolving uncomplicated acute pancreatitis. (Gastroenterology)

99232 Subsequent hospital visit for a patient with venous stasis ulcers who developed fever and red streaks adjacent to the ulcer. (Dermatology/Internal Medicine/Family Medicine)

Subsequent hospital visit for a 66-year-old male for dressing changes and observation. Patient has had a myocutaneous flap to close a pharyngeal fistula and now has a low-grade fever. (Plastic Surgery)

Subsequent hospital visit for a 54-year-old female admitted for myocardial infarction, but who is now having frequent premature ventricular contractions. (Internal Medicine)

Subsequent hospital visit for an 80-year-old patient with a pelvic rim fracture, inability to walk, and severe pain; now 36 hours post-injury, experiencing urinary retention. (Orthopaedic Surgery)

Subsequent hospital visit for a 17-year-old female with fever, pharyngitis, and airway obstruction, who after 48 hours develops a maculopapular rash. (Pediatrics/Family Medicine)

Follow-up hospital visit for a 32-year-old patient admitted the previous day for corneal ulcer. (Dermatology)

Follow-up visit for a 67-year-old male with congestive heart failure who has responded to antibiotics and diuretics, and has now developed a monoarthropathy. (Internal Medicine)

Follow-up hospital visit for a 58-year-old male receiving continuous opioids who is experiencing severe nausea and vomiting. (Pain Medicine)

Subsequent hospital visit for a patient after an auto accident who is slow to respond to ambulation training. (Physical Medicine & Rehabilitation)

Subsequent hospital visit for a 14-year-old with unstable bronchial asthma complicated by pneumonia. (Allergy & Immunology)

Subsequent hospital visit for a 50-year-old diabetic, hypertensive male with back pain not responding to conservative inpatient management with continued radiation of pain to the lower left extremity. (Orthopaedic Surgery)

Subsequent hospital visit for a 37-year-old female on day five of antibiotics for bacterial endocarditis, who still has low-grade fever.

Subsequent hospital visit for a 54-year-old patient, post MI (myocardial infarction), who is out of the CCU (coronary care unit) but is now having frequent premature ventricular contractions on telemetry. (Cardiology/Internal Medicine)

Subsequent hospital visit for a patient with neutropenia, a fever responding to antibiotics, and continued slow gastrointestinal bleeding on platelet support. (Hematology/Oncology)

Subsequent hospital visit for a 50-year-old male admitted two days ago for sub-acute renal allograft rejection. (Nephrology)

Subsequent hospital visit for a 35-year-old drug addict, not responding to initial antibiotic therapy for pyelonephritis. (Urology)

Subsequent hospital visit of an 81-year-old male with abdominal distention, nausea, and vomiting. (General Surgery)

Subsequent hospital care for a 62-year-old female with congestive heart failure, who remains dyspneic and febrile. (Internal Medicine)

Subsequent hospital visit for a 73-year-old female with recently diagnosed lung cancer, who complains of unsteady gait. (Pulmonary Medicine)

Subsequent hospital visit for a 20-month-old male with bacterial meningitis treated one week with antibiotic therapy; has now developed a temperature of 101.0. (Pediatrics)

Subsequent hospital visit for 13-year-old male admitted with left lower quadrant abdominal pain and fever, not responding to therapy. (General Surgery)

Subsequent hospital visit for a 65-year-old male with hemiplegia and painful paretic shoulder. (Physical Medicine & Rehabilitation)

99233 Subsequent hospital visit for a 38-year-old male, quadriplegic with acute autonomic hyperreflexia, who is not responsive to initial care. (Physical Medicine & Rehabilitation)

Follow-up hospital visit for a teenage female who continues to experience severely disruptive, violent and life-threatening symptoms in a complicated multi-system illness. Family/social circumstances also a contributing factor. (Psychiatry)

Subsequent hospital visit for a 42-year-old female with progressive systemic sclerosis (scleroderma), renal failure on dialysis, congestive heart failure, cardiac arrhythmias, and digital ulcers. (Allergy & Immunology)

Subsequent hospital visit for a 50-year-old diabetic, hypertensive male with nonresponding back pain and radiating pain to the lower left extremity, who develops chest pain, cough, and bloody sputum. (Orthopaedic Surgery)

Subsequent hospital visit for a 64-year-old female, status post-abdominal aortic aneurysm resection, with non-responsive coagulopathy, who has now developed lower GI bleeding. (Abdominal Surgery/Colon & Rectal Surgery/General Surgery)

Follow-up hospital care of a patient with pansinusitis infection complicated by a brain abscess and asthma; no response to current treatment. (Otolaryngology, Head & Neck Surgery)

Subsequent hospital visit for a patient with a laryngeal neoplasm who develops airway compromise, suspected metastasis. (Otolaryngology, Head & Neck Surgery)

Subsequent hospital visit for a 49-year-old male with significant rectal bleeding, etiology undetermined, not responding to treatment. (Abdominal Surgery/General Surgery/Colon & Rectal Surgery)

Subsequent hospital visit for a 50-year-old male, post-aortocoronary bypass surgery; now develops hypotension and oliguria. (Cardiology)

Subsequent hospital visit for an adolescent patient who is violent, unsafe, and noncompliant, with multiple expectations for participation in treatment plan and behavior on the treatment unit. (Psychiatry)

Subsequent hospital visit for an 18-year-old male being treated for presumed PCP psychosis. Patient is still moderately symptomatic with auditory hallucinations and is insisting on signing out against medical advice. (Psychiatry)

Subsequent hospital visit for an 8-year-old female with caustic ingestion, who now has fever, dyspnea, and dropping hemoglobin. (Gastroenterology)

Follow-up hospital visit for a chronic renal failure patient on dialysis who develops chest pain and shortness of breath and a new onset pericardial friction rub. (Nephrology)

Subsequent hospital visit for a 44-year-old patient with electrical burns to the left arm with ascending infection. (Orthopaedic Surgery)

Subsequent hospital visit for a patient with systemic sclerosis who has aspirated and is short of breath. (Dermatology)

Subsequent hospital visit for a 65-year-old female, status post-op resection of abdominal aortic aneurysm, with suspected ischemic bowel. (General Surgery)

Subsequent hospital visit for a 50-year-old male, post-aortocoronary bypass surgery, now develops hypotension and oliguria. (Cardiology)

Subsequent hospital visit for a 65-year-old male, following an acute myocardial infarction, who complains of shortness of breath and new chest pain. (Cardiology)

Subsequent hospital visit for a 65-year-old female with rheumatoid arthritis (stage 3, class 3) admitted for urosepsis. On the third hospital day, chest pain, dyspnea and fever develop. (Rheumatology)

Follow-up hospital care of a pediatric case with stridor, laryngomalcia, established tracheostomy, complicated by multiple medical problems in PICU. (Otolaryngology, Head & Neck Surgery)

Subsequent hospital visit for a 60-year-old female, four days post uncomplicated inferior myocardial infarction who has developed severe chest pain, dyspnea, diaphoresis and nausea. (Family Medicine)

Subsequent hospital visit for a patient with AML (acute myelogenous leukemia), fever, elevated white count and uric acid undergoing induction chemotherapy. (Hematology/Oncology)

Subsequent hospital visit for a 38-year-old quadriplegic male with acute autonomic hyperreflexia, who is not responsive to initial care. (Physical Medicine & Rehabilitation)

Subsequent hospital visit for a 65-year-old female post-op resection of abdominal aortic aneurysm, with suspected ischemic bowel. (General Surgery)

Subsequent hospital visit for a 60-year-old female with persistent leukocytosis and a fever seven days after a sigmoid colon resection for carcinoma. (Infectious Disease)

Subsequent hospital visit for a chronic renal failure patient on dialysis, who develops chest pain, shortness of breath and new onset of pericardial friction rub. (Nephrology)

Subsequent hospital visit for a 65-year-old male with acute myocardial infarction who now demonstrates complete heart block and congestive heart failure. (Cardiology)

Subsequent hospital visit for a 25-year-old female with hypertension and systemic lupus erythmatosus, admitted for fever and respiratory distress. On the third hospital day, the patient presented with purpuric skin lesions and acute renal failure. (Allergy & Immunology)

Subsequent hospital visit for a 55-year-old male with severe chronic obstructive pulmonary disease and bronchospasm; initially admitted for acute respiratory distress requiring ventilatory support in the ICU. The patient was stabilized, extubated and transferred to the floor, but has now developed acute fever, dyspnea, left lower lobe rhonchi and laboratory evidence of carbon dioxide retention and hypoxemia. (Family Medicine/Internal Medicine)

Subsequent hospital visit for 46-year-old female, known liver cirrhosis patient, with recent upper gastrointestinal hemorrhage from varices; now with worsening ascites and encephalopathy. (Gastroenterology)

Subsequent hospital visit for 62-year-old female admitted with acute subarachnoid hemorrhage, negative cerebral arteriogram, increased lethargy and hemiparesis with fever. (Neurosurgery)

Consultations

Office or Other Outpatient Consultations

New or Established Patient

99241 Initial office consultation for a 40-year-old female in pain from blister on lip following a cold. (Oral & Maxillofacial Surgery)

Initial office consultation for a 62-year-old construction worker with olecranon bursitis. (Orthopaedic Surgery)

Office consultation with 25-year-old postpartum female with severe symptomatic hemorrhoids. (Colon & Rectal Surgery)

Office consultation with 58-year-old male, referred for follow-up of creatinine level and evaluation of obstructive uropathy, relieved two months ago. (Nephrology)

Office consultation for 30-year-old female tennis player with sprain or contusion of the forearm. (Orthopaedic Surgery)

Office consultation for a 45-year-old male, requested by his internist, with asymptomatic torus palatinus requiring no further treatment. (Oral & Maxillofacial Surgery)

99242 Initial office consultation for a 20-year-old male with acute upper respiratory tract symptoms. (Allergy & Immunology)

Initial office consultation for a 29-year-old soccer player with painful proximal thigh/groin injury. (Orthopaedic Surgery)

Initial office consultation for a 66-year-old female with wrist and hand pain, numbness of finger tips, suspected median nerve compression by carpal tunnel syndrome. (Plastic Surgery)

Initial office consultation for a patient with a solitary lesion of discoid lupus erythematosus on left cheek to rule out malignancy of self-induced lesion. (Dermatology)

Office consultation for management of systolic hypertension in a 70-year-old male scheduled for elective prostate resection. (Geriatrics)

Office consultation with 27-year-old female, with old amputation, for evaluation of existing above-knee prosthesis. (Physical Medicine & Rehabilitation)

Office consultation with 66-year-old female with wrist and hand pain, and finger numbness, secondary to suspected carpal tunnel syndrome. (Orthopaedic Surgery)

Office consultation for 61-year-old female, recently on antibiotic therapy, now with diarrhea and leukocytosis. (Abdominal Surgery)

Office consultation for a patient with papulosquamous eruption of elbow with pitting of nails and itchy scalp. (Dermatology)

Office consultation for a 30-year-old female with single season allergic rhinitis. (Allergy & Immunology)

99243 Initial office consultation for a 60-year-old male with avascular necrosis of the left femoral head with increasing pain. (Orthopaedic Surgery)

Office consultation for a 31-year-old woman complaining of palpitations and chest pains. Her internist had described a mild systolic click. (Cardiology)

Office consultation for a 65-year-old female with persistent bronchitis. (Infectious Disease)

Office consultation for a 65-year-old man with chronic low-back pain radiating to the leg. (Neurosurgery)

Office consultation for 23-year-old female with Crohn's disease not responding to therapy. (Abdominal Surgery/Colon & Rectal Surgery)

Office consultation for 25-year-old patient with symptomatic knee pain and swelling, with torn anterior cruciate ligament and/or torn meniscus. (Orthopaedic Surgery)

Office consultation for a 67-year-old patient with osteoporosis and mandibular atrophy with regard to reconstructive alternatives. (Oral & Maxillofacial Surgery)

Office consultation for 39-year-old patient referred at a perimenopausal age for irregular menses and menopausal symptoms. (Obstetrics & Gynecology)

99244 Initial office consultation for a 28-year-old male, HIV+, with a recent change in visual acuity. (Ophthalmology)

Initial office consultation for a 15-year-old male with failing grades, suspected drug abuse. (Pediatrics)

Initial office consultation for a 36-year-old factory worker, status four months post-occupational low back injury and requires management of intractable low back pain. (Pain Medicine)

Initial office consultation for a 45-year-old female with a history of chronic arthralgia of TMJ and associated myalgia and sudden progressive symptomatology over last two to three months. (Oral & Maxillofacial Surgery)

Initial office consultation for evaluation of a 70-year-old male with appetite loss and diminished energy. (Psychiatry)

Initial office consultation for an elementary school-aged patient, referred by pediatrician, with multiple systematic complaints and recent onset of behavioral discontrol. (Psychiatry)

Initial office consultation for a 23-year-old female with developmental facial skeletal anomaly and subsequent abnormal relationship of jaw(s) to cranial base. (Oral & Maxillofacial Surgery)

Initial office consultation for a 45-year-old myopic patient with a one-week history of floaters and a partial retinal detachment. (Ophthalmology)

Initial office consultation for a 65-year-old female with moderate dementia, mild unsteadiness, back pain fatigue on ambulation, intermittent urinary incontinence. (Neurosurgery)

Initial office consultation for a 33-year-old female referred by endocrinologist with amenorrhea and galactorrhea, for evaluation of pituitary tumor. (Neurosurgery)

Initial office consultation for a 34-year-old male with new onset nephrotic syndrome. (Nephrology)

Initial office consultation for a 39-year-old female with intractable chest wall pain secondary to metastatic breast cancer. (Anesthesiology/Pain Medicine)

Initial office consultation for a patient with multiple giant tumors of jaws. (Oral & Maxillofacial Surgery)

Initial office consultation for a patient with a failed total hip replacement with loosening and pain upon walking. (Orthopaedic Surgery)

Initial office consultation for a 60-year-old female with three-year history of intermittent tic-like unilateral facial pain; now constant pain for six weeks without relief by adequate carbamazepine dosage. (Neurosurgery)

Initial office consultation for a 45-year-old male heavy construction worker with prior lumbar disk surgery two years earlier; now gradually recurring low back and unilateral leg pain for three months, unable to work for two weeks. (Neurosurgery)

Initial office consultation of a patient who presents with a 30-year history of smoking and right neck mass. (Otolaryngology, Head & Neck Surgery)

Office consultation with 38-year-old female, with inflammatory bowel disease, who now presents with right lower quadrant pain and suspected intra-abdominal abscess. (General Surgery/Colon & Rectal Surgery)

Office consultation with 72-year-old male with esophageal carcinoma, symptoms of dysphagia and reflux. (Thoracic Surgery)

Office consultation for discussion of treatment options for a 40-year-old female with a two-centimeter adenocarcinoma of the breast. (Radiation Oncology)

Office consultation for young patient referred by pediatrician because of patient's short attention span, easy distractibility and hyperactivity. (Psychiatry)

Office consultation for 66-year-old female, history of colon resection for adenocarcinoma six years earlier, now with severe mid-back pain; x-rays showing osteoporosis and multiple vertebral compression fractures. (Neurosurgery)

Office consultation for a patient with chronic pelvic inflammatory disease who now has left lower quadrant pain with a palpable pelvic mass. (Obstetrics & Gynecology)

Office consultation for a patient with long-standing psoriasis with acute onset of erythroderma, pustular lesions, chills and fever. Combinations of topical and systemic treatments discussed and instituted. (Dermatology)

99245 Initial office consultation for a 35-year-old multiple-trauma male patient with complex pelvic fractures, for evaluation and formulation of management plan. (Orthopaedic Surgery)

Initial emergency room consultation for 10-year-old male in status epilepticus, recent closed head injury, information about medication not available. (Neurosurgery)

Initial emergency room consultation for a 23-year-old patient with severe abdominal pain, guarding, febrile, and unstable vital signs. (Obstetrics & Gynecology)

Office consultation for a 67-year-old female longstanding uncontrolled diabetic who presents with retinopathy, nephropathy, and a foot ulcer. (Endocrinology)

Office consultation for a 37-year-old male for initial evaluation and management of Cushing's disease. (Endocrinology)

Office consultation for a 60-year-old male who presents with thyrotoxicosis, exophthalmos, frequent premature ventricular contractions and congestive heart failure. (Endocrinology)

Initial office consultation for a 36-year-old patient, one year status post occupational herniated cervical disk treated by laminectomy, requiring management of multiple sites of intractable pain, depression, and narcotic dependence. (Pain Medicine)

Office consultation for a 58-year-old man with a history of MI and CHF who complains of the recent onset of rest angina and shortness of breath. The patient has a systolic blood pressure of 90mmHG and is in Class IV heart failure. (Cardiology)

Emergency room consultation for a 1-year-old with a three-day history of fever with increasing respiratory distress who is thought to have cardiac tamponade by the ER physician. (Cardiology)

Office consultation in the emergency room for a 25-year-old male with severe, acute, closed head injury. (Neurosurgery)

Office consultation for a 23-year-old female with Stage II A Hodgkins disease with positive supraclavicular and mediastinal nodes. (Radiation Oncology)

Office consultation for a 27-year-old juvenile diabetic patient with severe diabetic retinopathy, gastric atony, nephrotic syndrome and progressive renal failure, now with a serum creatinine of 2.7, and a blood pressure of 170/114. (Nephrology)

Office consultation for independent medical evaluation of a patient with a history of complicated low back and neck problems with previous multiple failed back surgeries. (Orthopaedic Surgery)

Office consultation for an adolescent referred by pediatrician for recent onset of violent and self-injurious behavior. (Psychiatry)

Office consultation for a 6-year-old male for evaluation of severe muscle and joint pain and a diffuse rash. Well until four-six weeks earlier, when he developed arthralgia, myalgias, and a fever of 102 for one week. (Rheumatology)

Initial Inpatient Consultations

New or Established Patient

99251 Initial hospital consultation for a 27-year-old female with fractured incisor post-intubation. (Oral & Maxillofacial Surgery)

Initial hospital consultation for an orthopaedic patient on IV antibiotics who has developed an apparent candida infection of the oral cavity. (Oral & Maxillofacial Surgery)

Initial inpatient consultation for a 30-year-old female complaining of vaginal itching, post orthopaedic surgery. (Obstetrics & Gynecology)

Initial inpatient consultation for a 36-year-old male on orthopaedic service with complaint of localized dental pain. (Oral & Maxillofacial Surgery)

99252 Initial hospital consultation for a 45-year-old male, previously abstinent alcoholic, who relapsed and was admitted for management of gastritis. The patient readily accepts the need for further treatment. (Addiction Medicine)

Initial hospital consultation for a 35-year-old dialysis patient with episodic oral ulcerations. (Oral & Maxillofacial Surgery)

Initial inpatient preoperative consultation for a 43-year-old woman with cholecystitis and well-controlled hypertension. (Cardiology)

Initial inpatient consultation for recommendation of antibiotic prophylaxis for a patient with a synthetic heart valve who will undergo urologic surgery. (Internal Medicine)

Initial inpatient consultation for possible drug induced skin eruption in 50-year-old male. (Dermatology)

Preoperative inpatient consultation for evaluation of hypertension in a 60-year-old male who will undergo a cholecystectomy. Patient had a normal annual check-up in your office four months ago. (Internal Medicine)

Initial inpatient consultation for 66-year-old patient with wrist and hand pain and finger numbness, secondary to carpal tunnel syndrome. (Orthopaedic Surgery/Plastic Surgery)

Initial inpatient consultation for a 66-year-old male smoker referred for pain management immediately status post-biliary tract surgery done via sub-costal incision. (Anesthesiology/Pain Medicine)

99253 Initial hospital consultation for a 50-year-old female with incapacitating knee pain due to generalized rheumatoid arthritis. (Orthopaedic Surgery)

Initial hospital consultation for a 60-year-old male with avascular necrosis of the left femoral heel with increasing pain. (Orthopaedic Surgery)

Initial hospital consultation for a 45-year-old female with compound mandibular fracture and concurrent head, abdominal and/or orthopaedic injuries. (Oral & Maxillofacial Surgery)

Initial hospital consultation for a 22-year-old female, paraplegic, to evaluate wrist and hand pain. (Orthopaedic Surgery)

Initial hospital consultation for a 40-year-old male with 10-day history of incapacitating unilateral sciatica, unable to walk now, not improved by bed rest. (Neurosurgery)

Initial hospital consultation, requested by pediatrician, for treatment recommendations for a patient admitted with persistent inability to walk following soft tissue injury to ankle. (Physiatry)

Initial hospital consultation for a 27-year-old previously healthy male who vomited during IV sedation and may have aspirated gastric contents. (Anesthesiology)

Initial hospital consultation for a 33-year-old female, post-abdominal surgery, who now has a fever. (Internal Medicine)

Initial inpatient consultation for a 57-year-old male, post lower endoscopy, for evaluation of abdominal pain and fever. (General Surgery)

Initial inpatient consultation for rehabilitation of a 73-year-old female one week after surgical management of a hip fracture. (Physical Medicine & Rehabilitation)

Initial inpatient consultation for diagnosis/management of fever following abdominal surgery. (Internal Medicine)

Initial inpatient consultation for a 35-year-old female with a fever and pulmonary infiltrate following cesarean section. (Pulmonary Medicine)

Initial inpatient consultation for a 42-year-old non-diabetic patient, post-op cholecystectomy, now with an acute urinary tract infection. (Nephrology)

Initial inpatient consultation for 53-year-old female with moderate uncomplicated pancreatitis. (Gastroenterology)

Initial inpatient consultation for 45-year-old patient with chronic neck pain with radicular pain of the left arm. (Orthopaedic Surgery)

Initial inpatient consultation for 8-year-old patient with new onset of seizures who has a normal examination and previous history. (Neurology)

99254 Initial hospital consultation for a 15-year-old patient with painless swelling of proximal humerus with lytic lesion by x-ray. (Orthopaedic Surgery)

Initial hospital consultation for evaluation of a 29-year-old female with a diffusely positive medical review of systems and history of multiple surgeries. (Psychiatry)

Initial hospital consultation for a 70-year-old diabetic female with gangrene of the foot. (Orthopaedic Surgery)

Initial inpatient consultation for a 47-year-old female with progressive pulmonary infiltrate, hypoxemia, and diminished urine output. (Anesthesiology)

Initial hospital consultation for a 13-month-old with spasmodic cough, respiratory distress, and fever. (Allergy & Immunology)

Initial hospital consultation for a patient with failed total hip replacement with loosening and pain upon walking. (Orthopaedic Surgery)

Initial hospital consultation for a 62-year-old female with metastatic breast cancer to the femoral neck and thoracic vertebra. (Orthopaedic Surgery)

Initial hospital consultation for a 39-year-old female with nephrolithiasis requiring extensive opioid analgesics, whose vital signs are now elevated. She initially denied any drug use, but today gives history of multiple substance abuse, including opioids and prior treatment for a personality disorder. (Psychiatry)

Initial hospital consultation for a 70-year-old female without previous psychiatric history, who is now experiencing nocturnal confusion and visual hallucinations following hip replacement surgery. (Psychiatry)

Initial inpatient consultation for evaluation of a 63-year-old in the ICU with diabetes and chronic renal failure who develops acute respiratory distress syndrome 36 hours after a mitral valve replacement. (Anesthesiology)

Initial inpatient consultation for a 66-year-old female with enlarged supraclavicular lymph nodes, found on biopsy to be malignant. (Hematology/Oncology)

Initial inpatient consultation for a 43-year-old female for evaluation of sudden painful visual loss, optic neuritis and episodic paresthesia. (Ophthalmology)

Initial inpatient consultation for evaluation of a 71-year-old male with hyponatremia (serum sodium 114) who was admitted to the hospital with pneumonia. (Nephrology)

Initial inpatient consultation for a 72-year-old male with emergency admission for possible bowel obstruction. (Internal Medicine/General Surgery)

Initial inpatient consultation for a 35-year-old female with fever, swollen joints, and rash of one-week duration. (Rheumatology)

99255 Initial inpatient consultation for a 76-year-old female with massive, life-threatening gastrointestinal hemorrhage and chest pain. (Gastroenterology)

Initial inpatient consultation for a 75-year-old female, admitted to intensive care with acute respiratory distress syndrome, who is hypersensitive, has a moderate metabolic acidosis, and a rising serum creatinine. (Nephrology)

Initial hospital consultation for patient with a history of complicated low back pain and neck problems with previous multiple failed back surgeries. (Orthopaedic Surgery/Neurosurgery)

Initial hospital consultation for a 66-year-old female, two days post-abdominal aneurysm repair, with oliguria and hypertension of one-day duration. (Nephrology/Internal Medicine)

Initial hospital consultation for a patient with shotgun wound to face with massive facial trauma and airway obstruction. (Oral & Maxillofacial Surgery)

Initial hospital consultation for patient with severe pancreatitis complicated by respiratory insufficiency, acute renal failure, and abscess formation. (General Surgery/Colon & Rectal Surgery)

Initial hospital consultation for a 35-year-old multiple-trauma male patient with complex pelvic fractures to evaluate and formulate management plan. (Orthopaedic Surgery)

Initial inpatient consultation for adolescent patient with fractured femur and pelvis who pulled out IVs and disconnected traction in attempt to elope from hospital. (Psychiatry)

Initial hospital consultation for a 16-year-old primigravida at 32 weeks gestation requested by a family practitioner for evaluation of severe hypertension, thrombocytopenia, and headache. (Obstetrics & Gynecology)

Initial hospital consultation for a 58-year-old insulin-dependent diabetic with multiple antibiotic allergies, now with multiple fascial plane abscesses and airway obstruction. (Oral & Maxillofacial Surgery)

Initial inpatient consultation for a 55-year-old male with known cirrhosis and ascites, now with jaundice, encephalopathy, and massive hematemesis. (Gastroenterology)

Initial hospital consultation for a 25-year-old male, seen in emergency room with severe, closed head injury. (Neurosurgery)

Initial hospital consultation for a 2-day-old male with single ventricle physiology and subaortic obstruction. Family counseling following evaluation for multiple, staged surgical procedures. (Thoracic Surgery)

Initial hospital consultation for a 45-year-old male admitted with subarachnoid hemorrhage and intracranial aneurysm on angiogram. (Neurosurgery)

Initial inpatient consultation for myxedematous patient who is hypoventilating and obtunded. (Endocrinology)

Initial hospital consultation for a 45-year-old patient with widely metastatic lung carcinoma, intractable back pain, and a history that includes substance dependence, NSAID allergy, and two prior laminectomies with fusion for low back pain. (Pain Medicine)

Initial hospital consultation for evaluation of treatment options in a 50-year-old patient with cirrhosis, known peptic ulcer disease, hypotension, encephalopathy, and massive acute upper gastrointestinal bleeding which cannot be localized by endoscopy. (Interventional Radiology)

Initial inpatient consultation in the ICU for a 70-year-old male who experienced a cardiac arrest during surgery and was resuscitated. (Cardiology)

Initial inpatient consultation for a patient with severe pancreatitis complicated by respiratory insufficiency, acute renal failure and abscess formation. (Gastroenterology)

Initial inpatient consultation for a 70-year-old cirrhotic male admitted with ascites, jaundice, encephalopathy, and massive hematemesis. (Gastroenterology)

Initial inpatient consultation in the ICU for a 51-year-old patient who is on a ventilator and has a fever two weeks after a renal transplantation. (Infectious Disease)

Initial inpatient consultation for evaluation and formulation of plan for management of multiple trauma patient with complex pelvic fracture, 35-year-old male. (General Surgery/Orthopaedic Surgery)

Initial inpatient consultation for a 50-year-old male with a history of previous myocardial infarction, now with acute pulmonary edema and hypotension. (Cardiology)

Initial inpatient consultation for 45-year-old male with recent, acute subarachnoid hemorrhage, hesitant speech, mildly confused, drowsy. High risk group for HIV+ status. (Neurosurgery)

Initial inpatient consultation for 36-year-old female referred by her internist to evaluate a patient being followed for abdominal pain and fever. The patient has developed diffuse abdominal pain, guarding, rigidity and increased fever. (Obstetrics & Gynecology)

Follow-up Inpatient Consultations

Established Patient

99261 Follow-up consultation for a 78-year-old female nursing home resident for evaluation of medical management of pruritus ani. (Colon & Rectal Surgery/Geriatrics/General Surgery)

Follow-up hospital consultation on first post-op day for a 64-year-old male who has undergone uneventful CABG. (Anesthesiology)

Follow-up inpatient consultation for a 67-year-old female admitted several days ago for bleeding ulcer; now stable. (Gastroenterology)

Follow-up hospital consultation for a 35-year-old female with history of mitral valve prolapse. (Cardiology)

Follow-up inpatient consultation to complete initial consultation for dental pain after review of radiographs. (Oral & Maxillofacial Surgery)

Follow-up inpatient consultation for evaluation of response to therapy for moniliasis. (Oral & Maxillofacial Surgery)

Follow-up inpatient consultation for a 22-year-old female with recurrent aphthous ulcers. (Oral & Maxillofacial Surgery)

Follow-up hospital consultation for a 37-year-old female to complete review of previously unavailable studies. (Therapeutic Radiology & Oncology)

Follow-up consultation for a highly functional 75-year-old female with urinary incontinence to review preliminary results of diagnostic evaluation. (Geriatrics)

Follow-up inpatient consultation for a 1-week-old premature female with patent ductus arteriosus. The murmur has disappeared. (Cardiology)

Follow-up hospital consultation to review the results of an audiogram. (Otolaryngology, Head & Neck Surgery)

Follow-up inpatient consultation with 35-year-old female with pulmonary embolism post-op cesarean section, now stable, for assessment of response to anticoagulation and recommended adjustment of heparin dose. (Pulmonary Medicine)

Follow-up inpatient consultation for a 74-year-old male whose postoperative facial paralysis after a cholecystectomy is now resolving. (Neurology)

Follow-up inpatient consultation with 67-year-old female, established patient, for review of diagnostic studies ordered at time of first contact. (Internal Medicine)

Follow-up inpatient consultation for 78-year-old female nursing home resident for evaluation of medical management of pruritis ani. (General Surgery/Colon & Rectal Surgery)

Follow-up inpatient consultation for a 36-year-old female two days after spontaneous passage of 3mm stone. (Urology)

Follow-up inpatient consultation for a 94-year-old male nursing home resident for re-evaluation of hemorrhoids following conservative therapy. (Colon & Rectal Surgery/General Surgery/Geriatrics)

Follow-up inpatient consultation for a 50-year-old male, asymptomatic with borderline ECG abnormality, needs preoperative opinion after a thallium exercise perfusion scan. (Cardiology)

99262 Follow-up inpatient consultation for a 6-year-old female, established patient, with endocarditis and changing heart murmur. (Cardiology)

Follow-up inpatient consultation on a 2-year-old male, one day postoperative ventricular septal defect closure with signs of tachycardia. (Cardiology)

Follow-up inpatient consultation for a 63-year-old man, established patient, with moderately severe pulmonary insufficiency, 10 days postoperative coronary artery bypass for unstable angina. Patient has developed severe dyspnea, fever, and a new exudative right pleural effusion. (Cardiology)

Follow-up inpatient consultation for a 67-year-old woman with lung cancer and syndrome of inappropriate secretion of antidiuretic hormone (SIADH) who has had a seizure following intravenous saline. (Endocrinology)

Follow-up inpatient consultation for a 22-year-old female, established patient, with steroid-dependent systemic lupus erythematosus, arthritis, and glomerulonephritis. Patient is re-evaluated for loss of consciousness and chest pain. (Rheumatology)

Follow-up inpatient consultation for a 75-year-old diabetic with fever, chills, a gangrenous heel ulcer, rhonchi, and dyspnea who appears lethargic and tachypneic. (Endocrinology)

Follow-up inpatient consultation for a 30-year-old, established patient, with intractable neck and low back pain, who is excessively sedated after institution of methadone therapy. (Pain Medicine)

Follow-up inpatient consultation for a 65-year-old man with a history of hypertension and MI who is five days post uncomplicated GI procedure with an unremarkable postoperative recovery. He has just been resuscitated from a cardiopulmonary arrest. (Cardiology)

Follow-up inpatient consultation with 72-year-old female, established patient with bullous pemphigoid on combined oral therapy steroids and immunosuppressive to evaluate progress of cutaneous care orders and adjustment of oral/parenteral therapy dosages. (Dermatology)

Follow-up inpatient consultation for a 71-year-old male who has developed a maculopapular skin rash while on antibiotics recommended for an uncomplicated pneumonia. (Infectious Disease)

Follow-up inpatient consultation with 68-year-old, incapacitated male with spinal stenosis and failure to respond to bedrest, analgesics, and PT. (Neurosurgery)

Follow-up inpatient consultation with 51-year-old male for evaluation and determination of the etiology of postoperative hyponatremia following TURP. (Family Medicine)

Follow-up inpatient consultation for re-evaluation of a stroke patient, and development of plan for initial rehabilitation services. (Neurology)

Follow-up inpatient consultation with 45-year-old male, established patient for discussion of CT scan which demonstrates a cavernous hemangioma. (Ophthalmology)

Follow-up inpatient consultation for an asymptomatic 35-year-old Type I diabetic patient with hyperkalemic, hyperchloremia acidosis, to review lab results. (Nephrology)

Follow-up inpatient consultation for an elderly male with a perioperative myocardial infarction requiring adjustment of vasoactive medications. (Anesthesiology)

99263 Follow-up hospital consultation of an AIDS patient admitted with a sore throat who now has enlarging neck mass. (Otolaryngology, Head & Neck Surgery)

Follow-up hospital consultation of a pansinusitis patient with sudden onset of proptosis. (Otolaryngology, Head & Neck Surgery)

Follow-up inpatient consultation for a 53-year-old man with known angina who develops crescendo angina post cholecystectomy. (Cardiology)

Follow-up inpatient consultation with 72-year-old male established patient admitted for management of alcohol withdrawal, now confused and febrile. (Addiction Medicine)

Follow-up inpatient consultation for an HIV+ patient with an increasing fever following 10 days of antibiotic therapy for pneumocystis carinii pneumonia. (Infectious Disease)

Follow-up inpatient consultation with 58-year-old diabetic female, with bacterial endocarditis, continued fever after two weeks of intravenous antibiotic therapy, and new onset ventricular ectopia. (Cardiology)

Follow-up inpatient consultation for a 90-year-old female with urinary incontinence who has a complicated medical history requiring reassessment of multiple medical problems, recommendations for placement, further recommendation for management of incontinence and reevaluation of cognitive status because of competency issues. (Geriatrics/Psychiatry)

Follow-up inpatient consultation for 42-year-old male with persistent gastrointestinal bleeding, etiology undetermined, not responding to conservative therapy of transfusions. (General Surgery/Colon & Rectal Surgery)

Follow-up inpatient consultation for a 62-year-old female with steroid-dependent asthma, diabetes mellitus, thyrotoxicosis, abdominal pain and possible vasculitis. (Rheumatology)

Follow-up inpatient consultation for a 62-year-old male, status post-op acute small bowel obstruction; now with acute renal failure. (Family Medicine)

Emergency Department Services

New or Established Patient

99281 Emergency department visit for a patient for removal of sutures from a well-healed, uncomplicated laceration. (Emergency Medicine)

Emergency department visit for a patient for tetanus toxoid immunization. (Emergency Medicine)

Emergency department visit for a patient with several uncomplicated insect bites. (Emergency Medicine)

99282 Emergency department visit for a 20-year-old student who presents with a painful sunburn with blister formation on the back. (Emergency Medicine)

Emergency department visit for a child presenting with impetigo localized to the face. (Emergency Medicine)

Emergency department visit for a patient with a minor traumatic injury of an extremity with localized pain, swelling, and bruising. (Emergency Medicine)

Emergency department visit for an otherwise healthy patient whose chief complaint is a red, swollen cystic lesion on his/her back. (Emergency Medicine)

Emergency department visit for a patient presenting with a rash on both legs after exposure to poison ivy. (Emergency Medicine)

Emergency department visit for a young adult patient with infected sclera and purulent discharge from both eyes without pain, visual disturbance or history of foreign body in either eye. (Emergency Medicine)

99283 Emergency department visit for a sexually active female complaining of vaginal discharge who is afebrile and denies experiencing abdominal or back pain. (Emergency Medicine)

Emergency department visit for a well-appearing 8-year-old who has a fever, diarrhea and abdominal cramps, is tolerating oral fluids and is not vomiting. (Emergency Medicine)

Emergency department visit for a patient with an inversion ankle injury, who is unable to bear weight on the injured foot and ankle. (Emergency Medicine)

Emergency department visit for a patient who has a complaint of acute pain associated with a suspected foreign body in the painful eye. (Emergency Medicine)

Emergency department visit for a healthy, young adult patient who sustained a blunt head injury with local swelling and bruising without subsequent confusion, loss of consciousness or memory deficit. (Emergency Medicine)

99284 Emergency department visit for a 4-year-old who fell off a bike sustaining a head injury with brief loss of consciousness. (Emergency Medicine)

Emergency department visit for an elderly female who has fallen and is now complaining of pain in her right hip and is unable to walk. (Emergency Medicine)

Emergency department visit for a patient with flank pain and hematuria. (Emergency Medicine)

Emergency department visit for a female presenting with lower abdominal pain and a vaginal discharge. (Emergency Medicine)

99285 Emergency department visit for a patient with a complicated overdose requiring aggressive management to prevent side effects from the ingested materials. (Emergency Medicine)

Emergency department visit for a patient with a new onset of rapid heart rate requiring IV drugs. (Emergency Medicine)

Emergency department visit for a patient exhibiting active, upper gastrointestinal bleeding. (Emergency Medicine)

Emergency department visit for a previously healthy young adult patient who is injured in an automobile accident and is brought to the emergency department immobilized and has symptoms compatible with intra-abdominal injuries or multiple extremity injuries. (Emergency Medicine)

Emergency department visit for a patient with an acute onset of chest pain compatible with symptoms of cardiac ischemia and/or pulmonary embolism. (Emergency Medicine)

Emergency department visit for a patient who presents with a sudden onset of "the worst headache of her life," and complains of a stiff neck, nausea, and inability to concentrate. (Emergency Medicine)

Emergency department visit for a patient with a new onset of a cerebral vascular accident. (Emergency Medicine)

Emergency department visit for acute febrile illness in an adult, associated with shortness of breath and an altered level of alertness. (Emergency Medicine)

Critical Care Services

99291 First hour of critical care of a 65-year-old man with septic shock following relief of ureteral obstruction caused by a stone.

First hour of critical care of a 15-year-old with acute respiratory failure from asthma.

First hour of critical care of a 45-year-old who sustained a liver laceration, cerebral hematoma, flailed chest, and pulmonary contusion after being struck by an automobile.

First hour of critical care of a 65-year-old woman who, following a hysterectomy, suffered a cardiac arrest associated with a pulmonary embolus.

First hour of critical care of a 6-month-old with hypovolemic shock secondary to diarrhea and dehydration.

First hour of critical care of a 3-year-old with respiratory failure secondary to pneumocystis carinii pneumonia.

Comprehensive Nursing Facility Assessments

New or Established Patient

99301 Annual nursing facility history and physical and MDS/RAI evaluation for a two-year nursing facility resident who is an 84-year-old female with multiple chronic health problems, including: stable controlled hypertension, chronic constipation, osteoarthritis, and moderated stable dementia.

Nursing facility visit for an assessment of a resident with non-insulin dependent diabetes, stable angina, and chronic obstructive pulmonary disease (COPD) one year after previous MDS/RAI.

99302 Nursing facility visit one year after previous MDS/RAI to assess an 80-year-old woman with Parkinson's disease, chronic hypertension, and degenerative arthritis. Visit reveals Stage II decubitus.

Nursing facility assessment of a 28-year-old diabetic, male resident with a new Stage IV pressure ulcer on his left lateral malleolus that is unresponsive to treatment, thus triggering the need for a new MDS/RAI and new medical plan of care.

Nursing facility assessment of an 88-year-old male resident with a permanent change in status following a new cerebral vascular accident (CVA) that has triggered the need for a new MDS/RAI and medical plan of care.

Nursing facility visit and assessment to take over the primary care of a 75-year-old diabetic, previously stable, who was on oral hypoglycemic agents, but who now requires initiation of insulin therapy, a new MDS/RAI, and medical plan of care.

Nursing facility visit and assessment for an 81-year-old female resident with dementia who under structured guidance and intensive nutritional support has regained significant levels of function in three activities of daily living and is now able to feed and dress herself and ambulate with appliance and who now thus requires a new MDS/RAI and medical plan of care.

99303 Initial nursing facility assessment (MDS/RAI and medical plan of care) of a 72-year-old insulin dependent diabetic amputee with hearing and visual impairments and possible dementia seen in the office the day before and judged to require nursing facility care.

Sub-acute nursing facility assessment of a previously independently living 90-year-old male who suffered a recent cerebral vascular accident (CVA) and is transferred to the hospital sub-acute rehabilitation unit for further rehabilitation supportive services.

Initial nursing facility visit to evaluate a 72-year-old woman found confused and wandering, admitted by Adult Protective Services without a qualifying hospital stay or inpatient diagnostic work. The patient lives alone and has no relatives or significant others in the community.

Nursing facility assessment and creation of medical plan of care upon readmission to the nursing facility of an 82-year-old male who was previously discharged. The patient has just been discharged from the hospital where he had been treated for an acute gastric ulcer bleed associated with transient delirium. The patient returns to the nursing facility debilitated, protein depleted, and with a Stage III coccygeal decubitus.

Subsequent Nursing Facility Care

New or Established Patient

99311 Scheduled follow-up visit for a known 70-year-old stable paraplegic with no status change noted during visit.

Scheduled monthly nursing home visit with a patient who has mild senile dementia, Alzheimers' type, with no change in status, stable hypertension, and who is ambulating with a walker one year past stroke.

Follow-up in skilled nursing facility with a 70-year-old patient following a 10-day treatment of a cellulitis of the foot.

99312 Scheduled follow-up visit to a resident with controlled dementia, hypertension, and diabetes. During visit, patient seems to exhibit flu symptoms.

Scheduled nursing facility visit with an afebrile demented resident who also has a mild cough, requiring no change in the medical plan of care.

Subsequent visit in a skilled nursing facility with a patient who is six months post stroke and now has a fever and mild cough.

Scheduled nursing facility visit for an 84-year-old male with chronic renal insufficiency, on digitalis and diuretics, requiring adjustment of medications and revision of medical plan of care.

Nursing facility visit of a resident with multiple chronic health problems who is six months post stroke and now has a fever and mild cough, to evaluate for possible pneumonia. Requires the development of a new medical plan of care, but not a revised MDS/RAI.

99313 Follow-up nursing facility visit to evaluate the reason for frequent falls by a 90-year-old ataxic resident, and to determine possible need for change in medications and medical care plan.

Re-admission of a 75-year-old man with stroke who was hospitalized with pneumonia for his illness and who returns to the nursing facility with no permanent change in status from his condition prior to hospitalization; no new MDS/RAI is required.

Nursing facility visit with a diabetic resident who has developed Stage II decubitus ulcers with cellulitis, requiring a revision in the medical plan of care.

Nursing facility visit to develop a new plan of care for an amputee with atherosclerosis obliterans who has refused to eat for three days and has developed decreased urinary output.

Nursing facility visit for a 78-year-old resident with chronic atrial fibrillation and a history of heart failure to evaluate an acute confusional state and to revise the medical plan of care.

Unscheduled nursing facility visit for evaluation of a patient with fever and obtundation who is determined not to require hospital admission or new MDS, but who does require workup and revision of medical plan of care.

Prolonged Services

Prolonged Physician Service With Direct (Face-to-Face) Patient Contact

Office or Other Outpatient

99354/ 99355 A 20-year-old female with history of asthma presents with acute bronchospasm and moderate respiratory distress. Initial evaluation shows respiratory rate 30, labored breathing and wheezing heard in all lung fields. Office treatment is initiated which includes intermittent bronchial dilation and subcutaneous epinephrine. Requires intermittent physician face-to-face time with patient over a period of two-three hours. (Family Medicine/Internal Medicine)

Inpatient

99356 A 34-year-old primigravida presents to hospital in early labor. Admission history and physical reveals severe preeclampsia. Physician supervises management of preeclampsia, IV magnesium initiation and maintenance, labor augmentation with pitocin, and close maternal-fetal monitoring. Physician face-to-face involvement includes 40 minutes of continuous bedside care until the patient is stable, then is intermittent over several hours until the delivery. (Family Medicine/Internal Medicine/Obstetrics & Gynecology)

Prolonged Physician Service Without Direct Patient (Face-to-Face) Contact

99358/
99359
A 65-year-old new patient with multiple problems is seen and evaluated. After the visit, the physician requires extensive time to talk with the patient's daughter, to review complex, detailed medical records transferred from previous physicians and to complete a comprehensive treatment plan. This plan also requires the physician to personally initiate and coordinate the care plan with a local home health agency and a dietician. (Family Medicine/Internal Medicine)

Physician Standby Services

99360
A 24-year-old patient is admitted to OB unit attempting VBAC. Fetal monitoring shows increasing fetal distress. Patient's blood pressure is rising and labor progressing slowly. A primary care physician is requested by the OB/GYN to standby in the unit for possible cesarean delivery and neonatal resuscitation. (Family Medicine/Internal Medicine)

Care Plan Oversight Services

99375
First month of care plan oversight for terminal care of a 58-year-old woman with advanced intraabdominal ovarian cancer. Care plan includes home oxygen, diuretics IV for edema and ascites control and pain control management involving IV morphine infusion when progressive ileus occurred. Physician phone contacts with nurse, family, and MSW. Discussion with MSW concerning plans to withdraw supportive measures per patient wishes. Documentation includes review and modification of care plan and certifications from nursing, MSW, pharmacy, and DME. (Family Medicine/Internal Medicine)

Appendix D

Summary of CPT Add-on Codes

This listing is a summary of CPT add-on codes for *CPT 2003*. The codes listed below are identified in *CPT 2003* with a **+** symbol.

0006T	22226	37208	63048	76085	96412
0036T	22328	37250	63057	76125	96423
01953	22522	37251	63066	76802	96567
01968	22585	38102	63076	76810	96570
01969	22614	38746	63078	76812	96571
11001	22632	38747	63082	78020	97546
11101	26125	43635	63086	78478	99100
11201	26861	44015	63088	78480	99116
11732	26863	44121	63091	78496	99135
11922	27358	44128	63308	87187	99140
13102	27692	44139	64472	87904	99290
13122	32501	44203	64476	88141	99292
13133	33141	44701	64480	88155	99354
13153	33225	44955	64484	88311	99355
15001	33508	47001	64623	88312	99356
15101	33530	47550	64627	88313	99357
15121	33572	48400	64727	88314	99358
15201	33924	49568	64778	90472	99359
15221	33961	49905	64783	90474	99569
15241	34808	56606	64787	90781	
15261	34813	58611	64832	92547	
15343	34826	59525	64837	92608	
15351	35390	60512	64859	92973	
15401	35400	61316	64872	92974	
15787	35500	61517	64874	92978	
16036	35572	61609	64876	92979	
17003	35681	61610	64901	92981	
17310	35682	61611	64902	92984	
19001	35683	61612	66990	92996	
19126	35685	61795	67225	92998	
19291	35686	62148	67320	93320	
19295	35700	62160	67331	93321	
22103	36218	63035	67332	93325	
22116	36248	63043	67334	93571	
22216	37206	63044	67335	93572	
			67340	93609	
			69990	93613	
			74301	93621	
			75774	93622	
			75946	93623	
			75964	93662	
			75968	95920	
			75993	95962	
			75996	95967	
			76006	95973	

Appendix E

Summary of CPT Codes Exempt from Modifier '-51'

This listing is a summary of CPT codes that are exempt from the use of modifier '-51' but have NOT been designated as CPT add-on procedures/services. The codes listed below are identified in *CPT 2003* with a ⊘ symbol.

17004	32000	90386	90703	93540
17304	32002	90389	90704	93541
17305	32020	90393	90705	93542
17306	33517	90396	90706	93543
17307	33518	90399	90707	93544
20660	33519	90476	90708	93545
20690	33521	90477	90710	93555
20692	33522	90581	90712	93556
20900	33523	90585	90713	93600
20902	35600	90586	90716	93602
20910	36488	90632	90717	93603
20912	36489	90633	90718	93610
20920	36490	90634	90719	93612
20922	36491	90636	90720	93615
20924	36620	90645	90721	93616
20926	36660	90646	90723	93618
20930	38792	90647	90725	93619
20931	44500	90648	90727	93620
20936	61107	90657	90732	93624
20937	61210	90658	90733	93631
20938	62284	90659	90735	93640
20974	90281	90660	90740	93641
20975	90283	90665	90743	93642
22840	90287	90669	90744	93650
22841	90288	90675	90746	93651
22842	90291	90676	90747	93652
22843	90296	90680	90748	93660
22844	90371	90690	90749	95900
22845	90375	90691	93501	95903
22846	90376	90692	93503	95904
22847	90378	90693	93505	99141
22848	90379	90700	93508	99142
22851	90384	90701	93510	
31500	90385	90702	93511	
			93514	
			93524	
			93526	
			93527	
			93528	
			93529	
			93530	
			93531	
			93532	
			93533	
			93539	

Index

Main Terms

The index is organized by main terms. Each main term can stand alone, or be followed by up to three modifying terms. There are four primary classes of main entries:

1. Procedure or service.
   For example: Endoscopy; Anastomosis; Splint

2. Organ or other anatomic site.
   For example: Tibia; Colon; Salivary Gland

3. Condition.
   For example: Abscess; Entropion; Tetralogy of Fallot

4. Synonyms, Eponyms and Abbreviations.
   For example: EEG; Bricker Operation; Clagett Procedure

Modifying Terms

A main term may be followed by a series of up to three indented terms that modify the main term. When modifying terms appear, one should review the list, as these subterms do have an effect on the selection of the appropriate code for the procedure.

Code Ranges

Whenever more than one code applies to a given index entry, a code range is listed. If several non-sequential codes apply, they will be separated by a comma. For example:

Esophagus
    Reconstruction 43300, 43310, 43113

If two or more sequential codes apply, they will be separated by a hyphen. For example:

Debridement
    Burns 01951-01953, 16010-16030

Conventions

As a space saving convention, certain words infer some meaning. This convention is primarily used when a procedure or service is listed as a subterm. For example:

Knee
    Incision (of)

In this example, the word in parentheses (of) does not appear in the index, but it is inferred. As another example:

Pancreas
    Anesthesia (for procedures on)

In this example, as there is no such entity as pancreas anesthesia, the words in parentheses are inferred. That is, anesthesia for procedures on the pancreas.

The alphabetic index is NOT a substitute for the main text of *CPT*. Even if only one code appears, the user must refer to the main text to ensure that the code selection is accurate.

A

A-II
See Angiotensin II

Abbe-Estlander Procedure
See Reconstruction; Repair, Cleft Lip

Abdomen
Abdominal Wall
  Repair
    Hernia 49491-49496, 49501, 49507, 49521, 49590
  Tumor
    Excision 22900
  Unlisted Services and Procedures 22999
Abscess
  Incision and Drainage 49020, 49040
    Open 49040
    Percutaneous 49021
Angiography 74175, 75635
Artery
  Ligation 37617
Biopsy 49000
Bypass Graft 35907
Cannula/Catheter
  Removal 49422
Celiotomy
  for Staging 49220
CT Scan 74150-74175, 75635
Cyst
  Destruction/Excision 49200-49201
Drainage
  Fluid 49080-49081
Ectopic Pregnancy 59130
Endometrioma
  Destruction/Excision 49200-49201
Exploration 49000-49002
  Blood Vessel 35840
  Staging 58960
Incision 49000
  Staging 58960
Incision and Drainage
  Pancreatitis 48000
Injection
  Air 49400
  Contrast Material 49400
Insertion
  Catheter 49419-49421
  Venous Shunt 49425
Intraperitoneal
  Catheter Removal 49422
  Shunt
    Ligation 49428
    Removal 49429
Laparotomy
  Staging 49220
Magnetic Resonance Imaging
(MRI) 74181-74183
Needle Biopsy
  Mass 49180
Peritoneocentesis 49080-49081
Radical Resection 51597

Repair
  Blood Vessel 35221
    with Other Graft 35281
    with Vein Graft 35251
  Hernia 49491-49525, 49560-49587
  Suture 49900
Revision
  Venous Shunt 49426
Suture 49900
Tumor
  Destruction/Excision 49200-49201
Ultrasound 76700-76705
Unlisted Services and Procedures 49999
Wound Exploration
  Penetrating 20102
X-Ray 74000-74022

Abdominal Aorta
See Aorta, Abdominal

Abdominal Aortic Aneurysm
See Aorta, Abdominal, Aneurysm

Abdominal Deliveries
See Cesarean Delivery

Abdominal Hysterectomy
See Hysterectomy, Abdominal

Abdominal Lymphangiogram
See Lymphangiography, Abdomen

Abdominal Paracentesis
See Abdomen, Drainage

Abdominal Radiographies
See Abdomen, X-Ray

Abdominal Wall
Reconstruction 49905
Surgery 22999
Tumor
  Excision 22900

Abdominohysterectomy
See Hysterectomy, Abdominal

Abdominopelvic Amputation
See Amputation, Interpelviabdominal

Abdominoplasty 15831

Ablation
Anal
  Polyp 46615
  Tumor 46615
Colon
  Tumor 45339
CT Scan Guidance 76362
Endometrial 0009T, 58353, 58563
Endometrium
  Ultrasound Guidance 0009T
Heart
  Arrhythmogenic Focus 93650-93652
    See Cardiology; Diagnostic, Intracardiac Pacing and Mapping
Liver
  Tumor 47380-47382
    Laparoscopic 47370-47371
Magnetic Resonance Guidance 76394
Prostate 55873

Renal Cyst 50541
Renal Mass 50542
Turbinate Mucosa 30801-30802
Ultrasound Guidance 76490

Abortion
See Obstetrical Care
Incomplete 59812
Induced
  by Dilation and Curettage 59840
  by Dilation and Evacuation 59841
  by Saline 59850-59851
  by Vaginal Suppositories 59855-59856
  with Hysterectomy 59100, 59852, 59857
Missed
  First Trimester 59820
  Second Trimester 59821
Septic 59830
Spontaneous 59812
Therapeutic
  by Saline 59850
    with Dilation and Curettage 59851
    with Hysterectomy 59852

Abrasion
Skin
  Chemical Peel 15788-15793
  Dermabrasion 15780-15783
  Lesion 15786-15787
  Salabrasion 15810-15811

Abscess
Abdomen 49040-49041
  Incision and Drainage
    Open 49040
    Percutaneous 49021
Anal
  Incision and Drainage 46045-46050
Ankle 27603
Appendix
  Incision and Drainage 44900
    Open 44900
    Percutaneous 44901
Arm, Lower 25028
  Excision 25145
  Incision and Drainage 25035
Arm, Upper
  Incision and Drainage 23930-23935
Auditory Canal, External 69020
Bartholin's Gland
  Incision and Drainage 56420
Bladder
  Incision and Drainage 51080
Brain
  Drainage 61150-61151
  Excision 61514, 61522
  Incision and Drainage 61320-61321
Breast
  Incision and Drainage 19020
Carpals
  Incision, Deep 25035
Clavicle
  Sequestrectomy 23170
Drainage
  with X-Ray 75989
Ear, External
  Complicated 69005
  Simple 69000

Elbow
   Incision and Drainage 23930-23935
Epididymis
   Incision and Drainage 54700
Excision
   Olecranon Process 24138
   Radius 24136
   Ulna 24138
Eyelid
   Incision and Drainage 67700
Facial Bones
   Excision 21026
Finger 26010-26011
   Incision and Drainage 26034
Foot
   Incision 28005
Gums
   Incision and Drainage 41800
Hand
   Incision and Drainage 26034
Hematoma
   Incision and Drainage 27603
Hip
   Incision and Drainage 26990-26992
Humeral Head 23174
Humerus
   Excision 24134
   Incision and Drainage 23935
Kidney
   Incision and Drainage 50020
    Open 50020
    Percutaneous 50021
Leg, Lower
   Incision and Drainage 27603
Liver 47010
   Drainage
    Open 47010
    Injection 47015
    Repair 47300
Localization
   Nuclear Medicine 78806-78807
Lung
   Percutaneous Drainage 32200-32201
Lymphocele Drainage 49062
Lymph Node
   Incision and Drainage 38300-38305
Mandible
   Excision 21025
Mouth
   Incision and Drainage 40800-40801,
      41005-41009, 41015-41018
Nasal Septum
   Incision and Drainage 30020
Neck
   Incision and Drainage 21501-21502
Ovarian
   Incision and Drainage 58820-58822
    Abdominal Approach 58822
    Vaginal Approach 58820
Ovary
   Drainage
    Percutaneous 58823
Palate
   Incision and Drainage 42000
Paraurethral Gland
   Incision and Drainage 53060
Parotid Gland Drainage 42300-42305

Pelvic
   Drainage
    Percutaneous 58823
Pelvis
   Incision and Drainage ...26990-26992, 45000
Pericolic
   Drainage
    Percutaneous 58823
Perineum
   Incision and Drainage 56405
Perirenal or Renal
   Drainage 50020-50021
    Percutaneous 50021
Peritoneum
   Incision and Drainage
    Open 49020
    Percutaneous 49021
Prostate
   Incision and Drainage 55720-55725
   Transurethral Drainage 52700
Radius
   Incision, Deep 25035
Rectum
   Incision and Drainage 45005-45020,
      46040, 46060
Retroperitoneal 49060-49061
   Drainage
    Open 49060
    Percutaneous 49061
Salivary Gland
   Drainage 42300-42320
Scapula
   Sequestrectomy 23172
Scrotum
   Incision and Drainage 54700, 55100
Shoulder
   Drainage 23030
Skene's Gland
   Incision and Drainage 53060
Skin
   Incision and Drainage 10060-10061
   Puncture Aspiration 10160
Soft Tissue
   Incision 20000-20005
Subdiaphragmatic 49040-49041
Sublingual Gland
   Drainage 42310-42320
Submaxillary Gland
   Drainage 42310-42320
Subphrenic 49040-49041
Testis
   Incision and Drainage 54700
Thoracostomy 32020
Thorax
   Incision and Drainage 21501-21502
Throat
   Incision and Drainage 42700-42725
Tongue
   Incision and Drainage 41000-41006
Tonsil
   Incision and Drainage 42700
Ulna
   Incision, Deep 25035
Urethra
   Incision and Drainage 53040
Uvula
   Incision and Drainage 42000

Vagina
   Incision and Drainage 57010
Vulva
   Incision and Drainage 56405
Wrist
   Excision 25145
   Incision and Drainage 25028, 25035
X-Ray 76080

Abscess, Nasal
See Nose, Abscess

Abscess, Parotid Gland
See Parotid Gland, Abscess

Absorptiometry
Dual Energy
   Body Composition 0028T
   Bone 76075
    Appendicular 76076
    Axial Skeleton 76075
Dual Photon
   Bone 78351
Radiographic
   Photodensity 76078
Single Photon
   Bone 78350

Absorption Spectrophotometry, Atomic
See Atomic Absorption Spectroscopy

Accessory, Toes
See Polydactyly, Toes

Accessory Nerve, Spinal
See Nerves, Spinal Accessory

ACE
See Angiotensin Converting Enzyme

Acetabuloplasty 27120-27122

Acetabulum
Fracture
   Closed Treatment 27220-27222
   Open Treatment 27226-27228
   without Manipulation 27220
   with Manipulation 27222
Reconstruction 27120
   with Resection, Femoral Head 27122
Tumor
   Excision 27076

Acetaldehyde
Blood 82000

Acetaminophen
Urine 82003

Acetic Anhydrides 84600

Acetone
Blood or Urine 82009-82010

Acetone Body 82009-82010

Acetylcholinesterase
Blood or Urine 82013

AcG
See Clotting Factor

Achilles Tendon
Incision .27605-27606
Lengthening 27612
Repair 27650-27654

Achillotomy
See Tenotomy, Achilles Tendon

Acid
Gastric 82926-82928

Acid, Adenylic
See Adenosine Monophosphate (AMP)

Acid, Aminolevulinic
See Aminolevulinic Acid (ALA)

Acid, Ascorbic
See Ascorbic Acid

Acid, Deoxyribonucleic
See Deoxyribonucleic Acid

Acid, Folic
See Folic Acid

Acid, Glycocholic
See Cholylglycine

Acid, Lactic
See Lactic Acid

Acid, N-Acetylneuraminic
See Sialic Acid

Acid, Phenylethylbarbituric
See Phenobarbital

Acid, Uric
See Uric Acid

Acidity /Alkalinity
See pH

Acids, Amino
See Amino Acids

Acids, Bile
See Bile Acids

Acids, Fatty
See Fatty Acid

Acids, Guanylic
See Guanosine Monophosphate

Acids, N-Acetylneuraminic
See Sialic Acid

Acid Diethylamide, Lysergic
See Lysergic Acid Diethylamide

Acid Fast Bacilli (AFB)
Culture 87116

Acid Fast Bacillus Culture
See Culture, Acid Fast Bacilli

Acid Fast Stain 88312

Acid Perfusion Test
Esophagus 91012, 91030

Acid Phosphatase 84060-84066

Acid Probes, Nucleic
See Nucleic Acid Probe

Acid Reflux Test
Esophagus 91032-91033

Acne Surgery
Incision and Drainage
    Abscess 10060-10061
    Comedones 10040
    Cyst 10040
    Milia, Multiple 10040
    Pustules .10040

Acne Treatment
Abrasion .15786-15787
Chemical Peel 15788-15793
Cryotherapy 17340
Dermabrasion 15780-15783
Exfoliation
    Chemical 17360
Salabrasion 15810-15811

Acoustic Evoked Brain Stem Potential
See Evoked Potential, Auditory Brainstem

Acoustic Neuroma
See Brain, Tumor, Excision; Brainstem; Mesencephalon; Skull Base Surgery

Acromioclavicular Joint
Arthrocentesis 20605
Arthrotomy .23044
    with Biopsy 23101
Dislocation 23540-23552
    Open Treatment 23550-23552
X-Ray 73050

Acromion
Excision
    Shoulder .23130

Acromionectomy
Partial 23130

Acromioplasty 23415-23420
Partial 23130

ACTH
See Adrenocorticotropic Hormone (ACTH)

ACTH Releasing Factor
See Corticotropic Releasing Hormone (CRH)

Actinomyces
Antibody 86602

Actinomycosis 86000

Actinomycotic Infection
See Actinomycosis

Actinotherapy 96900
See Dermatology

Activated Factor X
See Thrombokinase

Activated Partial Thromboplastin Time
See Thromboplastin, Partial, Time

Activation, Lymphocyte
See Blastogenesis

Activities of Daily Living
See Physical Medicine/Therapy/Occupational Therapy

Activity, Glomerular Procoagulant
See Thromboplastin

Acupuncture
One or More Needles
    Electrical Stimulation 97781
    without Electric Stimulation 97780

Acute Poliomyelitis
See Polio

Acylcarnitines 82016-82017

Adamantinoma, Pituitary
See Craniopharyngioma

Addam Operation
See Dupuytren's Contracture

Adductor Tenotomy of Hip
See Tenotomy, Hip, Adductor

Adenoidectomy 42820-42821,
42830-42836

Adenoids
Excision 42830-42836
    with Tonsils 42820-42821
Unlisted Services and Procedures 42999

Adenoma
Pancreas
    Excision .48120
Thyroid Gland Excision 60200

Adenosine 3'5' Monophosphate
See Cyclic AMP

Adenosine Diphosphate
Blood 82030

Adenosine Monophosphate (AMP)
Blood 82030

Adenovirus
Antibody 86603
Antigen Detection
    Enzyme Immunoassay 87301
    Immunofluorescense 87260

Adenovirus Vaccine
See Vaccines

Adenylic Acid
See Adenosine Monophosphate (AMP)

ADH
See Antidiuretic Hormone

Adhesions
Epidural 0027T, 62263-62264
Eye
    Corneovitreal 65880
    Incision
      Anterior Segment 65860-65870
      Posterior Segment 65875

Intermarginal
    Construction 67880
        Transposition of Tarsal Plate 67882
Intestinal
    Enterolysis .44005
        Laparoscopic 44200
Intracranial
    Lysis 62161
Intrauterine
    Lysis 58559
Labial
    Lysis 56441
Lungs
    Lysis 32124
Pelvic
    Lysis 58660, 58662, 58740
Penile
    Lysis
        Post-circumcision 54162
Preputial
    Lysis 54450

Adipectomy
See Lipectomy

ADL
See Activities of Daily Living

Administration
Immunization
    Each Additional Vaccine/Toxoid 90472,
                                90474
    One Vaccine/Toxoid 90471, 90473

ADP
See Adenosine Diphosphate

ADP Phosphocreatine Phosphotransferase
See CPK

Adrenalectomy 60540
Anesthesia 00866
Laparoscopic 50545

Adrenalin
See Catecholamines
Blood 82383
Urine 82384

Adrenaline-Noradrenaline
Testing .82382-82384

Adrenal Cortex Hormone
See Corticosteroids

Adrenal Gland
Biopsy .60540-60545
Excision
    Laparoscopy 60650
    Retroperitoneal Tumor 60545
Exploration 60540-60545
Nuclear Medicine
    Imaging 78075

Adrenal Medulla
See Medulla

Adrenocorticotropic Hormone (ACTH) 80400-80406,
                          80412, 80418, 82024
Blood or Urine 82024
Stimulation Panel 80400-80406

Adrenogenital Syndrome .56805, 57335

Adult T Cell Leukemia Lymphoma Virus I
See HTLV I

Advanced Life Support
See Emergency Department Services
Physician Direction 99288

Advancement
Tendon
    Foot 28238
    Genioglossus 21199

Advancement Flap
See Skin, Adjacent Tissue Transfer

Aerosol Inhalation
See Pulmonology, Therapeutic
Pentamidine 94642, 99563

AFB
See Acid Fast Bacilli (AFB)

Afferent Nerve
See Sensory Nerve

AFP
See Alpha-Fetoprotein

After Hours Medical Services 99050-99054

Agents, Anticoagulant
See Clotting Inhibitors

Agglutinin
Cold .86156-86157
Febrile 86000

Aggregation
Platelet 85576

AHG
See Clotting Factor

AICD (Pacing Cardioverter-Defibrillator)
See Defibrillator, Heart; Pacemaker, Heart

Aid, Hearing
See Hearing Aid

AIDS Antibodies
See Antibody, HIV

AIDS Virus
See HIV-1

Akin Operation
See Bunion Repair

ALA
See Aminolevulinic Acid (ALA)

Alanine 2 Oxoglutarate Aminotransferase
See Transaminase, Glutamic Pyruvic

Alanine Amino (ALT) 84460

Alanine Transaminase
See Transaminase, Glutamic Pyruvic

Albarran Test
See Water Load Test

Albumin
Serum 82040
Urine 82042

Alcohol
Breath 82075
Ethyl
    Blood 82055
    Urine 82055
Ethylene Glycol 82693

Alcohol, Isopropyl
See Isopropyl Alcohol

Alcohol, Methyl
See Methanol

Alcohol Dehydrogenase
See Antidiuretic Hormone

Aldolase
Blood 82085

Aldosterone
Blood 82088
Suppression Evaluation 80408
Urine 82088

Alimentary Canal
See Gastrointestinal Tract

Alkaline Phosphatase 84075-84080
Leukocyte 85540
WBC 85540

Alkaloids
See Specific Drug
Urine 82101

Allergen Bronchial Provocation Tests
See Allergy Tests; Bronchial Challenge Test

Allergen Challenge, Endobronchial
See Bronchial Challenge Test

Allergen Immunotherapy
Allergen
    Prescription/Supply/Injection . .95120-95125
    with Extract Supply 95144
        Injection 95115-95117
Antigens 95144
IgE 86003-86005
IgG 86001
Insect Venom
    Prescription/Supply 95145-95149
    Prescription/Supply/Injection . .95130-95134
Prescription/Supply 95165
    Insect, Whole Body 95170
Rapid Desensitization 95180

ANA
See Antinuclear Antibodies (ANA)

Anabolic Steroid
See Androstenedione

Analgesia 99141-99142
See Anesthesia; Sedation

Analgesic Cutaneous Electrostimulation
See Application, Neurostimulation

Analysis
Computer Data 99090
Electroencephalogram
   Digital 95957
Electronic
   Drug Infusion Pump 62367-62368
   Pacing Cardioverter-
   Defibrillator 93741-93744
     See Pacemaker, Heart
   Pulse Generator 95970-95971
Physiologic Data, Remote 99091
Protein
   Tissue
     Western Blot 88372
Semen
   Sperm Isolation 89260-89261

Analysis, Spectrum
See Spectrophotometry

Anal Abscess
See Abscess, Anal

Anal Bleeding
See Anus, Hemorrhage

Anal Fistula
See Fistula, Anal

Anal Fistulectomy
See Excision, Fistula, Anal

Anal Fistulotomy
See Fistulotomy, Anal

Anal Sphincter
Dilation 45905
Incision 46080

Anal Ulceration
See Anus, Fissure

Anaspadias
See Epispadias

Anastomosis
Arteriovenous Fistula
   Direct 36821
   with Bypass Graft 35686
   with Graft 36825-36830, 36832
Artery
   to Aorta 33606
   to Artery
     Cranial 61711
Bile Duct
   to Bile Duct 47800
   to Intestines 47760, 47780
Bile Duct to Gastrointestinal 47785
Broncho-Bronchial 32486

Caval to Mesenteric 37160
Colorectal 44620
Epididymis
   to Vas Deferens
     Bilateral 54901
     Unilateral 54900
Excision
   Trachea 31780-31781
Fallopian Tube 58750
Gallbladder to Intestines 47720-47740
Hepatic Duct to Intestines 47765, 47802
Ileo-Anal 45113
Intestines
   Colo-anal 45119
   Cystectomy 51590
   Enterocystoplasty 51960
   Resection
     Laparoscopic 44202-44205
Intestine to Intestine 44130
Intrahepatic Portosystemic 37182-37183
Jejunum 43825
Microvascular
   Free Transfer
     Jejunum 43496
Nerve
   Facial to Hypoglossal 64868
   Facial to Phrenic 64870
Oviduct 58750
Pancreas to Intestines 48180, 48520-48540
Portocaval 37140
Pulmonary 33606
Renoportal 37145
Splenorenal 37180-37181
Stomach 43825
   to Duodenum 43810, 43855
   Revision 43850
   to Jejunum 43820, 43860-43865
Tubotubal 58750
Ureter
   to Bladder 50780-50785
   to Colon 50810-50815
   Removal 50830
   to Intestine 50800, 50820-50825
   Removal 50830
   to Kidney 50727-50750
   to Ureter 50727, 50760-50770
Vein
   Saphenopopliteal 34530
Vein to Vein 37140-37160, 37182-37183

Anastomosis, Aorta-Pulmonary Artery
See Aorta, Anastomosis, to Pulmonary Artery

Anastomosis, Bladder, to Intestine
See Enterocystoplasty

Anastomosis, Hepatic Duct
See Hepatic Duct, Anastomosis

Anastomosis of Lacrimal Sac to Conjunctival Sac
See Conjunctivorhinostomy

Anastomosis of Pancreas
See Pancreas, Anastomosis

Anderson Tibial Lengthening 27715
See Ankle; Tibia, Osteoplasty, Lengthening

Androstanediol Glucuronide ...82154

Androstanolone
See Dihydrotestosterone

Androstenedione
Blood or Urine 82157

Androstenolone
See Dehydroepiandrosterone

Androsterone
Blood or Urine 82160

Anesthesia
See Analgesia
Abbe-Estlander Procedure 00102
Abdomen
   Abdominal Wall 00700-00730,
          00800-00802, 00820-00836
     Halsted Repair 00750-00756
   Blood Vessels 00770, 00880-00882
   Endoscopy 00740, 00810
   Extraperitoneal 00860-00862,
          00866-00868, 00870
   Hernia Repair 00830-00836
     Halsted Repair 00750-00756
   Intraperitoneal ..00790-00797, 00840-00842
Abdominoperineal Resection 00844
Abortion
   Induced 01964
Achilles Tendon Repair 01472
Acromioclavicular Joint 01620
Adrenalectomy 00866
Amniocentesis 00842
Aneurysm
   Axillary-Brachial 01652
   Knee 01444
   Popliteal Artery 01444
Angiography 01920
Ankle 00400, 01462-01522
Anorectal Procedure 00902
Anus 00902
Arm
   Lower ...00400, 01810-01820, 01830-01860
   Upper 00400, 01710-01782
Arrhythmias 00410
Arteriography 01916
Arteriovenous Fistula 01432
Arthroplasty
   Hip 01214-01215
   Knee 01402
Arthroscopic Procedures
   Ankle 01464
   Elbow 01732-01740
   Foot 01464
   Hip 01202
   Knee 01382, 01400
   Shoulder 01622-01630
   Wrist 01829-01830
Auditory Canal, External
   Removal Foreign Body 69205
Axilla 00400, 01610-01682
Back Skin 00300
Batch-Spittler-McFaddin Operation 01404
Biopsy 00100
   Liver 00702
Bladder 00870, 00912
Brain 00210-00218, 00220-00222

Orchiectomy 00926-00928
Orchiopexy 00930
   Torek Procedure 00930
Organ Harvesting
   Brain-Dead Patient 01990
Osteoplasty
   Tibia/Fibula 01484
Osteotomy
   Humerus .01742
   Tibia/Fibula 01484
Other Procedures 01990, 01995-01999
Otoscopy 00124
Pacemaker Insertion 00530
Pacing Cardioverter/Defibrillator 00534
Pancreas 00794
Pancreatectomy .00794
Panniculectomy .00802
Patella 01390-01392
Pectus Excavatum 00474
Pelvic Exenteration 00848
Pelvis 00400, 00865, 01112-01190
   Amputation 01140
   Bone 01120
   Bone Marrow 01112
   Examination 57400
   Extraperitoneal 00864
   Intraperitoneal 00844-00848
   Skin 00300, 00400
Penis 00932-00938
Pericardial Sac 00560-00563
Perineum 00904-00908
Pharynx .00174-00176
Phleborrhaphy
   Arm, Upper 01782
   Forearm, Wrist and Hand 01852
Pleura 00540-00541
   Needle Biopsy 00522
Pleurectomy 00544
Pneumocentesis 00524
Popliteal Area 00400, 01320, 01430-01444
Prognathism 00192
Prostate 00865, 00908, 00914
Prostatectomy
   Perineal 00908
   Radical 00865
   Walsh Modified Radical 00865
Radiological Procedures 01905-01922
   Arterial
      Therapeutic 01924-01926
   Venous/Lymphatic
      Therapeutic 01930-01933
Renal Procedures 00862
Repair of Skull .00215
Replacement
   Ankle 01486
   Elbow 01760
   Hip .01212-01215
   Knee 01402
   Shoulder 01638
   Wrist 01832
Restriction
   Gastric
      for Obesity 00797
Retropharyngeal Tumor Excision 00174
Rib Resection 00470-00474
Sacroiliac Joint 01160-01170, 27096
Salivary Glands 00100
Scheie Procedure 00147

Sedation
   Analgesia 99141-99142
Seminal Vesicles 00922
Shoulder 00400, 00450-00454, 01610-01682
   Dislocation
      Closed Treatment 23655
Shunt
   Spinal Fluid 00220
Sinuses
   Accessory 00160-00164
Skull 00190
Skull Fracture
   Elevation .00215
Special Circumstances
   Emergency 99140
   Extreme Age 99100
   Hypotension 99135
   Hypothermia 99116
Spinal Instrumentation 00670
Spinal Manipulation 00640
Spine and Spinal Cord 00600-00670
   Cervical 00600-00604, 00640-00670
   Injection 62310-62319
   Lumbar 00630-00670
   Thoracic 00620-00622, 00640-00670
   Vascular 00670
Sternoclavicular Joint 01620
Sternum 00550
Stomach
   Restriction
      for Obesity 00797
Strayer Procedure 01474
Subdural Taps .00212
Suture Removal 15850-15851
Sympathectomy
   Lumbar 00632
   Thoracolumbar 00622
Symphysis Pubis 01160-01170
Tenodesis 01716
Tenoplasty 01714
Tenotomy 01712
Testis 00924-00930
Thoracoplasty .00472
Thoracoscopy 00528, 00540-00541
Thoracotomy 00540-00541
Thorax 00400-00406, 00410,
                00450-00454, 00470-00474
Thromboendarterectomy 01442
Thyroid .00320-00322
Tibia 01390-01392, 01484
Trachea 00320, 00326, 00542
   Reconstruction 00539
Transplantation
   Cornea 00144
   Heart 00580
   Kidney 00868
   Liver 00796, 01990
   Lungs 00580
   Organ Harvesting 01990
Transurethral Procedures 00910-00918
Tubal Ligation .00851
Tuffier Vaginal Hysterectomy 00944
TURP 00914
Tympanostomy 69436
Tympanotomy .00126
Unlisted Services and Procedures 01999
Urethra 00910, 00918-00920, 00942
Urethrocystoscopy 00910

Urinary Bladder 00864, 00870, 00912
Urinary Tract 00860
Uterus 00952
Vagina 00940-00942, 00950
   Dilation 57400
   Removal
      Foreign Body 57415
Vaginal Delivery 01960
Vascular Access 00532
Vascular Shunt .01844
Vascular Surgery
   Abdomen, Lower 00880-00882
   Abdomen, Upper 00770
   Arm, Lower 01840-01852
   Arm, Upper 01770-01782
   Brain 00216
   Elbow 01770-01782
   Hand 01840-01852
   Knee 01430-01444
   Leg, Lower 01500-01522
   Leg, Upper 01260-01274
   Neck 00350-00352
   Shoulder 01650-01670
   Wrist 01840-01852
Vasectomy 00921
Vas Deferens
   Excision 00921
Venography 01916
Ventriculography 00214, 01920
Vertebral Process
   Fracture/Dislocation
      Closed Treatment 22315
Vertebroplasty .01905
Vitrectomy 00145
Vitreoretinal Surgery 00145
Vitreous Body .00145
Vulva 00906
Vulvectomy 00906
Wertheim Operation 00846
Wrist 00400, 01810-01860

Anesthesia Local
See Anesthesia, Local

Aneurysm, Aorta, Abdominal
See Aorta, Abdominal, Aneurysm

Aneurysm, Basilar Artery
See Artery, Basilar, Aneurysm

Aneurysm Artery, Femoral
See Artery, Femoral, Aneurysm

Aneurysm Artery, Radial
See Artery, Radial, Aneurysm

Aneurysm Artery, Renal
See Artery, Renal, Aneurysm

Aneurysm Repair
Abdominal Aorta 0001T-0002T, 34800-34804,
      34825-34832, 35081-35103, 75952-75953
Axillary Artery 35011-35013
Basilar Artery 61698, 61702
Brachial Artery 35011-35013
Carotid Artery 35001-35002,
           61613, 61697, 61700, 61703
Celiac Artery 35121-35122
Femoral Artery 35141-35142

Hepatic Artery 35121-35122
Iliac Artery . . .34900, 35131-35132, 75953-75954
Innominate Artery 35021-35022
Intracranial Artery 61705-61708
Mesenteric Artery 35121-35122
Other Artery 35161-35162
Popliteal Artery 35151-35152
Radial Artery .35045
Renal Artery 35121-35122
Splenic Artery 35111-35112
Subclavian Artery . . .35001-35002, 35021-35022
Thoracic Aorta 0033T-0034T,
　　　　　　　　　　　　0035T-0039T, 0040T
Thoracoabdominal Aorta 33877
Ulnar Artery .35045
Vascular Malformation or Carotid-Cavernous
Fistula 61710
Vertebral Artery 61698, 61702

Angel Dust
See Phencyclidine

Angiocardiographies
See Heart, Angiography

Angiography
See Aortography
Abdomen 74175, 74185, 75635, 75726
Abdominal Aorta 75635, 75952-75953
Adrenal 75731-75733
Aorta
　Injection .93544
Arm Artery 73206, 75710-75716
Arteriovenous Shunt 75790
Brachial Artery 75658
Brain 70496
Carotid Artery 75660-75671
　Cervical
　　Bilateral 75680
　　Unilateral 75676
Chest 71275, 71555
Coronary Artery 93556
　Flow Velocity Measurement During
　Angiography 93571-93572
Coronary Bypass 93556
Endovascular Repair 75952-75953
Extremity, Lower 73725
Extremity, Upper 73225
Fluorescein .92235
Head 70496, 70544-70546
　Artery 75650
Heart Vessels
　Injection .93545
Indocyanine-green 92240
Left Heart
　Injection .93543
Leg Artery 73706, 75635, 75710-75716
Lung
　Injection .93541
　　See Cardiac Catheterization, Injection
Mammary Artery 75756
　　See Aortography
Neck 70498, 70547-70549
　Artery 75650
Nuclear Medicine 78445
Other Artery 75774
Pelvic Artery 72198, 75736
Pelvis 72191

Pulmonary 75741-75746
Renal Artery 75722-75724
Right Heart
　Injection .93542
Spinal Artery 75705
Spinal Canal 72159
Thorax 71275
Transcatheter Therapy
　Embolization 75894, 75898
　Infusion 75894, 75898
Vertebral 75685

Angioma
See Lesion, Skin

Angioplasties, Coronary Balloon
See Percutaneous Transluminal Angioplasty

Angioplasty
Aorta
　Intraoperative 35452
　Percutaneous 35472
Axillary Artery
　Intraoperative 35458
Brachiocephalic Artery
　Intraoperative 35458
　Percutaneous 35475
Coronary Artery
　Percutaneous Transluminal 92982-92984
Femoral Artery
　Intraoperative 35456
　Percutaneous 35474
Iliac Artery
　Intraoperative 35454
　Percutaneous 35473
Percutaneous Transluminal
Angioplasty 92982-92984
　　See Angioplasty; Percutaneous, Transluminal
Popliteal Artery
　Intraoperative 35456
　Percutaneous 35474
Pulmonary Artery
　Percutaneous Transluminal 92997-92998
Renal Artery
　Intraoperative 35450
　Percutaneous 35471
Subclavian Artery
　Intraoperative 35458
Tibioperoneal Artery
　Intraoperative 35459
　Percutaneous 35470
Transluminal
　Arterial 75962-75968
　Venous .75978
Venous
　Intraoperative 35460
　Percutaneous 35476
Visceral Artery
　Intraoperative 35450
　Percutaneous 35471

Angioscopy
Non-Coronary Vessels 35400

**Angiotensin Converting Enzyme
(ACE)** 82164

Angiotensin Forming Enzyme
See Renin

Angiotensin I 84244
Riboflavin 84252

Angiotensin II
Blood or Urine 82163

Angle Deformity
Reconstruction
　Toe 28313

Anhydride, Carbonic
See Carbon Dioxide

Anhydrides, Acetic
See Acetic Anhydrides

Animal Inoculation 87001-87003,
　　　　　　　　　　　　　　　　　87250

Ankle
See Fibula; Leg, Lower; Tibia; Tibiofibular Joint
Abscess
　Incision and Drainage 27603
Amputation .27888
Arthrocentesis 20605
Arthrodesis .27870
Arthrography 73615
Arthroplasty 27700-27703
Arthroscopy
　Surgical 29891-29899
Arthrotomy 27610-27612, 27620-27626
Biopsy 27613-27614, 27620
Bursa
　Incision and Drainage 27604
Disarticulation 27889
Dislocation
　Closed Treatment 27840-27842
　Open Treatment 27846-27848
Exploration 27610, 27620
Fracture
　Lateral 27786-27814
　Medial 27760-27766, 27808-27814
　Trimalleolar 27816-27823
Fusion 27870
Hematoma
　Incision and Drainage 27603
Incision 27607
Injection
　Radiologic 27648
Lesion
　Excision .27630
Magnetic Resonance Imaging
(MRI) 73721-73723
Manipulation 27860
Removal
　Foreign Body 27610, 27620
　Implant .27704
　Loose Body 27620
Repair
　Achilles Tendon 27650-27654
　Ligament 27695-27698
　Tendon 27612, 27680-27687
Strapping .29540
Synovium
　Excision 27625-27626
Tenotomy 27605-27606
Tumor
　Excision 27615-27619

Unlisted Services and Procedures 27899
X-Ray 73600-73610
   with Contrast .73615

Ankylosis (Surgical)
See Arthrodesis

Anogenital Region
See Perineum

Anoplasty
Stricture .46700-46705

Anorectal Myectomy
See Myomectomy, Anorectal

Anorectal Procedure
Biofeedback 90911

Anorectovaginoplasty 46744-46746

Anoscopy
Ablation
   Polyp 46615
   Tumor 46615
Biopsy 46606
Dilation 46604
Exploration 46600
Hemorrhage 46614
Removal
   Foreign Body 46608
   Polyp 46610-46612
   Tumor 46610-46612

Antebrachium
See Forearm

Antecedent, Plasma Thromboplastin
See Plasma Thromboplastin, Antecedent

Antepartum Care
Cesarean Delivery 59510
   Previous 59610, 59618
Vaginal Delivery 59425-59426

Anterior Ramus of Thoracic Nerve
See Intercostal Nerve

Anthrax Vaccine
See Vaccines

Anthrogon
See Follicle Stimulating Hormone (FSH)

Anti-Human Globulin Consumption Test
See Coombs Test

Anti-Phospholipid Antibody
See Antibody, Phospholipid

Antiactivator, Plasmin
See Alpha-2 Antiplasmin

Antibiotic Administration
Home Infusion Procedures 99556
Injection 90788

Antibiotic Sensitivity 87181-87184, 87188
Enzyme Detection 87185

Minimum Bactericidal Concentration 87187
Minimum Inhibitory Concentration 87186

Antibodies, Thyroid-Stimulating
See Immunoglobulin, Thyroid Stimulating

Antibodies, Viral
See Viral Antibodies

Antibody
See Antibody Identification; Microsomal Antibody
Actinomyces 86602
Adenovirus 86603
Antinuclear 86038-86039
Antiphosphatidylserine (Phospholipid) 86148
Antiprothrombin 0030T
Antistreptolysin O 86060-86063
Aspergillus 86606
Bacterium 86609
Bartonella 86611
Beta 2 Glycoprotein I 86146
Blastomyces 86612
Blood Crossmatch 86920-86922
Bordetella 86615
Borrelia 86618-86619
Brucella 86622
Campylobacter .86625
Candida 86628
Cardiolipin 86147
Chlamydia 86631-86632
Coccidioides 86635
Coxiella Burnetii 86638
Cryptococcus .86641
Cytomegalovirus 86644-86645
Cytotoxic Screen 86807-86808
Deoxyribonuclease 86215
Deoxyribonucleic Acid (DNA) 86225-86226
Diphtheria 86648
Ehrlichia 86666
Encephalitis 86651-86654
Enterovirus 86658
Epstein-Barr Virus 86663-86665
Fluorescent 86255-86256
Francisella Tularensis 86668
Fungus 86671
Giardia Lamblia 86674
Growth Hormone 86277
Helicobacter Pylori 86677
Helminth 86682
Hemoglobin, Fecal 86683
Hemophilus Influenza 86684
Hepatitis
   Delta Agent 86692
Hepatitis A 86708-86709
Hepatitis B
   Core 86704
   IgM 86705
   Surface 86706
Hepatitis Be 86707
Hepatitis C 86803-86804
Herpes Simplex 86694-86696
Heterophile 86308-86310
Histoplasma 86698
HIV 86689, 86701-86703
HIV-1 . . . . .86701, 86703
HIV-2 86702-86703
HTLV-I 86687, 86689
HTLV-II 86688
Influenza Virus 86710

Insulin 86337
Intrinsic Factor 86340
Islet Cell 86341
Legionella 86713
Leishmania 86717
Leptospira 86720
Listeria Monocytogenes 86723
Lyme Disease .86617
Lymphocytic Choriomeningitis 86727
Lymphogranuloma Venereum 86729
Microsomal 86376
Mucormycosis 86732
Mumps 86735
Mycoplasma 86738
Neisseria Meningitidis 86741
Nocardia 86744
Nuclear Antigen 86235
Other Virus 86790
Parvovirus 86747
Phospholipid .86147
Phospholipid Cofactor 0030T
Plasmodium 86750
Platelet 86022-86023
Protozoa 86753
Red Blood Cell 86850-86870
Respiratory Syncytial Virus 86756
Rickettsia 86757
Rotavirus 86759
Rubella 86762
Rubeola 86765
Salmonella 86768
Shigella 86771
Sperm 89325
Streptokinase .86590
Tetanus 86774
Thyroglobulin .86800
Toxoplasma 86777-86778
Treponema Pallidum 86781
Trichinella 86784
Varicella-Zoster 86787
White Blood Cell 86021
Yersinia 86793

Antibody Identification
Leukocyte Antibodies 86021
Platelet 86022-86023
Red Blood Cell
   Pretreatment 86970-86972
Serum
   Pretreatment 86975-86978

Antibody Neutralization Test
See Neutralization Test

Antibody Receptor
See FC Receptor

Anticoagulant
See Clotting Inhibitors

Antidiabetic Hormone
See Glucagon

Antidiuretic Hormone 84588

Antidiuretic Hormone Measurement
See Vasopressin

AntiDNA Autoantibody
See Antinuclear Antibodies (ANA)

Antigen
Allergen Immunotherapy 95144
Carcinoembryonic 82378
Prostate Specific 84152-84153

Antigen, Australia
See Hepatitis Antigen, B Surface

Antigen, CD4
See CD4

Antigen, CD8
See CD8

Antigens, CD142
See Thromboplastin

Antigens, CD143
See Angiotensin Converting Enzyme (ACE)

Antigens, E
See Hepatitis Antigen, Be

Antigens, Hepatitis
See Hepatitis Antigen

Antigens, Hepatitis B
See Hepatitis Antigen, B

Antigen Bronchial Provocation Tests
See Bronchial Challenge Test

Antigen Detection
Direct Fluorescence .87198-87199, 87265-87272,
       87276, 87278, 87280, 87285-87290
   Bordetella 87265
   Chlamydia Trachomatis 87270
   Cryptosporidium/Giardia 87272
   Cytomegalovirus 87198
   Enterovirus 87199
   Influenza A 87276
   Legionella Pneumophila 87278
   Not Otherwise Specified 87299
   Respiratory Syncytial Virus 87280
   Treponema Pallidum 87285
   Varicella-Zoster 87290
Enzyme Immunoassay
   Adenovirus 87301
   Chlamydia Trachomatis 87320
   Clostridium Difficile 87324
   Cryptococcus Neoformans 87327
   Cryptosporidium/Giardia 87328
   Cytomegalovirus 87332
   Entamoeba Histolytica Dispar Group . .87336
   Entamoeba Histolytica Group 87337
   Escherichia coli 0157 87335
   Helicobacter Pylori 87338-87339
   Hepatitis Be Antigen (HBeAg) 87350
   Hepatitis B Surface Antigen (HBsAg) . .87340
   Hepatitis B Surface Antigen (HBsAg)
   Neutralization 87341
   Hepatitis Delta Agent 87380
   Histoplasma capsulatum 87385
   HIV-1 87390
   HIV-2 87391
   Influenza A 87400
   Influenza B 87400
   Multiple Step Method 87301-87449
      Polyvalent 87451

Not Otherwise Specified 87449, 87451
Respiratory Syncytial Virus 87420
Rotavirus 87425
Shigella-like Toxin 87427
Single Step Method 87450
Streptococcus, Group A 87430
Immunofluorescence 87260, 87273-87275,
     87277, 87279, 87281-87283, 87299-87300
   Adenovirus 87260
   Herpes Simplex 87273-87274
   Influenza B 87275
   Legionella Micdadei 87277
   Not Otherwise Specified 87299
   Parainfluenza Virus 87279
   Pneumocystis Carinii 87281
   Polyvalent 87300
   Rubeola 87283

Antihemophilic Factor B
See Christmas Factor

Antihemophilic Factor C
See Plasma Thromboplastin, Antecedent

Antihemophilic Globulin (AHG) 85240

Antihuman Globulin 86880-86886

Antimony 83015

Antinuclear Antibodies (ANA) 86038-86039

Antiplasmin, Alpha-2 85410

Antiprotease, Alpha 1
See Alpha-1 Antitrypsin

Antiprothrombin Antibody 0030T

Antistreptococcal Antibody 86215

Antistreptokinase Titer 86590

Antistreptolysin O 86060-86063

Antithrombin III 85300-85301

Antithrombin VI
See Fibrin Degradation Products

Antitoxin Assay 87230

Antiviral Antibody
See Viral Antibodies

Anti Australia Antigens
See Antibody, Hepatitis B

Anti D Immunoglobulin
See Immune Globulins, Rho (D)

Antrostomy
Sinus
   Maxillary 31256-31267

Antrotomy
Sinus
   Maxillary 31020-31032
Transmastoid 69501

Antrum of Highmore
See Sinus, Maxillary

Antrum Puncture
Sinus
   Maxillary 31000
   Sphenoid 31002

Anus
See Hemorrhoids; Rectum
Ablation 46615
Abscess
   Incision and Drainage 46045-46050
Biofeedback 90911
Biopsy
   Endoscopy 46606
Crypt
   Excision 46210-46211
Dilation
   Endoscopy 46604
Endoscopy
   Biopsy 46606
   Dilation 46604
   Exploration 46600
   Hemorrhage .46614
   Removal
     Foreign Body 46608
     Polyp 46610, 46612
     Tumor 46610, 46612
Excision
   Tag 46220, 46230
Exploration
   Endoscopy 46600
Fissure
   Destruction 46940-46942
   Excision 46200
Fistula
   Excision 46270-46285
   Repair 46706
Hemorrhage
   Endoscopic Control 46614
Hemorrhoids
   Clot Excision 46320
   Destruction 46934-46936
   Excision 46250-46262
   Injection 46500
   Ligation 46221, 46945-46946
   Suture 46945-46946
Imperforated
   Repair 46715-46742
Incision
   Septum 46070
Lesion
   Destruction 46900-46917, 46924
   Excision 45108, 46922
Manometry 91122
Placement
   Seton 46020
Reconstruction .46742
   Congenital Absence 46730-46740
   Sphincter 46750-46751, 46760-46762
   with Graft 46753
   with Implant .46762
Removal
   Foreign Body 46608
   Seton 46030
   Suture 46754
   Wire 46754

Repair
　　Anovaginal Fistula 46715-46716
　　Cloacal Anomaly 46748
　　Fistula 46706
　　Stricture 46700-46705
Sphincter
　　Electromyography 51784-51785
　　Needle 51785
Unlisted Services and Procedures 46999

Aorta
Abdominal
　　Aneurysm 0001T-0002T, 34800-34804,
　　　　34825-34832, 35081-35103, 75952-75953
　　Thromboendarterectomy 35331
Anastomosis
　　to Pulmonary Artery 33606
Angiogram
　　Radiologic Injection 93544
　　　　See Cardiac Catheterization, Injection
Angioplasty 35452
Aortography 75600-75630
Balloon 33967, 33970
Catheterization
　　Catheter 36200
　　Intracatheter/Needle 36160
Circulation Assist 33967, 33970
Conduit to Heart 33404
Excision
　　Coarctation 33840-33851
Insertion
　　Balloon Device 33967
　　Graft 33330-33335
　　Intracatheter/Needle 36160
Removal
　　Balloon Assist Device 33968, 33971
Repair 33320-33322, 33802-33803
　　Coarctation 33840-33851
　　Graft 33860-33877
　　Hypoplastic or Interrupted Aortic Arch
　　　　without Cardiopulmonary Bypass . . .33852
　　　　with Cardiopulmonary Bypass 33853
　　Sinus of Valsalva 33702-33720
Suspension 33800
Suture 33320-33322
Thoracic
　　Aneurysm 0033T-0034T,
　　　　　　　　　　　　　0035T-0039T, 0040T
Valve
　　Incision 33415
　　Repair 33400-33403
　　　　Left Ventricle 33414
　　　　Supravalvular Stenosis 33417
　　Replacement 33405-33413
X-Ray with Contrast 75600-75630

Aorta-Pulmonary ART Transposition
See Transposition, Great Arteries

Aortic Sinus
See Sinus of Valsalva

Aortic Stenosis
Repair 33415
　　Supravalvular 33417

Aortic Valve
See Heart, Aortic Valve

Aortic Valve Replacement
See Replacement, Aortic Valve

Aortocoronary Bypass
See Coronary Artery Bypass Graft (CABG)

Aortocoronary Bypass for Heart Revascularization
See Artery, Coronary, Bypass

Aortography 75600-75605,
　　　　　　　　　　　　　　75630, 93544
See Angiography
Serial 75625
with Iliofemoral Artery 75630

Aortoiliac
Embolectomy 34151-34201
Thrombectomy 34151-34201

Aortopexy 33800

Aortoplasty
Supravalvular Stenosis 33417

AP
See Voiding Pressure Studies

Apert-Gallais Syndrome
See Adrenogenital Syndrome

Aphasia Testing 96105
See Neurology, Diagnostic

Apheresis
Therapeutic 36511-36516

Apical-Aortic Conduit 33404

Apicectomy
with Mastoidectomy 69605
　　Petrous 69530

Apoaminotransferase, Aspartate
See Transaminase, Glutamic Oxaloacetic

Apolipoprotein
Blood or Urine 82172

Appendectomy 44950-44960
Laparoscopic .44970

Appendiceal Abscess
See Abscess, Appendix

Appendico-Vesicostomy
Cutaneous 50845

Appendix
Abscess
　　Incision and Drainage
　　　　Open 44900
　　　　Percutaneous 44901
Excision 44950-44960

Application
Allergy Tests .95044
Bone Fixation Device
　　Multiplane .20692
　　Uniplane 20690
Caliper 20660
Cranial Tongs .20660

Fixation Device
　　Shoulder 23700
Halo
　　Cranial 20661
　　　　Thin Skull Osteology 20664
　　Femoral 20663
　　Maxillofacial Fixation 21100
　　Pelvic 20662
Interdental Fixation Device 21110
Neurostimulation 64550
Radioelement 77761-77778
　　Surface 77789
　　with Ultrasound 76965
Stereotactic Frame 20660

Application of External Fixation Device
See Fixation Device, Application, External

APPT
See Thromboplastin, Partial, Time

APTT
See Thromboplastin, Partial, Time

Aquatic Therapy
See Physical Medicine/Therapy/Occupational Therapy

Aqueous Shunt
to Extraocular Reservoir 66180
　　Revision 66185

Arch, Zygomatic
See Zygomatic Arch

Arm
See Radius; Ulna; Wrist
Lower
　　Abscess 25028
　　Amputation 24900-24920, 25900-25905,
　　　　　　　　　　　　　　　　　　　25915
　　　　Cineplasty 24940
　　　　Revision 25907-25909
　　Angiography 73206
　　Artery
　　　　Ligation 37618
　　Biopsy 25065-25066
　　Bursa
　　　　Incision and Drainage 25031
　　Bypass Graft 35903
　　Cast 29075
　　CT Scan 73200-73206
　　Decompression 25020-25025
　　Exploration
　　　　Blood Vessel 35860
　　Fasciotomy 24495, 25020-25025
　　Hematoma .25028
　　Lesion, Tendon Sheath
　　　　Excision 25110
　　Magnetic Resonance Imaging
　　(MRI) 73218-73220, 73223
　　Reconstruction
　　　　Ulna 25337
　　Removal
　　　　Foreign Body 25248
　　Repair
　　　　Blood Vessel with Other Graft 35266
　　　　Blood Vessel with Vein Graft 35236
　　　　Decompression 24495

Arthrotomy for Removal of Prosthesis of Ankle
See Ankle, Removal, Implant

Arthrotomy for Removal of Prosthesis of Hip
See Hip, Removal, Prosthesis

Arthrotomy for Removal of Prosthesis of Wrist
See Prosthesis, Wrist, Removal

Articular Ligament
See Ligament

Artificial Abortion
See Abortion

Artificial Cardiac Pacemaker
See Heart, Pacemaker

Artificial Eye
See Prosthesis

Artificial Genitourinary Sphincter
See Prosthesis, Urethral Sphincter

Artificial Knee Joints
See Prosthesis, Knee

Artificial Penis
See Penile Prosthesis

Artificial Pneumothorax
See Pneumothorax, Therapeutic

Aspartate Aminotransferase
See Transaminase, Glutamic Oxaloacetic

Aspiration, Chest
See Thoracentesis

Aspiration, Lung Puncture
See Pneumocentesis

Aspiration, Nail
See Evacuation, Hematoma, Subungual

Aspiration, Spinal Puncture
See Spinal Tap

Aspiration Lipectomies
See Liposuction

Aspiration of Bone Marrow from Donor for Transplant
See Bone Marrow, Harvesting

Assay, Very Long Chain Fatty Acids
See Fatty Acid, Very Long Chain

Assay Tobramycin
See Tobramycin

Assisted Circulation
See Circulation Assist

AST
See Transaminase, Glutamic Oxaloacetic

Astragalectomy 28130

Astragalus
See Talus

Asymmetry, Face
See Hemifacial Microsomia

Ataxia Telangiectasia
Chromosome Analysis 88248

Ataxy, Telangiectasia
See Ataxia Telangiectasia

Atherectomies, Coronary
See Artery, Coronary, Atherectomy

Atherectomy
See X-Ray, Artery
Open
    Aorta 35481
    Brachiocephalic 35484
    Femoral 35483
    Iliac 35482
    Popliteal 35483
    Renal 35480
    Tibioperoneal 35485
    Visceral 35480
Percutaneous
    Aorta 35491
    Brachiocephalic 35494
    Coronary 92995-92996
       See Artery, Coronary
    Femoral 35493
    Iliac 35492
    Popliteal 35493
    Renal 35490
    Tibioperoneal 35495
    Visceral 35490
X-Ray
    Peripheral Artery 75992-75993
    Renal Artery 75994
    Visceral Artery 75995-75996

ATLV
See HTLV I

ATLV Antibodies
See Antibody, HTLV-I

Atomic Absorption
Spectroscopy 82190

ATP Creatine Phosphotransferase
See CPK

Atresia, Choanal
See Choanal Atresia

Atresia, Congenital
Auditory Canal, External
    Reconstruction 69320

Atria
Reconstruction .33253

Atrial Electrogram
See Cardiology, Diagnostic
Esophageal Recording 93615-93616

Atrial Fibrillation
See Fibrillation, Atrial

Atrioseptopexy
See Heart, Repair, Atrial Septum

Atrioseptoplasty
See Heart, Repair, Atrial Septum

Attachment
See Fixation

Atticotomy 69631, 69635

Audiologic Function Tests
See Ear, Nose and Throat; Hearing Evaluation
Acoustic Reflex 92568
Acoustic Reflex Decay 92569

Audiometry
  Bekesy 92560-92561
  Comprehensive 92557
  Conditioning Play 92582
  Groups .92559
  Pure Tone 92552-92553
  Select Picture 92583
  Speech 92555-92556
  Visual Reinforcement 92579
Central Auditory Function 92589
Electrocochleography 92584
Evoked Otoacoustic Emission 92587-92588
Filtered Speech 92571
Lombard Test 92573
Loudness Balance 92562
Screening 92551
Sensorineural Acuity 92575
Short Increment Sensitivity Index 92564
Staggered Spondaic Word Test 92572
Stenger Test 92565, 92577
Synthetic Sentence Test 92576
Tone Decay .92563

Audiometry
Bekesy 92560-92561
Brainstem Evoked Response 92585-92586
Comprehensive 92557
Conditioning Play 92582
Groups 92559
    See Ear, Nose and Throat
Pure Tone 92552-92553
Select Picture 92583
Speech 92555-92556
Tympanometry 92567

Auditory Brain Stem Evoked Response
See Evoked Potential, Auditory Brainstem

Auditory Canal
Decompression 61591
External
  Abscess
    Incision and Drainage 69020
  Biopsy .69105
  Lesion
    Excision 69140-69155
  Reconstruction
    for Congenital Atresia 69320
    for Stenosis 69310
  Removal
    Cerumen 69210
    Ear Wax 69210
    Foreign Body 69200-69205
Internal
  Decompression 69960

Auditory Canal Atresia, External
See Atresia, Congenital, Auditory Canal, External

Auditory Evoked Otoacoustic Emission 92587-92588

Auditory Evoked Potentials 92585-92586
See Audiologic Function Tests

Auditory Labyrinth
See Ear, Inner

Auditory Meatus
X-Ray 70134

Auditory Tube
See Eustachian Tube

Augmentation
Chin 21120, 21123
Malar 21270
Mandibular Body
  with Bone Graft 21127
  with Prosthesis 21125
Osteoplasty
  Facial Bones 21208

Augmentation Mammoplasty
See Breast, Augmentation

Augmented Histamine Test 91052
See Gastric Analysis Test

Aural Rehabilitation 92510

Auricle (Heart)
See Atria

Auricular Fibrillation
See Fibrillation, Atrial

Auricular Prosthesis 21086

Australia Antigen
See Hepatitis Antigen, B Surface

Autograft
Bone
  Local 20936
  Morselized 20937
  Structural 20938
for Spine Surgery
  Local 20936
  Morselized 20937
  Structural 20938

Autologous Blood Transfusion
See Autotransfusion

Autologous Transplantation
See Autograft

Automated Data
Nuclear Medicine 78890-78891

Autonomic Nervous System Function
See Neurology, Diagnostic; Neurophysiologic Testing

Autoprothrombin C
See Thrombokinase

Autoprothrombin I
See Proconvertin

Autoprothrombin II
See Christmas Factor

Autoprothrombin III
See Stuart-Prower Factor

Autopsy
Coroner's Exam 88045
Forensic Exam 88040

Gross and Micro Exam 88020-88029
Gross Exam 88000-88016
Organ 88037
Regional 88036
Unlisted Services and Procedures 88099

Autotransfusion
Blood 86890-86891

Autotransplant
See Autograft

Autotransplantation
Renal 50380

Avulsion
Nails 11730-11732
Nerve 64732-64772

AV Fistula
See Arteriovenous Fistula

AV Shunt
See Arteriovenous Shunt

Axillary Arteries
See Artery, Axillary

Axillary Nerve
Injection
      Anesthetic 64417

Axis, Dens
See Odontoid Process

A Vitamin
See Vitamin, A

B

B-DNA
See Deoxyribonucleic Acid

b-Hexosaminidase 83080

B1 Vitamin
See Thiamine

B6 Vitamin
See Vitamin, B-6

Babcock Operation
See Ligation, Vein, Saphenous

Bacillus Calmette Guerin Vaccine
See BCG Vaccine

Back/Flank
Biopsy 21920-21925
Repair
      Hernia 49540
Strapping 29220
Tumor
      Excision 21930
      Radical Resection 21935
Wound Exploration
      Penetrating .20102

Backbone
See Spine
Bacterial Endotoxins 87176

Bacteria Culture
Additional Methods 87077
Anaerobic 87073-87076
Blood 87040
Feces 87045-87046
Other Source 87070-87073
Screening 87081
Urine 87086-87088

Bactericidal Titer, Serum 87197

Bacterium
Antibody 86609

BAER
See Evoked Potential, Auditory Brainstem

Baker's Cyst 27345

Baker Tube
Intestine Decompression 44021

Balanoplasty
See Penis, Repair

Baldy-Webster Operation
See Uterus, Repair, Suspension

Balkan Grippe
See Q Fever

Balloon Angioplasties, Coronary
See Percutaneous Transluminal Angioplasty

Balloon Angioplasty
See Angioplasty

Balloon Assisted Device
Aorta 33967-33974, 93727

Band, Pulmonary Artery
See Banding, Artery, Pulmonary

Banding
Artery
      Fistula 37607
      Pulmonary .33690

Bank, Blood
See Blood Banking

Bankart Procedure
See Capsulorrhaphy, Anterior

Barany Caloric Test
See Caloric Vestibular Test

Barbiturates
Blood or Urine .82205

Bardenheurer Operation
See Ligation, Artery, Chest

Barium 83015

Barium Enema 74270-74280

Barker Operation
See Talus, Excision

Barr Bodies 88130

Barr Procedure
See Tendon, Transfer, Leg, Lower

Bartholin's Gland
Abscess
      Incision and Drainage 56420
Cyst
      Repair 56440
Excision 56740
Marsupialization 56440

Bartonella
Antibody 86611

Bartonella Detection 87470-87472

Basic Life Services 99450

Basic Proteins, Myelin
See Myelin Basic Protein

Basilar Arteries
See Artery, Basilar

Batch-Spittler-McFaddin Operation
See Disarticulation, Knee

BCG Vaccine
See Vaccines

Bed Sores
See Debridement; Pressure Ulcer (Decubitus);
Skin Graft and Flap

Bekesy Audiometry
See Audiometry, Bekesy

Belsey IV Procedure
See Fundoplasty

Bender-Gestalt Test 96100

Benedict Test for Urea
See Urinalysis, Qualitative

Benign Cystic Mucinous Tumor
See Ganglion

Benign Neoplasm of Cranial
Nerves
See Cranial Nerve

Bennett Fracture
See Phalanx; Thumb, Fracture

Bennett Procedure
See Repair, Leg, Upper, Muscle; Revision

Benzidine Test
See Blood, Feces

Benzodiazepine
Assay 80154

Benzoyl Cholinesterase
See Cholinesterase

Bernstein Test
See Acid Perfusion Test, Esophagus

Beryllium 83015

Cornea .... .65410
Duodenum .... .44010
Ear
　External .... .69100
Elbow 24065-24066, 24101
　Synovium .... .24100
Endometrium .... .58100, 58558
Epididymis 54800-54820
Esophagus
　Endoscopy .... .43202
Eyelid .... .67810
Eye Muscle .... .67350
Forearm
　Soft Tissue 25065-25066
Gallbladder
　Endoscopy .... .43261
Gastrointestinal, Upper
　Endoscopy .... .43239
Hand Joint
　Synovium .... .26100
Heart .... .93505
Hip 27040-27041
　Joint .... .27052
Hypopharynx .... .42802
Ileum
　Endoscopy .... .44382
Interphalangeal Joint
　Finger .... .26110
　Toe .... .28054
Intertarsal Joint
　Toe .... .28050
Intestines, Small .... .44020, 44100
　Endoscopy .... .44361, 44377
Kidney 50200-50205
　Endoscopic 50555-50559,
　　　　　　　　　50574-50578, 52354
Knee 27323-27324
　Synovium .... .27330
Knee Joint
　Synovium .... .27330
Lacrimal Gland .... .68510
Lacrimal Sac .... .68525
Larynx
　Endoscopy .... .31510, 31576
Leg
　Lower 27613-27614
　Upper 27323-27324
Lip .... .40490
Liver 47000-47001, 47100
　Percutaneous .... .00702
Lung
　Needle .... .32405
　Thoracotomy 32095-32100
Lymph Nodes 38500-38530
　Injection Procedure
　　for Identification of Sentinel Node ..38792
　Laparoscopic 38570-38572
　Needle .... .38505
　Open .... .38500, 38510-38530
　　Superficial .... .38500
Mediastinum .... .39400
　Needle .... .32405
Metacarpophalangeal Joint .... .26105
Metatarsophalangeal Joint .... .28052
Mouth .... .40808, 41108
Muscle 20200-20206
Nail .... .11755
Nasopharynx 42804-42806

Neck .... .21550
Nerve .... .64795
Nose
　Endoscopic .... .31237
　Intranasal .... .30100
Orbit .... .61332
　Exploration .... .67400, 67450
　Fine Needle Aspiration .... .67415
Oropharynx .... .42800
Ovary .... .58900
Palate .... .42100
Pancreas .... .48100
Pelvis 27040-27041
Penis .... .54100
　Deep Structures .... .54105
Percutaneous Needle
　Spinal Cord .... .62269
Perineum 56605-56606
Peritoneum
　Endoscopic .... .47561
Pharynx 42800-42806
Pleura
　Needle 32400-32402
　Thoracotomy 32095-32100
Pleural
　Open .... .32402
Prostate 55700-55705
Rectum .... .45100
Retroperitoneal Area .... .49010
Sacroiliac Joint .... .27050
Salivary Gland .... .42405
Shoulder
　Deep .... .23066
　Soft Tissue .... .23065
Shoulder Joint 23100-23101
Sinus
　Sphenoid 31050-31051
Skin Lesion 11100-11101
Spinal Cord 63275-63290
　Percutaneous .... .62269
　Stereotaxis .... .63615
Stomach 43600-43605
Tarsometatarsal Joint
　Synovial .... .28050
Testis 54500-54505
Thorax .... .21550
Throat 42800-42806
Tongue 41100-41105
Transcatheter .... .37200
Ureter .... .52354
　Endoscopic 50955-50959, 50974-50978
Urethra .... .52204, 52354, 53200
Uterus
　Endometrial .... .58100
　Endoscopic .... .58558
Uvula .... .42100
Vagina 57100-57105, 57421
Vertebral Body 20250-20251
Vulva 56605-56606, 56821
with Arthrotomy
　Acromioclavicular Joint .... .23101
　Glenohumeral Joint .... .23100
　Sternoclavicular Joint .... .23101
with Cystourethroscopy .... .52354
Wrist 25065-25066, 25100-25101

Biopsy, Skin
See Skin, Biopsy

Biopsy, Vein
See Vein, Biopsy

Biostatistics
See Biometry

Biosterol
See Vitamin, A

Biotinidase .... .82261

Birthing Room
Newborn Care .... .99431

Bischof Procedure
See Laminectomy, Surgical

Bismuth .... .83015

Bizzozero's Corpuscle/Cell
See Blood, Platelet

Bladder
Abscess
　Incision and Drainage .... .51080
Anastomosis .... .51960
Aspiration 51000-51010
Biopsy .... .52204
Catheterization .... .51045, 51701-51703
Change Tube 51705-51710
Creation
　Stoma .... .51980
Cyst
　Urachal
　　Excision .... .51500
Destruction
　Endoscopic 52214-52224, 52354
Dilation
　Ureter 52260-52265, 52341-52342,
　　　　　　　　　　52344-52345
Diverticulum
　Excision .... .51525
　Incision .... .52305
　Resection .... .52305
Endoscopy .... .52000
　Biopsy .... .52204, 52354
　Catheterization .... .52005, 52010
　Destruction 52214-52224, 52400
　Dilation 52260-52265
　Diverticulum .... .52305
　Evacuation
　　Clot .... .52001
　Excision
　　Tumor 52234-52240, 52355
　Exploration .... .52351
　Injection .... .52283
　Lithotripsy .... .52353
　Radiotracer .... .52250
　Removal
　　Calculus 52310-52315, 52352
　　Foreign Body 52310-52315
　Sphincter Surgery .... .52277
　Tumor
　　Excision .... .52355
　Ureter Surgery 52290-52300
　Urethral Syndrome .... .52285
　with Urethrotomy 52270-52276

Bone Healing
Electrical Stimulation
　Invasive 20975
　Noninvasive 20974
Ultrasound Stimulation 20979

Bone Infection
See Osteomyelitis

Bone Marrow
Aspiration 38220
Harvesting 38230
Magnetic Resonance Imaging (MRI) 76400
Needle Biopsy 38221
Nuclear Medicine
　Imaging 78102-78104
Smear 85097
T-Cell
Transplantation 38240-38242
Trocar Biopsy 38221

Bone Plate
Mandible 21244

Bone Scan
See Bone, Nuclear Medicine; Nuclear Medicine

Bone Spur
See Exostosis

Bone Wedge Reversal
Osteotomy 21122

Bordetella
Antibody 86615
Antigen Detection
　Direct Fluorescence 87265

Borrelia
Antibody 86618-86619

Borrelia burgdorferi ab
See Antibody, Lyme Disease

Borreliosis, Lyme
See Lyme Disease

Borthen Operation
See Iridotasis

Bost Fusion
See Arthrodesis, Wrist

Bosworth Operation
See Acromioclavicular Joint, Dislocation;
Arthrodesis, Vertebrae; Fasciotomy, Elbow

Bottle Type Procedure 55060

Botulinum Toxin
See Chemodenervation

Boutonniere Deformity 26426-26428

Bowel
See Intestine

Bowleg Repair 27455-27457

Boyce Operation
See Nephrotomy

Boyd Hip Disarticulation
See Amputation, Leg, Upper; Radical Resection;
Replantation

Brace
See Cast
for Leg Cast 29358

Brachial Arteries
See Artery, Brachial

Brachial Plexus
Decompression 64713
Injection
　Anesthetic 64415-64416
Neuroplasty 64713
Release 64713
Repair/Suture 64861

Brachiocephalic Artery
See Artery, Brachiocephalic

Brachycephaly 21175

Brachytherapy 77761-77778, 77789
Dose Plan 77326-77328
Remote Afterloading
　1-4 Positions 77781
　5-8 Positions 77782
　9-12 Positions 77783
　Over 12 Positions 77784
　Over 4 Positions 77781-77784
Unlisted Services and Procedures 77799

Bradykinin
Blood or Urine 82286

Brain
See Brainstem; Mesencephalon; Skull Base
Surgery
Abscess
　Drainage 61150-61151
　Excision 61514, 61522
　Incision and Drainage 61320-61321
Adhesions
　Lysis 62161
Anesthesia 00210-00218, 00220-00222
Angiography 70496
Biopsy 61140
　Stereotactic 61750-61751
Catheter
　Irrigation 62194, 62225
　Replacement 62160, 62194, 62225
Cisternography 70015
Computer Assisted
　Surgery 61795
Cortex
　Magnetic Stimulation 0018T
Craniopharyngioma
　Excision 61545
CT Scan 0042T, 70450-70470, 70496
Cyst
　Drainage 61150-61151, 62161-62162
　Excision 61516, 61524, 62162
Epileptogenic Focus
　Excision 61534, 61536

Excision
　Choroid Plexus 61544
　Hemisphere 61542-61543
　Other Lobe 61323, 61539
　Temporal Lobe 61538
Exploration
　Infratentorial 61305
　Supratentorial 61304
Hematoma
　Drainage 61154
　Incision and Drainage 61312-61315
Implantation
　Chemotherapy Agent 61517
　Electrode 61850-61875
　Pulse Generator 61885-61886
　Receiver 61885-61886
Incision
　Corpus Callosum 61541
　Frontal Lobe 61490
　Mesencephalic Tract 61480
Insertion
　Catheter 61210
　Electrode 61531-61533, 61850-61875
　Pulse Generator 61885-61886
　Receiver 61885-61886
　Reservoir 61210-61215
Lesion
　Aspiration Stereotactic 61750-61751
　Excision 61534, 61536,
　　　　　　　61600-61608, 61615-61616
Magnetic Resonance Imaging
(MRI) 70551-70553
Meningioma
　Excision 61512, 61519
Myelography 70010
Nuclear Medicine
　Blood Flow 78610-78615
　Cerebrospinal Fluid 78630-78650
　Imaging 78600-78607
　　Vascular Flow 78610
Positron Emission Tomography 78608-78609
Removal
　Electrode 61535, 61880
　Foreign Body 61570, 62163
　Pulse Generator 61888
　Receiver 61888
　Shunt 62256-62258
Repair
　Dura 61618
　Wound 61571
Shunt
　Creation 62180-62192, 62200-62223
　Removal 62256-62258
　Replacement ...62160, 62194, 62225-62230,
　　　　　　　　　　　　62256-62258
　Reprogramming 62252
Skull
　Transcochlear Approach 61596
　Transcondylar Approach 61597
　Transpetrosal Approach 61598
　Transtemporal Approach 61595
Skull Base
　Craniofacial Approach 61580-61585
　Infratemporal Approach 61590-61591
　Orbitocranial Zygomatic Approach 61592

Bronchial Challenge Test
See Allergy Tests
with Antigens, Gases 95070
with Chemicals 95071

Bronchial Provocation Tests
See Bronchial Challenge Test

Bronchioalveolar Lavage
See Lung, Lavage

Broncho-Bronchial Anastomosis 32486

Bronchoalveolar Lavage
See Lung, Lavage

Bronchography 71040-71060
Catheterization 31710
Injection
    Transtracheal 31715
Instillation
    Contrast Material 31708
Segmental
    Injection 31656

Bronchoplasty 32501
See Reconstruction, Bronchi
Excision Stenosis and Anastomosis 31775
Graft Repair 31770

Bronchopneumonia, Hiberno-Vernal
See Q Fever

Bronchopulmonary Lavage
See Lung, Lavage

Bronchoscopy
Alveolar Lavage 31624
Aspiration 31645-31646
Biopsy 31625-31629
Brushing/Protected Brushing 31623
Catheter Placement
    Intracavitary Radioelement 31643
Dilation 31630-31631
Exploration 31622
Fracture 31630
Injection 31656
Needle Biopsy 31629
Removal
    Foreign Body 31635
    Tumor 31640-31641
Stenosis 31641
Stent Placement 31631
X-Ray Contrast 31656

Bronchospasm Evaluation
See Pulmonology, Diagnostic, Spirometry

Bronkodyl
See Theophylline

Brow Pyrosis
Repair 67900

Brucella 86000
Antibody 86622

Bruise
See Hematoma

Brunschwig Operation 58240
See Hip; Pelvis, Exenteration

Brush Biopsy
See Biopsy; Needle Biopsy
Bronchi 31717

Brush Border ab
See Antibody, Heterophile

Bucca
See Cheek

Buccal Mucosa
See Mouth, Mucosa

Bulbourethral Gland
Excision 53250

Bulla
Incision and Drainage
    Puncture Aspiration 10160
Lung
    Excision-Plication 32141
        Endoscopic 32655

BUN
See Blood Urea Nitrogen; Urea Nitrogen

Bunion Repair 28296-28299
Chevron Procedure 28296
Concentric Procedure 28296
Joplin Procedure 28294
Keller Procedure 28292
Lapidus Procedure 28297
Mayo Procedure 28292
McBride Procedure 28292
Mitchell Procedure 28296
Silver Procedure 28290
with Implant 28293

Burgess Amputation
See Disarticulation, Ankle

Burhenne Procedure
See Bile Duct, Removal, Calculi (Stone); Gallbladder

Burkitt Herpesvirus
See Epstein-Barr Virus

Burns
Allograft 15350-15351
Debridement 01951-01953,
         15000-15001, 16010-16030
Dressings 16010-16030
Escharotomy 16035-16036
Excision 01951-01953, 15000-15001
Initial Treatment 16000
Tissue Culture Skin Grafts 15100-15121,
                  15342-15343
Xenograft 15400-15401

Burrow's Operation
See Skin, Adjacent Tissue Transfer

Burr Hole
Anesthesia 00214
Skull
    Biopsy Brain 61140
    Catheterization 61210

Drainage
    Abscess 61150-61151
    Cyst 61150-61151
    Hematoma 61154-61156
Exploration
    Infratentorial 61253
    Supratentorial 61250
for Implant of Neurostimulator
    Array 61862
    Injection, Contrast Media 61120
Insertion
    Catheter 61210
    Reservoir 61210

Bursa
Ankle 27604
Arm, Lower 25031
Elbow
    Excision 24105
    Incision and Drainage 23931
Femur
    Excision 27062
Foot
    Incision and Drainage 28001
Hip
    Incision and Drainage 26991
Injection 20600-20610
Ischial
    Excision 27060
Joint
    Aspiration 20600-20610
    Drainage 20600-20610
    Injection 20600-20610
Knee
    Excision 27340
Leg, Lower 27604
Palm
    Incision and Drainage 26025-26030
Pelvis
    Incision and Drainage 26991
Shoulder
    Drainage 23031
Wrist 25031
    Excision 25115-25116

Bursectomy
See Excision, Bursa

Bursitis, Radiohumeral
See Tennis Elbow

Bursocentesis
See Aspiration, Bursa

Button
Nasal Septal Prosthesis
    Insertion 30220

Butyrylcholine Esterase
See Cholinesterase

Bypass, Cardiopulmonary
See Cardiopulmonary Bypass

Bypass Graft
Axillary Artery 35516-35521, 35533,
        35616-35623, 35650, 35654
Carotid Artery 35501-35509, 35526,
        35601-35606, 35626, 35642
Celiac Artery 35531, 35631

Coronary Artery
 Angiography .93556
 Arterial 33533-33536
 Venous Graft 33510-33516
Excision
 Abdomen .35907
 Extremity 35903
 Neck 35901
 Thorax 35905
Femoral Artery 35521, 35533, 35546,
    35551-35558, 35566, 35621, 35646-35647,
        35651-35661, 35666, 35700
Harvest
 Endoscopic 33508
 Upper Extremity Vein 35500
Iliac Artery 35541, 35563, 35641, 35663
Iliofemoral Artery . . .35548-35549, 35565, 35665
Mesenteric Artery 35531, 35631
Peroneal Artery 35566-35571, 35666-35671
Placement
 Vein Patch 35685
Popliteal Artery 35551-35558, 35571, 35623,
        35651, 35656, 35671, 35700
Renal Artery 35536, 35560, 35631-35636
Reoperation .35700
Repair
 Abdomen .35907
 Extremity 35903
 Lower Extremity
  with Composite Graft 35681-35683
 Neck 35901
 Thorax 35905
Revascularization
 Extremity 35903
 Neck 35901
 Thorax 35905
Revision
 Lower Extremity
  with Angioplasty 35879
  with Vein Interposition 35881
Secondary Repair 35870
Splenic Artery 35536, 35636
Subclavian Artery . . .35506-35507, 35511-35516,
        35526, 35606-35616, 35626, 35645
Thrombectomy
 Other than Hemodialysis Graft
 or Fistula 35875-35876
Tibial Artery . .35566-35571, 35623, 35666-35671
Vertebral Artery 35508, 35515, 35642-35645
with Composite Graft 35681

Bypass In-Situ
Femoral Artery 35582-35585
Peroneal Artery 35585-35587
Popliteal Artery 35582-35583, 35587
Tibial Artery 35585-35587

B 12, Vitamin
See Cyanocobalamin

B Antibodies, Hepatitis
See Antibody, Hepatitis B

B Antigens, Hepatitis
See Hepatitis Antigen, B

B Complex Vitamins
B-12 Absorption 78270-78272

C

C-13
Urease Activity 83013-83014
Urea Breath Test 83013-83014

C-14
Urease Activity 83013-83014
Urea Breath Test 78267-78268

C-Peptide 80432, 84681

C-Reactive Protein 86140-86141

C-Section
See Cesarean Delivery

CABG
See Coronary Artery Bypass Graft (CABG)

Cadmium
Urine 82300

Calcaneal Spur
See Heel Spur

Calcaneus
Craterization .28120
Cyst
 Excision 28100-28103
Diaphysectomy 28120
Excision 28118-28120
Fracture
 Open Treatment 28415-28420
 Percutaneous Fixation 28406
 without Manipulation 28400
 with Manipulation 28405-28406
Repair
 Osteotomy 28300
Saucerization 28120
Tumor
 Excision 27647, 28100-28103
X-Ray 73650

Calcareous Deposits
Subdeltoid
 Removal 23000

Calcifediol
Blood or Urine 82306

Calcifediol Assay
See Calciferol

Calciferol
Blood or Urine 82307

Calcification
See Calcium, Deposits

Calciol
See Vitamin, D-3

Calcitonin
Blood or Urine 82308
Stimulation Panel 80410

Calcium
Blood
 Infusion Test 82331
Deposits
 See Removal, Calculi (Stone); Removal,
 Foreign Bodies
Ionized 82330
Total 82310
Urine 82340

Calcium-Binding Protein, Vitamin K-Dependent
See Osteocalcin

Calcium-Pentagastrin Stimulation 80410

Calculus
Analysis 82355-82370
Destruction
 Bile Duct .43265
 Pancreatic Duct 43265
Removal
 Bile Duct 43264, 47554, 74327
 Bladder 51050, 52310-52318, 52352
 Kidney 50060-50081, 50130, 50561,
        50580, 52352
 Pancreatic Duct 43264
 Ureter 50610-50630, 50961, 50980,
    51060-51065, 52320-52325, 52352
 Urethra 52310-52315, 52352

Calculus of Kidney
See Calculus, Removal, Kidney

Caldwell-Luc Procedure
See Sinus, Maxillary; Sinusotomy; Sternum,
Fracture
Orbital Floor Blowout Fracture 21385
Sinusotomy 31030-31032

Caliper
Application/Removal 20660

Callander Knee Disarticulation
See Disarticulation, Knee

Callosum, Corpus
See Corpus Callosum

Calmette Guerin Bacillus Vaccine
See BCG Vaccine

Caloric Vestibular Test 92533

Calycoplasty 50405

Camey Enterocystoplasty 50825

CAMP
See Cyclic AMP

Campbell Procedure 27422

Campylobacter
Antibody 86625

Campylobacter Pylori
See Helicobacter Pylori

Canal, Ear
See Auditory Canal

Canal, Semicircular
See Semicircular Canal

Canaloplasty 69631, 69635

Candida
Antibody 86628
Skin Test 86485

Cannulation 36821
Arterial 36620-36625
Sinus
    Maxillary 31000
    Sphenoid 31002
Thoracic Duct 38794

Cannulation, Renoportal
See Anastomosis, Renoportal

Cannulization
See Catheterization
Arteriovenous 36145, 36810-36815
Declotting 36550, 36860-36861
ECMO 36822
External
    Declotting 36860-36861
Vas Deferens 55200
Vein to Vein 36800

Canthocystostomy
See Conjunctivorhinostomy

Canthopexy
Lateral 21282
Medial 21280

Canthoplasty 67950

Canthorrhaphy 67880-67882

Canthotomy 67715

Canthus
Reconstruction 67950

Cap, Cervical
See Cervical Cap

Capsule
See Capsulodesis
Elbow
    Arthrotomy 24006
    Excision 24006
Foot 28264
Interphalangeal Joint
    Excision 26525
    Incision 26525
Knee 27435
Metacarpophalangeal Joint
    Excision 26520
    Incision 26520
Metatarsophalangeal Joint
    Release 28289
Shoulder
    Incision 23020
Wrist
    Excision 25320

Capsulectomy
Breast
    Periprosthetic 19371

Capsulodesis
Metacarpophalangeal Joint 26516-26518

Capsulorrhaphy
Anterior 23450-23462
Multi-Directional Instability 23466
Posterior 23465
Wrist 25320

Capsulotomy
Breast
    Periprosthetic 19370
Foot 28260-28262
Hip
    with Release, Flexor Muscles 27036
Interphalangeal Joint 28272
Knee 27435
Metacarpophalangeal Joint 26520
Metatarsophalangeal Joint 28270
Toe 28270-28272
Wrist 25085

Captopril 80416-80417

Carbamazepine
Assay 80156-80157

Carbazepin
See Carbamazepine

Carbinol
See Methanol

Carbohydrate Deficient Transferrin 82373

Carbon Dioxide
Blood or Urine 82374

Carbon Monoxide
Blood 82375-82376

Carbon Tetrachloride 84600

Carboxycathepsin
See Angiotensin Converting Enzyme (ACE)

Carboxyhemoglobin 82375-82376

Carbuncle
Incision and Drainage 10060-10061

Carcinoembryonal Antigen
See Antigen, Carcinoembryonic

Carcinoembryonic Antigen 82378

Cardiac
See Coronary

Cardiac Arrhythmia, Tachycardia
See Tachycardia

Cardiac Atria
See Atria

Cardiac Catheterization
Combined Left and Right Heart 93526-93529
Combined Right and Retrograde Left
    Congenital Cardiac Anomalies 93531
Combined Right and Transseptal Left
    Congenital Cardiac Anomalies .93532-93533
for Biopsy 93505
for Dilution Studies 93561-93562
Imaging 93555-93556
Injection 93539-93545
    See Catheterization, Cardiac
Left Heart 93510-93524
Pacemaker 33210
Right
    Congenital Cardiac Anomalies 93530
Right Heart 93501-93503

Cardiac Electroversion
See Cardioversion

Cardiac Event Recorder
Implantation 33282
Removal 33284

Cardiac Magnetic Resonance Imaging (CMRI)
Complete Study 75554
Limited Study 75555
Morphology 75553
Velocity Flow Mapping 75556

Cardiac Massage
Thoracotomy 32160

Cardiac Muscle
See Myocardium

Cardiac Neoplasm
See Heart, Tumor

Cardiac Output
Indicator Dilution 93561-93562

Cardiac Pacemaker
See Heart, Pacemaker

Cardiac Rehabilitation 93797-93798

Cardiac Septal Defect
See Septal Defect

Cardiac Transplantation
See Heart, Transplantation

Cardiectomy
Donor 33930, 33940

Cardioassist 92970-92971

Cardiolipin Antibody 86147

Cardiology
See Electrocardiography
Diagnostic
    Atrial Electrogram
        Esophageal Recording 93615-93616
    Cardio-Defibrillator
        Evaluation and Testing 93640-93642,
                    93741-93744
    Echocardiography
        Doppler 93303-93321, 93662
        Intracardiac 93662
        Transesophageal 93318
        Transthoracic 93303-93317, 93350

Citrate
Blood or Urine 82507

Clagett Procedure
See Chest Wall, Repair, Closure

Clavicle
Craterization 23180
Cyst
 Excision 23140
  with Allograft 23146
  with Autograft 23145
Diaphysectomy 23180
Dislocation
 Acromioclavicular Joint
  Closed Treatment 23540-23545
  Open Treatment 23550-23552
 Sternoclavicular Joint
  Closed Treatment 23520-23525
  Open Treatment 23530-23532
  without Manipulation 23540
Excision 23170
 Partial 23120, 23180
 Total 23125
Fracture
 Closed Treatment
  without Manipulation 23500
  with Manipulation 23505
 Open Treatment 23515
Pinning, Wiring 23490
Prophylactic Treatment 23490
Repair Osteotomy 23480-23485
Saucerization 23180
Sequestrectomy 23170
Tumor
 Excision 23140, 23146, 23200
  with Autograft 23145
 Radical Resection 23200
X-Ray 73000

Clavicula
See Clavicle

Claviculectomy
Partial 23120
Total 23125

Claw Finger Repair 26499

Cleft, Branchial
See Branchial Cleft

Cleft Cyst, Branchial
See Branchial Cleft, Cyst

Cleft Foot
Reconstruction 28360

Cleft Hand
Repair 26580

Cleft Lip
Repair 40700-40761
Rhinoplasty 30460-30462

Cleft Palate
Repair 42200-42225
Rhinoplasty 30460-30462

Clinical Act of Insertion
See Insertion

Clinical Chemistry Test
See Chemistry Tests, Clinical

Clinical Pathology
See Pathology, Clinical

Clitoroplasty
Intersex State 56805

Closed [Transurethral] Biopsy of Bladder
See Biopsy, Bladder, Cystourethroscopy

Clostridial Tetanus
See Tetanus

Clostridium Botulinum Toxin
See Chemodenervation

Clostridium Difficile
Antigen Detection
 Enzyme Immunoassay 87324
by Immunoassay
 with Direct Optical Observation 87803

Clostridium Tetani ab
See Antibody, Tetanus

Closure 12001-13160
Anal Fistula 46288
Atrioventricular Valve 33600
Cystostomy 51880
Enterostomy 44625-44626
Lacrimal Fistula 68770
Lacrimal Punctum
 Plug 68761
 Thermocauterization, Ligation or Laser
 Surgery 68760
Rectovaginal Fistula 57300-57308
Semilunar Valve 33602
Septal Defect 33615
Sternotomy 21750
Ventricular Tunnel 33722

Closure, Atrial Septal Defect
See Heart, Repair, Atrial Septum

Closure, Cranial Sutures, Premature
See Craniosynostosis

Closure, Fistula, Vesicouterine
See Fistula, Vesicouterine, Closure

Closure, Meningocele Spinal
See Meningocele Repair

Closure, Vagina
See Vagina, Closure

Closure of Esophagostomy
See Esophagostomy, Closure

Closure of Gastrostomy
See Gastrostomy, Closure

Clot 34401-34490, 35875-35876, 50230
See Thrombectomy; Thromboendarterectomy

Clotting Disorder
See Coagulopathy

Clotting Factor 85210-85293

Clotting Inhibitors 85300-85305,
 85307, 99557

Clotting Operation
See Excision, Nail Fold

Clotting Test
Protein C 85303, 85307
Protein S 85306

Clotting Time
See Coagulation Time

Clot Lysis Time 85175

Clot Retraction 85170

Clubfoot Cast 29450
Wedging 29750

CMG
See Cystometrogram

CMRI
See Cardiac Magnetic Resonance Imaging

CMV
See Cytomegalovirus

CNPB
See Continuous Negative Pressure Breathing (CNPB); Pulmonology, Therapeutic

Co-Factor I, Heparin
See Antithrombin III

CO2
See Carbon Dioxide

Coagulation
Unlisted Services and Procedures 85999

Coagulation, Blood
See Blood Clot

Coagulation, Light
See Photocoagulation

Coagulation Defect
See Coagulopathy

Coagulation Factor
See Clotting Factor

Coagulation Factor I
See Fibrinogen

Coagulation Factor II
See Prothrombin

Coagulation Factor III
See Thromboplastin

Coagulation Factor IV
See Calcium

Coagulation Factor VII
See Proconvertin

Coagulation Factor VIII
See Clotting Factor

Surgical Pathology 88321-88325
    Intraoperation 88329-88332
X-Ray 76140

Consumption Test, Antiglobulin
See Coombs Test

Contact Lens Services
Fittings and Prescription 92070, 92310-92313
Modification 92325
Prescription 92314-92317
Replacement 92326
Supply .92391, 92396

Continuous Negative Pressure Breathing (CNPB) 94662

Continuous Positive Airway Pressure (CPAP) 94660
See Pulmonology, Therapeutic

Contouring
Silicone Injections 11950-11954
Tumor
    Facial Bone .21029

Contraception
Cervical Cap
    Fitting 57170
Diaphragm
    Fitting 57170
Intrauterine Device (IUD)
    See Insertion, Intrauterine Device (IUD);
    Intrauterine Device (IUD); Removal,
    Intrauterine Device (IUD)
    Insertion 58300
    Removal 58301

Contraceptive Capsules, Implantable
Insertion 11975
Removal 11976
    with Reinsertion 11977

Contraceptive Device, Intrauterine
See Intrauterine Device (IUD)

Contracture
Elbow
    Release
        with Radical Resection of Capsule . .24149
Palm
    Release 26121-26125
Thumb
    Release 26508

Contracture of Palmar Fascia
See Dupuytren's Contracture

Contralateral Ligament
Repair
    Knee 27405

Contrast Aortogram
See Aortography

Contrast Bath Therapy 97034
See Physical Medicine/Therapy/Occupational Therapy

Contrast Material
Injection
    via Peritoneal Catheter 49424
Instillation
    Bronchography 31708
    Laryngography 31708

Contrast Phlebogram
See Venography

Contusion
See Hematoma

Converting Enzyme, Angiotensin
See Angiotensin Converting Enzyme (ACE)

Coombs Test 86880

Copper 82525

Coprobilinogen
Feces 84577

Coproporphyrin 84120

Coracoacromial Ligament Release 23415

Coracoid Process Transfer 23462

Cord, Spermatic
See Spermatic Cord

Cord, Spinal
See Spinal Cord

Cord, Vocal
See Vocal Cords

Cordectomy 31300

Cordocenteses
See Cordocentesis

Cordocentesis 59012

Cordotomy 63194-63199

Corectomy
See Excision, Iris

Coreoplasty 66762

Cornea
Biopsy 65410
Curettage 65435-65436
    with Chelating Agent 65436
Epithelium
    Excision 65435-65436
        with Chelating Agent 65436
Lesion
    Destruction 65450
    Excision 65400
        without Graft 65420
        with Graft 65426
Prosthesis 65770
Pterygium
    Excision 65420
Puncture 65600
Relaxing Incisions 65772-65775

Repair
    Astigmatism 65772-65775
    Wedge Resection 65775
    with Glue 65286
    Wound
        Nonperforating 65275
        Perforating 65280-65285
        Tissue Glue 65286
Reshape
    Epikeratoplasty 65765
    Keratomileusis 65760
    Keratoprosthesis 65767
Scraping
    Smear 65430
Tattoo 65600
Thickness Measurement 0025T
Transplantation
    Autograft or Homograft
        Lamellar 65710
        Penetrating 65730-65755
    for Aphakia 65750

Coronary
Atherectomy
    Percutaneous 92995-92996
Thrombectomy
    Percutaneous 92973

Coronary Angioplasty, Transluminal Balloon
See Percutaneous Transluminal Angioplasty

Coronary Artery
Insertion
    Stent 92980-92981
Ligation 33502
Placement
    Radiation Delivery Device 92974
Repair 33500-33506

Coronary Artery Bypass Graft (CABG) 33503-33505, 33510-33516
Arterial 33533-33536
Arterial-Venous 33517-33523
Harvest
    Upper Extremity Artery 35600
Reoperation 33530
Venous .33510-33516

Coronary Endarterectomy 33572

Coroner's Exam 88045

Coronoidectomy
Temporomandibular Joint 21070

Corpora Cavernosa
Corpus Spongiosum Shunt 54430
Glans Penis Fistulization 54435
Injection 54235
Irrigation
    Priapism 54220
Saphenous Vein Shunt 54420
X-Ray with Contrast 74445

Corpora Cavernosa, Plastic Induration
See Peyronie Disease

Cranioplasty 62120
Encephalocele Repair 62120
for Defect 62140-62141, 62145
with Autograft 62146-62147
with Bone Graft 61316, 62146-62147

Craniostenosis
See Craniosynostosis

Craniosynostosis
Bifrontal Craniotomy 61557
Extensive Craniectomy 61558-61559

Craniotomy
See Burr Hole; Craniectomy; Drill Hole; Puncture
Bifrontal 61557
Decompression 61322-61323
Exploratory 61304-61305
for Craniosynostosis 61556-61557
for Encephalocele 62121
for Implant of Neurostimulators 61850-61875
Frontal 61556
Parietal 61556
Surgery 61312-61315, 61320-61323, 61440,
        61490, 61546, 61570-61571, 61582-61583,
        61590, 61592, 61760, 62120
with Bone Flap 61510-61516, 61526-61530,
        61533-61545

Cranium
See Skull

Craterization
Calcaneus 28120
Clavicle 23180
Femur 27070-27071, 27360
Fibula 27360, 27641
Hip 27070
Humerus 23184, 24140
Ileum 27070
Metacarpal 26230
Metatarsal 28122
Olecranon Process 24147
Phalanges
    Finger 26235-26236
    Toe 28124
Pubis 27070
Radius 24145, 25151
Scapula 23182
Talus 28120
Tarsal 28122
Tibia 27360, 27640
Ulna 24147, 25150

Creatine 82553-82554
Blood or Urine 82540

Creatine Kinase
Total 82550

Creatine Phosphokinase
Blood 82552
Total 82550

Creatinine
Blood 82565
Clearance 82575
Other Source 82570
Urine 82570-82575

Creation
Arteriovenous
    Fistula/Autogenous Graft 36825
Colonic Reservoir 45119
Complete Heart Block 93650
Defect 40720
Ileal Reservoir 44153, 45113
Lesion 61790, 63600
Mucofistula 44144
Pericardial Window 32659
Recipient Site 15000
Shunt
    Cerebrospinal Fluid 62200
    Subarachnoid
        Lumbar-Peritoneal 63740
        Subarachnoid-Subdural 62190
        Ventriculo 62220
Sigmoid Bladder 50810
Speech Prosthesis 31611
Stoma
    Bladder 51980
    Kidney 50395
    Renal Pelvis 50395
    Tympanic Membrane 69433-69436
    Ureter 50860
Ventral Hernia 39503

CRF
See Corticotropic Releasing Hormone (CRH)

CRH
See Corticotropic Releasing Hormone (CRH)

Cricoid Cartilage Split
Larynx 31587

Cricothyroid Membrane
Incision 31605

Cristobalite
See Silica

Critical Care Services 99289-99292
See Emergency Department Services; Prolonged
Attendance
Evaluation and Management 99291-99292
Gastric Intubation 91105
Interfacility Transport 99289-99290
Ipecac Administration for Poison 99175
Neonatal
    Initial 99295
    Low Birth Weight Infant 99298-99299
    Subsequent 99296
Pediatric
    Initial 99293
    Interfacility Transport 99289-99290
    Subsequent 99294, 99299

Crossmatch 86920-86922

Crossmatching, Tissue
See Tissue Typing

Cross Finger Flap 15574

Cruciate Ligament
Arthroscopic Repair 29888-29889
Repair 27407-27409
    Knee
        with Collateral Ligament 27409

Cryoablation
See Cryosurgery

Cryofibrinogen 82585

Cryofixation
See Cryopreservation

Cryoglobulin 82595

Cryopreservation
Cells 38207-38208, 88240-88241
Embryo 89258
Freezing and Storage 38207, 88240
Sperm 89259

Cryosurgery 17000-17286, 47371, 47381
See Destruction
Labyrinthotomy 69801
Lesion
    Mouth 40820
    Penis 54056, 54065
    Vagina 57061-57065
    Vulva 56501-56515

Cryotherapy
Acne 17340
Destruction
    Ciliary Body 66720
Lesion
    Cornea 65450
    Retina 67208, 67227
Retinal Detachment
    Prophylaxis 67141
    Repair 67101
Trichiasis
    Correction 67825

Cryptectomy 46210-46211

Cryptococcus
Antibody 86641
Antigen Detection
    Enzyme Immunoassay 87327

Cryptococcus Neoformans
Antigen Detection
    Enzyme Immunoassay 87327

Cryptorchism
See Testis, Undescended

Cryptosporidium
Antigen Detection
    Direct Fluorescence 87272
    Enzyme Immunoassay 87328

Crystal Identification
Any Body Fluid 89060

CSF
See Cerebrospinal Fluid Leak

CT Scan
Bone
    Density Study 76070-76071
Drainage 75989
Follow-up Study 76380

Cuff, Rotator
See Rotator Cuff

Culdocentesis
See Colpocentesis

Culture

Curettage
See Dilation and Curettage

Curettage, Uterus
See Uterus, Curettage

Curettage and Dilatation
See Dilation and Curettage

Curettement

Curietherapy
See Brachytherapy

Custodial Care
See Domiciliary Services; Nursing Facility
Services

Cutaneolipectomy
See Lipectomy

Cutaneous-Vesicostomy
See Vesicostomy, Cutaneous

**Cutaneous Electrostimulation,
Analgesic**
See Application, Neurostimulation

Cutaneous Tag
See Skin, Tags

Cutaneous Tissue
See Integumentary System

CVS
See Biopsy, Chorionic Villus

Cyanacobalamin
See Cyanocobalamin

Cyanide

Cyclic Somatostatin
See Somatostatin

Cyclocryotherapy
See Cryotherapy, Destruction, Ciliary Body

Cyclodialysis

Cyclophotocoagulation

Cyclosporine

Cyst

Bone
　Drainage 20615
　Injection 20615
Brain
　Drainage 61150-61151, 61156,
　　　　　　　　　　　　 62161-62162
　Excision 61516, 61524, 62162
Branchial Cleft
　Excision 42810-42815
Breast
　Incision and Drainage 19020
　Puncture Aspiration 19000-19001
Calcaneus 28100-28103
Carpal 25130-25136
Choledochal 47715-47716
Ciliary Body
　Destruction 66770
Clavicle
　Excision 23140-23146
Conjunctiva 68020
Dermoid
　Nose
　　Excision 30124-30125
Drainage
　Contrast Injection 49424
　　with X-Ray 76080
Excision
　Cheekbone 21030
　Clavicle 23140
　　with Allograft 23146
　　with Autograft 23145
　Femur 27355-27358
　Ganglion
　　See Ganglion
　Humerus
　　with Allograft 23156
　　with Autograft 23155
　Hydatid
　　See Echinococcosis
　Lymphatic
　　See Lymphocele
　Maxilla 21030
　Mediastinum 32662
　Olecranon Process
　　with Allograft 24126
　　with Autograft 24125
　Pericardial 32661
　Pilonidal 11770-11772
　Radius
　　with Allograft 24126
　　with Autograft 24125
　Scapula .23140
　　with Allograft 23146
　　with Autograft 23145
　Ulna
　　with Allograft 24126
　　with Autograft 24125
　Zygoma 21030
Facial Bones
　Excision 21030
Femur 27065-27067
Fibula .27635-27638
Ganglion
　Aspiration/Injection 20612
Gums
　Incision and Drainage 41800
Hip 27065-27067

Humerus
　Excision 23150-23156, 24110
　　with Allograft 24116
　　with Autograft 24115
Ileum .27065-27067
Incision and Drainage 10060-10061
　Pilonidal 10080-10081
Iris
　Destruction 66770
Kidney
　Ablation .50541
　Aspiration 50390
　Excision 50280-50290
　Injection .50390
　X-Ray 74470
Knee
　Baker's 27345
　Excision .27347
Leg, Lower
　Capsule 27630
　Tendon Sheath 27630
Liver 47010
　Drainage .47010
　Open 47010
　Repair 47300
Lung
　Incision and Drainage 32200
　Removal .32140
Lymph Node
　Axillary/Cervical
　　Excision 38550-38555
Mandible
　Excision 21040, 21046-21047
Maxilla
　Excision 21030, 21048-21049
Mediastinal
　Excision .39200
Metacarpal 26200-26205
Metatarsal 28104-28107
Mouth 41005-41009, 41015-41018
　Incision and Drainage 40800-40801
Mullerian Duct
　Excision .55680
Nose
　Excision 30124-30125
Olecranon 24120
Ovarian
　Excision .58925
　Incision and Drainage 58800-58805
Pancreas 48500
　Anastomosis 48520-48540
　Excision .48120
Pelvis
　Aspiration 50390
　Injection .50390
Pericardial
　Excision .33050
Phalanges
　Finger 26210-26215
　Toe 28108
Pilonidal
　Excision 11770-11772
　Incision and Drainage 10080-10081
Pubis .27065-27067
Radius 24120, 25120-25126
Rathke's Pouch
　See Craniopharyngioma

Removal
　Skin 10040
Retroperitoneal
　Destruction/Excision 49200-49201
Salivary Gland Creation
　Destruction/Excision
　　Fistula 42325-42326
　Drainage 42409
　Excision 42408
Scapula
　Excision 23140-23146
Seminal Vesicle
　Excision 55680
Skin
　Puncture Aspiration 10160
Spinal Cord
　Aspiration 62268
　Incision and Drainage 63172-63173
Sublingual Gland Drainage 42409
　Excision 42408
Talus 28100-28103
Tarsal 28104-28107
Thyroglossal Duct
　Excision 60280-60281
　Incision and Drainage 60000
Thyroid Gland Aspiration 60001
　Excision 60200
　Injection 60001
Tibia 27635-27638
Tongue 41000-41006, 41015
Ulna 24120, 25120-25126
Urachal
　Bladder
　　Excision 51500
Vaginal
　Excision 57135
Wrist 25130-25136
　Excision 25111-25112
Zygoma
　Excision 21030

Cystatins, Kininogen
See Kininogen

Cystectomy
Complete 51570
　with Bilateral Pelvic
　　Lymphadenectomy 51575, 51585, 51595
　　with Continent Diversion 51596
　　with Ureteroileal Conduit 51590
　　with Ureterosigmoidostomy 51580
Ovarian 58925
　Laparoscopic 58661
Partial
　Complicated 51555
　Reimplantation of Ureters 51565
　Simple .51550

Cystic Hygroma
See Hygroma

Cystine
Urine 82615

Cystitis
Interstitial 52260-52265

Cystography 74430
Injection .52281
　Radiologic 51600

Debridement

Brain 62010
Burns 01951-01953, 16010-16030
Mastoid Cavity
    Complex 69222
    Simple 69220
Metatarsophalangeal Joint 28289
Nails 11720-11721
Nose
    Endoscopic 31237
Pancreatic Tissue 48005
Skin
    Eczematous 11000-11001
    Full Thickness 11041
    Infected 11000-11001
    Partial Thickness 11040
    Subcutaneous Tissue 11042-11044
    with Open Fracture and/or
    Dislocation 11010-11012
Sternum 21627
Wound
    Non-Selective 97602
    Selective 97601

Debulking Procedure

Ovary/Pelvis 58952-58954

Decompression

See Section
Arm, Lower 24495, 25020-25025
Auditory Canal, Internal 69960
Brainstem 61575-61576
Cauda Equina 63011, 63017, 63047-63048,
            63056-63057, 63087-63091
Cranial Nerve 61458
Esophagogastric Varices 37181
Facial Nerve 61590
    Intratemporal
      Lateral to Geniculate Ganglion 69720,
                  69740
      Medial to Geniculate Ganglion 69725,
                  69745
    Total 69955
Finger 26035
Gasserian Ganglion
    Sensory Root 61450
Hand 26035-26037
Intestines
    Small 44021
Jejunostomy
    Laparoscopic 44201
Leg
    Fasciotomy 27600-27602
Nerve 64702-64727
    Root 63020-63091
Nucleus of Disk
    Lumbar 62287
Optic Nerve 67570
Orbit 61330
    Removal of Bone 67414, 67445
Skull 61322-61323, 61340-61345
Spinal Cord 63001-63017, 63045-63091
    Cauda Equina 63005
Tarsal Tunnel Release 28035
Volvulus 45321, 45337
with Nasal/Sinus Endoscopy
    Optic Nerve 31294
    Orbit Wall 31292-31293
Wrist 25020-25025

Decortication

Lung
    Endoscopic 32651-32652
    Partial 32225
    Total 32220
    with Parietal Pleurectomy 32320

Decubiti
See Pressure Ulcer (Decubitus)

Decubitus Ulcers
See Debridement; Pressure Ulcer (Decubitus);
Skin Graft and Flap

Deetjeen's Body
See Blood, Platelet

Defect, Coagulation
See Coagulopathy

Defect, Heart Septal
See Septal Defect

Defect, Septal Closure, Atrial
See Heart, Repair, Atrial Septum

Deferens, Ductus
See Vas Deferens

Defibrillation
See Cardioversion

Defibrillator, Heart
See Pacemaker, Heart
Evaluation and Testing 93640-93642
Insertion Single/Dual Chamber
    Electrodes 33216-33217,
            33224-33225, 33245-33249
    Pulse Generator 33240, 33246
Removal Single/Dual Chamber
    Electrodes 33243-33244
    Pulse Generator 33241
Repair 33218-33220
Repositioning Single/Dual Chamber
    Electrodes 33215, 33226
Revise Pocket Chest 33223

Deformity, Boutonniere
See Boutonniere Deformity

Deformity, Sprengel's
See Sprengel's Deformity

Degenerative, Articular Cartilage, Patella
See Chondromalacia Patella

Degradation Products, Fibrin
See Fibrin Degradation Products

Dehydroepiandrosterone 82626

Dehydroepiandrosterone Sulfate 82627

Dehydrogenase, 6-Phosphogluconate
See Phosphogluconate-6, Dehydrogenase

Dehydrogenase, Alcohol
See Antidiuretic Hormone

Dehydrogenase, Glucose-6-Phosphate
See Glucose-6-Phosphate, Dehydrogenase

Dehydrogenase, Glutamate
See Glutamate Dehydrogenase

Dehydrogenase, Isocitrate
See Isocitric Dehydrogenase

Dehydrogenase, Lactate
See Lactic Dehydrogenase

Dehydrogenase, Malate
See Malate Dehydrogenase

Dehydroisoandrosterone Sulfate
See Dehydroepiandrosterone Sulfate

Delay of Flap
Skin Graft 15600-15630

Deligation
Ureter 50940

Deliveries, Abdominal
See Cesarean Delivery

Delivery
See Cesarean Delivery; Vaginal Delivery

Delorme Operation
See Pericardiectomy

Denervation
Hip
    Femoral 27035
    Obturator 27035
    Sciatic 27035

Denervation, Sympathetic
See Excision, Nerve, Sympathetic

Denis-Browne Splint 29590

Dens Axis
See Odontoid Process

Denver-Krupin Procedure 66180

Denver Developmental Screening Test 96100

Denver Krupic Procedure
See Aqueous Shunt, to Extraocular Reservoir

Denver Shunt
Patency Test 78291

Deoxycorticosterone
See Desoxycorticosterone

Deoxycortisol 80436, 82634

Deoxyephedrine
See Methamphetamine

Deoxyribonuclease
Antibody 86215

Deoxyribonuclease I
See DNAse

Deoxyribonucleic Acid
Antibody 86225-86226

Clavicle
  Closed Treatment 23540-23545
  Open Treatment 23550-23552
  without Manipulation 23540
  with Manipulation 23545
Closed Treatment
  Carpometacarpal Joint 26670-26675
  Metacarpophalangeal 26700-26706
  Thumb 26641
Elbow
  Closed Treatment 24600-24605, 24640
  Open Treatment 24615
Hip Joint
  Closed Treatment 27250-27252, 27265-27266
  Congenital 27256-27259
  Open Treatment .27253-27254, 27258-27259
  without Trauma 27265-27266
Interphalangeal Joint
  Closed Treatment 26770-26775
  Open Treatment 26785
  Percutaneous Fixation 26776
  Toe
    Closed Treatment 28660-28665
    Open Treatment 28675
    Percutaneous Fixation 26770-26776, 28666
    with Manipulation 26770
Knee .27560-27562
  Closed Treatment 27550-27727,
                                                 27732-27752
  Open Treatment 27556-27558,
                                                 27566, 27730
  Recurrent 27420-27424
Lunate
  Closed Treatment 25690
  Open Treatment 25695
  with Manipulation 25690, 26670-26676,
                                                 26700-26706
Metacarpophalangeal Joint
  Closed Treatment 26700-26706
  Open Treatment 26715
Metatarsophalangeal Joint
  Closed Treatment 28630-28635
  Open Treatment 28645
  Percutaneous Fixation 28636
Open Treatment 26685-26686
Patella
  Closed Treatment 27560-27562
  Open Treatment 27566
  Recurrent 27420-27424
Pelvic Ring
  Closed Treatment 27193-27194
  Open Treatment 27217-27218
  Percutaneous Fixation 27216
  without Manipulation 27193-27194
Percutaneous Fixation
  Metacarpophalangeal 26705
Peroneal Tendons 27675-27676
Radio-Ulnar Joint 25520-25526
Radius
  Closed Treatment 24640
  with Fracture
    Closed Treatment 24620
    Open Treatment 24635

Shoulder
  Closed Treatment
    with Manipulation 23650-23655
  Open Treatment with Surgical or
  Anatomical Neck Fracture 23660
    Closed Treatment with Manipulation 23675
    Open Treatment 23680
  with Greater Tuberosity Fracture
    Closed Treatment 23665
    Open Treatment 23670
Skin
  Debridement 11010-11012
Sternoclavicular Joint
  Closed Treatment
    without Manipulation 23520
    with Manipulation 23525
  Open Treatment 23530-23532
Talotarsal Joint
  Closed Treatment 28570-28575
  Open Treatment 28546
  Percutaneous Fixation 28576
Tarsal
  Closed Treatment 28540-28545
  Open Treatment 28555
  Percutaneous Fixation 28546
Tarsometatarsal Joint
  Closed Treatment 28600-28605
  Open Treatment 28615
  Percutaneous Fixation 28606
Temporomandibular Joint
  Closed Treatment 21480-21485
  Open Treatment 21490
Thumb
  Closed Treatment 26641-26645
  Open Treatment 26665
  Percutaneous Fixation 26650
  with Fracture 26645
    Open Treatment 26665
    Percutaneous Fixation 26650-26665
  with Manipulation 26641-26650
Tibiofibular Joint
  Closed Treatment 27830-27831
  Open Treatment 27832
Vertebra
  Additional Segment
    Open Treatment 22328
  Cervical
    Open Treatment 22326
    Closed Treatment 22305
    without Manipulation 22310
    with Manipulation, Casting
    and/or Bracing 22315
  Lumbar
    Open Treatment 22325
  Thoracic
    Open Treatment 22327
Wrist
  Closed Treatment 25660, 25675, 25680
  Intercarpal .25660
    Open Treatment 25670
  Open Treatment 25670, 25685
  Percutaneous Fixation 25671
  Radiocarpal 25660
    Open Treatment 25670
  Radioulnar
    Closed Treatment 25675
    Open Treatment 25676
    Percutaneous Fixation 25671

  with Fracture
    Closed Treatment 25680
    Open Treatment 25685
    with Manipulation 25660, 25675, 25680

Dislocation, Radiocarpal Joint
See Radiocarpal Joint, Dislocation

Disorder
Blood Coagulation
  See Coagulopathy
Penis
  See Penis
Retinal
  See Retina

Displacement Therapy
Nose 30210

Dissection
Hygroma, Cystic
  Axillary/Cervical 38550-38555
Lymph Nodes 38542

Dissection, Neck, Radical
See Radical Neck Dissection

Distention
See Dilation

Diverticula, Meckel's
See Diverticulum, Meckel's

Diverticulectomy 44800
Esophagus 43130-43135

Diverticulectomy, Meckel's
See Meckel's Diverticulum, Excision

Diverticulum
Bladder
  See Bladder, Diverticulum
Meckel's
  Excision 44800
Repair
  Urethra 53400-53405

Division
Muscle
  Foot 28250
Plantar Fascia
  Foot 28250

Division, Isthmus, Horseshoe Kidney
See Symphysiotomy, Horseshoe Kidney

Division, Scalenus Anticus Muscle
See Muscle Division, Scalenus Anticus

DI-Amphetamine
See Amphetamine

DMO
See Dimethadione

DNA
Antibody 86225-86226

DNAse
Antibody 86215

Electrostimulation, Analgesic Cutaneous
See Application, Neurostimulation

Electrosurgery
Trichiasis
    Correction 67825

Electroversion, Cardiac
See Cardioversion

Elevation, Scapula, Congenital
See Sprengel's Deformity

Elliot Operation
See Excision, Lesion, Sclera

Eloesser Procedure
See Thoracostomy, Empyema

Eloesser Thoracoplasty
See Thoracoplasty

Embolectomy
Aortoiliac Artery 34151-34201
Axillary Artery 34101
Brachial Artery 34101
Carotid Artery 34001
Celiac Artery 34151
Femoral 34201
Iliac 34151-34201
Innominate Artery 34001-34101
Mesentery Artery 34151
Peroneal Artery 34203
Popliteal Artery 34203
Pulmonary Artery 33910-33916
Radial Artery 34111
Renal Artery 34151
Subclavian Artery 34001-34101
Tibial Artery 34203
Ulnar Artery 34111

Embryo
Cryopreservation 89258
Cryopreserved
  Preparation
    Transfer 89256
Culture
  with Culture
    Fertilized Oocyte 89251
Hatching
  Assisted
    Microtechnique 89253
Preparation
  for Transfer 89255

Embryonated Eggs
Inoculation 87250

Embryo /Fetus Monitoring
See Monitoring, Fetal

Embryo Implantation
See Implantation

Embryo Transfer
In Vitro Fertilization 58974-58976
  Intrafallopian Transfer 58976
  Intrauterine Transfer 58974

Emergency Department Services 99281-99288
See Critical Care; Emergency Department Services
Anesthesia 99140
Physician Direction of Advanced
Life Support 99288

Emesis Induction 99175

EMG
See Electromyography, Needle

Emission-Computed Tomography, Single-Photon
See SPECT

Emission Computerized Tomography 78607

EMI Scan
See CT Scan

Emmet Operation
See Vagina, Repair, Obstetric

Empyema
Closure
    Chest Wall 32810
Thoracostomy 32020-32036

Empyema, Lung
See Abscess, Thorax

Empyemectomy 32540

Encephalitis
Antibody 86651-86654

Encephalitis Virus Vaccine 90735

Encephalocele
Repair 62120
    Craniotomy 62121

Encephalon
See Brain

End-Expiratory Pressure, Positive
See Pressure Breathing, Positive

Endarterectomy
Coronary Artery 33572
Pulmonary..........................33916

Endemic Flea-Borne Typhus
See Murine Typhus

Endobronchial Challenge Tests
See Bronchial Challenge Test

Endocavitary Fulguration
See Electrocautery

Endocrine, Pancreas
See Islet Cell

Endocrine System
Unlisted Services and Procedures ..60699, 78099

Endolymphatic Sac
Exploration
    without Shunt 69805
    with Shunt 69806

Endometrial Ablation 0009T, 58353
Exploration
  via Hysteroscopy 58563

Endometrioma
Abdomen
  Destruction/Excision 49200-49201
Retroperitoneal
  Destruction/Excision 49200-49201

Endometriosis, Adhesive
See Adhesions, Intrauterine

Endometrium
Biopsy 58100, 58558

Endonuclease, DNA
See DNAse

Endoscopic Retrograde Cannulation of Pancreatic Duct (ERCP)
See Cholangiopancreatography

Endoscopies, Pleural
See Thoracoscopy

Endoscopy
See Arthroscopy; Thoracoscopy
Adrenal Gland
  Biopsy 60650
  Excision 60650
Anus
  Biopsy 46606
  Dilation 46604
  Exploration 46600
  Hemorrhage 46614
  Removal
    Foreign Body 46608
    Polyp 46610, 46612
    Tumor 46610, 46612
Bile Duct
  Biopsy 47553
  Destruction
    Calculi (Stone) 43265
    Tumor 43272
  Dilation 43271, 47555-47556
  Exploration 47552
  Intraoperative 47550
  Percutaneous 47552-47555
  Removal
    Calculi (Stone) 43264, 47554
    Foreign Body 43269
    Stent 43269
  Specimen Collection 43260
  Sphincterotomy 43262
  Sphincter Pressure 43263
  Tube Placement 43267-43268
Bladder 52000
  Biopsy 52204, 52354
  Catheterization 52005, 52010
  Destruction 52354
    Lesion 52400
  Evacuation
    Clot 52001
  Excision
    Tumor 52355
  Exploration 52351
  Lithotripsy 52353

Biopsy 54800-54820
Epididymography 74440
Excision
    Bilateral 54861
    Unilateral 54860
Exploration
    Biopsy 54820
Hematoma
    Incision and Drainage 54700
Lesion
    Excision
        Local 54830
        Spermatocele 54840
Needle Biopsy 54800
Spermatocele
    Excision 54840
Unlisted Services and Procedures 55899
X-Ray with Contrast 74440

Epididymograms 55300

Epididymography 74440

Epididymoplasty
See Repair, Epididymis

Epididymovasostomy
Bilateral 54901
Unilateral 54900

Epidural
Electrode
    Insertion 61531
    Removal 61535
Injection 62281-62282, 62310-62319,
                        64479-64484
Lysis 0027T, 62263-62264

Epidural Anesthesia
See Anesthesia, Epidural

Epidurography 72275

Epigastric
Hernia Repair 49572

Epiglottidectomy 31420

Epiglottis
Excision 31420

Epikeratoplasty 65767

Epilation
See Removal, Hair

Epinephrine
See Catecholamines
Blood 82383-82384
Urine 82384

Epiphyseal Arrest
Femur 20150, 27185, 27475, 27479-27485, 27742
Fibula 20150, 27477-27485, 27730-27742
Radius 20150, 25450-25455
Tibia .. 20150, 27477-27485, 27730, 27734-27742
Ulna 20150, 25450-25455

Epiphyseal Separation
Radius
    Closed Treatment 25600
    Open Treatment 25620

Epiphysiodesis
See Epiphyseal Arrest

Epiphysis
See Bone; Specific Bone

Epiploectomy 49255

Episiotomy 59300

Epispadias
Penis
    Reconstruction 54385
Repair 54380-54390
    with Exstrophy of Bladder 54390
    with Incontinence 54380-54390

Epistaxis 30901-30906
with Nasal/Sinus Endoscopy 31238

EPO
See Erythropoietin

Epstein-Barr Virus
Antibody 86663-86665

Equina, Cauda
See Cauda Equina

ERCP
See Bile Duct; Cholangiopancreatography;
Pancreatic Duct

ERG
See Electroretinography

Ergocalciferol
See Calciferol

Ergocalciferols
See Calciferol

Ergonovine Provocation Test ... 93024

Erythrocyte
See Red Blood Cell (RBC)

Erythrocyte ab
See Antibody, Red Blood Cell

Erythrocyte Count
See Red Blood Cell (RBC), Count

Erythropoietin 82668, 99554

Escharotomy
Burns 16035-16036

Escherichia coli 0157
Antigen Detection
    Enzyme Immunoassay 87335

ESD
See Endoscopy, Gastrointestinal, Upper

Esophageal Acid Infusion Test
See Acid Perfusion Test

Esophageal Polyp
See Polyp, Esophagus

Esophageal Tumor
See Tumor, Esophagus

Esophageal Varices
Ligation 43205, 43400
Transection/Repair 43401

Esophagectomy
Partial 43116-43124
Total 43107-43113, 43124

Esophagoenterostomy
with Total Gastrectomy 43620

Esophagogastroduodenoscopies
See Endoscopy, Gastrointestinal, Upper

Esophagogastromyotomy
See Esophagomyotomy

Esophagogastrostomy 43320

Esophagojejunostomy 43340-43341

Esophagomyotomy .. 32665, 43330-43331

Esophagorrhaphy
See Esophagus, Suture

Esophagoscopies
See Endoscopy, Esophagus

Esophagostomy 43350-43352
Closure 43420-43425

Esophagotomy 43020, 43045

Esophagotracheal Fistula
See Fistula, Tracheoesophageal

Esophagus
Acid Perfusion Test 91030
Acid Reflux Tests 91032-91033
Biopsy
    Endoscopy 43202
Cineradiography 74230
Dilation 43450-43458
    Endoscopic 43220-43226, 43248-43249
    Surgical 43510
Endoscopy
    Biopsy 43202
    Dilation 43220-43226
    Exploration 43200
    Hemorrhage 43227
    Injection 43201, 43204
    Insertion Stent 43219
    Needle Biopsy 43232
    Removal
        Foreign Body 43215
        Polyp 43216-43217, 43228
        Tumor 43216, 43228
    Ultrasound 43231-43232
    Vein Ligation 43205
Excision
    Diverticula 43130-43135
    Partial 43116-43124
    Total 43107-43113, 43124
Exploration
    Endoscopy 43200
Hemorrhage 43227
Incision 43020, 43045
    Muscle 43030

Tumor
Resection 58950, 58952-58954
Unlisted Services and Procedures 58999
X-Ray 74742

Fallopian Tube Pregnancy
See Ectopic Pregnancy, Tubal

Fallot, Tetralogy of
See Tetralogy of Fallot

Family Psychotherapy
See Psychotherapy, Family

Fanconi Anemia
Chromosome Analysis 88248

Farnsworth-Munsell Color Test
See Color Vision Examination

Farr Test
See Gammaglobulin, Blood

Fasanella-Servat Procedure . . .67908

Fascial Defect
Repair 50728

Fascial Graft
Free
　Microvascular Anastomosis 15758
Open Treatment
　Sternoclavicular Dislocation 23532

Fascia Graft 15840

Fascia Lata Graft
Harvesting .20920-20922

Fasciectomy
Foot 28060
　Radical 28060-28062
Palm 26121-26125

Fasciocutaneous Flaps . . .15732-15738

Fasciotomy
Arm, Lower 24495, 25020-25025
Elbow 24350-24356
Foot 28008
Hand Decompression 26037
Hip 27025
Knee 27305, 27496-27499
Leg, Lower 27600-27602, 27892-27894
Leg, Upper . . .27305, 27496-27499, 27892-27894
Palm 26040-26045
Plantar
　Endoscopic 29893
Thigh 27025
Toe 28008
Wrist 25020-25025

FAST
See Allergen Immunotherapy

Fat
Feces 82705-82715
Removal
　Lipectomy 15876-15879

Fatty Acid
Blood 82725
Very Long Chain .82726

Fat Stain
Feces 89125
Respiratory Secretions 89125
Sputum 89125
Urine 89125

Favre-Durand Disease
See Lymphogranuloma Venereum

FC Receptor 86243

FDP
See Fibrin Degradation Products

Feedback, Psychophysiologic
See Biofeedback; Training, Biofeedback

Female Castration
See Oophorectomy

Female Gonad
See Ovary

Femoral Arteries
See Artery, Femoral

Femoral Nerve
Injection
　Anesthetic 64447-64448

Femoral Stem Prosthesis
See Arthroplasty, Hip

Femoral Vein
See Vein, Femoral

Femur
See Hip; Knee; Leg, Upper
Abscess
　Incision 27303
Bursa
　Excision 27062
Craterization 27070, 27360
Cyst
　Excision 27065-27067, 27355-27358
Diaphysectomy 27360
Drainage 27303
Excision .27070, 27360
　Epiphyseal Bar 20150
Fracture 27244
Fracture
　Closed Treatment 27501-27503
　Distal 27508, 27510, 27514
　Distal, Medial or Lateral Condyle 27509
　Epiphysis 27516-27519
　Intertrochanteric 27244
　Intertrochanteric
　　Closed Treatment 27238
　　Treatment with Implant 27244
　　with Implant 27245
　　with Manipulation 27240
　Neck
　　Closed Treatment 27230-27232
　　Open Treatment 27236
　　Percutaneous Fixation 27235
　Open Treatment 27245, 27506-27507,
　　　　　　　　　　　　　　　27511-27513
　Percutaneous Fixation 27509
　Pertrochanteric 27244
　Pertrochanteric
　　Closed Treatment 27238
　　Treatment with Implant 27244

Fertility Control (continued)
　with Implant 27245
　with Manipulation 27240
Shaft 27500, 27502, 27506-27507
Subtrochanteric 27244
Subtrochanteric
　Closed Treatment 27238
　Treatment with Implant 27244
　with Implant 27245
　with Manipulation 27240
Supracondylar 27501-27503, 27509,
　　　　　　　　　　　　　　　　27511-27513
Transcondylar 27501-27503, 27509,
　　　　　　　　　　　　　　　　27511-27513
Trochanteric
　Closed Treatment 27246
　Open Treatment 27248
　without Manipulation 27501
　with Manipulation 27503
Halo 20663
Lesion
　Excision 27062
Osteoplasty
　Lengthening 27466-27468
　Shortening 27465, 27468
Osteotomy
　without Fixation 27448
Prophylactic Treatment 27187, 27495
Realignment .27454
Reconstruction 27468
　at Knee 27442-27443, 27446
　Lengthening 27466-27468
　Shortening 27465, 27468
Repair 27470-27472
　Epiphysis 27181, 27475, 27742
　　Arrest 27185
　Muscle Transfer 27110
　Osteotomy 27140, 27151-27156,
　　　　　　　　　27161-27165, 27450-27454
　with Graft .27170
Saucerization 27070, 27360
Tumor
　Excision . .27065-27067, 27355-27358, 27365
X-Ray 73550

Fenestration, Pericardium
See Pericardiostomy

Fenestration Procedure
Semicircular Canal 69820
　Revision 69840
Tracheostomy 31610

Fern Test 87210
See Smear and Stain, Wet Mount

Ferric Chloride
Urine 81005

Ferrihemoglobin
See Methemoglobin

Ferritin
Blood or Urine 82728

Ferroxidase
See Ceruloplasmin

Fertility Control
See Contraception

Finney Operation
See Gastroduodenostomy

Fishberg Concentration Test
See Water Load Test

Fissurectomy 46200

Fissurectomy, Anal
See Anus, Fissure, Excision

Fissure in Ano
See Anus, Fissure

Fistula
Anal
　　Repair 46288, 46706
Autogenous Graft 36825
Bronchi
　　Repair 32815
Carotid-Cavernous
　　Repair 61710
Chest Wall
　　Repair 32906
Conjunctiva
　　without Tube 68745
　　with Tube or Stent 68750
Enterovesical
　　Closure 44660-44661
Kidney 50520-50526
Lacrimal Gland Closure 68770
　　Dacryocystorhinostomy 68720
Nose
　　Repair 30580-30600
Oval Window 69666
Postauricular 69700
Rectovaginal
　　Abdominal Approach 57305
　　Transperineal Approach 57308
　　with Concomitant Colostomy 57307
Round Window 69667
Sclera
　　Iridencleisis or Iridotasis 66165
　　Sclerectomy with Punch or Scissors
　　with Iridectomy 66160
　　Thermocauterization with Iridectomy ..66155
　　Trabeculectomy ab Externo in
　　Absence Previous Surgery 66170
　　Trabeculectomy ab Externo with
　　Scarring 66172
　　Trephination with Iridectomy 66150
Suture
　　Kidney 50520-50526
　　Ureter 50920-50930
Trachea 31755
Tracheoesophageal
　　Repair 43305, 43312, 43314
　　Speech Prosthesis 31611
Ureter 50920-50930
Urethra 53400-53405
Urethrovaginal 57310
　　with Bulbocavernosus Transplant 57311
Vesicouterine
　　Closure 51920-51925
Vesicovaginal
　　Closure.........................51900
　　Transvesical and Vaginal Approach ..57330
　　Vaginal Approach 57320
X-Ray 76080

Fistula Arteriovenous
See Arteriovenous Fistula

Fistulectomy
Anal 46060, 46270-46285
　　See Hemorrhoids

Fistulization
Conjunction
　　to Nasal Cavity 68745
Esophagus 43350-43352
Intestines 44300-44346
Lacrimal Sac
　　to Nasal Cavity 68720
Penis 54435
Pharynx 42955
Repair Salivary Cyst
　　Sublingual 42325-42326
Tracheopharyngeal 31755

Fistulization, Interatrial
See Septostomy, Atrial

Fistulotomy
Anal 46270, 46280

Fitting
Cervical Cap 57170
Contact Lens 92070, 92310-92313
　　See Contact Lens Services
Diaphragm 57170
Low Vision Aid 92354-92355
　　See Spectacle Services
Ocular Prosthesis 92330
Spectacles 92340-92342
Spectacle Prosthesis 92352-92353

Fitzgerald Factor 85293

Fixation
Interdental
　　without Fracture 21497

Fixation, External
See External Fixation

Fixation, Kidney
See Nephropexy

Fixation, Rectum
See Proctopexy

Fixation, Tongue
See Tongue, Fixation

Fixation (Device)
See Application; Bone, Fixation; Spinal
Instrumentation
Application
　　External 20690-20692
Pelvic
　　Insertion 22848
Removal
　　External 20694
　　Internal 20670-20680
Sacrospinous Ligament
　　Vaginal Prolapse 57282
Shoulder 23700
Skeletal
　　Humeral Epycondyle
　　　Percutaneous 24566

Spinal
　　Insertion 22841-22847
　　Prosthetic.....................22851
　　Reinsertion 22849

Fixation Test, Complement
See Complement, Fixation Test

Flank
See Back/Flank

Flap
See Skin Graft and Flap
Free
　　Breast Reconstruction 19364
Grafts 15574-15650, 15842
Latissimus Dorsi
　　Breast Reconstruction 19361
Omentum 49905
Omentum
　　Free
　　　with Microvascular Anastomosis ...49906
Transverse Rectus Abdominis Myocutaneous
　　Breast Reconstruction 19367-19369

Flatfoot Correction 28735

Flea Typhus
See Murine Typhus

Fletcher Factor 85292

Flow-Volume Loop
See Pulmonology, Diagnostic
Pulmonary.........................94375

Flow Cytometry 88180-88182

Fluid, Amniotic
See Amniotic Fluid

Fluid, Body
See Body Fluid

Fluid, Cerebrospinal
See Cerebrospinal Fluid

Fluid Collection
Incision and Drainage
　　Skin 10140

Fluorescein
Angiography, Ocular 92287
Intravenous Injection
　　Vascular Flow Check, Graft 15860

Fluorescein Angiography
See Angiography, Fluorescein

Fluoride
Blood 82735
Urine 82735

Fluoroscopy
Bile Duct
　　Calculus Removal 74327
　　Guide Catheter 74328, 74330
Chest 31628
　　Complete (Four Views) 71034
　　Partial (Two Views) 71023
Drain Abscess 75989
GI Tract
　　Guide Intubation 74340

Frenum
Lip
   Incision 40806
     See Lip

Frenumectomy 40819

Frickman Operation
See Proctopexy

Frontal Craniotomy 61556

Frontal Sinus
See Sinus, Frontal

Frontal Sinusotomy
See Exploration, Sinus, Frontal

Frost Suture 67875

Frozen Blood
Preparation 86930-86932

Fructose 84375
Semen 82757

Fruit Sugar
See Fructose

FSF 85290-85291

FSH
See Follicle Stimulating Hormone (FSH)

FSP
See Fibrin Degradation Products

FT-4 84439

Fulguration
See Destruction
Bladder 51020
Cystourethroscopy with 52214
   Lesion 52224
   Tumor 52234-52240
Ureter 50957-50959, 50976-50978
Ureterocele
   Ectopic 52301
   Orthotopic 52300

Fulguration, Endocavitary
See Electrocautery

Full Thickness Graft 15200-15261

Function, Study, Nasal
See Nasal Function Study

Functional Ability
See Activities of Daily Living

Function Test, Lung
See Pulmonology, Diagnostic

Function Test, Vestibular
See Vestibular Function Tests

Fundoplasty
Esophagogastric 43324-43325
   Laparoscopic 43280
   with Gastroplasty 43326

Fundoplication
See Fundoplasty, Esophagogastric

Fungus
Antibody 86671
Culture
   Blood 87103
   Identification 87106
   Other 87102
   Skin 87101
Tissue Exam 87220

Funnel Chest
See Pectus Excavatum

Furuncle
Incision and Drainage 10060-10061

Furuncle, Vulva
See Abscess, Vulva

Fusion
See Arthrodesis
Pleural Cavity 32005
Thumb
   in Opposition 26820

Fusion, Epiphyseal-Diaphyseal
See Epiphyseal Arrest

Fusion, Joint
See Arthrodesis

Fusion, Joint, Ankle
See Ankle, Arthrodesis

Fusion, Joint, Interphalangeal, Finger
See Arthrodesis, Finger Joint, Interphalangeal

G

Gago Procedure
See Repair, Tricuspid Valve; Revision

Gait Training 97116
See Physical Medicine/Therapy/Occupational Therapy

Galactogram 76086-76088
Injection 19030

Galactokinase
Blood 82759

Galactose
Blood 82760
Urine 82760

Galactose-1-Phosphate
Uridyl Transferase 82775-82776

Gallbladder
See Bile Duct
Anastomosis
   with Intestines 47720-47741
Excision 47562-47564, 47600-47620
Exploration 47480
Incision 47490

Incision and Drainage 47480
Nuclear Medicine
   Imaging 78223
Removal
   Calculi (Stone) 47480
Repair
   with Gastroenterostomy 47741
   with Intestines 47720-47740
Unlisted Services and Procedures 47999
X-Ray with Contrast 74290-74291

Gall Bladder
See Gallbladder

Galvanocautery
See Electrocautery

Galvanoionization
See Iontophoresis

Gamete Intrafallopian Transfer
See GIFT

Gamete Transfer
In Vitro Fertilization 58976

Gammacorten
See Dexamethasone

Gammaglobulin
Blood 82784-82787

Gamma Camera Imaging
See Nuclear Medicine

Gamma Glutamyl Transferase 82977

Gamma Seminoprotein
See Antigen, Prostate Specific

Gamulin Rh
See Immune Globulins, Rho (D)

Ganglia, Trigeminal
See Gasserian Ganglion

Ganglion
See Gasserian Ganglion
Cyst
   Aspiration/Injection 20612
   Drainage 20612
   Wrist
    Excision 25111-25112
Injection
   Anesthetic 64505, 64510

Ganglion, Gasser's
See Gasserian Ganglion

Ganglion Cervicothoracicum
See Stellate Ganglion

Ganglion Pterygopalatinum
See Sphenopalatine Ganglion

Gardnerella Vaginalis Detection 87510-87512

Gardner Operation
See Meningocele Repair

Gasserian Ganglion
Sensory Root
Decompression 61450
Section 61450
Stereotactic 61790

Gasser Ganglion
See Gasserian Ganglion

Gastrectomy
Partial 43631-43639
    with Gastrojejunostomy 43632
Total 43621-43622
    with Esophagoenterostomy 43620
with Gastroduodenostomy 43631

Gastric Acid 82926-82928

Gastric Analysis Test 91052

Gastric Intubation ...89130-89141, 91105

Gastric Lavage, Therapeutic ...91105

Gastric Tests
Manometry 91020

Gastric Ulcer Disease
See Stomach, Ulcer

Gastrin 82938-82941

Gastrocnemius Recession
Leg, Lower 27687

Gastroduodenostomy 43810, 43850-43855

Gastroenterology, Diagnostic
Breath Hydrogen Test 91065
Esophagus Tests
    Acid Perfusion 91030
    Acid Reflux 91032-91033
    Intubation with Specimen Collection ..91000
    Motility Study 91010-91012
Gastric Tests
    Manometry 91020
Intestine
    Bleeding Tube 91100
Manometry 91020
Rectum/Anus
    Manometry 91122
Stomach
    Intubation with Specimen Prep 91055
    Saline Load Test 91060
    Stimulation of Secretion 91052
Unlisted Services and Procedures 91299

Gastroenterostomy
for Obesity 43846

Gastrointestinal, Upper
Biopsy
    Endoscopy 43239
Dilation
    Endoscopy 43245
    Esophagus 43248
Endoscopy
    Catheterization 43241
    Destruction
        Lesion 43258

Dilation 43245
Drainage
    Pseudocyst 43240
Exploration 43234-43235
Hemorrhage 43255
Injection 43236
Inject Varices 43243
Needle Biopsy 43242
Removal
    Foreign Body 43247
    Lesion 43251
    Polyp 43251
    Tumor 43251
Stent Placement 43256
Suturing
    Esophagogastric junction 0008T
Tube Placement 43246
Ultrasound 43242, 76975
Exploration
    Endoscopy 43234-43235
Hemorrhage
    Endoscopic Control 43255
Injection
    Submucosal 43236
    Varices 43243
Lesion
    Destruction 43258
Ligation of Vein 43244
Needle Biopsy
    Endoscopy 43242
Removal
    Foreign Body 43247
    Lesion 43250
    Polyp 43250-43251
    Tumor 43250
Tube Placement
    Endoscopy 43246
Ultrasound
    Endoscopy 43242, 43259

Gastrointestinal Endoscopies
See Endoscopy, Gastrointestinal

Gastrointestinal Exam
Nuclear Medicine
    Blood Loss Study 78278
    Protein Loss Study 78282
    Shunt Testing 78291
    Unlisted Services and Procedures 78299

Gastrointestinal Tract
Reconstruction 43360-43361
Upper
    Dilation 43249
X-Ray 74240-74245
    Guide Dilator 74360
    Guide Intubation 74340-74350
    with Contrast 74246-74249

Gastrojejunostomy 43860-43865
without Vagotomy 43820
with Duodenal Exclusion 48547
with Partial Gastrectomy 43632
with Vagotomy 43825

Gastroplasty
Revision
    for Obesity 43848

Gastroplasty with Esophagogastric Fundoplasty 43326, 43842-43843

Gastrorrhaphy 43840

Gastroschises
See Gastroschisis

Gastroschisis 49605

Gastrostomy
Closure 43870
Laparoscopic
    Temporary 43653
Temporary 43830
    Laparoscopic 43653
    Neonatal 43831
with Pancreatic Drain 48001
with Pyloroplasty 43640
with Vagotomy 43640

Gastrostomy Tube
Change of 43760
Directed Placement
    Endoscopic 43246
Insertion
    Percutaneous 43750
Percutaneous 43750
Repositioning 43761

Gastrotomy 43500-43501, 43510

GDH
See Glutamate Dehydrogenase

Gel Diffusion 86331

Gel Diffusion Test
See Immunodiffusion

Gene Product
See Protein

Genioplasty 21120-21123
Augmentation 21120, 21123
Osteotomy 21121-21123

Genitourinary Sphincter, Artificial
See Prosthesis, Urethral Sphincter

Genotype Analysis
by Nucleic Acid
    Infectious Agent
        Hepatitis C Virus 87902
        HIV-1 Protease/Reverse
        Transcriptase 87901

Gentamicin 80170
Assay 80170

Gentamycin Level
See Gentamicin

Gentiobiase
See Beta Glucosidase

Genus: Human Cytomegalovirus Group
See Cytomegalovirus

German Measles
See Rubella

Gestational Trophoblastic Tumor
See Hydatidiform Mole

GGT
See Gamma Glutamyl Transferase

Giardia Lamblia
Antibody 86674

Gibbons Stent 52332

GIF
See Somatostatin

GIFT 89250

Gillies Approach
Fracture
    Zygomatic Arch 21356

Gill Operation 63012

Gingiva
See Gums

Gingiva, Abcess
See Abscess
Fracture
  See Abscess, Gums; Gums
    Zygomatic Arch
      See Abscess, Gums; Gums, Abscess

Gingivectomy 41820

Gingivoplasty 41872

Girdlestone Laminectomy
See Laminectomy

Girdlestone Procedure
See Acetabulum, Reconstruction

GI Tract
See Gastrointestinal Tract

Gland
See Specific Gland

Gland, Adrenal
See Adrenal Gland

Gland, Bartholin's
See Bartholin's Gland

Gland, Bulbourethral
See Bulbourethral Gland

Gland, Lacrimal
See Lacrimal Gland

Gland, Mammary
See Breast

Gland, Parathyroid
See Parathyroid Gland

Gland, Parotid
See Parotid Gland

Gland, Pituitary
See Pituitary Gland

Gland, Salivary
See Salivary Glands

Gland, Sublingual
See Sublingual Gland

Gland, Sweat
See Sweat Glands

Gland, Thymus
See Thymus Gland

Gland, Thyroid
See Thyroid Gland

Glasses
See Spectacle Services

Glaucoma
Fistulization of Sclera 66150
Provocative Test .92140

Glaucoma Drainage Implant
See Aqueous Shunt

Gla Protein (Bone)
See Osteocalcin

Glenn Procedure 33766-33767

Glenohumeral Joint
Arthrotomy 23040
  with Biopsy 23100
  with Synovectomy 23105
Exploration 23107
Removal
  Foreign or Loose Body 23107

Glenoid Fossa
Reconstruction 21255

GLN
See Glutamine

Globulin
Antihuman 86880-86886
Immune 90281-90399
Sex Hormone Binding 84270

Globulin, Corticosteroid-Binding
See Transcortin

Globulin, Rh Immune
See Immune Globulins, Rho (D)

Globulin, Thyroxine-Binding
See Thyroxine Binding Globulin

Glomerular Procoagulant Activity
See Thromboplastin

Glomus Caroticum
See Carotid Body

Glossectomies
See Excision, Tongue

Glossopexy
See Tongue, Fixation

Glossorrhaphy
See Suture, Tongue

Glucagon 82943
Tolerance Panel 80422-80424
Tolerance Test 82946

Glucose . .80422-80424, 80430-80435, 95250
Blood Test 82947-82950, 82962
Body Fluid 82945
Interstitial Fluid
  Continuous Monitoring 95250
Tolerance Test 82951-82952
  with Tolbutamide 82953

Glucose-6-Phosphate
Dehydrogenase 82955-82960

Glucose Phosphate Isomerase
See Phosphohexose Isomerase

Glucose Phosphate Isomerase Measurement
See Phosphohexose Isomerase

Glucosidase 82963

Glucuronide Androstanediol . . .82154

Glue
Cornea Wound 65286
Sclera Wound 65286

Glukagon
See Glucagon

Glutamate Dehydrogenase
Blood 82965

Glutamate Pyruvate Transaminase
See Transaminase, Glutamic Pyruvic

Glutamic Alanine Transaminase
See Transaminase, Glutamic Pyruvic

Glutamic Aspartic Transaminase
See Transaminase, Glutamic Oxaloacetic

Glutamic Dehydrogenase
See Glutamate Dehydrogenase

Glutamine 82975

Glutamyltransferase, Gamma 82977

Glutathione 82978

Glutathione Reductase 82979

Glutethimide 82980

Glycanhydrolase, N-Acetylmuramide
See Lysozyme

Glycated Hemoglobins
See Glycohemoglobin

Glycated Protein 82985

Glycerol, Phosphatidyl
See Phosphatidylglycerol

Glycerol Phosphoglycerides
See Phosphatidylglycerol

Glycerophosphatase
See Alkaline Phosphatase

Glycinate, Theophylline Sodium
See Theophylline

Glycocholic Acid
See Cholylglycine

Glycohemoglobin 83036

Glycol, Ethylene
See Ethylene Glycol

Glycols, Ethylene
See Ethylene Glycol

Glycosaminoglycan
See Mucopolysaccharides

GMP
See Guanosine Monophosphate

GMP, Cyclic
See Cyclic GMP

**Goeckerman
Treatment** 96910-96913

Gol-Vernet Operation
See Pyelotomy, Exploration

Gold
Assay 80172

Goldwaite Procedure 27422

Golfer's Elbow
See Tennis Elbow

Gonadectomy, Female
See Oophorectomy

Gonadectomy, Male
See Excision, Testis

Gonadotropin
Chorionic 84702-84703
FSH 83001
ICSH 83002
LH 83002

Gonadotropin Panel 80426

Gonioscopy 92020

Goniotomy .65820

Gonococcus
See Neisseria Gonorrhoeae

**Goodenough Harris
Drawing Test** 96100

GOTT
See Transaminase, Glutamic Oxaloacetic

GPUT
See Galactose-1-Phosphate, Uridyl Transferase

Graft
See Bone Graft; Bypass Graft
Anal 46753
Aorta 33840-33851, 33860-33877
Artery
    Coronary 33503-33505
Bone
    See Bone Marrow, Transplantation
    Harvesting 20900-20902
    Microvascular Anastomosis 20955-20962

Osteocutaneous Flap with Microvascular
    Anastomosis 20969-20973
    Vascular Pedicle 25430
Bone and Skin 20969-20973
Cartilage
    Ear to Face 21235
    Harvesting 20910-20912
        See Cartilage Graft
    Rib to Face 21230
Cornea
    with Lesion Excision 65426
Cornea Transplant
    in Aphakia 65750
    in Pseudophakia 65755
    Lamellar 65710
    Penetrating 65730
Dura
    Spinal Cord 63710
Endovascular 34900
Facial Nerve Paralysis 15840-15845
Fascia
    Cheek 15840
Fascia Lata
    Harvesting 20920-20922
Gum Mucosa 41870
Heart
    See Heart, Transplantation
Heart Lung
    See Transplantation, Heart-Lung
Kidney
    See Kidney, Transplantation
Liver
    See Liver, Transplantation
Lung
    See Lung, Transplantation
Muscle
    Cheek 15841-15845
Nail Bed
    Reconstruction 11762
Nerve .64885-64907
Oral Mucosa 40818
Organ
    See Transplantation
Pancreas
    See Pancreas, Transplantation
Skin
    Biological
        See Allograft, Skin
    Blood Flow Check, Graft 15860
        See Skin Graft and Flap
    Vascular Flow Check, Graft 15860
Tendon
    Finger 26392
    Hand 26392
    Harvesting 20924
Tissue
    Harvesting 20926
Vein
    Cross-Over 34520

Grain Alcohol
See Alcohol, Ethyl

Granulation Tissue
Cauterization, Chemical 17250

Gravi, Myasthenia
See Myasthenia Gravis

Gravities, Specific
See Specific Gravity

Greater Tuberosity Fracture
with Shoulder Dislocation
    Closed Treatment 23665
    Open Treatment 23670

Greater Vestibular Gland
See Bartholin's Gland

Great Toe
Free Osteocutaneous Flap with
Microvascular Anastomosis 20973

Great Vessels
Shunt
    Aorta to Pulmonary Artery
        Ascending 33755
        Descending 33762
        Central 33764
        Subclavian to Pulmonary Artery 33750
        Vena Cava to Pulmonary
        Artery 33766-33767
Unlisted Services and Procedures 33999

Great Vessels Transposition
See Transposition, Great Arteries

Green Operation
See Scapulopexy

Gridley Stain 88312

Grippe, Balkan
See Q Fever

Gritti Operation
See Amputation, Leg, Upper; Radical Resection;
Replantation

Groin Area
Repair
    Hernia 49550-49557

Grouping, Blood
See Blood Typing

Group Health Education 99078

Growth Factors, Insulin-Like
See Somatomedin

Growth Hormone 83003
Human 80418, 80428-80430, 86277

**Growth Hormone Release
Inhibiting Factor**
See Somatostatin

GTT
See Hydatidiform Mole

Guaiac Test
See Blood, Feces

Guanosine Monophosphate 83008

Guanosine Monophosphate, Cyclic
See Cyclic GMP

Guanylic Acids
See Guanosine Monophosphate

Guard Stain 88313

Gullet
See Esophagus

Gums
Abscess
　　Incision and Drainage 41800
Alveolus
　　Excision 41830
Cyst
　　Incision and Drainage 41800
Excision
　　Gingiva 41820
　　Operculum .41821
Graft
　　Mucosa 41870
Hematoma
　　Incision and Drainage 41800
Lesion
　　Destruction 41850
　　Excision 41822-41828
Mucosa
　　Excision 41828
Reconstruction
　　Alveolus 41874
　　Gingiva 41872
Removal
　　Foreign Body 41805
Tumor
　　Excision 41825-41827
Unlisted Services and Procedures 41899

Gunning-Lieben Test
See Acetone, Blood or Urine

Guthrie Test 84030

H

H-Reflex Study 95934-95936

HAAb
See Antibody, Hepatitis

HAA (Hepatitis Associated Antigen)
See Hepatitis Antigen, B Surface

Haemoglobin F
See Fetal Hemoglobin

Haemorrhage
See Hemorrhage

Haemorrhage Rectum
See Hemorrhage, Rectum

Hageman Factor 85280

Hair
Electrolysis 17380
KOH Examination 87220
Microscopic Evaluation 96902
Transplant
　　Punch Graft 15775-15776
　　Strip Graft 15220-15221

Hair Removal
See Removal, Hair

HAI Test
See Hemagglutination Inhibition Test

Hallux
See Great Toe

Halo
Body Cast 29000
Cranial 20661
　　for Thin Skull Osteology 20664
Femur 20663
Maxillofacial .21100
Pelvic 20662
Removal 20665

Haloperidol
Assay 80173

Halsted Mastectomy
See Mastectomy, Radical

Halsted Repair
See Hernia, Repair, Inguinal

Hammertoe Repair 28285-28286

Hamster Penetration Test 89329

Ham Test
See Hemolysins

Hand
See Carpometacarpal Joint; Intercarpal Joint
Amputation
　　at Metacarpal 25927
　　at Wrist 25920
　　　　Revision 25922
　　Revision 25924, 25929-25931
Arthrodesis
　　Carpometacarpal Joint 26843-26844
　　Intercarpal Joint 25820-25825
Bone
　　Incision and Drainage 26034
Cast 29085
Decompression 26035-26037
Fracture
　　Metacarpal 26600
Insertion
　　Tendon Graft 26392
Magnetic Resonance Imaging
(MRI) .73218-73223
Reconstruction
　　Tendon Pulley 26500-26504
Removal
　　Implantation 26320
　　　　Tube/Rod 26390-26392, 26416
Repair
　　Blood Vessel 35207
　　Cleft Hand 26580
　　Muscle 26591-26593
　　Tendon
　　　　Extensor 26410-26416, 26426-26428,
　　　　　　　　　　　　　　　　　　 26433-26437
　　　　Flexor 26350-26358, 26440
　　　　Profundus 26370-26373
Replantation .20808
Strapping 29280

Tendon
　　Excision 26390
　　　　Extensor 26415
Tenotomy 26450, 26460
Tumor
　　Excision 26115-26117
Unlisted Services and Procedures 26989
X-Ray .73120-73130

Hand(s) Dupuytrens Contracture(s)
See Dupuytren's Contracture

Handling
Device 99002
Radioelement .77790
Specimen 99000-99001

Hand Abscess
See Abscess, Hand

Hand Phalange
See Finger, Bone

Hanganutziu Deicher Antibodies
See Antibody, Heterophile

Haptoglobin 83010-83012

Hard Palate
See Palate

Harelip Operation
See Cleft Lip, Repair

Harii Procedure 25430

Harrington Rod
Insertion 22840
Removal 22850

Hartmann Procedure 44143
Laparoscopy
　　Partial Colectomy with Colostomy 44206

Harvesting
Bone Graft 20900-20902
Bone Marrow .38230
Cartilage Graft 20910-20912
Eggs
　　In Vitro Fertilization 58970
Endoscopic
　　Vein for Bypass Graft 33508
Fascia Lata Graft 20920-20922
Intestines 44132-44133
Kidney 50300-50320, 50547
Liver .47133-47134
Lower Extremity Vein
　　for Vascular Reconstruction 35572
Stem Cell 38205-38206
Tendon Graft .20924
Tissue Grafts .20926
Upper Extremity Artery
　　for Coronary Artery Bypass Graft 35600
Upper Extremity Vein
　　for Bypass Graft 35500

Hauser Procedure 27420

Hayem's Elementary Corpuscle
See Blood, Platelet

Haygroves Procedure
See Reconstruction, Acetabulum; Revision

HBcAb
See Antibody, Hepatitis

HBeAb
See Antibody, Hepatitis

HBeAg
See Hepatitis Antigen, Be

HBsAb
See Antibody, Hepatitis

HBsAg (Hepatitis B Surface Antigen)
See Hepatitis Antigen, B Surface

HCG
See Chorionic Gonadotropin

HCO3
See Bicarbonate

HCV Antibodies
See Antibody, Hepatitis C

HDL
See Lipoprotein

Head
Angiography 70496, 70544-70546
CT Scan 70450-70470, 70496
Excision 21015-21040, 21044-21070
Fracture and/or Dislocation 21300-21497
Incision 21010, 61316, 62148
Introduction or Removal 21076-21116
Lipectomy, Suction Assisted 15876
Magnetic Resonance Angiography
(MRA) 70544-70546
Nerve
    Graft 64885-64886
Other Procedures 21299, 21499
Repair/Revision and/or
Reconstruction 21120-21296
Ultrasound Exam 76506, 76536
Unlisted Services and Procedures 21499
X-Ray 70350

Headbrace
Application 21100
Application/Removal 20661

Head Rings, Stereotactic
See Stereotactic Frame

Heaf Test
See TB Test

Health Behavior
See Evaluation and Management, Health Behavior

Health Risk Assessment Instrument
See Preventive Medicine

Hearing Aid
Bone Conduction
    Implantation 69710
    Removal 69711
    Repair 69711
    Replacement 69710

Hearing Aid Check 92592-92593

Hearing Aid Services
Electroacoustic Test 92594-92595
Examination 92590-92591

Hearing Evaluation 92510

Hearing Tests
See Audiologic Function Tests; Hearing Evaluation

Hearing Therapy 92507-92510,
                              92601-92604

Heart
Ablation
    Ventricular Septum
        Non-surgical 0024T
Angiography
    Injection 93542-93543
        See Cardiac Catheterization; Injection
Aortic Arch
    without Cardiopulmonary Bypass 33852
    with Cardiopulmonary Bypass 33853
Aortic Valve
    Repair
        Left Ventricle 33414
    Replacement 33405-33413
Arrhythmogenic Focus
    Catheter Ablation 93650-93652
    Destruction 33250-33251, 33261
Atria
    See Atria
Biopsy 93505
    Imaging Guidance 76932
    Ultrasound
        Imaging Guidance 76932
Blood Vessel
    Repair 33320-33322
Cardiac Output Measurements 93561-93562
Cardiac Rehabilitation 93797-93798
Cardioassist 92970-92971
Cardiopulmonary Bypass
    with Lung Transplant 32852, 32854
Catheterization 93501, 93510-93533
    Combined Right and Retrograde Left
        for Congenital Cardiac Anomalies ...93531
    Combined Right and Transseptal Left
        for Congenital Cardiac
        Anomalies 93532-93533
    Flow Directed 93503
    Right
        for Congenital Cardiac Anomalies ...93530
        See Catheterization, Cardiac
Closure
    Septal Defect 33615
Valve
    Atrioventricular 33600
    Semilunar 33602
Commissurotomy
    Right Ventricle 33476-33478
Destruction
    Arrhythmogenic Focus 33250, 33261
Electrical Recording
    3-D Mapping 93613
    Atria 93602
    Atrial Electrogram, Esophageal
    (or Trans-esophageal) 93615-93616

Bundle of His 93600
Comprehensive 93619-93622
Right Ventricle 93603
Tachycardia Sites 93609
Electroconversion 92960-92961
Electrophysiologic Follow-up Study 93624
Excision
    Donor 33930, 33940
    Tricuspid Valve 33460
Fibrillation
    Atrial 33253
Great Vessels
    See Great Vessels
Heart-Lung Bypass
    See Cardiopulmonary Bypass
Heart-Lung Transplantation
    See Transplantation, Heart-Lung
Implantation
    Ventricular Assist Device 33976
        Intracorporeal 33979
Incision
    Atrial 33253
    Exploration 33310-33315
Injection
    Radiologic 93542-93543
        See Cardiac Catheterization, Injection
Insertion
    Balloon Device 33973
    Defibrillator 33246
    Electrode 33210-33211, 33216-33217,
                              33224-33225
    Pacemaker 33200-33208
        Catheter 33210
        Pulse Generator 33212-33213
    Ventricular Assist Device 33975
Intraoperative Pacing and Mapping 93631
Ligation
    Fistula 37607
Magnetic Resonance Imaging
(MRI) 75552-75553
Mitral Valve
    See Mitral Valve
Muscle
    See Myocardium
Myocardium
    Imaging 78466-78469
    Perfusion Study 78460-78465
Nuclear Medicine
    Blood Flow Study 78414
    Blood Pool Imaging 78472-78473,
                      78481-78483, 78494-78496
    Myocardial Imaging 78466-78469
    Myocardial Perfusion 78460-78465
    Shunt Detection 78428
    Unlisted Services and Procedures 78499
Open Chest Massage 32160
Output
    See Cardiac Output
Pacemaker
    Conversion 33214
    Insertion 33200-33208
        Pulse Generator 33212-33213
    Removal 33233-33237
    Replacement 33206-33208
        Catheter 33210
    Upgrade 33214

Pacing
    Arrhythmia Induction 93618
    Atria 93610
    Transcutaneous
        Temporary 92953
    Ventricular 93612
Pacing Cardioverter-Defibrillator
    Evaluation and Testing 93640-93642,
                      93740-93744
    Insertion Single/Dual Chamber
        Electrodes 33216-33217,
              33224-33225, 33245-33249
        Pulse Generator 33240, 33246
    Repositioning Single/Dual Chamber
        Electrodes 33215, 33226
Positron Emission Tomography (PET) 78459
    Perfusion Study 78491-78492
Pulmonary Valve
    See Pulmonary Valve
Rate Increase
    See Tachycardia
Reconstruction
    Atrial Septum 33735-33737
    Vena Cava 34502
Reduction
    Ventricular Septum
        Non-surgical 0024T
Removal
    Balloon Device 33974
    Electrode 33238
    Ventricular Assist Device 33977-33978
        Intracorporeal 33980
Removal Single/Dual Chamber
    Electrodes 33243-33244
    Pulse Generator 33241
    Repair 33218-33220
Repair
    Anomaly 33615-33617
    Aortic Sinus 33702-33722
    Atrial Septum 33253, 33641, 33647
    Atrioventricular Canal 33660-33665
        Complete .33670
        Prosthetic Valve 33670
    Atrioventricular Valve 33660-33665
    Cor Triatriatum 33732
    Electrode 33218
    Fenestration 93580
    Infundibular 33476-33478
    Mitral Valve 33420-33430
    Myocardium 33542
    Outflow Tract 33476-33478
    Postinfarction 33542-33545
    Prosthetic Valve Dysfunction 33496
    Septal Defect 33608-33610, 33660,
                33813-33814, 93581
    Sinus of Valsalva 33702-33722
    Sinus Venosus 33645
    Tetralogy of Fallot 33692-33697, 33924
    Tricuspid Valve 33463-33468
    Ventricle 33611-33612
        Obstruction 33619
    Ventricular Septum 33545, 33647,
          33681-33688, 33692-33697, 93581
    Ventricular Tunnel 33722
    Wound 33300-33305

Replacement
    Electrode 33210-33211, 33217
    Mitral Valve 33430
    Tricuspid Valve 33465
Repositioning
    Electrode 33215, 33217, 33226
    Tricuspid Valve 33468
Resuscitation 92950
Septal Defect
    See Septal Defect
Stimulation and Pacing 93623
Transplantation 33935, 33945
Tricuspid Valve
    See Tricuspid Valve
Tumor
    Excision 33120-33130
Unlisted Services and Procedures 33999
Ventriculography
    See Ventriculography
Ventriculomyectomy 33416
Wound
    Repair 33300-33305

Heart Vessels
Angioplasty
    Percutaneous 92982-92984
        See Angioplasty; Percutaneous
        Transluminal Angioplasty
Insertion
    Graft 33330-33335
Thrombolysis 92975-92977
Valvuloplasty
    See Valvuloplasty
    Percutaneous 92986-92990

Heat Unstable Haemoglobin
See Hemoglobin, Thermolabile

Heavy Lipoproteins
See Lipoprotein

Heavy Metal 83015-83018

Heel
See Calcaneus
Collection of Blood 36415-36416
X-Ray 73650

Heel Bone
See Calcaneus

Heel Fracture
See Calcaneus, Fracture

Heel Spur
Excision 28119

Heine-Medin Disease
See Polio

Heine Operation
See Cyclodialysis

Heinz Bodies 85441-85445

Helicobacter Pylori
Antibody 86677
Antigen Detection
    Enzyme Immunoassay 87338-87339
Breath Test 78267-78268, 83013-83014
Stool 87338
Urease Activity 83013-83014

Heller Operation
See Esophagomyotomy

Heller Procedure 32665, 43330-43331

Helminth
Antibody 86682

Hemagglutination Inhibition
Test 86280

Hemangioma
See Lesion, Skin; Tumor

Hemapheresis
See Apheresis

Hematochezia
See Blood, Feces

Hematologic Test
See Blood Tests

Hematology
Unlisted Services and Procedures 85999

Hematoma
Ankle 27603
Arm, Lower 25028
Arm, Upper
    Incision and Drainage 23930
Brain
    Drainage 61154-61156
    Evacuation 61312-61315
    Incision and Drainage 61312-61315
Drain 61108
Ear, External
    Complicated 69005
    Simple 69000
Elbow
    Incision and Drainage 23930
Epididymis
    Incision and Drainage 54700
Gums
    Incision and Drainage 41800
Hip 26990
Incision and Drainage
    Neck 21501-21502
    Skin 10140
    Thorax 21501-21502
Knee 27301
Leg, Lower 27603
Leg, Upper 27301
Mouth 41005-41009, 41015-41018
    Incision and Drainage 40800-40801
Nasal Septum
    Incision and Drainage 30020
Nose
    Incision and Drainage 30000-30020
Pelvis 26990
Scrotum
    Incision and Drainage 54700
Shoulder
    Drainage 23030
Skin
    Puncture Aspiration 10160
Subdural 61108
Subungual
    Evacuation .11740

Testis
Incision and Drainage 54700
Tongue 41000-41006, 41015
Vagina
Incision and Drainage 57022-57023
Wrist 25028

Hematopoietic Stem Cell Transplantation
See Stem Cell, Transplantation

Hematopoietin
See Erythropoietin

Hematuria
See Blood, Urine

Hemic System
Unlisted Procedure 38999

Hemiepiphyseal Arrest
Elbow 24470

Hemifacial Microsomia
Reconstruction
Mandibular Condyle 21247

Hemilaminectomy 63020-63044

Hemilaryngectomy 31370-31382

Hemipelvectomies
See Amputation, Interpelviabdominal

Hemiphalangectomy
Toe 28160

Hemispherectomy
Partial 61543
Total 61542

Hemocytoblast
See Stem Cell

Hemodialyses
See Hemodialysis

Hemodialysis 90935-90937, 99512
Blood Flow Study 90939-90940
Duplex Scan of Access 93990

Hemofiltration 90945-90947

Hemoglobin 83036
Analysis
O2 Affinity 82820
Antibody
Carboxyhemoglobin 82375-82376
Chromatography 83021
Concentration 85046
Electrophoresis 83020
Fetal 83030-83033, 85460-85461
Fractionation and Quantitation 83020
Methemoglobin 83045-83050
Non-Automated 83026
Plasma 83051
Sulfhemoglobin 83055-83060
Thermolabile 83065-83068
Urine 83069

Hemoglobin, Glycosylated
See Glycohemoglobin

Hemoglobin F
Fetal
Chemical 83030
Qualitative .83033

Hemogram
Added Indices 85025-85027
Automated 85025-85027
Manual 85014, 85018, 85032

Hemolysins 85475
with Agglutinins 86940-86941

Hemolytic Complement
See Complement, Hemolytic

Hemolytic Complement, Total
See Complement, Hemolytic, Total

Hemoperfusion 90997

Hemophil
See Clotting Factor

Hemophilus Influenza
Antibody 86684

Hemorrhage
Abdomen 49002
Anal
Endoscopic Control 46614
Bladder
Postoperative 52606
Chest Cavity
Endoscopic Control 32654
Colon
Endoscopic Control 44391, 45382
Colon-Sigmoid
Endoscopic Control 45334
Esophagus
Endoscopic Control 43227
Gastrointestinal, Upper
Endoscopic Control 43255
Intestines, Small
Endoscopic Control 44366, 44378
Liver
Control 47350
Lung 32110
Nasal
Cauterization 30901-30906
Endoscopic Control 31238
Nasopharynx 42970-42972
Oropharynx 42960-42962
Rectum
Endoscopic Control 45317
Throat .42960-42962
Uterus
Postpartum .59160
Vagina 57180

Hemorrhoidectomy
Complex 46260
with Fissurectomy 46261-46262
External Complete 46250
Ligature 46221
Simple 46255
with Fissurectomy 46257-46258

Hemorrhoids
Destruction 46934-46936
Incision
External 46083
Injection
Sclerosing Solution 46500
Ligation 46945-46946
Suture .46945-46946

Hemosiderin 83070-83071

Hemothorax
Thoracostomy .32020

Heparin 85520
See Clotting Inhibitors
Neutralization .85525
Protamine Tolerance Test 85530

Heparin Cofactor I
See Antithrombin III

Hepatectomy
Extensive 47122
Left Lobe 47125
Partial
Donor 47134
Lobe 47120
Right Lobe 47130
Total
Donor 47133

Hepaticodochotomy
See Hepaticostomy

Hepaticoenterostomy 47802

Hepaticostomy 47400

Hepaticotomy 47400

Hepatic Abscess
See Abscess, Liver

Hepatic Arteries
See Artery, Hepatic

Hepatic Artery Aneurysm
See Artery, Hepatic, Aneurysm

Hepatic Duct
Anastomosis
with Intestines 47765, 47802
Exploration 47400
Incision and Drainage 47400
Nuclear Medicine
Imaging 78223
Removal
Calculi (Stone) 47400
Repair
with Intestines 47765, 47802
Unlisted Services and Procedures 47999

Hepatic Haemorrhage
See Hemorrhage, Liver

Hepatic Portal Vein
See Vein, Hepatic Portal

Hepatic Portoenterostomies
See Hepaticoenterostomy

Hepatic Transplantation
See Liver, Transplantation

Hepatitis Antibody
A 86708-86709
B
   Be 86707
   B Core 86704-86705
   B Surface 86706
C 86803-86804
Delta Agent 86692
IgG 86704, 86708
IgM 86704-86705, 86708-86709

Hepatitis Antigen
B 87515-87517
Be 87350
B Surface 87340-87341
C 87520-87522
Delta Agent 87380
G 87525-87527

Hepatitis A and Hepatitis B 90636

Hepatitis A Vaccine
Adolescent/Pediatric
   2 Dose Schedule 90633
   3 Dose Schedule 90634
Adult Dosage 90632

Hepatitis B and Hib 90748

Hepatitis B Vaccine
Dosage
   Adolescent 90743
   Adult 90746
   Immunosuppressed 90740, 90747
   Pediatric/Adolescent 90744

Hepatitis B Virus E Antibody
See Antibody, Hepatitis

Hepatitis B Virus Surface ab
See Antibody, Hepatitis B, Surface

Hepatorrhaphy
See Liver, Repair

Hepatotomy
Abscess 47010-47011
   Percutaneous 47011
Cyst 47010-47011
   Percutaneous 47011

Hernia
Repair
   Abdominal 49590
     Incisional 49560
     Recurrent 49565
   Diaphragmatic 39502-39541
   Epigastric 49570
     Incarcerated 49572
   Femoral 49550
     Incarcerated 49553
     Recurrent 49555
     Recurrent Incarcerated 49557
   Incisional
     Incarcerated 49561

   Inguinal 49491, 49495-49500, 49505
     Incarcerated 49492, 49496, 49501,
            49507, 49521
     Laparoscopic 49650-49651
     Recurrent 49520
     Sliding 49525
     Strangulated 49492
   Lumbar 49540
   Lung 32800
   Orchiopexy 54640
   Recurrent Incisional
     Incarcerated 49566
   Umbilicus 49580, 49585
     Incarcerated 49582, 49587
   with Spermatic Cord 55540
Spigelian 49590

Hernia, Cerebral
See Encephalocele

Hernia, Rectovaginal
See Rectocele

Hernia, Umbilical
See Omphalocele

Heroin, Alkaloid Screening 82101

Heroin Screen 82486

Herpesvirus 4 (Gamma), Human
See Epstein-Barr Virus

Herpes Simplex
Antibody 86696
Antigen Detection
   Immunofluorescence 87273-87274
   Nucleic Acid 87528-87530

Herpes Smear 87207
Herpes Virus-6 Detection 87531-87533

Herpes Virus-6
Detection 87531-87533

Herpetic Vesicle
Destruction 54050-54065

Heteroantibodies
See Antibody, Heterophile

Heterograft
Skin 15400

Heterologous Transplant
See Xenograft

Heterologous Transplantation
See Heterograft

Heterophile Antibody 86308-86310

Heterotropia
See Strabismus

Hexadecadrol
See Dexamethasone

Hexosephosphate Isomerase
See Phosphohexose Isomerase

Hex B
See b-Hexosaminidase

Heyman Procedure 27179, 28264

HGB
See Hemoglobin, Concentration

HGH
See Growth Hormone, Human

Hg Factor
See Glucagon

HHV-4
See Epstein-Barr Virus

HIAA
See Hydroxyindolacetic Acid, Urine

Hibb Operation
See Spinal Cord; Spine, Fusion; Vertebra;
Vertebral Body; Vertebral Process

Hib Vaccine
4 Dose Schedule
   HbOC 90645
   PRP-T 90648
PRP-D
   Booster 90646
PRP-OMP
   3 Dose Schedule 90647

Hickmann Catheterization
See Cannulization; Catheterization, Venous;
Central Line; Venipuncture

Hidradenitis
See Sweat Gland
Excision 11450-11471
Suppurative
   Incision and Drainage 10060-10061

Highly Selective Vagotomy
See Vagotomy, Highly Selective

Highmore Antrum
See Sinus, Maxillary

High Density Lipoprotein
See Lipoprotein

High Molecular Weight Kininogen
See Fitzgerald Factor

Hill Procedure 43324
Laparoscopic 43280

Hinton Positive
See RPR

Hip
See Femur; Pelvis
Abscess
   Incision and Drainage 26990
Arthrocentesis 20610
Arthrodesis 27284-27286
Arthrography 73525
Arthroplasty 27130-27132
Arthroscopy 29860-29863
Arthrotomy 27030-27033
Biopsy 27040-27041
Bone
   Drainage 26992
Bursa
   Incision and Drainage 26991

Capsulectomy
   with Release, Flexor Muscles 27036
Cast 29305-29325
Craterization 27070
Cyst
   Excision 27065-27067
Denervation 27035
Echography
   Infant 76885-76886
Endoprosthesis
   See Prosthesis, Hip
Excision 27070
Exploration 27033
Fasciotomy 27025
Fusion .27284-27286
Hematoma
   Incision and Drainage 26990
Injection
   Radiologic 27093-27096
Reconstruction
   Total Replacement 27130
Removal
   Cast 29710
   Foreign Body 27033, 27086-27087
     Arthroscopic 29861
   Loose Body
     Arthroscopic 29861
   Prosthesis 27090-27091
Repair
   Muscle Transfer 27100-27105, 27111
   Osteotomy 27146-27156
   Tendon 27097
Saucerization 27070
Stem Prostheses
   See Arthroplasty, Hip
Strapping 29520
Tenotomy
   Abductor Tendon 27006
   Adductor Tendon 27000-27003
   Iliopsoas 27005
Total Replacement 27130-27132
Tumor
   Excision 27047-27049, 27065-27067
     Radical 27075-27076
Ultrasound
   Infant 76885-76886
X-Ray 73500-73520, 73540
   Intraoperative 73530
   with Contrast 73525

Hip Joint

Arthroplasty 27132
   Revision 27134-27138
Arthrotomy 27052
Biopsy 27052
Capsulotomy
   with Release, Flexor Muscles 27036
Dislocation 27250-27252
   Congenital 27256-27259
   Open Treatment 27253-27254
   without Trauma 27265-27266
Manipulation .27275
Reconstruction
   Revision 27134-27138
Synovium
   Excision 27054
     Arthroscopic 29863
Total Replacement 27132

Hip Stem Prostheses
See Arthroplasty, Hip

Histamine 83088

Histamine Release Test 86343

Histochemistry 88318-88319

Histocompatibility Testing
See Tissue Typing

Histoplasma
Antibody 86698
Antigen 87385

Histoplasma capsulatum
Antigen Detection
   Enzyme Immunoassay 87385

Histoplasmin Test
See Histoplasmosis, Skin Test

Histoplasmoses
See Histoplasmosis

Histoplasmosis
Skin Test 86510

History and Physical
See Evaluation and Management, Office and/or
Other Outpatient Services
Pelvic Exam 57410

HIV
Antibody 86701-86703
   Confirmation Test 86689

HIV-1
Antigen Detection
   Enzyme Immunoassay 87390

HIV-2
Antigen Detection
   Enzyme Immunoassay 87391

HK3 Kallikrein
See Antigen, Prostate Specific

HLA Typing 86812-86817

HMRK
See Fitzgerald Factor

HMW Kininogen
See Fitzgerald Factor

Hoffman Apparatus 20690

Hofmeister Operation
See Gastrectomy, Total

Holographic Imaging 76375

Holten Test
See Creatinine, Urine, Clearance

Home Services
Activities of Daily Living 99509
Catheter Care 99507
Enema Administration 99511
Established Patient 99347-99350
Hemodialysis 99512

Home Infusion Procedures 99551-99560,
                  99562, 99564-99569
Individual or Family Counseling 99510
Inhalation Therapy 99563
Intramuscular Injections 99506
Mechanical Ventilation 99504
Newborn Care 99502
New Patient 99341-99345
Postnatal Assessment 99501
Prenatal Monitoring 99500
Respiratory Therapy 99503
Sleep Studies 95805-95811
Stoma Care 99505
Unlisted Services and Procedures 99600

Home Visit
See House Calls

Homocystine 83090
Urine 82615

Homogenization, Tissue 87176

Homograft
Skin 15350

Homologous Grafts
See Graft

Homologous Transplantation
See Homograft

Homovanillic Acid
Urine 83150

Hormone, Adrenocorticotrophic
See Adrenocorticotropic Hormone (ACTH)

Hormone, Corticotropin-Releasing
See Corticotropic Releasing Hormone (CRH)

Hormone, Growth
See Growth Hormone

Hormone, Human Growth
See Growth Hormone, Human

Hormone, Interstitial Cell-Stimulating
See Luteinizing Hormone (LH)

Hormone, Parathyroid
See Parathormone

Hormone, Pituitary Lactogenic
See Prolactin

Hormone, Placental Lactogen
See Lactogen, Human Placental

Hormone, Somatotropin Release-Inhibiting
See Somatostatin

Hormone, Thyroid-Stimulating
See Thyroid Stimulating Hormone (TSH)

Hormone-Binding Globulin, Sex
See Globulin, Sex Hormone Binding

Hormones, Adrenal Cortex
See Corticosteroids

Hormones, Antidiuretic
See Antidiuretic Hormone

Hormone Assay
ACTH 82024
Aldosterone
    Blood or Urine 82088
Androstenedione
    Blood or Urine 82157
Androsterone
    Blood or Urine 82160
Angiotensin II 82163
Corticosterone 82528
Cortisol
    Total 82533
Dehydroepiandrosterone 82626
Dihydroelestosterone 82651
Dihydrotestosterone 82651
Epiandrosterone 82666
Estradiol 82670
Estriol 82677
Estrogen 82671-82672
Estrone 82679
Follicle Stimulating Hormone 83001
Growth Hormone 83003
Hydroxyprogesterone 83498-83499
Luteinizing Hormone 83002
Somatotropin 83003
Testosterone 84403
Vasopressin 84588

Hormone Pellet
Implantation 11980

Hospital Discharge Services
See Discharge Services, Hospital

Hospital Services
Inpatient Services 99238-99239
    Discharge Services 99238-99239
    Initial Care
      New or Established Patient ..99221-99233
    Initial Hospital Care 99221-99223
    Newborn 99431-99433
    Prolonged Services 99356-99357
    Subsequent Hospital Care 99231-99233
Observation
    Discharge Services 99234-99236
    Initial Care 99218-99220
      New or Established Patient ..99218-99220
Same Day Admission
    Discharge Services 99234-99236
Subsequent Newborn Care 99433

Hot Pack Treatment 97010
See Physical Medicine and Rehabilitation

House Calls 99341-99350

Howard Test
See Cystourethroscopy, Catheterization, Ureter

HPL
See Lactogen, Human Placental

HTLV-IV
See HIV-2

HTLV I
Antibody
    Confirmatory Test 86689
    Detection 86687

HTLV II
Antibody 86688

HTLV III
See HIV

HTLV III Antibodies
See Antibody, HIV

Hubbard Tank Therapy 97036
See Physical Medicine/Therapy/Occupational Therapy

Hue Test 92283

Huggin Operation
See Orchiectomy, Simple

Huhner Test 89300, 89320

Human Chorionic Gonadotropin
See Chorionic Gonadotropin

Human Chorionic Somatomammotropin
See Lactogen, Human Placental

Human Cytomegalovirus Group
See Cytomegalovirus

Human Growth Hormone (HGH) 80418, 80428-80430

Human Herpes Virus 4
See Epstein-Barr Virus

Human Immunodeficiency Virus
See HIV

Human Immunodeficiency Virus 1
See HIV-1

Human Immunodeficiency Virus 2
See HIV-2

Human Papillomavirus Detection 87620-87622

Human Placental Lactogen
See Lactogen, Human Placental

Human T Cell Leukemia Virus I
See HTLV I

Human T Cell Leukemia Virus II
See HTLV II

Human T Cell Leukemia Virus II Antibodies
See Antibody, HTLV-II

Human T Cell Leukemia Virus I Antibodies
See Antibody, HTLV-I

Humeral Epicondylitides, Lateral
See Tennis Elbow

Humeral Fracture
See Fracture, Humerus

Humerus
See Arm, Upper; Shoulder
Abscess
    Incision and Drainage 23935
Craterization 23184, 24140
Cyst
    Excision 23150, 24110
    with Allograft 23156, 24116
    with Autograft 23155, 24115
Diaphysectomy 23184, 24140
Excision 23174, 23184, 23195, 24134, 24140,
                         24150-24151
Fracture
    Closed Treatment 24500-24505
      without Manipulation 23600
      with Manipulation 23605
    Condyle
      Closed Treatment 24576-24577
      Open Treatment 24579
      Percutaneous Fixation 24582
    Epicondyle
      Closed Treatment 24560-24565
      Open Treatment 24575
      Skeletal Fixation
        Percutaneous 24566
    Greater Tuberosity Fracture
      Closed Treatment without
        Manipulation 23620
      Closed Treatment with
        Manipulation 23625
      Open Treatment 23630
    Open Treatment 23615-23616
    Shaft 24500-24505, 24516
      Open Treatment 24515
    Supracondylar
      Closed Treatment 24530-24535
      Open Treatment 24545-24546
      Percutaneous Fixation 24538
    Transcondylar
      Closed Treatment 24530-24535
      Open Treatment 24545-24546
      Percutaneous Fixation 24538
    with Dislocation 23665-23670
Osteomyelitis 24134
Pinning, Wiring 23491, 24498
Prophylactic Treatment 23491, 24498
Radical Resection 23220-23222
Repair 24430
    Nonunion, Malunion 24430-24435
    Osteoplasty 24420
    Osteotomy 24400-24410
    with Graft 24435
Resection Head 23195
Saucerization 23184, 24140
Sequestrectomy 23174, 24134
Tumor
    Excision 23150, 23220-23222, 24110
    with Allograft 23156, 24116
    with Autograft 23155, 24115
X-Ray 73060

Hummelshein Operation
See Strabismus, Repair

Humor Shunt, Aqueous
See Aqueous Shunt

HVA
See Homovanillic Acid

Hysterotomy 59100
See Ligation, Uterus
Induced Abortion
    with Amniotic Injections 59852
    with Vaginal Suppositories 59857

Hysterotrachelectomy
See Amputation, Cervix

H Flu
See Hemophilus Influenza

I

I, Angiotensin
See Angiotensin I

I, Coagulation Factor
See Fibrinogen

I, Heparin Co-Factor
See Antithrombin III

ICCE
See Extraction, Lens, Intracapsular

Ichthyosis, Sex Linked
See Syphilis Test

ICSH
See Luteinizing Hormone (LH)

Identification
Oocyte
    from Follicular Fluid 89254
Sperm
    from Aspiration 89257
    from Tissue 89264

IDH
See Isocitric Dehydrogenase, Blood

IG
See Immune Globulins

IgE 86003-86005

IgG 86001

II, Coagulation Factor
See Prothrombin

II, Cranial Nerve
See Optic Nerve

Ileal Conduit
Visualization 50690

Ileoscopy
via Stoma 44383

Ileostomy 44310, 45136
Continent (Kock Procedure) 44316
Revision 44312-44314

Iliac Arteries
See Artery, Iliac

Iliac Crest
Free Osteocutaneous Flap with Microvascular
Anastomosis 20970

Iliohypogastric Nerve
Injection
    Anesthetic 64425

Ilioinguinal Nerve
Injection
    Anesthetic 64425

Ilium
Craterization 27070
Cyst
    Excision 27065-27067
Excision 27070
Fracture
    Open Treatment 27215, 27218
Saucerization 27070
Tumor
    Excision 27065-27067

Ilizarov Procedure
Monticelli Type 20692
    See Application, Bone Fixation Device

Imaging
See Vascular Studies

Imaging, Gamma Camera
See Nuclear Medicine

Imaging, Magnetic Resonance
See Magnetic Resonance Imaging (MRI)

Imaging, Ultrasonic
See Echography

Imbrication
Diaphragm 39545

Imidobenzyle
See Imipramine

Imipramine
Assay 80174

Immune Complex Assay 86332

Immune Globulins
Antitoxin
    Botulinum 90287
    Diphtheria 90296
Botulism 90288
Cytomegalovirus 90291
Hepatitis B 90371
Human 90281-90283
Rabies 90375-90376
Respiratory Syncytial Virus 90378-90379
Rho (D) 90384-90386
Tetanus 90389
Unlisted Immune Globulin 90399
Vaccinia 90393
Varicella-Zoster 90396

Immune Globulin Administration 90780-90784

Immune Globulin E
See IgE

Immunization, Mumps
See Mumps, Immunization

Immunization Administration
Each Additional Vaccine/Toxoid 90472, 90474
One Vaccine/Toxoid 90471, 90473

Immunoassay
Analyte 83519-83520
Infectious Agent 86317-86318, 87449-87451
Nonantibody 83516-83519
Tumor Antigen 86294, 86316
    CA 125 86304
    CA 15-3 86300
    CA 19-9 86301

Immunoblotting, Western
See Western Blot

Immunochemical, Lysozyme (Muramidase)
See Lysozyme

Immunocytochemistry 88342

Immunodeficiency Virus, Human
See HIV

Immunodeficiency Virus Type 1, Human
See HIV-1

Immunodeficiency Virus Type 2, Human
See HIV-2

Immunodiffusion 86329-86331

Immunoelectrophoresis 86320-86327, 86334

Immunofixation Electrophoresis 86334

Immunofluorescent Study 88346-88347

Immunogen
See Antigen

Immunoglobulin 82787
Platelet Associated 86023
Thyroid Stimulating 84445

Immunoglobulin E
See IgE

Immunoglobulin Receptor Assay 86243

Immunologic Skin Test
See Skin, Tests

Immunology
Unlisted Services and Procedures ..86849, 99558

Immunotherapies, Allergen
See Allergen Immunotherapy

Impedance Testing 92567
See Audiologic Function Tests

Imperfectly Descended Testis
See Testis, Undescended

Intercarpal Joint
    Dislocation 25670
Interphalangeal Joint
    Capsule 26525
Intestines, Small 44010
    Biopsy 44020
    Creation
        Pouch .44316
        Stoma 44300-44310, 44314
    Decompression 44021
    Exploration 44020
    Incision 44020
    Removal
        Foreign Body 44020
    Revision
        Stoma .44312
Intestines (Except Rectum)
    See Enterotomy
Iris 66500-66505
Kidney 50010, 50045
Knee
    Capsule 27435
    Exploration 27310
    Fasciotomy 27305
    Removal of Foreign Body 27310
Lacrimal Punctum 68440
Lacrimal Sac
    See Dacryocystotomy
Larynx .31300-31320
Leg, Lower
    Fasciotomy 27600-27602
Leg, Upper
    Fasciotomy 27305
    Tenotomy 27306-27307, 27390-27392
Lip
    Frenum 40806
Liver
    See Hepatotomy
Lung
    Biopsy 32095-32100
    Decortication
        Partial 32225
        Total .32220
Lymphatic Channels 38308
Mastoid
    See Mastoidotomy
Medullary Tract 61470
Mesencephalic Tract 61480
Metacarpophalangeal Joint
    Capsule 26520
Mitral Valve 33420-33422
Muscle
    See Myotomy
Nerve 64573-64580,
            64585-64595, 64702-64772
    Foot 28035
    Root 63185-63190
    Sacral 64581
    Vagus 43640-43641
Nose
    See Rhinotomy
Orbit
    See Orbitotomy
Palm
    Fasciotomy 26040-26045
Pancreas
    Sphincter .43262

Penis
    Prepuce 54000-54001
        Newborn 54000
Pericardium
    with Clot Removal 33020
    with Foreign Body Removal 33020
    with Tube .33015
Pharynx
    Stoma 42955
Pleura
    Biopsy 32095-32100
Pleural Cavity
    Empyema 32035-32036
    Pneumothorax 32020
Prostate
    Exposure
        Bilateral Pelvic Lymphadenectomy . .55865
        Insertion Radioactive Substance 55860
        Lymph Node Biopsy 55862
        Transurethral 52450
Pterygomaxillary Fossa 31040
Pulmonary Valve 33470-33474
Pyloric Sphincter 43520
Retina
    Encircling Material 67115
Sclera
    Fistulization
        Iridencleisis or Iridotasis 66165
        Sclerectomy with Punch or Scissors
          with Iridectomy 66160
        Thermocauterization with
          Iridectomy 66155
        Trabeculectomy ab Externo in Absence
          Previous Surgery 66170
        Trephination with Iridectomy 66150
Semicircular Canal
    Fenestration 69820
    Revision .69840
Seminal Vesicle 55600-55605
    Complicated 55605
Shoulder
    Bone 23035
    Capsular Contracture Release 23020
    Removal
        Calcareous Deposits 23000
    Tenomyotomy 23405-23406
Shoulder Joint 23040-23044
Sinus
    Frontal 31070-31087
    Maxillary 31020-31032
        Endoscopic 31256-31267
    Multiple .31090
    Sphenoid
        Sinusotomy 31050-31051
Skin .10040-10180
Skull .61316, 62148
Skull
    Suture 61550-61552
Spinal Cord .63200
    Tract 63170, 63194-63199
Stomach
    Creation
        Stoma 43830-43832
    Exploration 43500
    Pyloric Sphincter 43520
    Synovectomy 26140
Temporomandibular Joint 21010

Tendon
    Arm, Upper 24310
Thigh
    Fasciotomy 27025
Thorax
    Empyema 32035-32036
    Pneumothorax 32020
Thyroid Gland
    See Thyrotomy
Tibia 27607
Toe
    Capsule 28270-28272
    Fasciotomy 28008
    Tendon 28232-28234
    Tenotomy 28010-28011
Tongue
    Frenum 41010
Trachea
    Emergency 31603-31605
    Planned 31600-31601
    with Flaps 31610
Tympanic Membrane 69420
    with Anesthesia 69421
Ureter 50600
Ureterocele 51535
Urethra 53000-53010
    Meatus 53020-53025
Uterus
    Remove Lesion 59100
Vagina
    Exploration 57000
Vas Deferens 55200
    for X-Ray .55300
Vestibule of the Mouth
    See Mouth, Vestibule of, Incision
Vitreous Strands
    Laser Surgery 67031
    Pars Plana Approach 67030
Wrist 25100-25105
    Capsule 25085
    Decompression 25020-25025
    Tendon Sheath 25000-25001

Incisional Hernia Repair
See Hernia, Repair, Incisional

Incision and Drainage
See Drainage; Incision
Abdomen
    Fluid 49080-49081
    Pancreatitis 48000
Abscess
    Abdomen 49020, 49040
        Open .49040
        Percutaneous 49021
    Anal 46045-46050
    Ankle 27603
    Appendix .44900
        Open .44900
        Percutaneous 44901
    Arm, Lower 25028
    Arm, Upper 23930-23931
    Auditory Canal, External 69020
    Bartholin's Gland 56420
    Bladder 51080
    Brain 61320-61321
    Breast 19020

Incomplete Abortion
See Abortion, Incomplete

Indicator Dilution
Studies 93561-93562

Induced Abortion
See Abortion

Induced Hyperthermia
See Thermotherapy

Induced Hypothermia
See Hypothermia

Induratio Penis Plastica
See Peyronie Disease

Infant, Newborn, Intensive Care
See Intensive Care, Neonatal

Infantile Paralysis
See Polio

Infection
Immunoassay 86317-86318
Rapid Test 86403-86406

Infection, Actinomyces
See Actinomycosis

Infection, Bone
See Osteomyelitis

Infection, Filarioidea
See Filariasis

Infection, Postoperative Wound
See Postoperative Wound Infection

Infection, Wound
See Wound, Infection

Infectious Agent
Antigen Detection
    Direct Fluorescence ...87198-87199, 87265-
      87272, 87276, 87278, 87280, 87285-87290
      Bordetella 87265
      Chlamydia Trachomatis 87270
      Cryptosporidium/Giardia 87272
      Cytomegalovirus 87198
      Enterovirus 87199
      Influenza A 87276
      Legionella Pneumophila 87278
      Respiratory Syncytial Virus 87280
      Treponema Pallidum 87285
      Varicella-Zoster 87290
    Enzyme Immunoassay
      Adenovirus 87301
      Chlamydia Trachomatis 87320
      Clostridium Difficile 87324
      Cryptococcus Neoformans 87327
      Cryptosporidium/Giardia 87328
      Cytomegalovirus 87332
      Entamoeba Histolytica Dispar
      Group 87336
      Entamoeba Histolytica Group ...87337
      Escherichia coli O157 87335
      Helicobacter Pylori 87338-87339
      Hepatitis, Delta Agent 87380
      Hepatitis Be Antigen (HBeAg) 87350

Hepatitis B Surface Antigen
(HBsAg) 87340
Hepatitis B Surface Antigen (HBsAg)
  Neutralization 87341
Histoplasma capsulatum 87385
HIV-1 87390
HIV-2 87391
Influenza A 87400
Influenza B 87400
Multiple Step Method 87301-87449,
                    87451
    See specific agent
Not Otherwise Specified 87449, 87451
Respiratory Syncytial Virus 87420
Rotavirus 87425
Shiga-like Toxin 87427
Single Step Method 87450
Streptococcus, Group A 87430
Immunofluorescence ...87260, 87273-87275,
    87277, 87279, 87281-87283, 87299-87300
  Adenovirus 87260
  Herpes Simplex 87273-87274
  Influenza B 87275
  Legionella Micdadei 87277
  Not Otherwise Specified 87299
  Parainfluenza Virus 87279
  Pneumocystis Carinii 87281
  Polyvalent 87300
  Rubeola 87283
Concentration 87015
Detection
  by Immunoassay with Direct Optical
    Observation 87802-87899
    Chlamydia Trachomatis 87810
    Clostridium difficile 87803
    Influenza 87804
    Neisseria gonorrheae 87850
    Not Otherwise Specified 87899
    Streptococcus, Group A 87880
    Streptococcus, Group B 87802
  by Nucleic Acid
    Bartonella henselae 87470-87472
    Bartonella quintana 87470-87472
    Borrelia burgdorferi 87475-87477
    Candida species 87480-87482
    Chlamydia pneumoniae 87485-87487
    Chlamydia Trachomatis 87490-87492
    Cytomegalovirus 87495-87497
    Gardnerella Vaginalis 87510-87512
    Hepatitis B Virus 87515-87517
    Hepatitis C 87520-87522
    Hepatitis G 87525-87527
    Herpes Simplex Virus 87528-87530
    Herpes Virus-6 87531-87533
    HIV-1 87534-87536
    HIV-2 87537-87539
    Legionella Pneumophila 87540-87542
    Multiple Organisms 87800-87801
    Mycobacteria
    avium-intracellulare 87560-87562
    Mycobacteria species 87550-87552
    Mycobacteria tuberculosis ..87555-87557
    Mycoplasma pneumoniae ...87580-87582
    Neisseria gonorrheae 87590-87592
    Not Otherwise Specified ...87797-87799
    Papillomavirus, Human 87620-87622
    Streptococcus, Group A 87650-87652
Urinalysis 0041T

Genotype Analysis
  by Nucleic acid
    Hepatitis C Virus 87902
    HIV-1 Protease/Reverse
    Transcriptase 87901
Phenotype Analysis
  by Nucleic acid
    HIV-1 Drug Resistance 87903-87904
Phenotype Prediction
  by Genetic Database
    HIV-1 Drug Resistance 0023T

Infectious Mononucleosis Virus
See Epstein-Barr Virus

Inflammatory Process
Localization
    Nuclear Medicine 78805-78807

Inflation
Ear, Middle
  Eustachian Tube
    without Catheterization 69401
    with Catheterization 69400
Eustachian Tube
  Myringotomy 69420
  Anesthesia 69424

Influenza A
Antigen Detection
  Direct Fluorescence 87276
  Enzyme Immunoassay 87400

Influenza B
Antigen Detection
  Enzyme Immunoassay 87400
  Immunofluorescence 87275

Influenza Vaccine
See Vaccines

Influenza Virus
Antibody 86710
by Immunoassay
  with Direct Optical Observation 87804

Infraorbital Nerve
Avulsion 64734
Incision 64734
Transection 64734

Infrared Light Treatment 97026
See Physical Medicine/Therapy/Occupational
Therapy

Infratentorial
Craniectomy 61520-61521

Infusion
Cerebral
  Intravenous
    for Thrombolysis 37195
Intraosseous 36680
Radioelement 77750
Transcatheter Therapy 37201-37202

Infusion Pump
Electronic Analysis
  Spinal Cord 62367-62368
Insertion
  Intra-arterial 36260

Inspiratory Positive Pressure Breathing

See Intermittent Positive Pressure Breathing (IPPB)

Instillation

Instillation, Bladder

See Bladder, Instillation

Instrumentation

See Application; Bone, Fixation; Spinal Instrumentation

Insufflation, Eustachian Tube

See Eustachian Tube, Inflation

Insulin 80422, 80432-80435

Insulin C-Peptide Measurement

See C-Peptide

Insulin Like Growth Factors

See Somatomedin

Insurance

Integumentary System

Kidney Stone
See Calculus, Removal, Kidney

Killian Operation
See Sinusotomy, Frontal

Kinase, Creatine
See CPK

Kineplasty
See Cineplasty

Kinetic Therapy
See Physical Medicine/Therapy/Occupational Therapy

Kininase A
See Angiotensin Converting Enzyme (ACE)

Kininogen

Kininogen, High Molecular Weight
See Fitzgerald Factor

Kleihauer-Betke Test

Kloramfenikol
See Chloramphenicol

Knee
See Femur; Fibula; Patella; Tibia

Kneecap

Knee Joint

Knee Prosthesis
See Prosthesis, Knee

Knock-Knee Repair

Kocher Operation
See Clavicle; Scapula; Shoulder, Dislocation, Closed Treatment

Kocher Pylorectomy
See Gastrectomy, Partial

Kock Pouch

Kock Procedure

KOH
See Hair, Nails, Tissue, Examination for Fungi

Kraske Procedure

Krause Operation
See Gasserian Ganglion, Sensory Root, Decompression

Kroenlein Procedure

Orchiopexy 54692
Oviduct Surgery 58670-58671, 58679
Pelvis 49320
Prostatectomy 55866
Pyeloplasty 50544
Removal
    Fallopian Tube 58661
    Leiomyomata 58545-58546
    Ovaries 58661
    Spleen 38120
    Testis 54690
Resection
    Intestines
       with Anastomosis 44202-44203
Salpingostomy 58673
Splenectomy 38120-38129
Surgical 38570-38572, 43651-43653, 44200-
      44206, 44970, 47370-47371, 49321-49323,
      49650-49651, 50541-50543, 50545, 50945-50948,
      51990-51992, 54690-54692, 55550, 55866,
          58545-58546, 58552-58554
    Anastomosis 44207
    Colostomy 44208
    with Guided Transhepatic
    Cholangiography 47560-47561
Unlisted Services and Procedures 38129,
      38589, 43289, 43659, 44238-44239, 44979,
      47379, 47579, 49329, 49659, 50549, 50949,
      54699, 55559, 58578-58579, 58679, 59898
Ureterolithotomy 50945
Ureteroneocystostomy 50947-50948
Urethral Suspension 51990
Vaginal Hysterectomy 58550
Vagus Nerves
    Transection 43651-43652
with X-Ray 47560

Laparotomy
Exploration 47015, 49000-49002, 58960
for Staging 49220
Hemorrhage Control 49002
Second Look 58960
Staging 58960
with Biopsy 49000

Laparotomy, Exploratory
See Abdomen, Exploration

Lapidus Procedure 28297

Large Bowel
See Anus; Cecum; Rectum

Laroyenne Operation
See Vagina, Abscess, Incision and Drainage

Laryngeal Function Study 92520

Laryngeal Sensory Testing 92614-92617

Laryngectomy 31360-31382
Partial 31367-31382
Subtotal 31367-31368

Laryngocele
Removal 31300

Laryngofissure 31300

Laryngography 70373
Instillation
    Contrast Material 31708

Laryngopharyngectomy
See Excision, Larynx, with Pharynx

Laryngopharynx
See Hypopharynx

Laryngoplasty
Burns 31588
Cricoid Split 31587
Laryngeal Stenosis 31582
Laryngeal Web 31580
Open Reduction of Fracture 31584

Laryngoscopy
Diagnostic 31505
Direct 31515-31571
Exploration 31505, 31520-31526, 31575
Fiberoptic 31575-31579
    with Stroboscopy 31579
Indirect 31505-31513
Newborn 31520
Operative 31530-31561

Laryngotomy 31300
Diagnostic 31320
Total 31360-31368

Larynx
Aspiration
    Endoscopy 31515
Biopsy
    Endoscopy 31510, 31535-31536, 31576
Dilation
    Endoscopic 31528-31529
Endoscopy
    Direct 31515-31571
    Exploration 31505, 31520-31526, 31575
    Fiberoptic 31575-31579
      with Stroboscopy 31579
    Indirect 31505-31513
    Operative 31530-31561
Excision
    Lesion 31512, 31578
    Partial 31367-31382
    Total 31360-31365
    with Pharynx 31390-31395
Exploration
    Endoscopic 31505, 31520-31526, 31575
Fracture
    Closed Treatment
      without Manipulation 31585
      with Manipulation 31586
    Open Treatment 31584
Insertion
    Obturator 31527
Nerve
    Destruction 31595
Reconstruction
    Burns 31588
    Cricoid Split 31587
    Other 31588
    Stenosis 31582
    Web 31580
Removal
    Foreign Body
      Endoscopic ...31511, 31530-31531, 31577

Lesion
    Endoscopic 31512, 31578
Repair
    Reinnervation Neuromuscular
    Pedicle 31590
Stroboscopy 31579
Tumor
    Excision 31300
    Endoscopic 31540-31541
Unlisted Services and Procedures 31599
Vocal Cord(s)
    Injection 31513, 31570-31571
X-Ray 70370
    with Contrast 70373

Laser Surgery
Anal 46917
Lesion
    Mouth 40820
    Nose 30117-30118
    Penis 54057

Laser Treatment 17000-17286, 96920-96922
See Destruction

Lateral Epicondylitis
See Tennis Elbow

Latex Fixation 86403-86406

LATS
See Thyrotropin Releasing Hormone (TRH)

Latzko Operation
See Repair, Vagina, Fistula; Revision

LAV
See HIV

LAV-2
See HIV-2

Lavage, Bronchioalveolar
See Lung, Lavage

Lavage, Colonic
See Colon, Lavage

Lavage, Peritoneal
See Peritoneal Lavage

Lav Antibodies
See Antibody, HIV

LCM
See Lymphocytic Choriomeningitis

LD
See Lactic Dehydrogenase

LDH 83615-83625

LDL
See Lipoprotein, LDL

Lead 83655

Leadbetter Procedure 53431

Lecithin-Sphingomyelin Ratio .83661

Lecithinase C
See Tissue Typing

Colon
 Destruction 44393, 45383
 Excision 44110-44111
Conjunctiva
 Destruction 68135
 Excision 68110-68130
  Over 1 cm 68115
  with Adjacent Sclera 68130
 Expression 68040
Cornea
 Destruction 65450
 Excision 65400
  of Pterygium 65420-65426
Destruction
 Ureter ...52341-52342, 52344-52345, 52354
Ear, Middle
 Excision 69540
Epididymis
 Excision 54830
Esophagus
 Ablation 43228
 Excision 43100-43101
 Removal 43216
Excision 59100
 Bladder 52224
 Urethra 52224, 53265
Eye
 Excision 65900
Eyelid
 Destruction 67850
 Excision
  Multiple, Different Lids 67805
  Multiple, Same Lid 67801
  Single 67800
  Under Anesthesia 67808
  without Closure 67840
Facial
 Destruction 17000-17004, 17280-17286
Femur
 Excision 27062
Finger
 Tendon Sheath 26160
Foot
 Excision 28080, 28090
Gums
 Destruction 41850
 Excision 41822-41828
Hand Tendon Sheath 26160
Intestines
 Excision 44110
Intestines, Small
 Destruction 44369
 Excision 44111
Iris
 Destruction 66770
Leg, Lower
 Tendon Sheath 27630
Lymph Node
 Incision and Drainage 38300-38305
Mesentery
 Excision 44820
Mouth
 Destruction 40820
 Excision 40810-40816, 41116
 Vestibule
  Destruction 40820
  Repair 40830

Nerve
 Excision 64774-64792
Nose
 Intranasal
  External Approach 30118
  Internal Approach 30117
Orbit
 Excision 61333, 67412
Palate
 Destruction 42160
 Excision 42104-42120
Pancreas
 Excision 48120
Pelvis
 Destruction 58662
Penis
 Destruction
  Cryosurgery 54056
  Electrodesiccation 54055
  Extensive 54065
  Laser Surgery 54057
  Simple 54050-54060
  Surgical Excision 54060
 Excision 54060
  Penile Plaque 54110-54112
Pharynx
 Destruction 42808
 Excision 42808
Rectum
 Excision 45108
Removal
 Larynx 31512, 31578
Resection 52354
Retina
 Destruction
  Extensive 67227-67228
  Localized 0017T, 67208-67210
  Radiation by Implantation of Source ...67218
Sclera
 Excision 66130
Skin
 Abrasion 15786-15787
 Biopsy 11100-11101
 Destruction
  Benign 17000-17250
  Malignant 17260-17286
   by Photodynamic Therapy 96567
 Excision
  Benign 11400-11471
  Malignant 11600-11646
 Injection 11900-11901
 Paring or Curettement 11055-11057
 Shaving 11300-11313
Skin Tags
 Removal 11200-11201
Skull
 Excision ..61500, 61600-61608, 61615-61616
Spermatic Cord
 Excision 55520
Spinal Cord
 Destruction 62280-62282
 Excision 63265-63273
Stomach
 Excision 43611
Testis
 Excision 54512
Toe
 Excision 28092

Tongue
 Excision 41110-41114
Uvula
 Destruction 42145
 Excision 42104-42107
Vagina
 Destruction 57061-57065
Vulva
 Destruction
  Extensive 56515
  Simple 56501
Wrist Tendon
 Excision 25110

Lesion of Sciatic Nerve
See Sciatic Nerve, Lesion

Leucine Aminopeptidase 83670

Leukemia Lymphoma Virus I, Adult T Cell
See HTLV I

Leukemia Lymphoma Virus II Antibodies, Human T Cell
See Antibody, HTLV-II

Leukemia Lymphoma Virus I Antibodies, Human T Cell
See Antibody, HTLV-I

Leukemia Virus II, Hairy Cell Associated, Human T Cell
See HTLV II

Leukoagglutinins 86021

Leukocyte
See White Blood Cell
Alkaline Phosphatase 85540
Antibody 86021
Histamine Release Test 86343
Phagocytosis 86344
Transfusion 86950

Leukocyte Count
See White Blood Cell, Count

Leu 2 Antigens
See CD8

Levarterenol
See Noradrenalin

Levator Muscle Rep
See Blepharoptosis, Repair

LeVeen Shunt
Insertion 49425
Patency Test 78291
Revision 49426

Levulose
See Fructose

LGV
See Lymphogranuloma Venereum

LH
See Luteinizing Hormone (LH)

LHR
See Leukocyte Histamine Release Test

Nuclear Medicine
Function Study .78220
Imaging 78201-78216
Vascular Flow 78206
Repair
Abscess 47300
Cyst 47300
Wound 47350-47362
Suture
Wound 47350-47362
Transplantation 47135-47136
Trisegmentectomy 47122
Unlisted Services and Procedures . .47379, 47399

Living Activities, Daily
See Activities of Daily Living

Lobectomy
Brain .61323, 61539
Contralateral Subtotal
Thyroid Gland 60212, 60225
Liver .47120-47130
Lung 32480-32482
Sleeve 32486
Parotid Gland 42410-42415
Segmental 32663
Sleeve 32486
Temporal Lobe 61538
Thyroid Gland Partial 60210-60212
Total 60220-60225
Total 32663

Lobotomy
Frontal 61490

Localization of Nodule
Radiographic
Breast 76096

Local Excision Mastectomies
See Breast, Excision, Lesion

Local Excision of Lesion or Tissue of Femur
See Excision, Lesion, Femur

Log Hydrogen Ion Concentration
See pH

Lombard Test
See Audiologic Function Test

Longmire Operation
See Anastomosis, Hepatic Duct to Intestines

Long Acting Thyroid Stimulator
See Thyrotropin Releasing Hormone (TRH)

Long Term Care Facility Visits
See Nursing Facility Services

Loopogram
See Urography, Antegrade

Loose Body
Removal
Ankle 27620
Carpometacarpal Joint 26070
Elbow 24101
Interphalangeal Joint 28020
Toe 28024

Knee Joint .27331
Metatarsophalangeal Joint 28022
Tarsometatarsal Joint 28020
Toe 28022
Wrist 25101

Lord Procedure
See Anal Sphincter, Dilation

Louis Bar Syndrome
See Ataxia Telangiectasia

Low Birth Weight Intensive Care Services 99298-99299

Lower Extremities
See Extremity, Lower

Lower GI Series
See Barium Enema

Low Density Lipoprotein
See Lipoprotein, LDL

Low Vision Aids
See Spectacle Services
Fitting 92354-92355
Supply 92392

LRH
See Luteinizing Releasing Factor

LSD
See Lysergic Acid Diethylamide

LTH
See Prolactin

Lumbar
See Spine
Aspiration, Disk
Percutaneous 62287

Lumbar Plexus
Decompression 64714
Neuroplasty .64714
Release 64714
Repair/Suture 64862

Lumbar Puncture
See Spinal Tap

Lumbar Spine Fracture
See Fracture, Vertebra, Lumbar

Lumbar Sympathectomy
See Sympathectomy, Lumbar

Lumbar Vertebra
See Vertebra, Lumbar

Lumen Dilation 74360

Lumpectomies
See Breast, Excision, Lesion

Lunate
Arthroplasty
with Implant 25444
Dislocation
Closed Treatment 25690
Open Treatment 25695

Lung
Abscess
Incision and Drainage
Open 32200
Percutaneous 32200-32201
Aspiration 32420
Biopsy 32095-32100
Bullae
Excision 32141
Endoscopic 32655
Cyst
Incision and Drainage
Open 32200
Removal 32140
Decortication
Endoscopic 32651-32652
Partial 32225
Total 32220
with Parietal Pleurectomy 32320
Empyema
Excision 32540
Excision
Bronchus Resection 32486
Chest Resection 32520-32525
Completion 32488
Donor 33930
Emphysematous 32491
Lobe 32480-32482
Segment .32484
Total 32440-32445
Wedge Resection 32500
Endoscopic 32657
Foreign Body
Removal 32151
Hemorrhage .32110
Lavage
Bronchial .31624
Total 32997
Lysis
Adhesions 32124
Needle Biopsy 32405
Nuclear Medicine
Imaging, Perfusion 78580-78585
Imaging, Ventilation 78586-78594
Unlisted Services and Procedures 78599
Pneumocentesis 32420
Pneumolysis .32940
Pneumothorax 32960
Puncture 32420
Removal
Bronchoplasty 32501
Completion Pneumonectomy 32488
Extrapleural 32445
Single Lobe 32480
Single Segment 32484
Sleeve Lobectomy 32486
Sleeve Pneumonectomy 32442
Total Pneumonectomy 32440-32445
Two Lobes 32482
Volume Reduction 32491
Wedge Resection 32500
Repair
Hernia 32800
Segmentectomy 32484
Tear
Repair 32110

Lysis
Adhesions
  Epidural 0027T, 62263-62264
  Fallopian Tube 58740
  Foreskin 54450
  Intestinal .44005
  Labial 56441
  Lung 32124
  Nose 30560
  Ovary 58740
  Oviduct 58740
  Penile
    Post-circumcision 54162
  Ureter 50715-50725
  Uterus 58559
Euglobulin 85360
Labial
  Adhesions .56441
Nose
  Intranasal Synechia 30560

Lysozyme 85549

L Ascorbic Acid
See Ascorbic Acid

L Aspartate 2 Oxoglutarate Aminotransferase
See Transaminase, Glutamic Oxaloacetic

L Glutamine
See Glutamine

M

MacEwen Operation
See Hernia, Repair, Inguinal

Machado Test
See Complement, Fixation Test

MacLean-De Wesselow Test
See Blood Urea Nitrogen; Urea Nitrogen, Clearance

Macrodactylia
Repair 26590

Madlener Operation
See Tubal Ligation

Magnesium 83735

Magnetic Resonance
Unlisted Services and Procedures 76498

Magnetic Resonance Angiography (MRA)
Abdomen 74185
Arm 73225
Chest 71555
Head 70544-70546
Leg 73725
Neck 70547-70549
Pelvis 72198
Spine 72159

Magnetic Resonance Imaging (MRI)
Abdomen 74181-74183
Ankle 73721-73723
Arm 73218-73220, 73223
Bone Marrow Study 76400
Brain 70551-70553
Breast 76093-76094
Chest 71550-71552
Elbow 73221
Face 70540-70543
Finger Joint 73221
Foot 73718-73719
Foot Joints 73721-73723
Guidance
  Needle Placement 76393
  Tissue Ablation 76394
Hand 73218-73220, 73223
Heart 75552
  Complete Study 75554
  Flow Mapping 75556
  Limited Study 75555
  Morphology 75553
Joint
  Lower Extremity 73721-73723
  Upper Extremity 73221-73223
Knee 73721-73723
Leg 73718-73720
Neck 70540-70543
Orbit 70540-70543
Pelvis 72195-72197
Radiology
  Diagnostic
    Procedures 76499
Spectroscopy 76390
Spine
  Cervical 72141-72142, 72156-72158
  Lumbar 72148-72158
  Thoracic 72146-72147, 72156-72158
Temporomandibular Joint (TMJ) 70336
Toe 73721-73723
Wrist 73221

Magnetic Resonance Spectroscopy 76390

Magnetic Stimulation
Brain Cortex 0018T

Magnetoencephalography (MEG) 95965-95967

Magnet Operation
See Ciliary Body; Cornea; Eye, Removal, Foreign Body; Iris; Lens; Retina; Sclera; Vitreous

Magnuson Procedure 23450

Magpi Operation 54322

Magpi Procedure
See Hypospadias, Repair

Major Vestibular Gland
See Bartholin's Gland

Malaria Antibody 86750

Malaria Smear 87207

Malar Area
Augmentation 21270
Bone Graft .21210
Fracture
  Open Treatment 21360-21366
  with Bone Graft 21366
  with Manipulation 21355
Reconstruction 21270

Malar Bone
See Cheekbone

Malate Dehydrogenase 83775

Maldescent, Testis
See Testis, Undescended

Male Circumcision
See Circumcision

Malformation, Arteriovenous
See Arteriovenous Malformation

Malic Dehydrogenase
See Malate Dehydrogenase

Malleolus
See Ankle; Fibula; Leg, Lower; Tibia; Tibiofibular Joint
Metatarsophalangeal Joint 27889

Mallet Finger Repair 26432

Maltose
Tolerance Test 82951-82952

Malunion Repair
Femur
  without Graft 27470
  with Graft 27472
Metatarsal .28322
Tarsal Joint 28320

Mammalian Oviduct
See Fallopian Tube

Mammaplasties
See Breast, Reconstruction

Mammary Abscess
See Abscess, Breast

Mammary Arteries
See Artery, Mammary

Mammary Duct
X-Ray with Contrast 76086-76088

Mammary Ductogram
Injection 19030

Mammary Stimulating Hormone
See Prolactin

Mammilliplasty
See Nipples, Reconstruction

Mammogram
Breast
  Localization Nodule 76096

Mammography 76090-76092
Screening .76092
with Computer-aided Detection 76085

Mastectomy
Gynecomastia 19140
Modified Radical 19240
Partial 19160-19162
Radical .19200-19220
Simple, Complete 19180
Subcutaneous 19182

Mastectomy, Halsted
See Mastectomy, Radical

Mastoid
Excision
    Complete 69502
    Radical 69511
       Modified 69505
       Petrous Apicectomy 69530
    Simple 69501
Obliteration 69670
Repair
    by Excision 69601-69603
    Fistula 69700
    with Apicectomy 69605
    with Tympanoplasty 69604

Mastoidectomy
Osseointegrated Implant
    for External Speech Processor/Cochlear
    Stimulator 69715, 69718
with Apicectomy 69605
with Skull Base Surgery 61590, 61597
    Decompression 61595
    Facial Nerve 61595
with Tympanoplasty 69604, 69641-69646
    Cochlear Device Implantation 69930
    Complete 69502
       Revision 69601
    Ossicular Chain Reconstruction 69605
    Radical 69511
       Modified 69505
       Revision 69602-69603
    Simple 69501
    with Labyrinthectomy 69910
    with Labyrinthotomy 69802
    with Petrous Apicectomy 69530

Mastoidotomy 69635-69637
with Tympanoplasty 69635
    Ossicular Chain Reconstruction 69636
    and Synthetic Prosthesis 69636

Mastoids
Polytomography 76101-76102
X-Ray 70120-70130

Mastoid Cavity
Debridement 69220-69222

Mastopexy 19316

Mastotomy 19020

Maternity Care
See Abortion; Cesarean Delivery; Ectopic
Pregnancy; Obstetrical Care

Maternity Care and
Delivery 59612-59622, 59898

Maxilla
See Facial Bones; Mandible
Bone Graft 21210
CT Scan 70486-70488
Cyst
    Excision 21048-21049
Excision 21030, 21032-21034
Fracture
    Closed Treatment 21345, 21421
    Open Treatment .21346-21348, 21422-21423
    with Fixation 21345-21347
Osteotomy 21206
Reconstruction
    with Implant 21245-21246, 21248-21249
Tumor
    Excision 21048-21049

Maxillary Arteries
See Artery, Maxillary

Maxillary Sinus
See Sinus, Maxillary

Maxillary Torus Palatinus
Tumor Excision .21032

Maxillectomy 31225-31230

Maxillofacial Fixation
Application
    Halo Type Appliance 21100

Maxillofacial Impressions
Auricular Prosthesis 21086
Definitive Obturator Prosthesis 21080
Facial Prosthesis 21088
Interim Obturator Prosthesis 21079
Mandibular Resection Prosthesis 21081
Nasal Prosthesis 21087
Oral Surgical Splint 21085
Orbital Prosthesis 21077
Palatal Augmentation Prosthesis 21082
Palatal Lift Prosthesis 21083
Speech Aid Prosthesis 21084
Surgical Obturator Prosthesis 21076

Maxillofacial Procedures
Unlisted Services and Procedures 21299

Maxillofacial
Prosthetics 21076-21089
Unlisted Services and Procedures 21089

Maydl Operation 45563, 50810
See Colostomy

Mayo Hernia Repair
See Hernia, Repair, Umbilicus

Mayo Operation
See Varicose Vein, Removal

Mayo Procedure 28292

MBC
See Minimum Bactericidal Concentration

McBride Procedure 28292

McBurney Operation
See Hernia, Repair, Inguinal

McCannel Procedure 66682

McDonald Operation
See Repair, Cervix, Cerclage, Abdominal; Revision

McIndoe Procedure
See Vagina, Construction

McKissock Surgery
See Breast, Reduction

McVay Operation
See Hernia, Repair, Inguinal

Measles, German
See Rubella

Measles Uncomplicated
See Rubeola

Measles Vaccine
See Vaccines

Meatoplasty 69310

Meatotomy 53020-53025
Contact Laser Vaporization with/without
    Transurethral Resection of Prostate . . .52648
    with Cystourethroscopy 52281
Infant 53025
Non-Contact Laser Coagulation Prostate . .52647
Transurethral Electrosurgical Resection
    Prostate 52601
Ureter 52290
Ureteral
    Cystourethroscopy 52290-52305

Meat Fibers
Feces 89160

Meckel's Diverticulum
Excision 44800
Unlisted Services and Procedures 44899

Median Nerve
Decompression .64721
Neuroplasty 64721
Release 64721
Repair/Suture
    Motor 64835
Transposition 64721

Median Nerve Compression
See Carpal Tunnel Syndrome

Mediastinal Cyst
See Cyst, Mediastinal

Mediastinoscopy 39400

Mediastinotomy
Cervical Approach 39000
Transthoracic Approach 39010

Mediastinum
See Chest; Thorax
Cyst
    Excision 32662, 39200
Endoscopy
    Biopsy 39400
    Exploration .39400
Exploration 39000-39010

Repair
Hallux Rigidus 28289
Synovial
Biopsy 28052
Excision .28072
Toe 28270

Methadone 83840

Methaemoglobin
See Methemoglobin

Methamphetamine
Blood or Urine .82145

Methanol 84600

Methbipyranone
See Metyrapone

Methemalbumin 83857

Methemoglobin 83045-83050

Methenamine Silver Stain 88312

Methopyrapone
See Metyrapone

Methoxyhydroxymandelic Acid
See Vanillylmandelic Acid

Methsuximide 83858

Methylamphetamine
See Methamphetamine

Methylene Bichloride
See Dichloromethane

Methylfluorprednisolone
See Dexamethasone

Methylmorphine
See Codeine

Methyl Alcohol
See Methanol

Metroplasty
See Hysteroplasty

Metyrapone 80436

MIC
See Minimum Inhibitory Concentration

Micro-Ophthalmia
Orbit Reconstruction 21256

Microalbumin
Urine .82043-82044

Microbiology 0023T, 87001-87999

Microdissection 88380

Microfluorometries, Flow
See Flow Cytometry

Microglobulin, Beta 2
Blood 82232
Urine 82232

Micrographic Surgery
Mohs Technique 17304-17310

Micrographic Surgery, Mohs
See Mohs Micrographic Surgery

Micropigmentation
Correction 11920-11922

Microscope, Surgical
See Operating Microscope

Microscopic Evaluation
Hair 96902

Microscopies, Electron
See Electron Microscopy

Microscopy
Ear Exam 92504

Microsomal Antibody 86376

Microsomia, Hemifacial
See Hemifacial Microsomia

Microsurgery
Operating Microscope 69990

Microvascular Anastomosis
Bone Graft
Fibula 20955
Other 20962
Fascial Flap, Free 15758
Muscle Flap, Free 15756
Osteocutaneous Flap with 20969-20973
Skin Flap, Free 15757

Microvite A
See Vitamin, A

Microwave Therapy 97020
See Physical Medicine/Therapy/Occupational
Therapy

Midbrain
See Brain; Brainstem; Mesencephalon; Skull
Base Surgery

Midcarpal Medioccipital Joint
Arthrotomy 25040

Middle Ear
See Ear, Middle

Midface
Reconstruction
Forehead Advancement 21159-21160
without Bone Graft 21141-21143
with Bone Graft 21145-21160, 21188

**Migration Inhibitory Factor
(MIF)** 86378

Mile Operation
See Colectomy, Total, with Proctectomy

Milia, Multiple
Removal 10040

**Miller-Abbott
Intubation** 44500, 74340

Miller Procedure 28737

Minerva Cast 29035
Removal 29710

**Minimum Inhibitory
Concentration** 87186

**Minimum Lethal
Concentration** 87187

**Minnesota Multiphasic Personality
Inventory**
See MMPI

Miscarriage
Incomplete Abortion 59812
Missed Abortion
First Trimester 59820
Second Trimester 59821
Septic Abortion 59830

Missed Abortion
See Abortion

Mitchell Procedure 28296

Mitogen Blastogenesis 86353

Mitral Valve
Incision 33420-33422
Repair 33420-33427
Incision 33420-33422
Replacement 33430

Mitrofanoff Operation 50845
See Appendico-Vesicostomy

Miyagawanella
See Chlamydia

MMPI 96100

MMR Shots 90707
See Vaccines

Mobilization
Splenic Flexure 44139
Stapes 69650

Modified Radical Mastectomy
See Mastectomy, Modified Radical

**Mohs Micrographic
Surgery** 17304-17310

Molar Pregnancy
See Hydatidiform Mole

Mold
Culture 87107

Mole, Carneous
See Abortion

Mole, Hydatid
See Hydatidiform Mole

**Molecular
Cytogenetics** 88271-88275
Interpretation and Report 88291

Molecular Diagnostics . . .83890-83898
Amplification 83898-83901
Dot/Slot Production 83893
Enzymatic Digestion 83892
Extraction 83890-83891
Interpretation 83912

Molecular Isolation (Extraction) 83890
Mutation Identification 83904-83906
Mutation Scanning .83903
Nucleic Acid Probe .83896
Nucleic Acid Transfer 83897
Polymerase Reaction Chain 83898
Reverse Transcription 83902
Separation 83894

Molecular Oxygen Saturation
See Oxygen Saturation

Molluscum Contagiosum
Destruction 17110-17111, 54050-54065

Molteno Procedure 66180

Monilia
See Candida

Monitoring
Blood Pressure, 24 Hour 93784-93790
Electrocardiogram 93224-93237
　　See Electrocardiography
Electroencephalogram 95812-95813,
　　　　　　　　　　　　95950-95953, 95956
　　　with Drug Activation 95954
　　　with Physical Activation 95954
　　　with WADA Activation 95958
Fetal
　　During Labor 59050-59051, 99500
　　　Interpretation Only 59051
Glucose
　　Interstitial Fluid 95250
Interstitial Fluid Pressure 20950
Seizure 61531, 61760

Monitoring, Sleep
See Polysomnography

Monoethylene Glycol
See Ethylene Glycol

Mononucleosis Virus, Infectious
See Epstein-Barr Virus

Monophosphate, Adenosine
See Adenosine Monophosphate (AMP)

Monophosphate, Adenosine Cyclic
See Cyclic AMP

Monophosphate, Guanosine
See Guanosine Monophosphate

Monophosphate, Guanosine Cyclic
See Cyclic GMP

Monospot Test
See Rapid Test for Infection

Monoxide, Carbon
See Carbon Monoxide

Monteggia Fracture 24620-24635

Monticelli Procedure
See Application, Bone Fixation Device

Morbilli
See Rubeola

Morphine Methyl Ether
See Codeine

Morphometric Analysis
Nerve 88356
Skeletal Muscle 88355
Tumor 88358

Morton's Neuroma
Excision 28080

Moschcowitz Operation
See Repair, Hernia, Femoral; Revision

Mosenthal Test
See Urinalysis, Routine

Mother Cell
See Stem Cell

Motility Study
Esophagus .91010-91012

Motion Analysis
by Video and 3-D Kinematics 96000, 96004
Computer-based 96000, 96004

Mouth
Abscess
　　Incision and Drainage 40800-40801,
　　　　　　　　　41005-41009, 41015-41018
Biopsy 40808, 41108
Cyst
　　Incision and Drainage 40800-40801,
　　　　　　　　　41005-41009, 41015-41018
Excision
　　Frenum 40819
Hematoma
　　Incision and Drainage 40800-40801,
　　　　　　　　　41005-41009, 41015-41018
Lesion
　　Destruction 40820
　　Excision 40810-40816, 41116
　　Vestibule of
　　　Destruction 40820
　　　Repair 40830
Mucosa
　　Excision 40818
Reconstruction 40840-40845
Removal
　　Foreign Body 40804-40805
Repair
　　Laceration 40830-40831
Unlisted Services and Procedures . .40899, 41599
Vestibule of
　　Excision
　　　Destruction 40808-40820
　　　Incision 40800-40806
　　　Other Procedures 40899
　　Removal
　　　Foreign Body 40804
　　　Repair 40830-40845

Move
See Transfer
Finger 26555
Toe Joint 26556
Toe to Hand 26551-26554

Moynihan Test
See Gastrointestinal Tract, X-Ray, with Contrast

MPD Syndrome
See Temporomandibular Joint (TMJ)

MPR
See Multifetal Pregnancy Reduction

MRA
See Magnetic Resonance Angiography

MRI
See Magnetic Resonance Imaging (MRI)

MR Spectroscopy
See Magnetic Resonance Spectroscopy

MSLT
See Multiple Sleep Latency Testing (MSLT)

Mucin
Synovial Fluid 83872

Mucocele
Sinusotomy
　　Frontal 31075

Mucopolysaccharides 83864-83866

Mucormycoses
See Mucormycosis

Mucormycosis
Antibody 86732

Mucosa
Ectopic Gastric Imaging 78290
Excision of Lesion
　　Alveolar, Hyperplastic 41828
　　Vestibule of Mouth 40810-40818
　　via Esophagoscopy 43228
　　via Small Intestinal Endoscopy 44369
　　via Upper GI Endoscopy 43258
Periodontal Grafting 41870
Urethra, Mucosal Advancement 53450
Vaginal Biopsy 57100-57105

Mucosa, Buccal
See Mouth, Mucosa

Mucous Cyst
Antibody
　　Hand or Finger 26160

Mucous Membrane
See Mouth, Mucosa
Cutaneous
　　Biopsy .11100-11101
　　Excision
　　　Benign Lesion 11440-11446
　　　Malignant Lesion 11640-11646
　　Layer Closure, Wounds 12051-12057
　　Simple Repair, Wounds 12011-12018
Excision
　　Sphenoid Sinus 31288
Lid Margin
　　Correction of Trichiasis 67835
　　Nasal Test 95065
　　Ophthalmic Test 95060
Rectum
　　Proctoplasty for Prolapse 45505

Mucus Cyst
See Mucous Cyst

MUGA (Multiple Gated Acquisition) 78472-78478, 78483

Muller Procedure
See Sleep Study

Multifetal Pregnancy Reduction 59866

Multiple Sleep Latency Testing (MSLT) 95805

Multiple Valve Procedures
See Valvuloplasty

Mumford Operation
See Claviculectomy, Partial

Mumford Procedure 29824

Mumps
Antibody 86735
Immunization 90704, 90707, 90710
Vaccine 90704
    MMR 90707
    MMRV 90710

Muramidase 85549

Murine Typhus 86000

Muscle
See Specific Muscle
Abdomen
    See Abdominal Wall
Biopsy 20200-20206
Heart
    See Myocardium
Neck
    See Neck Muscle
Removal
    Foreign Body 20520-20525
Repair
    Forearm 25260-25274
    Wrist.....................25260-25274
Revision
    Arm, Upper 24330-24331
Transfer
    Arm, Upper 24301, 24320
    Elbow 24301
    Femur 27110
    Hip 27100-27105, 27111
    Shoulder 23395-23397, 24301, 24320

Muscle, Oculomotor
See Eye Muscles

Muscles
Repair
    Extraocular 65290

Muscle Compartment Syndrome
Detection 20950

Muscle Denervation
See Denervation

Muscle Division
Scalenus Anticus 21700-21705
Sternocleidomastoid 21720-21725

Muscle Flaps 15732-15738
Free 15756

Muscle Grafts 15841-15845

Muscle Testing
Dynamometry, Eye 92260
Extraocular Multiple Muscles 92265
Manual 95831-95834

Musculo-Skeletal System
See Musculoskeletal System

Musculoplasty
See Muscle, Repair

Musculoskeletal System
Unlisted Services and Procedures 20999, 24999, 25999, 26989, 27299, 27599, 27899
Unlisted Services and Procedures, Head ...21499

Musculotendinous (Rotator) Cuff
Repair 23410-23412

Mustard Procedure
See Repair, Great Arteries; Revision

Myasthenia Gravis
Tensilon Test 95857-95858

Myasthenic, Gravis
See Myasthenia Gravis

Mycobacteria
Culture 87116
    Identification 87118
Detection 87550-87562
Sensitivity Studies 87190

Mycoplasma
Antibody 86738
Culture 87109
Detection 87580-87582

Mycota
See Fungus

Myectomy, Anorectal
See Myomectomy, Anorectal

Myelencephalon
See Medulla

Myelin Basic Protein
Cerebrospinal Fluid 83873

Myelography
Brain 70010
Spine
    Cervical 72240
    Lumbosacral 72265
    Thoracic 72255
    Total 72270

Myelomeningocele
Repair 63704-63706

Myelotomy 63170

Myocardial
Perfusion Imaging ...78460-78465, 78478-78480
    See Nuclear Medicine
Positron Emission Tomography (PET) 78459

Myocardial Imaging 78466-78469
Positron Emission Tomography
    Perfusion Study 78491-78492
Repair
    Postinfarction 33542

Myocutaneous Flaps 15732-15738, 15756

Myofascial Pain Dysfunction Syndrome
See Temporomandibular Joint (TMJ)

Myofibroma
See Leiomyomata

Myoglobin 83874

Myomectomy
Anorectal 45108
Uterus 58140-58146, 58545-58546

Myoplasty
See Muscle, Repair

Myotomy
Esophagus 43030

Myringoplasty 69620

Myringostomy
See Myringotomy

Myringotomy 69420-69421

Myxoid Cyst
See Ganglion

N

N. Meningitidis
See Neisseria Meningitidis

Naffziger Operation
See Decompression, Orbit; Section

Nagel Test
See Color Vision Examination

Nails
Avulsion 11730-11732
Biopsy 11755
Debridement 11720-11721
Evacuation
    Hematoma, Subungual 11740
Excision 11750-11752
    Cyst
        Pilonidal 11770-11772
KOH Examination 87220
Removal 11730-11732, 11750-11752
Trimming 11719

Nail Bed
Reconstruction 11762
Repair 11760

Nail Fold
Excision
    Wedge 11765

Nail Plate Separation
See Onychia

Narcosynthesis
Diagnostic and Therapeutic 90865

Nasal Abscess
See Nose, Abscess

Nasal Area
Bone Graft 21210

Nasal Bleeding
See Epistaxis

Nasal Bone
Fracture
    Closed Treatment 21310-21320
    Open Treatment 21325-21335
    without Manipulation 21310
    with Manipulation 21315-21320
X-Ray 70160

Nasal Deformity
Repair 40700-40761

Nasal Function Study 92512

Nasal Polyp
See Nose, Polyp

Nasal Prosthesis
Impression 21087

Nasal Septum
Abscess
    Incision and Drainage 30020
Fracture
    Closed Treatment 21337
    Open Treatment 21336
Hematoma
    Incision and Drainage 30020
Repair 30630
Submucous Resection 30520

Nasal Sinuses
See Sinus; Sinuses

Nasal Smear
Eosinophils 89190

Nasal Turbinate
Fracture
    Therapeutic 30930

Nasoethmoid Complex
Fracture
    Open Treatment 21338-21339
    Percutaneous Treatment 21340
Reconstruction 21182-21184

Nasogastric Tube
Placement 43752

Nasolacrimal Duct
Exploration 68810
    with Anesthesia 68811
Insertion
    Stent 68815

X-Ray
    with Contrast 70170

Nasomaxillary
Fracture
    Closed Treatment 21345
    Open Treatment 21346-21348
    with Bone Grafting 21348

Nasopharynges
See Nasopharynx

Nasopharyngoscopy 92511

Nasopharynx
See Pharynx
Biopsy 42804-42806
Hemorrhage 42970-42972
Unlisted Services and Procedures 42999

Natriuretic Peptide 83880

Natural Ostium
Sinus
    Maxillary 31000
    Sphenoid 31002

Navicular
Arthroplasty
    with Implant 25443
Fracture
    Closed Treatment 25622
    Open Treatment 25628
    with Manipulation 25624
Repair 25440

Neck
Angiography 70498, 70547-70549
Artery
    Ligation 37615
Biopsy 21550
Bypass Graft 35901
CT Scan 70490-70492, 70498
Dissection, Radical
    See Radical Neck Dissection
Exploration
    Blood Vessel 35800
    Lymph Nodes 38542
Incision and Drainage
    Abscess 21501-21502
    Hematoma 21501-21502
Lipectomy, Suction Assisted 15876
Magnetic Resonance Angiography
(MRA) 70547-70549
Magnetic Resonance Imaging
(MRI) 70540-70543
Nerve
    Graft 64885-64886
Repair
    Blood Vessel 35201
    with Other Graft 35261
    with Vein Graft 35231
Skin
    Revision 15819
Tumor
    Excision 21555-21556
    Excision/Resection 21557
Ultrasound Exam 76536
Unlisted Services and Procedures,
Surgery 21899

Urinary Bladder
    See Bladder, Neck
Wound Exploration
    Penetrating 20100
X-Ray 70360

Neck Muscle
Division
    Scalenus Anticus 21700-21705
    Sternocleidomastoid 21720-21725

Necropsy
Coroner's Exam 88045
Forensic Exam 88040
Gross and Micro Exam 88020-88029
Gross Exam 88000-88016
Organ 88037
Regional 88036
Unlisted Services and Procedures 88099

Needle Biopsy
See Biopsy
Abdomen Mass 49180
Bone 20220-20225
Bone Marrow 38221
Breast 19100
Colon-Sigmoid
    Endoscopy 45342
CT Scan Guidance 76360
Epididymis 54800
Esophagus
    Endoscopy 43232
Fluoroscopic Guidance 76003
Gastrointestinal, Upper
    Endoscopy 43242
Kidney 50200
Liver 47000-47001
Lung 32405
Lymph Nodes 38505
Mediastinum 32405
Muscle 20206
Pancreas 48102
Pleura 32400
Prostate 55700
Retroperitoneal Mass 49180
Salivary Gland 42400
Spinal Cord 62269
Testis 54500
Thyroid Gland 60100
Transbronchial 31629

Needle Localization
Breast
    Placement 19290-19291
    with Lesion Excision 19125-19126
Magnetic Resonance Guidance 76393

Needle Manometer
Technique 20950

Needle Wire
Introduction
    Trachea 31730
Placement
    Breast 19290-19291

Neer Procedure 23470

Neisseria gonorrheae 87590-87592,
87850

Neisseria Meningitidis
Antibody 86741

Neobladder
Construction 51596

Neonatal Critical Care
See Newborn Care
Initial 99295
Subsequent 99296

Neoplasm
Cancer Photoradiation Therapy
   See Photochemotherapy
Cardiac
   See Heart, Tumor
Colon
   See Colon, Tumor
Esophageal
   See Tumor, Esophagus
Spinal Cord
   See Spinal Cord, Neoplasm
Unspecified Nature of Brain
   See Brain, Tumor

Neoplastic Growth
See Tumor

Nephelometry 83883

Nephrectomy
Donor 50300-50320, 50547
Laparoscopic 50545-50548
Partial 50240
   Laparoscopic 50543
Recipient 50340
with Ureters 50220-50236, 50546, 50548

Nephrolith
See Calculus, Removal, Kidney

Nephrolithotomy 50060-50075

Nephropexy 50400-50405

Nephroplasty
See Kidney, Repair

Nephropyeloplasty
See Pyeloplasty

Nephrorrhaphy 50500

Nephroscopy
See Endoscopy, Kidney

Nephrostogram 50394

Nephrostolithotomy
Percutaneous 50080-50081

Nephrostomy 50040
Change Tube 50398
Endoscopic 50562-50570
Percutaneous 52334
with Drainage 50040
X-Ray with Contrast
   Guide Dilation 74485

Nephrostomy Tract
Establishment 50395

Nephrotomogram
See Nephrotomography

Nephrotomography 74415

Nephrotomy 50040-50045
with Exploration 50045

Nerve
Cranial
   See Cranial Nerve
Facial
   See Facial Nerve
Intercostal
   See Intercostal Nerve
Lingual
   See Lingual Nerve
Median
   See Median Nerve
Obturator
   See Obturator Nerve
Peripheral
   See Peripheral Nerve
Phrenic
   See Phrenic Nerve
Sciatic
   See Sciatic Nerve
Spinal
   See Spinal Nerve
Tibial
   See Tibial Nerve
Ulnar
   See Ulnar Nerve
Vestibular
   See Vestibular Nerve

Nerves
Anastomosis
   Facial to Hypoglossal 64868
   Facial to Phrenic 64870
   Facial to Spinal Accessory 64866
Avulsion 64732-64772
Biopsy 64795
Decompression 64702-64727
Destruction 64600-64680
   Laryngeal, Recurrent 31595
Foot
   Excision 28030
   Incision 28035
Graft 64885-64907
Implantation
   Electrode 64553-64581
   to Bone 64787
   to Muscle 64787
Incision 43640-43641, 64732-64772
Injection
   Anesthetic 01991-01992, 64400-64530
   Neurolytic Agent 64600-64680
Insertion
   Electrode 64553-64581
Lesion
   Excision 64774-64792
Neurofibroma
   Excision 64788-64792
Neurolemmoma
   Excision 64788-64792
Neurolytic
   Internal 64727

Neuroma
   Excision 64774-64786
Neuroplasty 64702-64721
Removal
   Electrode 64585
Repair
   Graft 64885-64907
   Microdissection 69990
   Suture 64831-64876
Spinal Accessory
   Incision 63191
   Section 63191
Suture 64831-64876
Sympathectomy
   Excision 64802-64818
Transection 43640-43641, 64732-64772
Transposition 64718-64721
Unlisted Services and Procedures 64999

Nerve Conduction
Motor Nerve 95900-95903
Sensory Nerve or Mixed 95904

Nerve II, Cranial
See Optic Nerve

Nerve Root
See Cauda Equina; Spinal Cord
Decompression 63020-63091
Incision 63185-63190
Section 63185-63190

Nerve Stimulation, Transcutaneous
See Application, Neurostimulation

Nerve Teasing 88362

Nerve V, Cranial
See Trigeminal Nerve

Nerve VII, Cranial
See Facial Nerve

Nerve X, Cranial
See Vagus Nerve

Nerve XI, Cranial
See Accessory Nerve

Nerve XII, Cranial
See Hypoglossal Nerve

Nervous System
Nuclear Medicine
   Unlisted Services and Procedures 78699

Nesidioblast
See Islet Cell

Neural Conduction
See Nerve Conduction

Neural Ganglion
See Ganglion

Neurectomy
Foot 28030
Gastrocnemius 27320
Hamstring Muscle 27315
Leg, Upper 27315-27320
Popliteal 27320
Tympanic 69676

Nipples
See Breast
Inverted 19355
Reconstruction 19350

Nissen Operation
See Fundoplasty, Esophagogastric

Nissen Procedure 43324
Laparoscopic 43280

Nitrate Reduction Test
See Urinalysis

Nitroblue Tetrazolium Dye Test 86384

Nitrogen, Blood Urea
See Blood Urea Nitrogen

NMR Imaging
See Magnetic Resonance Imaging (MRI)

NMR Spectroscopies
See Magnetic Resonance Spectroscopy

Noble Procedure
See Repair; Suture

Nocardia
Antibody 86744

Nocturnal Penile Rigidity Test 54250

Nocturnal Penile Tumescence Test 54250

Node, Lymph
See Lymph Nodes

Nodes
See Lymph Nodes

Node Dissection, Lymph
See Dissection, Lymph Nodes

Non-Invasive Vascular Imaging
See Vascular Studies

Non-Office Medical Services ..99056

Non-Stress Test, Fetal 59025

Nonunion Repair
Femur
    without Graft 27470
    with Graft 27472
Metatarsal 28322
Tarsal Joint 28320

Noradrenalin
Blood 82383-82384
Urine 82384

Norchlorimipramine
See Imipramine

Norepinephrine
See Catecholamines
Blood 82383-82384
Urine 82384

Nortriptyline
Assay 80182

Norwood Procedure 33611-33612,
                              33619
See Repair, Heart, Ventricle; Revision

Nose
Abscess
    Incision and Drainage 30000-30020
Artery
    Incision 30915-30920
Biopsy
    Intranasal 30100
Dermoid Cyst
    Excision
        Complex 30125
        Simple 30124
Displacement Therapy 30210
Endoscopy
    Diagnostic 31231-31235
    Surgical 31237-31294
Excision
    Rhinectomy 30150-30160
Fracture
    Closed Treatment 21345
    Open Treatment 21325-21336,
           21338-21339, 21346-21347
    Percutaneous Treatment 21340
    with Fixation 21330, 21340, 21345-21347
Hematoma
    Incision and Drainage 30000-30020
Hemorrhage
    Cauterization 30901-30906
Insertion
    Septal Prosthesis 30220
Intranasal
    Lesion
        External Approach 30118
        Internal Approach 30117
Lysis of Adhesions 30560
Polyp
    Excision
        Extensive 30115
        Simple 30110
Reconstruction
    Cleft Lip/Cleft Palate 30460-30462
    Dermatoplasty 30620
    Primary 30400-30420
    Secondary 30430-30450
    Septum 30520
Removal
    Foreign Body 30300
        Anesthesia 30310
        Lateral Rhinotomy 30320
Repair
    Adhesions 30560
    Cleft Lip 40700-40761
    Fistula 30580-30600, 42260
    Rhinophyma 30120
    Septum 30540-30545, 30630
    Synechia 30560
    Vestibular Stenosis 30465
Skin
    Excision 30120
    Surgical Planing 30120
Submucous Resection Turbinate
    Excision 30140

Turbinate
    Excision 30130-30140
    Fracture 30930
    Injection 30200
Turbinate Mucosa
    Cauterization 30801-30802
Unlisted Services and Procedures 30999

Nose Bleed 30901-30906
See Hemorrhage, Nasal

No Man's Land
Tendon Repair 26356-26358

NTD 86384
See Nitroblue Tetrazolium Dye Test

Nuclear Antigen
Antibody 86235

Nuclear Imaging
See Nuclear Medicine

Nuclear Magnetic Resonance Imaging
See Magnetic Resonance Imaging (MRI)

Nuclear Magnetic Resonance Spectroscopy
See Magnetic Resonance Spectroscopy

Nuclear Medicine
Adrenal Gland Imaging 78075
Automated Data 78890-78891
Bile Duct
    Imaging 78223
Bladder
    Residual Study 78730
Blood
    Bone
        Density Study 78350-78351
        Imaging 78300-78320
        SPECT 78320
        Ultrasound 76977
        Unlisted Services and Procedures ...78399
    Flow Imaging 78445
    Iron
        Absorption 78162
        Chelatable 78172
        Plasma 78160
        Red Cells 78140
        Utilization 78170
    Platelet Survival 78190-78191
    Red Cells 78120-78121
    Red Cell Survival 78130-78135
    Unlisted Services and Procedures 78199
    Whole Blood Volume 78122
Bone Marrow
    Imaging 78102-78104
Brain
    Blood Flow 78610-78615
    Cerebrospinal Fluid 78630-78650
    Imaging 78600-78609
        Vascular Flow 78610
Endocrine System
    Unlisted Services and Procedures 78099
Esophagus
    Imaging (Motility) 78258
    Reflux Study 78262

Nucleases, DNA
See DNAse

Nutrition Therapy
Enteral 99560-99561
Group 97804
Initial Assessment 97802
Reassessment 97803
Total Parenteral 99562

Nystagmus Tests
See Vestibular Function Tests
Optokinetic 92534, 92544
Positional 92532, 92542
Spontaneous 92531, 92541

O

O2 Saturation
See Oxygen Saturation

Ober-Yount Procedure 27025
See Fasciotomy, Hip

Obliteration
Mastoid 69670

Obliteration, Total Excision of Vagina
See Excision, Vagina, Complete

Obliteration, Vaginal Vault
See Vagina, Closure

Oblongata, Medulla
See Medulla

Observation 99234-99236
See Evaluation and Management; Hospital Services

Obstetrical Care
Abortion
   Induced
      by Amniocentesis Injection . .59850-59852
        See Abortion; Cesarean Delivery;
        Ectopic Pregnancy
      by Dilation and Curettage 59840
      by Dilation and Evaluation 59841
   Missed
      First Trimester 59820
      Second Trimester 59821
   Spontaneous 59812
   Therapeutic 59840-59852
Antepartum Care 59425-59426
Cesarean Delivery 59618-59622
   Only 59514
   Postpartum Care 59515
   Routine .59510
   with Hysterectomy 59525
Curettage
   Hydatidiform Mole 59870
Evacuation
   Hydatidiform Mole 59870
External Cephalic Version 59412
Miscarriage
   Surgical Completion 59812-59821

Placenta Delivery 59414
Postpartum Care 59430, 59514
Septic Abortion 59830
Total (Global) 59400, 59610, 59618
Unlisted Services and Procedures . .59898-59899
Vaginal
      after Cesarean 59610-59614
Vaginal Delivery 59409-59410
   Delivery after Cesarean 59610-59614

Obstruction
See Occlusion

Obstruction Clearance
Venous Access Device 36536-36537

Obstruction Colon
See Colon, Obstruction

Obturator Nerve
Avulsion 64763-64766
Incision 64763-64766
Transection 64763-64766

Obturator Prosthesis 21076
Definitive .21080
Insertion
   Larynx 31527
Interim 21079

Occipital Nerve, Greater
Avulsion 64744
Incision 64744
Injection
   Anesthetic 64405
Transection 64744

Occlusion
Extracranial
   Intracranial 61623
Fallopian Tube
   Oviduct .58615
Penis
   Vein 37790

Occlusive Disease of Artery
See Repair, Artery; Revision

Occult Blood 82270
Penis
   by Hemoglobin Immunoassay 82274

Occupational Therapy
Evaluation 97003-97004

Ocular Implant 65175
See Orbital Implant
Insertion
      in Scleral Shell 65130
      Muscles, Not Attached 65135
      Muscles Attached 65140
Modification 65125
Reinsertion 65150
   with Foreign Material 65155
Removal 65175

Ocular Muscle
See Eye Muscles

Ocular Orbit
See Orbit

Ocular Prostheses
See Prosthesis, Ocular

Oculomotor Muscle
See Eye Muscles

Oddi Sphincter
See Sphincter of Oddi

Odontoid Dislocation
Open Treatment/Reduction 22318
   with Grafting 22319

Odontoid Fracture
Open Treatment/Reduction 22318
   with Grafting 22319

Odontoid Process
Excision 22548

Oesophageal Neoplasm
See Tumor, Esophagus

Oesophageal Varices
See Esophageal Varices

Oesophagus
See Esophagus

Oestradiol
See Estradiol

Office and/or Other Outpatient Services
See History and Physical
Consultation
   Confirmatory Consultations 99271-99275
Established Patient 99211-99215
New Patient 99201-99205
Normal Newborn 99432
Office Visit
   Established Patient 99211-99215
   New Patient 99201-99205
Outpatient Visit
   Established Patient 99211-99215
   New Patient 99201-99205
   Prolonged Services 99354-99355
with Surgical Procedure 99025

Office Medical Services
After Hours 99050-99054
Emergency Care 99058

Office or Other Outpatient Consultations
See Consultation, Office and/or Other Outpatient

Olecranon
See Elbow; Humerus; Radius; Ulna
Bursa
   Arthrocentesis 20605
Cyst
   Excision 24125-24126
Tumor
   Cyst 24120
   Excision 24125-24126

Olecranon Process
Craterization 24147
Diaphysectomy 24147
Excision 24147
   Abscess 24138

Fracture
  See Elbow; Humerus; Radius
    Closed Treatment 24670-24675
    Open Treatment 24685
Osteomyelitis 24138, 24147
Saucerization 24147
Sequestrectomy 24138

Oligoclonal Immunoglobulins .83916

Omentectomy 49255, 58950-58954
Laparotomy 58960
Oophorectomy 58943
Resection Ovarian Malignancy 58950-58954
Resection Peritoneal Malignancy . . .58950-58954
Resection Tubal Malignancy 58950-58954

Omentum
Excision 49255, 58950-58954
Flap 49904-49905
  Free
    with Microvascular Anastomosis . . .49906
Unlisted Services and Procedures 49999

Omphalectomy 49250

Omphalocele
Repair .49600-49611

Omphalomesenteric Duct
Excision 44800

Omphalomesenteric Duct, Persistent
See Diverticulum, Meckel's

Oncoprotein
HER-2/neu .83950

One Stage Prothrombin Time 85610-85611
See Prothrombin Time

Onychectomy
See Excision, Nails

Onychia
Drainage 10060-10061

Oocyte
Assisted Fertilization
  Microtechnique 89252
Culture
  for In Vitro Fertilization 89250
Identification
  Follicular Fluid 89254
Retrieval
  for In Vitro Fertilization 58970

Oophorectomy .58262-58263, 58291-58292,
      58552, 58554, 58661, 58940-58943
Ectopic Pregnancy
  Laparoscopic Treatment 59120
  Surgical Treatment 59120

Oophorectomy, Partial
See Excision, Ovary, Partial

Oophorocystectomy
See Cystectomy, Ovarian

Open Biopsy, Adrenal Gland
See Adrenal Gland, Biopsy

Operating Microscope 69990

Operation
Blalock-Hanlon
  See Septostomy, Atrial
Blalock-Taussig Subclavian-Pulmonary Anastomosis
  See Pulmonary Artery, Shunt, Subclavian
Borthen
  See Iridotasis
Dana
  See Rhizotomy
Dunn
  See Arthrodesis, Foot Joint
Duvries
  See Tenoplasty
Estes
  See Ovary, Transposition
Foley Pyeloplasty
  See Pyeloplasty
Fontan
  See Repair, Heart, Anomaly
Fox
  See Fox Operation
Gardner
  See Meningocele Repair
Green
  See Scapulopexy
Harelip
  See Cleft Lip, Repair
Heine
  See Cyclodialysis
Heller
  See Esophagomyotomy
Iris, Inclusion
  See Iridencleisis
Jaboulay Gastroduodenostomy
  See Gastroduodenostomy
Johanson
  See Reconstruction, Urethra
Keller
  See Keller Procedure
Krause
  See Gasserian Ganglion, Sensory Root, Decompression
Kuhnt-Szymanowski
  See Ectropion, Repair, Blepharoplasty
Mumford
  See Claviculectomy, Partial
Nissen
  See Fundoplasty, Esophagogastric
Peet
  See Nerves, Sympathectomy, Excision
Ramstedt
  See Pyloromyotomy
Richardson Hysterectomy
  See Hysterectomy, Abdominal, Total
Schanz
  See Femur, Osteotomy
Schlatter Total Gastrectomy
  See Excision, Stomach, Total
Smithwick
  See Excision, Nerve, Sympathetic
Winiwarter Cholecystoenterostomy
  See Anastomosis, Gallbladder to Intestines

Operation Microscopes
See Operating Microscope

Operculectomy 41821

Operculum
See Gums

Ophthalmic Mucous Membrane Test 95060
See Allergy Tests

Ophthalmology
Unlisted Services and Procedures 92499
  See Ophthalmology, Diagnostic

Ophthalmology, Diagnostic
Color Vision Exam 92283
Computerized Scanning 92135
Computerized Screening 99172
Dark Adaptation 92284
Electro-oculography 92270
Electromyography, Needle 92265
Electroretinography 92275
Endoscopy .66990
Eye Exam
  Established Patient 92012-92014
  New Patient 92002-92004
  with Anesthesia 92018-92019
Glaucoma Provocative Test 92140
Gonioscopy .92020
Ocular Photography
  External 92285
  Internal 92286-92287
Ophthalmoscopy 92225-92226
  with Dynamometry 92260
  with Fluorescein Angiography 92235
  with Fluorescein Angioscopy 92230
  with Fundus Photography 92250
  with Indocyanine-green Angiography . .92240
Refractive Determination 92015
Sensorimotor Exam 92060
Tonography .92120
  with Provocation 92130
Tonometry
  Serial .92100
Visual Acuity Screen 99172-99173
Visual Field Exam 92081-92083
Visual Function Screen 99172

Ophthalmoscopy 92225-92226
See Ophthalmology, Diagnostic

Opiates 83925

Opinion, Second
See Confirmatory Consultations

Optic Nerve
Decompression 67570
  with Nasal/Sinus Endoscopy 31294

Optokinetic Nystagmus Test
See Nystagmus Tests, Optokinetic

Oral Lactose Tolerance Test 82951-82953
See Glucose, Tolerance Test

Oral Mucosa
See Mouth, Mucosa

Tumor
    Resection 58950-58954
Unlisted Services and Procedures ..58679, 58999
Wedge Resection 58920

Oviduct
Anastomosis 58750
Chromotubation 58350
Ectopic Pregnancy 59120-59121
Excision 58700-58720
Fulguration
    Laparoscopic 58670
Hysterosalpingography 74740
Laparoscopy 58679
Ligation 58600-58611
Lysis
    Adhesions 58740
Occlusion 58615
    Laparoscopic 58671
Repair 58752
    Anastomosis 58750
    Create Stoma 58770
Unlisted Services and Procedures ..58679, 58999
X-Ray with Contrast 74740

Ovocyte
See Oocyte

Ovulation Tests 84830

Ovum Implantation
See Implantation

Ovum Transfer Surgery
See GIFT

Oxalate 83945

Oxidase, Ceruloplasmin
See Ceruloplasmin

Oxidoreductase, Alcohol-Nad+
See Antidiuretic Hormone

Oximetry (Noninvasive)
See Pulmonology, Diagnostic
Blood O2 Saturation
    Ear or Pulse 94760-94762

Oxoisomerase
See Phosphohexose Isomerase

Oxosteroids
See Ketosteroids

Oxycodinone 80102-80103, 83925

Oxygenation, Extracorporeal Membrane
See Extracorporeal Membrane Oxygenation

Oxygen Saturation 82805-82810

Oxyproline
See Hydroxyproline

Oxytocin Stress Test, Fetal 59020

P

P-Acetamidophenol
See Acetaminophen

Pacemaker, Heart
See Defibrillator, Heart
Conversion 33214
Electronic Analysis 93641-93642
    Antitachycardia System 93724
    Dual Chamber 33731-33732
    Single Chamber 93734-93735
Insertion 33200-33208
    Electrode 33210-33211, 33216-33217,
        33224-33225
    Pulse Generator Only 33212-33213
Removal 33233-33237
    via Thoracotomy 33236-33237
Repair
    Electrode 33218-33220
Replacement
    Catheter 33210
    Electrode 33210-33211, 33217
    Insertion 33200-33208
    Pulse Generator 33212-33213
Repositioning
    Electrode 33215, 33226
Revise Pocket
    Chest 33222
Telephonic Analysis 93733, 93736
Upgrade 33214

Pachymetry 0025T

Packing
Nasal Hemorrhage 30901-30906

Pain Management 99551
See Injection, Chemotherapy
Epidural/Intrathecal 62351, 62360-62362,
        99552
Intravenous Therapy 90783-90784

Palatal Augmentation Prosthesis 21082

Palatal Lift Prosthesis 21083

Palate
Abscess
    Incision and Drainage 42000
Biopsy 42100
Excision 42120, 42145
Fracture
    Closed Treatment 21421
    Open Treatment 21422-21423
Lesion
    Destruction 42160
    Excision 42104-42120
Prosthesis 42280-42281
Reconstruction
    Lengthening 42226-42227
Repair
    Cleft Palate 42200-42225
    Laceration 42180-42182
    Vomer Flap 42235
Unlisted Services and Procedures 42299

Palate, Cleft
See Cleft Palate

Palatoplasty 42200-42225

Palatoschisis
See Cleft Palate

Palm
Bursa
    Incision and Drainage 26025-26030
Fasciectomy 26121-26125
Fasciotomy 26040-26045
Tendon
    Excision 26170
Tendon Sheath
    Excision 26145
    Incision and Drainage 26020

Palsy, Seventh Nerve
See Facial Nerve Paralysis

Pancreas
Anastomosis
    to Intestines 48180
    with Intestines 48520-48540
Anesthesia 00794
Biopsy 48100
Cyst
    Anastomosis 48520-48540
    Repair 48500
Debridement
    Peripancreatic Tissue 48005
Excision
    Ampulla of Vater 48148
    Duct 48148
    Partial ...48140-48146, 48150, 48153-48154,
        48160
    Peripancreatic Tissue 48005
    Total 48155-48160
Lesion
    Excision 48120
Needle Biopsy 48102
Placement
    Drainage 48001
Pseudocyst
    Drainage
        Open 48510
        Percutaneous 48511
Removal
    Calculi (Stone) 48020
Removal Transplanted Allograft 48556
Repair
    Cyst 48500
    Suture 48545
Transplantation 48160, 48550-48556
Unlisted Services and Procedures 48999
X-Ray with Contrast 74300-74305
    Injection Procedure 48400

Pancreas, Endocrine Only
See Islet Cell

Pancreatectomy
Partial 48140-48146, 48150-48154, 48160
Total 48155-48160
with Transplantation 48160

Pancreaticojejunostomy 48180

Pancreatic DNAse
See DNAse

Pancreatic Duct
Destruction
    Calculi (Stone) 43265
Dilation
    Endoscopy 43271
Endoscopy
    Collection
        Specimen 43260
    Destruction
        Calculi (Stone) 43265
        Tumor 43272
    Dilation 43271
    Removal
        Calculi (Stone) 43264
        Foreign Body 43269
        Stent 43269
    Sphincterotomy 43262
    Sphincter Pressure 43263
    Tube Placement 43267-43268
Incision
    Sphincter 43262
Removal
    Calculi (Stone) 43264
    Foreign Body 43269
    Stent 43269
Tube Placement
    Nasopancreatic 43267
    Stent 43268
Tumor
    Destruction .43272
X-Ray with Contrast
    Guide Catheter 74329-74330

Pancreatic Islet Cell AB
See Antibody, Islet Cell

Pancreatography
Injection Procedure 48400
Intraoperative 74300-74301
Postoperative 74305

Pancreatojejunostomies
See Pancreaticojejunostomy

Pancreatorrhaphy 48545

Pancreatotomy
See Incision, Pancreas

Pancreozymin-Secretin Test . . .82938

Panel
See Organ or Disease Oriented Panel

Panniculectomy
See Lipectomy

Paper, Chromatography
See Chromatography, Paper

Paper Chromatographies
See Chromatography, Paper

Papilla, Interdental
See Gums

Papillectomy 46220

Papilloma
Destruction 54050-54065

PAPP D
See Lactogen, Human Placental

Pap Smears 88141-88143, 88147-88155,
88164-88167, 88174-88175

Para-Tyrosine
See Tyrosine

Paracentesis 49080
Eye
    Anterior Chamber
        with Diagnostic Aspiration of
        Aqueous 65800
        with Removal of Blood 65815
        with Removal Vitreous and/or Discission
        of Anterior Hyaloid Membrane 65810
        with Therapeutic Release of
        Aqueous 65805

Paracentesis, Abdominal
See Abdomen, Drainage

Paracentesis, Thoracic
See Thoracentesis

Paracervical Nerve
Injection
    Anesthetic .64435

Paraffin Bath Therapy 97018
See Physical Medicine/Therapy/Occupational
Therapy

Paraganglioma, Medullary
See Pheochromocytoma

Parainfluenza Virus
Antigen Detection
    Immunofluorescence 87279

Paralysis, Facial Nerve
See Facial Nerve Paralysis

Paralysis, Infantile
See Polio

Paranasal Sinuses
See Sinus; Sinuses

Parasites
Blood 87207
Examination .87169
Smear 87177

Parasitic Worms
See Helminth

Parathormone 83970

Parathyrin
See Parathormone

Parathyroidectomy 60500-60505

Parathyroid
Autotransplantation 60512

Parathyroid Gland
Autotransplant .60512
Excision .60500-60502
Exploration 60500-60505
Nuclear Medicine
    Imaging 78070

Parathyroid Hormone 83970

Parathyroid Hormone
Measurement
See Parathormone

Parathyroid Transplantation
See Transplantation, Parathyroid

Paraurethral Gland
Abscess
    Incision and Drainage 53060

Paravertebral Nerve
Destruction 64622-64627
Injection
    Anesthetic 64470-64484
    Neurolytic 64622-64627

Parietal Cell Vagotomies
See Vagotomy, Highly Selective

Parietal Craniotomy 61556

Paring
Skin Lesion
    Benign Hyperkeratotic
        More than Four Lesions 11057
        Single Lesion 11055
        Two to Four Lesions 11056

Paronychia
Incision and Drainage 10060-10061

Parotid Duct
Diversion 42507-42510
Reconstruction 42507-42510

Parotid Gland
Abscess
    Incision and Drainage 42300-42305
Calculi (Stone)
    Excision 42330, 42340
Excision
    Partial 42410-42415
    Total 42420-42426
Tumor
    Excision 42410-42426

Parotitides, Epidemic
See Mumps

Pars Abdominalis Aortae
See Aorta, Abdominal

Partial Colectomy
See Colectomy, Partial

Partial Cystectomy
See Cystectomy, Partial

Partial Esophagectomy
See Esophagectomy, Partial

Partial Gastrectomy
See Excision, Stomach, Partial

Partial Glossectomy
See Excision, Tongue, Partial

Partial Hepatectomy
See Excision, Liver, Partial

Partial Mastectomies
See Breast, Excision, Lesion

Partial Nephrectomy
See Excision, Kidney, Partial

Partial Pancreatectomy
See Pancreatectomy, Partial

Partial Splenectomy
See Splenectomy, Partial

Partial Thromboplastin Time
See Thromboplastin, Partial, Time

Partial Ureterectomy
See Ureterectomy, Partial

Particle Agglutination 86403-86406

Parvovirus
Antibody .... .86747

Patch
Allergy Tests .... .95044
   See Allergy Tests

Patella
See Knee
Dislocation 27560-27566
Excision .... .27350
   with Reconstruction .... .27424
Fracture 27520-27524
Reconstruction 27437-27438
Repair
   Chondromalacia .... .27418
   Instability 27420-27424

Patella, Chondromalacia
See Chondromalacia Patella

**Patellar Tendon Bearing
(PTB) Cast** .... .29435

Patellectomy
with Reconstruction .... .27424

Paternity Testing 86910-86911

Patey's Operation
See Mastectomy, Radical

Pathologic Dilatation
See Dilation

Pathology
Clinical
   Consultation 80500-80502
Surgical .... .88355
   Consultation 88321-88325
    Intraoperative 88329-88332
   Decalcification Procedure .... .88311
   Electron Microscopy 88348-88349
   Gross and Micro Exam
    Level II .... .88302
    Level III .... .88304
    Level IV .... .88305

    Level V .... .88307
    Level VI .... .88309
   Gross Exam
    Level I .... .88300
   Histochemistry 88318-88319
   Immunocytochemistry .... .88342
   Immunofluorescent Study 88346-88347
   Morphometry
    Nerve .... .88356
    Skeletal Muscle .... .88355
    Tumor .... .88358
   Nerve Teasing .... .88362
   Special Stain 88312-88314
   Staining 88312-88314
   Tissue Hybridization .... .88365
   Unlisted Services and
   Procedures .... .88399, 89399

Patterson's Test
See Blood Urea Nitrogen

Paul-Bunnell Test
See Antibody; Antibody Identification;
Microsomal Antibody

PBG
See Porphobilinogen

PCP
See Phencyclidine

PCR
See Polymerase Chain Reaction

Peans' Operation
See Amputation, Leg, Upper, at Hip; Radical
Resection; Replantation

Pectoral Cavity
See Chest Cavity

Pectus Carinatum
Reconstructive Repair 21740-21742
   with Thoracoscopy .... .21743

Pectus Excavatum
Reconstructive Repair 21740-21742
   with Thoracoscopy .... .21743

Pediatric Critical Care 99293-99294

Pediatric Intensive Care .... .99293

Pedicle Fixation
Insertion 22842-22844

Pedicle Flap
Formation 15570-15576
Island .... .15740
Neurovascular .... .15750
Transfer .... .15650

PEEP
See Pressure Breathing, Positive

Peet Operation
See Nerves, Sympathectomy, Excision

Pelvi-Ureteroplasty
See Pyeloplasty

Pelvic Adhesions
See Adhesions, Pelvic

Pelvic Exam .... .57410

Pelvic Exenteration .... .51597

Pelvic Fixation
Insertion .... .22848

Pelvic Lymphadenectomy ...... .58240

Pelvimetry .... .74710

Pelviolithotomy .... .50130

Pelvis
See Hip
Abscess
   Incision and Drainage .... .26990, 45000
Angiography .... .72191
Biopsy 27040-27041
Bone
   Drainage .... .26992
Brace Application .... .20662
Bursa
   Incision and Drainage .... .26991
CT Scan 72191-72194
Cyst
   Aspiration .... .50390
   Injection .... .50390
Destruction
   Lesion .... .58662
Endoscopy
   Destruction of Lesion .... .58662
   Lysis of Adhesions .... .58660
   Oviduct Surgery 58670-58671
Exclusion
   Small Intestine .... .44700
Exenteration .... .45126, 58240
Halo .... .20662
Hematoma
   Incision and Drainage .... .26990
Lysis
   Adhesions .... .58660
Magnetic Resonance Angiography .... .72198
Magnetic Resonance Imaging
(MRI) 72195-72197
Removal
   Foreign Body 27086-27087
Repair
   Osteotomy .... .27158
   Tendon .... .27098
Ring
   Dislocation 27193-27194, 27216-27218
   Fracture 27216-27218
    Closed Treatment 27193-27194
Tumor
   Excision 27047-27049
Ultrasound 76856-76857
Unlisted Services and Procedures for Hips and
Hip Joint .... .27299
X-Ray 72170-72190, 73540
   Manometry .... .74710

Pemberton Osteotomy of Pelvis
See Osteotomy, Pelvis

Penectomy
See Amputation, Penis

Penetrating Keratoplasties
See Keratoplasty, Penetrating

Pericardiectomy
Complete .33030-33031
Subtotal 33030-33031
Total
　　Endoscopic .32660

Pericardiocentesis 33010-33011
Ultrasound Guidance 76930

Pericardiostomy
Tube 33015

Pericardiotomy
Removal
　　Clot 33020
　　Foreign Body 33020

Pericardium
Cyst
　　Excision 32661, 33050
Excision 32659, 33030-33031
Incision
　　Removal
　　　　Clot 33020
　　　　Foreign Body 33020
　　　　with Tube 33015
　　Incision and Drainage 33025
Puncture Aspiration 33010-33011
Removal
　　Clot
　　　　Endoscopic 32658
　　Foreign Body
　　　　Endoscopic 32658
Tumor
　　Excision 32661, 33050

Peridural Anesthesia
See Anesthesia, Epidural

Peridural Injection
See Epidural, Injection

Perineal Prostatectomy
See Prostatectomy, Perineal

Perineoplasty 56810

Perineorrhaphy
Repair
　　Rectocele .57250

Perineum
Abscess
　　Incision and Drainage 56405
Colposcopy 99170
Removal
　　Prosthesis 53442
Repair 56810
X-Ray with Contrast 74775

Perionychia
See Paronychia

Periorbital Region
Reconstruction
　　Osteotomy with Graft 21267-21268
Repair-Osteotomy 21260-21263

**Peripheral Artery Disease (PAD)
Rehabilitation** 93668

Peripheral Nerve
Repair/Suture
　　Major 64856, 64859

Periprosthetic Capsulectomy
Breast 19371

Peristaltic Pumps
See Infusion Pump

Peritoneal Dialysis 90945-90947

Peritoneal Free Air
See Pneumoperitoneum

Peritoneal Lavage 49080

Peritoneocentesis 49080-49081

Peritoneoscopy
See Endoscopy, Peritoneum

Peritoneum
Abscess
　　Incision and Drainage 49020
　　　　Percutaneous 49021
Chemotherapy Administration 96445
　　See Chemotherapy
Endoscopy
　　Biopsy 47561
　　Drainage
　　　　Lymphocele 49323
　　　　X-Ray 47560
Exchange
　　Drainage Catheter 49423
Injection
　　Contrast
　　　　via Catheter 49424
Ligation
　　Shunt 49428
Removal
　　Cannula/Catheter 49422
　　Foreign Body 49085
　　Shunt 49429
Tumor
　　Resection 58950-58954
Unlisted Services and Procedures 49999
Venous Shunt
　　Injection .49427
X-Ray 74190

**Persistent, Omphalomesenteric
Duct**
See Diverticulum, Meckel's

Persistent Truncus Arteriosus
See Truncus Arteriosus

Personal Care
See Self Care

Pessary
Insertion 57160

Pesticides
Chlorinated Hydrocarbons 82441

PET
See Positron Emission Tomography

Petrous Temporal
Excision
　　Apex 69530

Peyronie Disease
Injection 54200
Surgical Exposure 54205
with Graft 54110-54112

pH
See Blood
Other Fluid 83986
Urine 83986

Phacoemulsification
Removal
　　Extracapsular Cataract 66982, 66984
　　Secondary Membranous Cataract 66850

Phagocytosis
White Blood Cells 86344

Phalangectomy
Toe 28150
　　Partial 28160

Phalanges (Hand)
See Finger, Bone

Phalanx, Finger
Craterization 26235-26236
Cyst
　　Excision 26210-26215
Diaphysectomy 26235-26236
Excision 26235-26236
　　Radical
　　　　for Tumor 26260-26262
Fracture
　　Articular
　　　　Closed Treatment 26740
　　　　Open Treatment 26746
　　　　with Manipulation 26742
　　Distal 26755-26756
　　　　Closed Treatment 26750
　　　　Open Treatment 26765
　　　　Percutaneous Fixation 26756
　　Open Treatment 26735
　　　　Distal 26765
　　Shaft 26720-26727
　　　　Open Treatment 26735
Incision and Drainage 26034
Ostectomy
　　Radical
　　　　for Tumor 26260-26262
Repair
　　Lengthening 26568
　　Nonunion 26546
　　Osteotomy 26567
Saucerization 26235-26236
Thumb
　　Fracture
　　　　Shaft 26720-26727
Tumor
　　Excision 26210-26215

Photopheresis
Extracorporeal 36522

Photophoresis
See Actinotherapy; Photochemotherapy

Photoradiation Therapies
See Actinotherapy

Photosensitivity Testing 95056
See Allergy Tests

Phototherapies
See Actinotherapy

Phototherapy, Ultraviolet
See Actinotherapy

Photo Patch
Allergy Test 95052
   See Allergy Tests

Phrenic Nerve
Anastomosis
   to Facial Nerve 64870
Avulsion 64746
Incision 64746
Injection
   Anesthetic 64410
Transection 64746

Physical Medicine/Therapy/Occupational Therapy
See Neurology, Diagnostic
Activities of Daily Living 97535, 99509
Aquatic Therapy
   with Exercises 97113
Athletic Training
   Evaluation 97005
   Re-evaluation 97006
Check-Out
   Orthotic/Prosthetic 97703
Cognitive Skills Development 97532
Community/Work Reintegration 97537
Evaluation 97001-97002
Kinetic Therapy 97530
Manual Therapy 97140
Modalities
   Contrast Baths 97034
   Diathermy Treatment 97024
   Electric Simulation
    Unattended 97014
   Electric Stimulation
    Attended, Manual 97032
   Hot or Cold Pack 97010
   Hydrotherapy (Hubbard Tank) 97036
   Infrared Light Treatment 97026
   Iontophoresis 97033
   Microwave Therapy 97020
   Paraffin Bath 97018
   Traction 97012
   Ultrasound 97035
   Ultraviolet Light 97028
   Unlisted Services and Procedures 97039
   Vasopneumatic Device 97016
   Whirlpool Therapy 97022
Orthotics Training 97504
Osteopathic Manipulation 98925-98929

Procedures
   Aquatic Therapy 97113
   Gait Training 97116
   Group Therapeutic 97150
   Massage Therapy 97124
   Neuromuscular Reeducation 97112
   Physical Performance Test 97750
   Therapeutic Exercises 97110
   Traction Therapy 97140
   Work Hardening 97545-97546
Prosthetic Training 97520
Sensory Integration 97533
Therapeutic Activities 97530
Unlisted Services and Procedures ..97139, 97799
Wheelchair Management/Propulsion 97542
Work Reintegration 97537

Physical Therapy
See Physical Medicine/Therapy/Occupational Therapy

Physician Services
Care Plan Oversight Services 99374-99380
   Home Health Agency Care 99374
   Hospice 99377-99378
   Nursing Facility 99379-99380
Direction, Advanced Life Support 99288
Prolonged
   without Direct Patient Contact .99358-99359
   with Direct Patient Contact ..99354-99357
    Outpatient/Office 99354-99355
   with Direct Patient Services
    Inpatient 99356-99357
Standby 99360
Supervision, Care Plan Oversight
Services 99374-99380

Pierce Ears 69090

Piercing of Ear Lobe
See Ear Lobes, Pierce

Piles
See Hemorrhoids

Pilonidal Cyst
Excision 11770-11772
Incision and Drainage 10080-10081

Pin
See Wire
Insertion/Removal
   Skeletal Traction 20650
Prophylactic Treatment
   Femur 27187
   Humerus 24498
   Shoulder 23490-23491

Pinch Graft 15050

Pinna
See Ear, External

Pinworms
Examination 87172

Pirogoff Procedure 27888

Pituitary Epidermoid Tumor
See Craniopharyngioma

Pituitary Gland
Excision 61546-61548
Tumor
   Excision 61546-61548, 62165

Pituitary Growth Hormone
See Growth Hormone

Pituitary Lactogenic Hormone
See Prolactin

Pituitectomy
See Excision, Pituitary Gland

PKU
See Phenylalanine

Placement
Catheter
   Bile Duct 75982
   Bronchus
    for Intracavitary Radioelement
    Application 31643
     See Catheterization
Catheter, Cardiac 93503
   See Catheterization, Cardiac
Colonic Stent 44397, 45327, 45345, 45387
Drainage
   Pancreas 48001
IVC Filter 75940
Jejunostomy Tube
   Endoscopic 44372
Metallic Localization Clip
   Breast 19295
Nasogastric Tube 43752
Needle
   Bone 36680
Needle Wire
   Breast 19290-19291
Orogastric Tube 43752
Radiation Delivery Device
   Intracoronary Artery 92974
Seton
   Anal 46020
Tracheal Stent 31631
Ureteral Stent 50947

Placenta
Delivery 59414

Placental Lactogen
See Lactogen, Human Placental

Placental Villi
See Chorionic Villus

Plagiocephaly 21175

Plague Vaccine 90727

Planing
Nose
   Skin 30120

Plantar Digital Nerve
Decompression 64726

Plantar Pressure Measurements
Dynamic 96001, 96004

Plasma
Frozen Preparation 86927

Plasma Prokallikrein
See Fletcher Factor

Plasma Test
Volume Determination 78110-78111

Plasma Thromboplastin
Antecedent 85270, 99564
Component 85250

Plasmin 85400

Plasminogen 85420-85421

Plasmin Antiactivator
See Alpha-2 Antiplasmin

Plasmodium
Antibody 86750

Plastic Repair of Mouth
See Mouth, Repair

Plate, Bone
See Bone Plate

Platelet
See Blood Cell Count, Complete Blood Count
Aggregation 85576
Antibody 86022-86023
Blood 85024-85025
Count 85032, 85049
Neutralization 85597

Platelet Cofactor I
See Clotting Factor

Platelet Test
Survival Test 78190-78191

Platysmal Flap 15825

PLC
See Tissue Typing

Pleoptic Training 92065

Plethysmography
See Vascular Studies
Extremities 93922-93923
Veins 93965
Penis 54240
Total Body 93720-93722

Pleura
Biopsy 32095-32100, 32400-32402
Decortication 32320
Empyema
Excision 32540
Excision 32310-32320
Endoscopic 32656
Foreign Body
Removal 32150-32151
Needle Biopsy 32400
Removal
Foreign Body 32653
Repair 32215
Thoracotomy 32095-32100
Unlisted Services and Procedures 32999

Pleural Cavity
Aspiration 32000-32002
Chemotherapy Administration 96440
See Chemotherapy

Fusion 32005
Incision
Empyema 32035-32036
Pneumothorax 32020
Puncture and Drainage 32000-32002
Thoracostomy 32035-32036

Pleural Endoscopies
See Thoracoscopy

Pleural Scarification
for Repeat Pneumothorax 32215

Pleural Tap
See Thoracentesis

Pleurectomy
Anesthesia 00544
Parietal 32310-32320
Endoscopic 32656

Pleuritis, Purulent
See Abscess, Thorax

Pleurocentesis
See Thoracentesis

Pleurodesis
Chemical 32005
Endoscopic 32650

Pleurosclerosis
See Pleurodesis

Pleurosclerosis, Chemical
See Pleurodesis, Chemical

Plexectomy, Choroid
See Choroid Plexus, Excision

Plexus, Choroid
See Choroid Plexus

Plexus Brachialis
See Brachial Plexus

Plexus Cervicalis
See Cervical Plexus

Plexus Coeliacus
See Celiac Plexus

Plexus Lumbalis
See Lumbar Plexus

PLGN
See Plasminogen

Plication, Sphincter, Urinary Bladder
See Bladder, Repair, Neck

Pneumocentesis
Lung 32420

Pneumocisternogram
See Cisternography

Pneumococcal Vaccine
See Vaccines

Pneumocystis Carinii
Antigen Detection
Immunofluorescence 87281

Pneumogastric Nerve
See Vagus Nerve

Pneumogram
Pediatric 94772

Pneumolysis 32940

Pneumonectomy 32440-32500
Completion 32488
Donor 32850, 33930
Sleeve 32442
Total 32440-32445

Pneumonology
See Pulmonology

Pneumonolysis 32940
Intrapleural 32652
Open Intrapleural 32124

Pneumonostomy 32200-32201

Pneumonotomy
See Incision, Lung

Pneumoperitoneum 49400

Pneumoplethysmography
Ocular 93875

Pneumothorax
Chemical Pleurodesis 32005
Pleural Scarification for Repeat 32215
Therapeutic
Injection Intrapleural Air 32960
Thoracentesis with Tube Insertion 32002

Polio
Antibody 86658
Vaccine 90712-90713

Poliovirus Vaccine, Inactivated
See Vaccines

Pollicization
Digit 26550

Polya Gastrectomy
See Gastrectomy, Partial

Polydactylism
See Supernumerary Digit

Polydactylous Digit
Reconstruction 26587
Repair 26587

Polydactyly, Toes 28344

Polymerase Chain Reaction 83898

Polyp
Antrochoanal
Removal .31032
Esophagus
Ablation .43228
Nose
Excision
Endoscopic 31237-31240
Extensive 30115
Simple 30110

Sphenoid Sinus
    Removal 31051
Urethra
    Excision 53260

Polypectomy
Nose
    Endoscopic 31237
Uterus 58558

Polypeptide, Vasoactive Intestinal
See Vasoactive Intestinal Peptide

Polysomnography 95808-95811

Polyuria Test
See Water Load Test

Pomeroy's Operation
See Tubal Ligation

Pooling
Blood Products 86965

Popliteal Arteries
See Artery, Popliteal

Popliteal Synovial Cyst
See Baker's Cyst

Poradenitistras
See Lymphogranuloma Venereum

Porphobilinogen
Urine 84106-84110

Porphyrins
Feces 84126-84127
Urine 84119-84120

Porphyrin Precursors 82135

PORP (Partial Ossicular Replacement Prosthesis) 69633, 69637

Portal Vein
See Vein, Hepatic Portal

Porter-Silber Test
See Corticosteroid, Blood

Portoenterostomies, Hepatic
See Hepaticoenterostomy

Portoenterostomy 47701

Port Film 77417

Posadas-Wernicke Disease
See Coccidioidomycosis

Positional Nystagmus Test
See Nystagmus Tests, Positional

Positive-Pressure Breathing, Inspiratory
See Intermittent Positive Pressure Breathing (IPPB)

Positive End Expiratory Pressure
See Pressure Breathing, Positive

Positron Emission Tomography (PET)
Brain 78608-78609
Heart 78459
Myocardial Imaging
    Perfusion Study 78491-78492
Tumor 78810

Post-Op Visit 99024

Postauricular Fistula
See Fistula, Postauricular

Postcaval Ureter
See Retrocaval Ureter

Postmortem
See Autopsy

Postoperative Wound Infection
Incision and Drainage 10180

Postop Vas Reconstruction
See Vasovasorrhaphy

Postpartum Care
Cesarean Delivery 59515
    after Attempted Vaginal Delivery 59622
    Previous 59610, 59614-59618, 59622
Vaginal Delivery 59430
    after Previous Cesarean Delivery 59614

Potassium 84132
Urine 84133

Potential, Auditory Evoked
See Auditory Evoked Potentials

Potential, Evoked
See Evoked Potential

Potts-Smith Procedure 33762

Pouch, Kock
See Kock Pouch

PPP
See Fibrin Degradation Products

PRA
See Cytotoxic Screen

Prealbumin 84134

Prebeta Lipoproteins
See Lipoprotein, Blood

Pregl's Test
See Cystourethroscopy, Catheterization, Urethral

Pregnancy
Abortion
    Induced 59855-59857
        by Amniocentesis Injection ..59850-59852
        by Dilation and Curettage 59840
        by Dilation and Evaluation 59841
    Septic 59830
    Therapeutic
        by Dilation and Curettage 59851
        by Hysterectomy 59852
        by Saline 59850

Cesarean Delivery 59618-59622
    Only 59514
    Postpartum Care 59514-59515
    Routine Care 59510
    Vaginal Birth After 59610-59614
    with Hysterectomy 59525
Ectopic
    Abdominal 59130
    Cervix 59140
    Interstitial
        Partial Resection Uterus 59136
        Total Hysterectomy 59135
    Laparoscopy
        without Salpingectomy and/or
        Oophorectomy 59150
        with Salpingectomy and/or
        Oophorectomy 59151
    Tubal 59121
        with Salpingectomy and/or
        Oophorectomy 59120
Miscarriage
    Surgical Completion
        Any Trimester 59812
        First Trimester 59820
        Second Trimester 59821
Molar
    See Hydatidiform Mole
Multifetal Reduction 59866
Placenta Delivery 59414
Vaginal Delivery 59409-59410
    after Cesarean Delivery 59610-59614
    Antepartum Care 59425-59426
    Postpartum Care 59430
    Total Obstetrical Care ..59400, 59610, 59618

Pregnancy Test 84702-84703
Urinalysis 81025

Pregnanediol 84135

Pregnanetriol 84138

Pregnenolone 84140

Prekallikrein
See Fletcher Factor

Prekallikrein Factor 85292

Premature, Closure, Cranial Suture
See Craniosynostosis

Prenatal Testing
Amniocentesis 59000
    with Amniotic Fluid Reduction 59001
Chorionic Villus Sampling 59015
Cordocentesis 59012
Fetal Blood Sample 59030
Fetal Monitoring 59050
    Interpretation Only 59051
Non-Stress Test, Fetal 59025, 99500
Oxytocin Stress Test 59020
Stress Test
    Oxytocin 59020
Ultrasound 76801-76817
    Fetal Biophysical Profile 76818-76819
    Fetal Heart 76825

Prentiss Operation
See Orchiopexy, Inguinal Approach

Prophylaxis
Retina
  Detachment
    Cryotherapy, Diathermy 67141
    Photocoagulation 67145

Prostaglandin 84150
Insertion 59200

Prostanoids
See Prostaglandin

Prostate
Ablation
  Cryosurgery 55873
Abscess
  Drainage 52700
  Incision and Drainage 55720-55725
Biopsy 55700-55705
Brachytherapy
  Needle Insertion 55859
Coagulation
  Laser 52647
Destruction
  Cryosurgery 55873
  Thermotherapy 53850-53853
    Microwave 53850
    Radio Frequency 53852
Excision
  Partial 55801, 55821-55831
  Perineal 55801-55815
  Radical 55810-55815, 55840-55845
  Retropubic 55831-55845
  Suprapubic 55821
  Transurethral 52601, 52612-52614
Exploration
  Exposure 55860
  with Nodes 55862-55865
Incision
  Exposure 55860-55865
  Transurethral 52450
Insertion
  Radioactive Substance 55860
Needle Biopsy .55700
Thermotherapy
  Transurethral 53850-53853
Ultrasound 76872-76873
Unlisted Services and Procedures 55899
  Urinary System 53899
Urethra
  Transurethral Balloon Dilation 52510
Vaporization
  Laser 52648

Prostatectomy 52601
Laparascopic 55866
Perineal
  Partial 55801
  Radical 55810-55815
Retropubic
  Partial 55831
  Radical 55840-55845, 55866
Suprapubic
  Partial 55821
Transurethral 52612-52614

Prostate Specific
Antigen 84152-84154

Prostatic Abscess
See Abscess, Prostate

Prostatotomy 55720-55725

Prosthesis
Augmentation
  Mandibular Body 21125
Auricular 21086
Breast
  Insertion 19340-19342
  Removal 19328-19330
  Supply 19396
Check-Out 97703
  See Physical Medicine/Therapy/Occupational
  Therapy
Cornea 65770
Facial 21088
Hernia
  Mesh 49568
Hip
  Removal 27090-27091
Intestines 44700
Knee
  Insertion 27438, 27445
Lens
  Insertion 66982-66985
  Manual or Mechanical
    Technique 66982-66984
  Not Associated with Concurrent Cataract
    Removal 66985
Mandibular Resection 21081
Nasal 21087
Nasal Septum
  Insertion 30220
Obturator 21076
  Definitive 21080
  Interim 21079
Ocular 21077, 65770, 66982-66985,
          92330-92335, 92358, 92393
  Fitting and Prescription 92330
  Loan 92358
  Prescription .92335
  Supply 92393
Orbital 21077
  Partial or Total 69633, 69637
Ossicle Reconstruction
  Chain 69633
Palatal Augmentation 21082
Palatal Lift 21083
Palate .42280-42281
Penile
  Insertion 54400-54405
  Removal 54406, 54410-54417
  Repair 54408
  Replacement 54410-54411, 54416-54417
Perineum
  Removal 53442
Skull Plate
  Removal 62142
  Replacement 62143
Spectacle
  Fitting 92352-92353
  Repair 92371
Speech Aid 21084
Spinal
  Insertion 22851
Synthetic 69633, 69637

Temporomandibular Joint
  Arthroplasty .21243
Testicular
  Insertion 54660
Training 97520
Urethral Sphincter
  Insertion 53444-53445
  Removal 53446-53447
  Repair 53449
  Replacement 53448
Wrist
  Removal 25250-25251

Protease F
See Plasmin

Protein
C-Reactive 86140-86141
Glycated 82985
Myelin Basic 83873
Osteocalcin 83937
Prealbumin 84134
Serum 84160-84165
Total 84155
Western Blot 84181-84182, 88372

Protein Analysis, Tissue
Western Blot 88371

Protein Blotting
See Western Blot

Protein C Activator 85337

Protein C Antigen 85302

Protein C Assay 85303

Protein C Resistance Assay 85307

Protein S
Assay 85306
Total 85305

Prothrombase
See Thrombokinase

Prothrombin 85210

Prothrombinase
See Thromboplastin

Prothrombin Time 85610-85611

Prothrombokinase 85230

Protime
See Prothrombin Time

Proton Treatment Delivery
Complex 77525
Intermediate 77523
Simple 77520-77522

Protoporphyrin 84202-84203

Protozoa
Antibody 86753

Provitamin A
See Vitamin, A

Pulse Generator
Electronic Analysis 95970-95971
Heart
    Insertion/Replacement 33212-33213

Pulse Rate Increased
See Tachycardia

Pump
See Chemotherapy, Pump Services; Infusion
Pump

Pump, Infusion
See Infusion Pump

Pump Services
Oxygenator/Heat Exchanger 99190-99192

Pump Stomach for Poison 91105

Punch Graft 15775-15776

Puncture
Artery 36600
Chest
    Drainage 32000-32002
Cisternal
    See Cisternal Puncture
Lumbar
    See Spinal Tap
Lung 32420
Pericardium 33010-33011
Pleural Cavity
    Drainage 32000-32002
Skull
    Drain Fluid 61000-61020
        Cistern 61050
    Inject Cistern 61055
    Inject Ventricle 61026
    Shunt
        Drain Fluid 61070
        Injection 61070
Spinal Cord
    Diagnostic 62270
    Drain Fluid 62272
    Lumbar 62270
Tracheal
    Aspiration and/or Injection 31612

Puncture Aspiration
Abscess
    Skin 10160
Bulla 10160
Cyst
    Breast 19000-19001
    Skin 10160
Hematoma 10160

Puncturing
See Puncture

Pure-Tone Audiometry
See Audiometry, Pure Tone

Pustules
Removal 10040

Putti-Platt Procedure 23450

PUVA
See Dermatology; Photochemotherapy;
Ultraviolet Light Therapy

Pyelogram
See Urography, Intravenous; Urography,
Retrograde

Pyelography 74400, 74425
Injection 50394

Pyelolithotomy 50130
Anatrophic 50075
Coagulum 50130

Pyeloplasty 50400-50405, 50544
Repair
    Horseshoe Kidney 50540
Secondary 50405

Pyeloscopy
with Cystourethroscopy 52351
    Biopsy 52354
    Destruction 52354
    Lithotripsy 52353
    Removal
        Calculus 52352
    Tumor Excision 52355

Pyelostogram 50394

Pyelostolithotomy
Percutaneous 50080-50081

Pyelostomy 50125, 50400-50405
Change Tube 50398

Pyelotomy
Complicated 50135
Endoscopic 50570
Exploration 50120
with Drainage 50125
with Removal Calculus 50130

Pyeloureterogram
Antegrade 50394

Pyeloureteroplasty
See Pyeloplasty

Pyloric Sphincter
Incision 43520
Reconstruction 43800

Pyloromyotomy 43520
with Gastrectomy 43639

Pyloroplasty 43800
with Gastrectomy 43639
with Vagotomy 43640

Pyothorax
See Abscess, Thorax

Pyridoxal Phosphate 84207

Pyrophosphate, Adenosine
See Adenosine Diphosphate

Pyrophosphorylase, Udp Galactose
See Galactose-1-Phosphate, Uridyl Transferase

Pyruvate 84210-84220

P & P
See Proconvertin

P B Antibodies
See Antibody, Heterophile

Q

Quadriceps Repair 27430

Quick Test
See Prothrombin Time

Quinidine
Assay 80194

Quinine 84228

Q Fever 86000, 86638

Q Fever ab
See Antibody, Coxiella Burnetii

R

Rabies Vaccine
See Vaccines

Rachicentesis
See Spinal Tap

Radial Arteries
See Artery, Radial

Radial Head, Subluxation
See Nursemaid Elbow

Radial Keratotomy 65771

Radiation
See Irradiation

Radiation, X
See X-Ray

Radiation Physics
Consultation 77336-77370
Unlisted Services and Procedures 77399

Radiation Therapy 77280-77295
Consultation
    Radiation Physics 77336-77370
CT Scan Guidance 76370
Dose Plan 77300, 77305-77331
    Brachytherapy 77326-77328
    Intensity Modulation 77301
    Teletherapy 77305-77321
Field Set-up 77280-77295
Planning 77261-77263, 77299
Special 77470
Stereotactic 77432

Radical Excision of Lymph Nodes

See Excision, Lymph Nodes, Radical

Radical Mastectomies, Modified

See Mastectomy, Modified Radical

Radical Neck Dissection

Radical Resection

See Resection, Radical

Radical Vaginal Hysterectomy

See Hysterectomy, Vaginal, Radical

Radical Vulvectomy

See Vulvectomy, Radical

Radio-Cobalt B12 Schilling Test

See Vitamin, B12, Absorption Study

Radioactive Colloid Therapy

Radioactive Substance

Radiocarpal Joint

Radiocinematographies

See Cineradiography

Radioelement

Radioelement Substance

Radiography

See Radiology, Diagnostic; X-Ray

Radioimmunosorbent Test

See Gammaglobulin, Blood

Radioisotope Brachytherapy

See Brachytherapy

Radioisotope Scan

See Nuclear Medicine

Radiological Marker

Radiology

Radionuclide CT Scan

See Emission Computerized Tomography

Radionuclide Imaging

See Nuclear Medicine

Radionuclide Therapy

Radionuclide Tomography, Single-Photon Emission-Computed

See SPECT

Radiopharmaceutical Therapy

Radiotherapeutic

See Radiation Therapy

Radiotherapies

See Irradiation

Radiotherapy, Surface

See Application, Radioelement, Surface

Radioulnar Joint

Radius

See Arm, Lower; Elbow; Ulna
Arthroplasty 24365
  with Implant 24366, 25441
Craterization 24145, 25151
Cyst
  Excision 24125-24126, 25120-25126
Diaphysectomy 24145, 25151
Dislocation
  Partial 24640
  Subluxate .24640
  with Fracture
    Closed Treatment 24620
    Open Treatment 24635
Excision 24130, 24136, 24145, 24152-24153
  Epiphyseal Bar 20150
  Partial 25145
  Styloid Process 25230
Fracture 25605
  Closed Treatment 25500-25505, 25520,
                      25600-25605
    without Manipulation 25600
    with Manipulation 25605
  Distal 25600-25611
    Open Treatment 25620
  Head/Neck
    Closed Treatment 24650-24655
    Open Treatment 24665-24666
  Open Treatment 25515, 25525-25526,
                      25574
  Percutaneous Fixation 25611
  Shaft 25500-25526
    Open Treatment 25574
  with Ulna 25560-25565
    Open Treatment 25575
Implant
  Removal 24164
Incision and Drainage 25035
Osteomyelitis 24136, 24145
Osteoplasty 25390-25393
Prophylactic Treatment 25490, 25492
Repair
  Epiphyseal Arrest 25450-25455
  Epiphyseal Separation
    Closed 25600
    Closed with Manipulation 25605
    Open Treatment 25620
    Percutaneous Fixation 25611
  Malunion or Nonunion 25400, 25415
  Osteotomy 25350-25355, 25370-25375
    and Ulna 25365
  with Graft 25405, 25420-25426
Saucerization 24145, 25151
Sequestrectomy 24136, 25145
Tumor
  Cyst 24120
  Excision . .24125-24126, 25120-25126, 25170

Ramstedt Operation
See Pyloromyotomy

Ramus Anterior, Nervus Thoracicus
See Intercostal Nerve

Range of Motion Test
Extremities or Trunk 95851
Eye 92018-92019
Hand 95852

Rapid Heart Rate
See Tachycardia

Rapid Plasma Reagin Test
. 86592-86593

Rapid Test for Infection
. . . . .86308, 86403-86406
Monospot Test 86308

Rapoport Test
. 52005

Raskind Procedure
. 33735-33737

Rathke Pouch Tumor
See Craniopharyngioma

Rat Typhus
See Murine Typhus

Rays, Roentgen
See X-Ray

Raz Procedure
. 51845
See Repair, Bladder, Neck

RBC
See Red Blood Cell (RBC)

RBC ab
See Antibody, Red Blood Cell

Reaction
Lip
  without Reconstruction 40530

Reaction, Polymerase Chain
See Polymerase Chain Reaction

Realignment
Femur
  with Osteotomy 27454
Knee
  Extensor .27422

Receptor
See CD4; Estrogen, Receptor; FC Receptor;
Progesterone Receptors

Receptor Assay
Hormone 84233-84235
Non Hormone 84238

Recession
Gastrocnemius
  Leg, Lower 27687

Reconstruction
See Revision
Abdominal Wall
  Omental Flap 49905
Acetabulum 27120-27122
Anal
  Congenital Absence 46730-46740
  Fistula 46742
  Graft 46753
  Sphincter 46750-46751, 46760-46762
  with Implant 46762
Ankle .27700-27703
Apical-Aortic Conduit 33404
Atrial 33253

Reconstruction (continued)
Auditory Canal, External 69310-69320
Bile Duct
  Anastomosis 47800
Bladder
  and Urethra 51800-51820
  from Colon 50810
  from Intestines 50820, 51960
Breast 19357-19369
  Augmentation 19324-19325
  Mammoplasty 19318-19325
  Nipple 19350-19355
  Revision .19380
  Transverse Rectus Abdominis Myocutaneous
    Flap 19367-19369
  with Free Flap 19364
  with Latissimus Dorsi Flap 19361
  with Other Techniques 19366
  with Tissue Expander 19357
Bronchi 32501
  Graft Repair 31770
  Stenosis .31775
Canthus 67950
Carpal 25443
Carpal Bone 25394, 25430
Cheekbone .21270
Chest Wall
  Omental Flap 49904
  Trauma .32820
Cleft Palate 42200-42225
Conduit
  Apical-Aortic 33404
Conjunctiva 68320-68335
  with Flap
    Bridge or Partial 68360
    Total .68362
Cranial Bone
  Extracranial 21181-21184
Ear, Middle
  Tympanoplasty without
    Mastoidectomy 69631
    with Ossicular Chain
      Reconstruction 69632-69633
  Tympanoplasty with Antrotomy or
    Mastoidotomy
    with Ossicular Chain
      Reconstruction 69636-69637
  Tympanoplasty with Mastoidectomy . .69641
    Radical or Complete 69644-69645
    with Intact or Reconstructed
      Wall 69643-69644
    with Ossicular Chain
      Reconstruction 69642
Elbow 24360
  Total Replacement 24363
  with Implant 24361-24362
Esophagus 43300, 43310, 43313
  Creation
    Stoma 43350-43352
  Esophagostomy 43350
  Fistula 43305, 43312, 43314
  Gastrointestinal 43360-43361
Eyelid
  Canthus .67950
  Second Stage 67975
  Total 67973-67975

Rectal Bleeding
See Hemorrhage, Rectum

Rectal Prolapse
See Procidentia, Rectum

Rectal Sphincter
Dilation 45910

Rectocele
Repair 45560

Rectopexy
See Proctopexy

Rectoplasty
See Proctoplasty

Rectorrhaphy
See Rectum, Suture

Rectovaginal Fistula
See Fistula, Rectovaginal

Rectovaginal Hernia
See Rectocele

Rectum
See Anus
Abscess
    Incision and Drainage 45005-45020,
                                46040, 46060
Biopsy 45100
Dilation
    Endoscopy 45303
Endoscopy
    Destruction
        Tumor 45320
    Dilation 45303
    Exploration .45300
    Hemorrhage 45317
    Removal
        Foreign Body 45307
        Polyp 45308-45315
        Tumor 45308-45315
    Volvulus 45321
Excision
    Partial 45111, 45113-45116, 45123
    Total 45110, 45112, 45119-45120
    with Colon .45121
Exploration
    Endoscopic 45300
Hemorrhage
    Endoscopic 45317
Injection
    Sclerosing Solution 45520
Lesion
    Excision 45108
Manometry 91122
Prolapse
    Excision 45130-45135
Pulsed Irrigation
    Fecal Impaction 91123
Removal
    Fecal Impaction 45915
        by Pulsed Irrigation 91123
    Foreign Body 45307, 45915
Repair
    Fistula 45800-45825
    Injury 45562-45563
    Prolapse 45505-45541, 45900
    Rectocele .45560
    Stenosis 45500
    with Sigmoid Excision 45550
Stricture
    Excision 45150
Suture
    Fistula 45800-45825
    Prolapse 45540-45541
Tumor
    Destruction 45190, 45320, 46937-46938
    Excision 45160-45170
Unlisted Services and Procedures . .44239, 45999

Reductase, Glutathione
See Glutathione Reductase

Reductase, Lactic Cytochrome
See Lactic Dehydrogenase

Reduction
Forehead 21137-21139
Lung Volume 32491
Mammoplasty 19318
Masseter Muscle/Bone 21295-21296
Osteoplasty
    Facial Bones 21209
Pregnancy
    Multifetal 59866
Skull
    Craniomegalic 62115-62117
Ventricular Septum
    Non-surgical 0024T

Red Blood Cell (RBC)
Antibody 86850-86870
    Pretreatment 86970-86972
Count .85032-85041
Fragility
    Mechanical 85547
    Osmotic 85555-85557
Hematocrit 85014
Iron Utilization 78170
Morphology 85007
Platelet Estimation 85007
Sedimentation Rate
    Automated 85652
    Manual 85651
Sequestration 78140
Sickling 85660
Survival Test 78130-78135
Volume Determination 78120-78121

Red Blood Cell ab
See Antibody, Red Blood Cell

Reflex Test
Blink Reflex 95933
H-Reflex 95934-95936

Reflux Study .78262

Refraction 92015

Rehabilitation
Artery
    Occlusive Disease 93668
Aural 92510
Cardiac 93797-93798

Rehabilitative
See Rehabilitation

Rehfuss Test
See Gastroenterology, Diagnostic, Stomach

Reichstein's Substance S
See Deoxycortisol

Reimplantation
Arteries
    Carotid 35691, 35694-35695
    Subclavian 35693-35695
    Vertebral 35691-35693
Kidney 50380
Ovary 58825

Pulmonary Artery 33788
Ureter, to Bladder 50780-50785
Ureters 51565

Reinnervation
Larynx
    Neuromuscular Pedicle 31590

Reinsch Test .83015

Reinsertion
Drug Delivery Implant 11983
Implantable Contraceptive Capsules 11977
Spinal Fixation Device 22849

Relative Density
See Specific Gravity

Release
Carpal Tunnel 64721
Elbow Contracture
    with Radical Release of Capsule 24149
Flexor Muscles
    Hip 27036
Muscle
    Knee 27422
Nerve .64702-64726
    Neurolytic .64727
Retina
    Encircling Material 67115
Spinal Cord 63200
Stapes 69650
Tarsal Tunnel 28035
Tendon 24332, 25295

Release-Inhibiting Hormone, Somatotropin
See Somatostatin

Removal
Balloon
    Intra-Aortic 33974
Balloon Assist Device
    Intra-Aortic 33968, 33971
Blood Clot
    Eye 65930
Blood Component
    Apheresis 36511-36516
Breast
    Capsules 19371
    Implants 19328-19330
    Modified Radical 19240
    Partial 19140-19162
    Radical 19200-19220
    Simple, Complete 19180
    Subcutaneous 19182
Calcareous Deposits
    Subdeltoid .23000
Calculi (Stone)
    Bile Duct 43264, 47420-47425
        Percutaneous 47554, 47630
    Bladder 51050, 52310-52318, 52352
    Gallbladder 47480
    Hepatic Duct 47400
    Kidney 50060-50081, 50130, 50561,
                               50580, 52352
    Pancreas 48020
    Pancreatic Duct 43264

Renal Abscess
See Abscess, Kidney

Renal Arteries
See Artery, Renal

Renal Autotransplantation
See Autotransplantation, Renal

Renal Calculus
See Calculus, Removal, Kidney

Renal Cyst
See Cyst, Kidney

Renal Dialyses
See Hemodialysis

Renal Disease Services
See Dialysis

Renal Transplantation
See Kidney, Transplantation

Renin-Converting Enzyme ..... .82164

Reoperation

Repair

Entropion
  Blepharoplasty 67923-67924
  Suture 67921-67924
  Thermocauterization 67922
  Excisional 67961-67966
Ptosis
  Conjunctivo-Tarso-Muller's
  Muscle-Levator Resection 67908
  Frontalis Muscle Technique ..67901-67902
  Levator Resection 67903-67904
  Reduction of Overcorrection 67909
  Superior Rectus Technique 67906
  Retraction 67911
Wound
  Suture 67930-67935
Eye Muscles
  Strabismus
    Adjustable Sutures 67335
    One Horizontal Muscle 67311
    One Vertical Muscle 67314
    Posterior Fixation Suture
    Technique 67334-67335
    Previous Surgery, Not Involving
    Extraocular Muscles 67331
    Release Extensive Scar Tissue 67343
    Superior Oblique Muscle 67318
    Two Horizontal Muscles..........67312
    Two or More Vertical Muscles......67316
  Wound
    Extraocular Muscle 65290
Facial Bones 21208-21209
Facial Nerve
  Paralysis 15840-15845
  Suture
    Intratemporal, Lateral to Geniculate
    Ganglion 69740
    Intratemporal, Medial to Geniculate
    Ganglion 69745
Fallopian Tube 58752
  Anastomosis 58750
  Create Stoma 58770
Fascial Defect 50728
Femur 27470-27472
  Epiphysis 27475-27485, 27742
    Arrest 27185
    by Pinning 27176
    by Traction 27175
    Open Treatment 27177-27178
    Osteoplasty 27179
    Osteotomy 27181
  Muscle Transfer 27110
  Osteotomy 27140, 27151, 27450-27454
  Femoral Neck 27161
    with Fixation 27165
    with Open Reduction 27156
  with Graft 27170
Fibula
  Epiphysis 27477-27485, 27730-27742
  Osteotomy 27707-27712
Finger
  Claw Finger 26499
  Macrodactylia 26590
  Polydactylous 26587
  Syndactyly 26560-26562

Tendon
  Extensor 26415-26434, 26445-26449
  Flexor 26356-26358, 26440-26442
  Joint Stabilization 26474
  PIP Joint 26471
  Toe Transfer 26551-26556
  Trigger 26055
  Volar Plate 26548
  Web Finger 26560-26562
Fistula
  Carotid-Cavernous 61710
  Mastoid 69700
  Rectovaginal 57308
Foot
  Fascia 28250
  Muscle 28250
  Tendon 28200-28226, 28238
Gallbladder
  with Gastroenterostomy 47741
  with Intestines 47720-47740
Great Arteries 33770-33781
Great Vessel 33320-33322
Hallux Valgus 28290-28299
Hamstring 27097
Hand
  Cleft Hand 26580
  Muscle 26591-26593
  Tendon
    Extensor 26410-26416, 26426-26428,
                          26433-26437
    Flexor 26350-26358, 26440
    Profundus 26370-26373
Hearing Aid
  Bone Conduction 69711
Heart
  Anomaly 33600-33617
  Aortic Sinus 33702-33722
  Atrial 33253
  Atrioventricular Canal 33660-33665
    Complete 33670
  Atrioventricular Valve 33660-33665
  Blood Vessel 33320-33322
  Cor Triatriatum 33732
  Fibrillation 33253
  Infundibular 33476-33478
  Mitral Valve 33420-33427
  Myocardium 33542
  Outflow Tract 33476-33478
  Postinfarction 33542-33545
  Prosthetic Valve 33670, 33852-33853
  Prosthetic Valve Dysfunction 33496
  Pulmonary Artery Shunt 33924
  Pulmonary Valve 33470-33474
  Septal Defect 33545, 33608-33610,
                    33681-33688, 33692-33697
    Atrial and Ventricular 33647
    Atrium 33641
    Sinus of Valsalva 33702-33722
    Sinus Venosus 33645
  Tetralogy of Fallot 33692-33697
  Tricuspid Valve 33465
  Ventricle 33611-33612
    Obstruction 33619
  Ventricular Tunnel 33722
  Wound 33300-33305
Hepatic Duct
  with Intestines 47765, 47802

Hernia 50728
  Abdomen 49565, 49590
    Incisional 49560
    Epigastric 49570
    Incarcerated 49572
  Femoral 49550
    Incarcerated 49553
    Recurrent 49555
    Recurrent Incarcerated 49557
    Reducible Recurrent 49555
  Incisional
    Incarcerated 49561
    Recurrent Incarcerated 49566
  Inguinal 49491-49521
    Initial 49650
    Recurrent 49651
    Sliding 49525
  Intestinal 44025-44050
  Lumbar 49540
  Lung 32800
  Orchiopexy 54640
  Reducible 49565, 49570
    Femoral 49550
    Incisional 49560
    Inguinal 49500, 49505
    Recurrent 49520
    Sliding 49525
    Spigelian 49590
    Umbilical 49580, 49585
    Incarcerated 49582, 49587
    Reducible 49580
  with Spermatic Cord 54640
Hip
  Muscle Transfer 27100-27105, 27111
  Osteotomy 27146-27156
  Tendon 27097
Humerus 24420-24430
  Osteotomy 24400-24410
  with Graft 24435
Ileostomy
  See Ileostomy, Repair
Interphalangeal Joint
  Volar Plate 26548
Intestine
  Large
    Ulcer 44605
    Wound 44605
Intestines
  Enterocele
    Abdominal Approach 57270
    Vaginal Approach 57268
  Large
    Closure Enterostomy 44620-44626
    Diverticula 44605
    Obstruction 44615
Intestines, Small
  Closure Enterostomy 44620-44626
  Diverticula 44602-44603
  Fistula 44640-44661
  Hernia 44050
  Malrotation 44055
  Obstruction 44025-44050
  Ulcer 44602-44603
  Wound 44602-44603
Introitus
  Vagina 56800
Iris, Ciliary Body 66680

Spine
  Osteotomy 22210-22226
Spleen 38115
Stomach
  Esophagogastrostomy 43320
  Fistula 43880
  Fundoplasty 43324-43325
  Laceration 43501-43502
  Stoma 43870
  Ulcer 43501
Talus
  Osteotomy 28302
Tarsal 28320
  Osteotomy 28304-28305
Testis
  Injury 54670
  Suspension 54620-54640
  Torsion 54600
Throat
  Pharyngoesophageal 42953
  Wound 42900
Thumb
  Muscle 26508
  Tendon 26510
Tibia 27720-27725
  Epiphysis 27477-27485, 27730-27742
  Osteotomy 27455-27457, 27705,
                          27709-27712
  Pseudoarthrosis 27727
Toe
  Bunion 28290-28299
  Muscle 28240
  Tendon 28240
  Webbing 28280, 28345
Toes
  Macrodactylia 26590
  Polydactylous 26587
Tongue 41250-41252
  Fixation 41500
  Laceration 41250-41252
  Mechanical .41500
  Suture 41510
Trachea
  Fistula 31755
    without Plastic Repair 31820
    with Plastic Repair 31825
  Stenosis 31780-31781
  Stoma 31613-31614
    Scar 31830
    without Plastic Repair 31820
    with Plastic Repair 31825
  Wound
    Cervical 31800
    Intrathoracic 31805
Tricuspid Valve 33463-33465
Truncus Arteriosus
  Rastelli Type 33786
Tunica Vaginalis
  Hydrocele 55060
Tympanic Membrane 69450, 69610
Ulna
  Epiphyseal 25450-25455
  Malunion or Nonunion 25400, 25415
  Osteotomy 25360, 25370-25375,
                          25425-25426
  with Graft 25405, 25420
Umbilicus
  Omphalocele 49600-49611

Ureter
  Anastomosis 50740-50825
  Continent Diversion 50825
  Deligation 50940
  Fistula 50920-50930
  Lysis Adhesions 50715-50725
  Suture 50900
  Urinary Undiversion 50830
Ureterocele 51535
Urethra
  Artificial Sphincter 53449
  Diverticulum 53240, 53400-53405
  Fistula . . .45820-45825, 53400-53405, 53520
  Stoma 53520
  Stricture 53400-53405
  Urethrocele .57230
  Wound 53502-53515
Urethral Sphincter 57220
Urinary Incontinence 53431-53440, 57284
Uterus
  Fistula 51920-51925
  Rupture 58520, 59350
  Suspension 58400-58410
Vagina
  Anterior
    See Colporrhaphy, Anterior
  Cystocele 57240, 57260
  Enterocele 57265
  Fistula 46715-46716, 51900
    Rectovaginal 57300-57307
    Transvesical and Vaginal Approach . .57330
    Urethrovaginal 57310-57311
    Vesicovaginal 57320-57330
  Hysterectomy 58267, 58293
  Incontinence 57284, 57288
  Pereyra Procedure 57289
  Postpartum .59300
  Prolapse 57282-57284
  Rectocele 57250-57260
  Suspension 57280, 57284
  Wound 57200-57210
Vaginal Wall Prolapse
  See Colporrhaphy
Vas Deferens
  Suture 55400
Vein
  Angioplasty 35460, 35476, 75978
  Femoral 34501
  Graft 34520
  Pulmonary 33730
  Transposition 34510
Vulva
  Postpartum .59300
Wound
  Complex 13100-13160
  Intermediate 12031-12057
  Simple 12001-12021
Wound Dehiscence
  Complex 13160
  Simple 12020-12021
Wrist 25260-25263, 25270, 25447
  Bone 25440
  Carpal Bone 25431
  Cartilage 25107
  Removal
    Implant 25449
    Secondary 25265, 25272-25274

Tendon 25280-25316
Tendon Sheath 25275
Total Replacement 25446

Repeat Surgeries
See Reoperation

Replacement
Aortic Valve 33405-33413
Arthroplasties, Hip
  See Arthroplasty, Hip
Cerebrospinal Fluid Shunt 62160, 62194,
                          62225-62230
Contact Lens
  See Contact Lens Services
Elbow
  Total 24363
Electrode
  Heart 33210-33211, 33216, 33217
Eye
  Drug Delivery System 67121
Gastrostomy Tube 43760
Hearing Aid
  Bone Conduction 69710
Hip 27130-27132
  Revision 27134-27138
Implant
  Bone
    for External Speech Processor/Cochlear
    Stimulator 69717-69718
Knee
  Total 27447
Mitral Valve .33430
Nephrostomy Tube
  See Nephrostomy, Change Tube
Nerve 64726
Ossicles
  with Prosthesis 69633, 69637
Ossicular Replacement
  See TORP (Total Ossicular Replacement
  Prosthesis)
Pacemaker 33206-33208
  Catheter 33210
  Electrode 33210-33211, 33216, 33217
Pacing Cardioverter-Defibrillator
  Leads 33243-33244
  Pulse Generator Only 33241
Penile
  Prosthesis 54410-54411, 54416-54417
Prosthesis
  Skull 62143
  Urethral Sphincter 53448
Pulmonary Valve 33475
Skull Plate 62143
Spinal Cord
  Reservoir 62360
Tissue Expanders
  Skin 11970
Total Replacement
  See Hip, Total Replacement
Tricuspid Valve 33465
Ureter
  with Intestines 50840

Replantation
Arm, Upper 20802
Digit .20816-20822
Foot 20838

Retropubic Prostatectomies
See Prostatectomy, Retropubic

Revascularization
Penis 37788
Transmyocardial 33140-33141

Reversal, Vasectomy
See Vasovasorrhaphy

Reverse T3
See Triiodothyronine, Reverse

Reverse Triiodothyronine
See Triiodothyronine, Reverse

Revision
See Reconstruction
Aorta 33404
Atrial 33253
Blepharoplasty 15820-15823
Bronchus 32501
Bypass Graft
　　Vein Patch 35685
Cervicoplasty 15819
Colostomy
　　See Colostomy, Revision
Cornea
　　Prosthesis 65770
　　Reshaping
　　　　Epikeratoplasty 65767
　　　　Keratomileusis 65760
　　　　Keratophakia 65765
Defibrillator Site
　　Chest 33223
Ear, Middle 69662
External Fixation System 20693
Eye
　　Aqueous Shunt 66185
Gastrostomy Tube 44373
Hip Replacement
　　See Replacement, Hip, Revision
Hymenal Ring 56700
Ileostomy
　　See Ileostomy, Revision
Infusion Pump
　　Intraarterial .36261
　　Intravenous .36531
Iris
　　Iridoplasty 66762
　　Iridotomy 66761
Jejunostomy Tube 44373
Lower Extremity Arterial Bypass . . .35879-35881
Pacemaker Site
　　Chest 33222
Rhytidectomy 15824-15829
Semicircular Canal
　　Fenestration 69840
Shunt
　　Intrahepatic Portosystemic 37183
Sling 53442
Stapedectomy
　　See Stapedectomy, Revsion
Stomach
　　for Obesity 43848
Tracheostomy
　　Scar 31830
Urinary-Cutaneous Anastomosis . . .50727-50728

Vagina
　　Sling
　　　　Stress Incontinence 57287
Venous Access Device 36534
Ventricle
　　Ventriculomyectomy 33416
　　Ventriculomyotomy 33416

Rheumatoid Factor 86430-86431

Rhinectomy
Partial 30150
Total 30160

Rhinomanometry 92512

Rhinopharynx
See Nasopharynx

Rhinophyma
Repair 30120

Rhinoplasty
Cleft Lip/Cleft Palate 30460-30462
Primary 30400-30420
Secondary 30430-30450

Rhinoscopy
See Endoscopy, Nose

Rhinotomy
Lateral .30118, 30320

Rhizotomy 63185-63190

Rho Variant Du 86905

Rhytidectomy 15824-15829

Rhytidoplasties
See Face Lift

Rh (D)
See Blood Typing

Rh Immune Globulin
See Immune Globulins, Rho (D)

Rib
Excision 21600-21616, 32900
Fracture
　　Closed Treatment 21800
　　External Fixation 21810
　　Open Treatment 21805
Graft
　　to Face 21230
Resection 32900
X-Ray 71100-71111

Riboflavin .84252

**Richardson Operation
Hysterectomy**
See Hysterectomy, Abdominal, Total

Richardson Procedure 53460

Rickettsia
Antibody 86757

Ridell Operation
See Sinusotomy, Frontal

Ridge, Alveolar
See Alveolar Ridge

Right Atrioventricular Valve
See Tricuspid Valve

Right Heart Cardiac Catheterization
See Cardiac Catheterization, Right Heart

Ripstein Operation
See Proctopexy

Risk Factor Reduction Intervention
See Preventive Medicine

Risser Jacket 29010-29015
Removal 29710

Rocky Mountain Spotted Fever 86000

Roentgenographic
See X-Ray

Roentgenography
See Radiology, Diagnostic

Roentgen Rays
See X-Ray

Ropes Test .83872

Rorschach Test 96100

Ross Procedure 33413

Rotation Flap
See Skin, Adjacent Tissue Transfer

Rotator Cuff
Repair .23410-23420

Rotavirus
Antibody 86759
Antigen Detection
　　Enzyme Immunoassay 87425

Rotavirus Vaccine 90680

Round Window
Repair Fistula 69667

Round Window Fistula
See Fistula, Round Window

Roux-En-Y Procedure 43621,
　　　43633-43634, 43846, 47740-47741,
　　　　　　47780-47785, 48540

RPR 86592-86593

RSV
See Immune Globulins; Respiratory Syncytial
Virus

RT3
See Triiodothyronine, Reverse

Rubbing Alcohol
See Isopropyl Alcohol

Rubella
Antibody 86762
Vaccine 90706

Rubella/Mumps
See Vaccines

Rubella HI Test
See Hemagglutination Inhibition Test

Rubeola
Antibody 86765
Antigen Detection
　Immunofluorescence 87283

Rubeolla
See Rubeola

**Russell Viper Venom
Time** 85612-85613

S

Sac, Endolymphatic
See Endolymphatic Sac

Saccomanno Technique 88108

Sacral Nerve
Implantation
　Electrode 64561, 64581
Insertion
　Electrode 64561, 64581

Sacroiliac Joint
Arthrodesis 27280
Arthrotomy 27050
Biopsy 27050
Dislocation
　Open Treatment 27218
Fusion 27280
Injection for Arthrography 27096
X-Ray 72200-72202, 73542

Sacrum
Tumor
　Excision 49215
X-Ray 72220

Sahli Test
See Gastroenterology, Diagnostic, Stomach

Salabrasion 15810-15811

Salicylate
Assay 80196

Saline-Solution Abortion
See Abortion, Induced, by Saline

Saline Load Test 91060

Salivary Duct
Catheterization 42660
Dilation .42650-42660
Ligation 42665
Repair .42500-42505
　Fistula 42600

Salivary Glands
Abscess
　Incision and Drainage 42310-42320
Biopsy 42405
Calculi (Stone)
　Excision 42330-42340
Cyst
　Creation
　　Fistula 42325-42326
　Drainage 42409
　Excision 42408
Injection
　X-Ray 42550
Needle Biopsy 42400
Nuclear Medicine
　Function Study 78232
　Imaging 78230-78231
Parotid
　Abscess 42300-42305
Unlisted Services and Procedures 42699
X-Ray 70380-70390
　with Contrast 70390

Salivary Gland Virus
See Cytomegalovirus

Salmonella
Antibody 86768

Salpingectomy 58262-58263,
　　58291-58292, 58552, 58554, 58661, 58700
Ectopic Pregnancy
　Laparoscopic Treatment 59151
　Surgical Treatment 59120
Oophorectomy 58943

Salpingo-Oophorectomy 58720
Resection Ovarian Malignancy 58950-58954
Resection Peritoneal Malignancy . . .58950-58954
Resection Tubal Malignancy 58950-58954

Salpingohysterostomy
See Implantation, Tubouterine

Salpingolysis 58740

Salpingoneostomy 58673, 58770

Salpingoplasty
See Fallopian Tube, Repair

Salpingostomy 58673, 58770
Laparoscopic 58673

Salter Osteotomy of the Pelvis
See Osteotomy, Pelvis

Sampling
See Biopsy; Brush Biopsy; Needle Biopsy

Sang-Park Procedure 33735-33737

Sao Paulo Typhus
See Rocky Mountain Spotted Fever

Saucerization
Calcaneus 28120
Clavicle 23180
Femur 27070, 27360
Fibula 27360, 27641
Hip 27070

Humerus .23184, 24140
Ileum 27070
Metacarpal 26230
Metatarsal 28122
Olecranon Process 24147
Phalanges
　Finger 26235-26236
　Toe 28124
Pubis 27070
Radius 24145, 25151
Scapula 23182
Talus 28120
Tarsal 28122
Tibia 27360, 27640
Ulna 24147, 25150

Saundby Test
See Blood, Feces

Scabies
See Tissue, Examination for Ectoparasites

Scalenotomy
See Muscle Division, Scalenus Anticus

Scalenus Anticus
Division .21700-21705

Scaling
See Exfoliation

Scalp
Tumor Resection
　Radical 21015

Scalp Blood Sampling 59030

Scan
See Specific Site, Nuclear Medicine
Abdomen
　See Abdomen, CT Scan
CT
　See CT Scan
MRI
　See Magnetic Resonance Imaging
PET
　See Positron Emission Tomography
Radionuclide
　See Emission Computerized Tomography

Scanning, Radioisotope
See Nuclear Medicine

Scanogram 76040

Scaphoid
Fracture
　Closed Treatment 25622
　Open Treatment 25628
　with Manipulation 25624

Scapula
Craterization 23182
Cyst
　Excision 23140
　　with Allograft 23146
　　with Autograft 23145
Diaphysectomy .23182
Excision 23172, 23190
　Partial 23182

Fracture
Closed Treatment
without Manipulation 23570
with Manipulation 23575
Open Treatment 23585
Ostectomy 23190
Repair
Fixation .23400
Scapulopexy 23400
Saucerization .23182
Sequestrectomy 23172
Tumor
Excision 23140, 23210
with Allograft 23146
with Autograft 23145
Radical Resection 23210
X-Ray 73010

Scapulopexy 23400

Scarification
Pleural 32215

Scarification of Pleura
See Pleurodesis

Schanz Operation
See Femur, Osteotomy

Schauta Operation
See Hysterectomy, Vaginal, Radical

Schede Procedure 32905-32906

Scheie Procedure
See Iridectomy

Schilling Test 78270
See Vitamin B-12 Absorption Study

Schlatter Operation Total Gastrectomy
See Excision, Stomach, Total

Schlicter Test 87197
See Bactericidal Titer, Serum

Schocket Procedure 66180
See Aqueous Shunt

Schonbein Test
See Blood, Feces

Schuchard Procedure
Osteotomy
Maxilla 21206

Schwannoma, Acoustic
See Brain, Tumor, Excision

Sciatic Nerve
Decompression 64712
Injection
Anesthetic 64445-64446
Lesion
Excision 64786
Neuroma
Excision 64786
Neuroplasty 64712
Release 64712
Repair/Suture .64858

Scintigraphy
See Nuclear Medicine
Computed Tomographic
See Emission Computerized Tomography

Scissoring
Skin Tags 11200-11201

Sclera
Excision
Sclerectomy with Punch or Scissors . . .66160
Fistulization
Iridencleisis or Iridotasis 66165
Sclerectomy with Punch or Scissors with
Iridectomy 66160
Thermocauterization with Iridectomy . .66155
Trabeculectomy ab Externo in Absence of
Previous Surgery 66170
Trephination with Iridectomy 66150
Incision
Fistulization
Iridencleisis or Iridotasis 66165
Sclerectomy with Punch or Scissors with
Iridectomy 66160
Thermocauterization with Iridectomy 66155
Trabeculectomy ab Externo in Absence of
Previous Surgery 66170
Trephination with Iridectomy 66150
Lesion
Excision 66130
Repair
Reinforcement
without Graft 67250
with Graft .67255
Staphyloma
without Graft 66220
with Graft .66225
with Glue .65286
Wound
Operative .66250
Tissue Glue 65286

Scleral Buckling Operation
See Retina, Repair, Detachment

Scleral Ectasia
See Staphyloma, Sclera

Sclerectomy 66160

Sclerotherapy
Venous 36468-36471

Sclerotomy
See Incision, Sclera

Screening, Drug
See Drug Screen

Scribner Cannulization 36810

Scrotal Varices
See Varicocele

Scrotoplasty 55175-55180

Scrotum
Abscess
Incision and Drainage 54700, 55100
Excision 55150
Exploration 55110

Hematoma
Incision and Drainage 54700
Removal
Foreign Body 55120
Repair 55175-55180
Ultrasound 76870
Unlisted Services and Procedures 55899

Scrub Typhus 86000

Second Look Surgery
See Reoperation

Second Opinion
See Confirmatory Consultations

Section
See Decompression
Cesarean
See Cesarean Delivery
Cranial Nerve .61460
Spinal Access 63191
Dentate Ligament 63180-63182
Gasserian Ganglion
Sensory Root 61450
Medullary Tract 61470
Mesencephalic Tract 61480
Nerve Root 63185-63190
Spinal Accessory Nerve 63191
Spinal Cord Tract 63194-63199
Tentorium Cerebelli 61440
Vestibular Nerve
Transcranial Approach 69950
Translabyrinthine Approach 69915

Sedation
with or without Analgesia 99141-99142

Seddon-Brookes Procedure . . .24320

Sedimentation Rate
Blood Cell
Automated .85652
Manual .85651

Segmentectomy
Lung 32484

Seidlitz Powder Test
See X-Ray, with Contrast

Selenium .84255

Self Care
See Physical Medicine/Therapy/Occupational
Therapy
Training .97535, 99509

Sella Turcica
CT Scan .70480-70482
X-Ray 70240

Semenogelase
See Antigen, Prostate Specific

Semen Analysis 89300-89321
Sperm Analysis
Antibodies .89325
with Sperm Isolation 89260-89261

Semicircular Canal
Incision
  Fenestration 69820
  Revised 69840

Semilunar
Bone
  See Lunate
Ganglion
  See Gasserian Ganglion

Seminal Vesicle
Cyst
  Excision 55680
Excision 55650
Incision 55600-55605
Mullerian Duct
  Excision 55680
Unlisted Services and Procedures 55899

Seminal Vesicles
Vesiculography 74440
X-Ray with Contrast 74440

Seminin
See Antigen, Prostate Specific

Semiquantitative 81005

Sengstaaken Tamponade
Esophagus 43460

Senning Procedure 33774-33777
See Repair, Great Arteries; Revision

Senning Type 33774-33777

Sensitivity Study
Antibiotic
  Agar 87181
  Disc 87184
  Enzyme Detection 87185
  Macrobroth .87188
  MIC 87186
  Microtiter 87186
  MLC 87187
  Mycobacteria 87190
Antiviral Drugs
  HIV-1
    Tissue Culture 87904

Sensor, Fetal Oximetry
Insertion
  Cervix 0021T
  Vagina 0021T

Sensorimotor Exam 92060

Sensory Nerve
Common
  Repair/Suture 64834

Sentinel Node
Injection Procedure 38792

Separation
Craniofacial
  Closed Treatment 21431
  Open Treatment 21432-21436

Septal Defect
Repair 33813-33814

Septectomy
Atrial 33735-33737
  Balloon (Rashkind Type) 92992
  Blade Method (Park) 92993
Closed
  See Septostomy, Atrial
Submucous Nasal
  See Nasal Septum, Submucous Resection

Septic Abortion
See Abortion, Septic

Septoplasty 30520

Septostomy
Atrial 33735-33737
  Balloon (Rashkind Type) 92992
  Blade Method (Park) 92993

Septum, Nasal
See Nasal Septum

Sequestrectomy
Carpal 25145
Clavicle 23170
Humeral Head 23174
Humerus 24134
Olecranon Process 24138
Radius .24136, 25145
Scapula 23172
Skull 61501
Ulna 24138, 25145

Serialography
Aorta 75625

Serodiagnosis, Syphilis
See Serologic Test for Syphilis

Serologic Test for
Syphilis 86592-86593

Seroma
Incision and Drainage
  Skin 10140

Serotonin 84260

Serum
Albumin
  See Albumin, Serum
Antibody Identification
  Pretreatment 86975-86978
CPK
  See Creatine Kinase, Total
Serum Immune Globulin 90281-90283

Sesamoidectomy
Toe 28315

Sesamoid Bone
Excision 28315
Finger
  Excision 26185
Foot
  Fracture 28530-28531
Thumb
  Excision 26185

Severing of Blepharorrhaphy
See Tarsorrhaphy, Severing

Sever Procedure
See Contracture, Palm, Release

Sex-Linked Ichthyoses
See Syphilis Test

Sex Change Operation
Female to Male 55980
Male to Female 55970

Sex Chromatin
See Barr Bodies

Sex Chromatin
Identification 88130-88140

Sex Hormone Binding
Globulin .84270

SGOT 84450

SGPT 84460

Shaving
Skin Lesion 11300-11313

SHBG
See Sex Hormone Binding Globulin

Shelf Procedure
See Osteotomy, Hip

Shiga-like Toxin
Antigen Detection
  Enzyme Immunoassay 87427

Shigella
Antibody 86771

Shirodkar Operation
See Repair, Cervix, Cerclage, Abdominal

Shock Wave, Ultrasonic
See Ultrasound

Shock Wave (Extracorporeal)
Therapy 0019T-0020T

Shock Wave Lithotripsy 50590

Shop Typhus of Malaya
See Murine Typhus

Shoulder
See Clavicle; Scapula
Abscess
  Drainage 23030
Amputation 23900-23921
Arthrocentesis 20610
Arthrodesis 23800
  with Autogenous Graft 23802
Arthrography
  Injection
    Radiologic 23350
Arthroscopy
  Diagnostic .29805
  Surgical 29806-29827
Arthrotomy
  with Removal Loose or Foreign Body . .23107
Biopsy
  Deep 23066
  Soft Tissue .23065

Blade
  See Scapula
Bone
  Excision
    Acromion 23130
    Clavicle 23120-23125
    Incision 23035
  Tumor
    Excision 23140-23146
Bursa
  Drainage 23031
Capsular Contracture Release 23020
Cast
  Figure Eight 29049
  Removal 29710
  Spica 29055
  Velpeau 29058
Disarticulation 23920-23921
Dislocation
  Closed Treatment
    with Manipulation 23650-23655
Exploration 23107
Hematoma
  Drainage 23030
Manipulation
  Application of Fixation Apparatus 23700
Prophylactic Treatment 23490-23491
Radical Resection 23077
Removal
  Calcareous Deposits 23000
  Cast 29710
  Foreign Body
    Complicated 23332
    Deep 23331
    Subcutaneous 23330
  Foreign or Loose Body 23107
Repair
  Capsule 23450-23466
  Ligament Release 23415
  Muscle Transfer 23395-23397
  Rotator Cuff 23410-23420
  Tendon 23410-23412, 23430-23440
  Tenomyotomy 23405-23406
Strapping 29240
Surgery
  Unlisted Services and Procedures 23929
Tumor
  Excision 23075-23077
Unlisted Services and Procedures 23929
X-Ray 73020-73030
X-Ray with Contrast 73040

Shoulder Joint
See Clavicle; Scapula
Arthroplasty
  with Implant 23470-23472
Arthrotomy
  with Biopsy 23100-23101
  with Synovectomy 23105-23106
Dislocation
  Open Treatment 23660
  with Greater Tuberosity Fracture
    Closed Treatment 23665
    Open Treatment 23670
  with Surgical or Anatomical Neck Fracture
    Closed Treatment with Manipulation 23675
    Open Treatment 23680

Excision
  Torn Cartilage 23101
Exploration 23040-23044
Incision and Drainage 23040-23044
Removal
  Foreign Body 23040-23044
X-Ray 73050

Shunt(s)
Aqueous
  to Extraocular Reservoir 66180
    Revision 66185
Arteriovenous
  See Arteriovenous Shunt
Brain
  Creation 62180-62223
  Removal 62256-62258
  Replacement 62160, 62194,
                        62225-62230, 62258
  Reprogramming 62252
Cerebrospinal Fluid
  See Cerebrospinal Fluid Shunt
Creation
  Arteriovenous
    Direct 36821
    ECMO 36822
    Thomas Shunt 36835
    Transposition 36820
    with Bypass Graft 35686
    with Graft 36825-36830
  Cerebrospinal Fluid 62200
  Thomas Shunt 36835
Great Vessel
  Aorta
    Pulmonary 33924
  Aorta to Pulmonary Artery
    Ascending 33755
    Descending 33762
    Central 33764
    Subclavian Pulmonary Artery 33750
    Vena Cava to Pulmonary Artery .33766-33767
  Intra-atrial 33735-33737
LeVeen
  See LeVeen Shunt
Nonvascular
  X-Ray 75809
Peritoneal
  Venous
    Injection 49427
    Ligation 49428
    Removal 49429
    X-Ray 75809
Pulmonary Artery
  See Pulmonary Artery, Shunt
Revision
  Arteriovenous 36832
Spinal Cord
  Creation 63740-63741
  Irrigation 63744
  Removal 63746
  Replacement 63744
Superior Mesenteric-Caval
  See Anastomosis, Caval to Mesenteric
Ureter to Colon 50815
Ventriculocisternal with Valve
  See Ventriculocisternostomy

Shuntogram 75809

Sialic Acid 84275

Sialodochoplasty 42500-42505

Sialogram
See Sialography

Sialography 70390

Sickling
Electrophoresis 83020

Siderocytes 85536

Siderophilin
See Transferrin

Sigmoid
See Colon-Sigmoid

Sigmoidoscopy
Ablation
  Polyp 45339
  Tumor 45339
Biopsy 45331
Collection
  Specimen 45331
Exploration 45330, 45335
Hemorrhage Control 45334
Injection
  Submucosal 45335
Needle Biopsy 45342
Placement
  Stent 45345
Removal
  Foreign Body 45332
  Polyp 45333, 45338
  Tumor 45333, 45338
Repair
  Volvulus 45337
Ultrasound 45341-45342

Sigmoid Bladder
Cystectomy 51590

Signal-Averaged Electrocardiography
See Electrocardiogram

Silica 84285

Silicone
Contouring Injections 11950-11954

Silicon Dioxide
See Silica

Silver Operation
See Keller Procedure

Silver Procedure 28290

Simple Mastectomies
See Mastectomy

Single Photon Absorptiometry
See Absorptiometry, Single Photon

Single Photon Emission Computed Tomography
See SPECT

Free Skin Graft
    Full Thickness 15200-15261
Island Pedicle Flap .15740
Muscle 15732-15738, 15842
    Free 15756
Myocutaneous 15732-15738, 15756
Pedicle Flap
    Formation 15570-15576
    Island 15740
    Neurovascular .15750
    Transfer 15650
Pinch Graft 15050
Platysmal 15825
Punch Graft 15775-15776
Punch Graft for Hair Transplant 15775-15776
Recipient Site Preparation 15000-15001
Skin
    Free 15757
Split Graft 15100-15121
Superficial Musculoaponeurotic System . . .15829
Tissue-Cultured 15100-15121, 15342-15343
Tissue Transfer 14000-14350
Transfer 15650
Vascular Flow Check 15860
Xenograft 15400-15401

Skull

Burr Hole
    Biopsy Brain 61140
    Drainage
        Abscess 61150-61151
        Cyst 61150-61151
        Hematoma 61154-61156
    Exploration
        Infratentorial 61253
        Supratentorial 61250
    Insertion
        Catheter 61210
        EEG Electrode 61210
        Reservoir 61210
    Intracranial
        Biopsy 61140
    with Injection 61120
Decompression 61322-61323, 61340-61345
    Orbit 61330
Drill Hole
    Catheter 61107
    Drainage Hematoma 61108
    Exploration 61105
Excision 61501
Exploration
    Drill Hole 61105
Fracture 62000-62010
    Closed Treatment 21300
Hematoma
    Drainage 61108
Incision
    Suture 61550-61552
Insertion
    Catheter 61107
Lesion
    Excision . .61500, 61600-61608, 61615-61616
Orbit
    Biopsy 61332
    Excision
        Lesion 61333
    Exploration 61332-61334
    Removal Foreign Body 61334

Puncture
    Cervical 61050
    Cisternal 61050
    Drain Fluid 61070
    Injection 61070
    Subdural 61000-61001
    Ventricular Fluid 61020
Reconstruction 21172-21180
    Defect 62140-62141, 62145
Reduction
    Craniomegalic 62115-62117
Removal
    Plate 62142
    Prosthesis 62142
Repair
    Cerebrospinal Fluid Leak 62100
    Encephalocele 62120
Replacement
    Plate 62143
    Prosthesis 62143
Tumor
    Excision 61500
X-Ray 70250-70260

Skull Base Surgery

Anterior Cranial Fossa
    Bicoronal Approach 61586
    Craniofacial Approach 61580-61583
    Extradural 61600-61601
    LeFort I Osteotomy Approach 61586
    Orbitocranial Approach 61584-61585
    Transzygomatic Approach 61586
Carotid Aneurysm 61613
Carotid Artery 61610
    Transection/Ligation 61609-61612
Craniotomy 62121
Dura
    Repair of Cerebrospinal Fluid
    Leak 61618-61619
Middle Cranial Fossa
    Extradural 61605, 61607
    Infratemporal Approach 61590-61591
    Intradural 61606, 61608
Orbitocranial Zygomatic Approach 61592
Posterior Cranial Fossa
    Extradural 61615
    Intradural 61616
    Transcondylar Approach 61596-61597
    Transpetrosal Approach 61598
    Transtemporal Approach 61595

Sleep Study 95806-95807

Sliding Inlay Graft, Tibia

See Ankle; Tibia, Repair

Sling Operation

Incontinence 53440
    Removal 53442
Stress Incontinence 51992, 57287
Vagina 57287-57288

Small Bowel

See Intestines, Small
Neoplasm
    See Tumor, Intestines, Small

SMAS Flap 15829

Smear

Cervical
    See Cervical Smears
Papanicolaou
    See Pap Smears

Smear and Stain

See Cytopathology, Smears
Cornea 65430
Fluorescent 87206
Gram or Giesma 87205
Ova
    Parasites 87177
Parasites 87207
Wet Mount 87210

Smith-Robinson Operation

See Arthrodesis, Vertebra

Smithwick Operation

See Excision, Nerve, Sympathetic

Smith Fracture 25600-25620

SO4

See Sulfate

Soave Procedure 45120

Sodium 84295, 84302

Urine 84300

Sodium Glycinate, Theophylline

See Theophylline

Sofield Procedure 24410

Soft Tissue

See Tissue, Soft

Solar Plexus

See Celiac Plexus

Solitary Cyst

See Bone, Cyst

Somatomammotropin, Chorionic 83632

Somatomedin 84305

Somatosensory Testing

Lower Limbs 95926
Trunk or Head .95927
Upper Limbs 95925

Somatostatin 84307

Somatotropin 83003

Somatotropin Release Inhibiting Hormone

See Somatostatin

Somatropin

See Growth Hormone, Human

Somnographies

See Polysomnography

Somophyllin T

See Theophylline

Sonography
See Echography

Sore, Bed
See Pressure Ulcer (Decubitus)

Spasm Eyelid
See Blepharospasm

Special Services
After Hours Medical Services 99050-99054
Analysis
    Remote Physiologic Data 99091
Computer Data Analysis 99090
Device Handling 99002
Emergency Care In Office 99058
Group Education 99078
Hyperbaric Oxygen 99183
Hypothermia 99185-99186
Medical Testimony 99075
Non-Office Medical Services 99056
Office Visit with Surgery 99025
On Call Services 99026-99027
Phlebotomy 99199
Post-Op Visit 99024
Pump Services 99190-99192
Reports and Forms
    Medical, Extended 99080
    Psychiatric .90889
Specimen Handling 99000-99001
Supply of Materials 99070
    Educational .99071
Unlisted Services and Procedures 99199
Unusual Travel .99082

Specific Gravity
Body Fluid 84315

Specimen Collection
Intestines 89100-89105
Stomach 89130-89141

Specimen Concentration 87015

Specimen Handling 99000-99001

SPECT 78607
See Emission Computerized Tomography
Abscess Localization 78807
Bone 78320
Cerebrospinal Fluid 78647
Heart
    Multiple 78465
    Single 78464
Kidney 78710
Liver 78205
Tumor Localization 78803

Spectacle Services
Fitting
    Low Vision Aid 92354-92355
    Spectacles 92340-92342
    Spectacle Prosthesis 92352-92353
Repair .92370-92371
Supply
    Low Vision Aids 92392
    Spectacles .92390
    Spectacle Prosthesis 92395

Spectrometry
Mass
    Analyte
        Qualitative 83788
        Quantitative 83789

Spectrophotometry 84311
Atomic Absorption
    See Atomic Absorption Spectroscopy

Spectroscopy
Atomic Absorption 82190
Magnetic Resonance 76390

Spectrum Analyses
See Spectrophotometry

Speculoscopy 0031T
with Direct Sampling 0032T

Speech Evaluation 92506
Cine 70371
for Prosthesis 92597, 92607-92608
Video 70371

Speech Prosthesis 21084, 92609
Creation 31611
Evaluation for Speech 92597, 92607-92608
Insertion 31611

Speech Therapy 92507-92508

Spermatic Cord
Hydrocele
    Excision 55500
Laparoscopy 55559
Lesion
    Excision 55520
Repair
    Veins 55530-55540
        Abdominal Approach 55535
        with Hernia Repair 55540
Varicocele
    Excision 55530-55540

Spermatic Veins
Excision 55530-55540
Ligation 55550

Spermatocele
Excision 54840

Spermatocystectomy
See Spermatocele, Excision

Sperm Analysis
Antibodies 89325
Cervical Mucus Penetration Test 89330
Cryopreservation 89259
Hamster Penetration Test 89329
Identification
    Aspiration .89257
    from Testis Tissue 89264
Isolation 89260-89261

Sperm Evaluation, Cervical Mucus Penetration Test
See Huhner Test

Sperm Washing 58323

Sphenoidotomy
Excision
    with Nasal/Sinus Endoscopy . . .31287-31288

Sphenoid Sinus
See Sinuses, Sphenoid

Sphenopalatine Ganglion
Injection
    Anesthetic .64505

Sphincter
See Specific Sphincter
Anal
    See Anal Sphincter
Artificial Genitourinary
    See Prosthesis, Urethral Sphincter
Pyloric
    See Pyloric Sphincter

Sphincteroplasty
Anal 46750-46751, 46760-46761
    with Implant 46762
Bile Duct 47460
Bladder Neck
    See Bladder, Repair, Neck

Sphincterotomy 52277
Anal 46080
Bile Duct 47460

Sphincter of Oddi
Pressure Measurement
    Endoscopy .43263

Spica Cast
Hip 29305-29325
Repair 29720
Shoulder 29055

Spinal Accessory Nerve
Anastomosis
    to Facial Nerve 64866
Incision 63191
Injection
    Anesthetic .64412
Section 63191

Spinal Column
See Spine

Spinal Cord
See Cauda Equina; Nerve Root
Biopsy .63275-63290
Cyst
    Aspiration .62268
    Incision and Drainage 63172-63173
Decompression 63001-63091
Drain Fluid 62272
Exploration 63001-63044
Graft
    Dura 63710
Implantation
    Electrode 63650-63655
    Pulse Generator 63685
    Receiver 63685
Incision 63200
    Dentate Ligament 63180-63182
    Tract 63170, 63194-63199

Splitting
Blood Products 86985

Split Grafts 15100-15121

Split Renal Function Test
See Cystourethroscopy, Catheterization, Ureteral

Spontaneous Abortion
See Abortion

Sprengel's Deformity 23400

Spring Water Cyst
See Cyst, Pericardial

Spur, Bone
See Exostosis
Calcaneal
　　See Heel Spur

Sputum Analysis 89350

SRIH
See Somatostatin

Ssabanejew-Frank Operation
See Incision, Stomach, Creation, Stoma; Incision
and Drainage

Stabilizing Factor, Fibrin
See Fibrin Stabilizing Factor

Stable Factor 85230

Stallard Procedure
See Conjunctivorhinostomy

Stamey Procedure 51845
See Repair, Bladder, Neck

Standby Services
Physician 99360

Stanford-Binet Test
See Psychiatric Diagnosis

Stanftan
See Binet Test

Stapedectomy
Revision 69662
without Foreign Material 69660
with Footplate Drill Out 69661

Stapedotomy
Revision 69662
without Foreign Material 69660
with Footplate Drill Out 69661

Stapes
Excision
　　without Foreign Material 69660
　　　with Footplate Drill Out 69661
Mobilization
　　See Mobilization, Stapes
Release 69650
Revision 69662

Staphyloma
Sclera
　　Repair
　　　without Graft 66220
　　　with Graft .66225

Starch Granules
Feces 89355

State Operation
See Proctectomy

Statistics /Biometry
See Biometry

Steindler Stripping 28250

Stellate Ganglion
Injection
　　Anesthetic .64510

Stem, Brain
See Brainstem

Stem Cell
Cell Concentration 38215
Cryopreservation 38207, 88240
Donor Search 38204
Harvesting 38205-38206
Plasma Depletion 38214
Platelet Depletion 38213
Red Blood Cell Depletion 38212
T-cell Depletion .38210
Thawing 38208, 88241
Transplantation 38240-38242
Tumor Cell Depletion 38211
Washing 38209

Stenger Test 92565, 92577
See Audiologic Function Test; Ear, Nose and
Throat

Stenosis
Aortic
　　See Aortic Stenosis
Bronchi 31641
　　Reconstruction 31775
Excision
　　Trachea 31780-31781
Laryngoplasty 31582
Reconstruction
　　Auditory Canal, External 69310
Repair
　　Trachea 31780-31781
Tracheal
　　See Trachea Stenosis
Urethral
　　See Urethral Stenosis

Stensen Duct
See Parotid Duct

Stent
Indwelling
　　Insertion
　　　Ureter 50605
Placement
　　Bronchoscopy 31631
　　Colonoscopy 45387
　　　via Stoma 44397
　　Endoscopy
　　　Gastrointestinal, Upper 43256
　　Enteroscopy 44370
　　Proctosigmoidoscopy 45327

Sigmoidoscopy 45345
Ureteroneocystomy 50947-50948
Urethra
　　Insertion 52282

Stent, Intravascular
See Transcatheter, Placement, Intravascular
Stents

Stents, Tracheal
See Tracheal Stent

Stereotactic Frame
Application/Removal 20660

Stereotaxis
Aspiration
　　Brain Lesion 61750
　　　with CT Scan and/or MRI 61751
　　Spinal Cord 63615
Biopsy
　　Aspiration
　　　Brain Lesion 61750
　　Brain 61750
　　　with CT Scan and/or MRI 61751
　　Breast 76095
　　Spinal Cord 63615
Computer Assisted
　　Brain Surgery 61795
Creation Lesion
　　Brain
　　　Deep 61720-61735
　　　Percutaneous 61790
　　Gasserian Ganglion 61790
　　Spinal Cord 63600
　　Trigeminal Tract 61791
CT Scan
　　Aspiration .61751
　　Biopsy 61751
Excision Lesion
　　Brain 61750
　　Spinal Cord 63615
Focus Beam
　　Radiosurgery 61793
Localization
　　Brain 61770
Radiation Therapy 77432
Stimulation
　　Spinal Cord 63610

Sterile Coverings
See Dressings

Sternal Fracture
See Fracture, Sternum

Sternoclavicular Joint
Arthrotomy 23044
　　with Biopsy 23101
　　with Synovectomy 23106
Dislocation
　　Closed Treatment
　　　without Manipulation 23520
　　　with Manipulation 23525
　　Open Treatment 23530-23532
　　　with Fascial Graft 23532

Sternocleidomastoid
Division .21720-21725

Sternotomy
Closure 21750

Sternum
Debridement 21627
Excision 21620, 21630-21632
Fracture
    Closed Treatment 21820
    Open Treatment 21825
Ostectomy 21620
Radical Resection 21630-21632
Reconstruction 21740-21742, 21750
    with Thoracoscopy 21743
X-Ray 71120-71130

Steroid-Binding Protein, Sex
See Globulin, Sex Hormone Binding

Steroids
Anabolic
    See Androstenedione
Injection
    Urethral Stricture 52283
Ketogenic
    Urine 83582

STH (Somatotropic Hormone)
See Growth Hormone

Stimulating Antibody, Thyroid
See Immunoglobulin, Thyroid Stimulating

Stimulation
Electric
    See Electrical Stimulation
Lymphocyte
    See Blastogenesis
Spinal Cord
    Stereotaxis 63610
Transcutaneous Electric
    See Application, Neurostimulation

Stimulator, Long-Acting Thyroid
See Thyrotropin Releasing Hormone (TRH)

Stimulators, Cardiac
See Heart, Pacemaker

Stimulus Evoked Response 51792

Stoffel Operation
See Rhizotomy

Stoma
Creation
    Bladder 51980
    Kidney 50551-50561
    Stomach
        Neonatal 43831
        Temporary 43830-43831
    Ureter 50860
Ureter
    Endoscopy via 50951-50961

Stomach
Anastomosis
    with Duodenum 43810, 43850-43855
    with Jejunum ..43820-43825, 43860-43865
Biopsy 43600-43605

Creation
    Stoma
        Temporary 43830-43831
    Temporary Stoma
        Laparoscopic 43653
Electrogastrography 91132-91133
Excision
    Partial 43631-43639
    Total 43620-43622
Exploration 43500
Gastric Bypass 43846
    Revision 43848
Incision 43830-43832
    Exploration 43500
    Pyloric Sphincter 43520
    Removal
        Foreign Body 43500
Intubation with Specimen Prep 91055
Nuclear Medicine
    Blood Loss Study 78278
    Emptying Study 78264
    Imaging 78261
    Protein Loss Study 78282
    Reflux Study 78262
    Vitamin B-12 Absorption 78270-78272
Reconstruction
    for Obesity 43842-43847
    Roux-En-Y 43846
Removal
    Foreign Body 43500
Repair 48547
    Fistula 43880
    Fundoplasty 43324-43325
        Laparoscopic 43280
    Laceration 43501-43502
    Stoma 43870
    Ulcer 43501
Saline Load Test 91060
Specimen Collection 89130-89141
Stimulation of Secretion 91052
Suture
    Fistula 43880
    for Obesity 43842-43843
    Stoma 43870
    Ulcer 43840
    Wound 43840
Tumor
    Excision 43610-43611
Ulcer
    Excision 43610
Unlisted Services and Procedures ..43659, 43999

Stomatoplasty
See Mouth, Repair

Stone, Kidney
See Calculus, Removal, Kidney

Stookey-Scarff Procedure
See Ventriculocisternostomy

Stool Blood
See Blood, Feces

Strabismus
Chemodenervation 67345
Repair
    Adjustable Sutures 67335
    Extraocular Muscles 67340

    One Horizontal Muscle 67311
    One Vertical Muscle 67314
    Posterior Fixation Suture
        Technique 67334-67335
    Previous Surgery, Not Involving Extraocular
        Muscles 67331
    Release Extensive Scar Tissue 67343
    Superior Oblique Muscle 67318
    Transposition 67320
    Two Horizontal Muscles 67312
    Two or More Vertical Muscles 67316

Strapping
See Cast; Splint
Ankle 29540
Back 29220
Chest 29200
Elbow 29260
Finger 29280
Foot 29540, 29590
Hand 29280
Hip 29520
Knee 29530
Shoulder 29240
Thorax 29200
Toes 29550
Unlisted Services and Procedures 29799
Unna Boot 29580
Wrist 29260

Strassman Procedure 58540

Strayer Procedure
Leg, Lower 27687

Streptococcus, Group A
Antigen Detection
    Enzyme Immunoassay 87430
    Nucleic Acid 87650-87652
Direct Optical Observation 87880

Streptococcus, Group B
by Immunoassay
    with Direct Optical Observation 87802

Streptococcus pneumoniae Vaccine
See Vaccines

Streptokinase, Antibody 86590

Stress Tests
Cardiovascular 93015-93024
Multiple Gated Acquisition
(MUGA) 78472-78473
Myocardial Perfusion Imaging 78460-78465
Pulmonary 94620-94621
    See Pulmonology, Diagnostic

Stricture
Repair
    Urethra 53400-53405
Urethra
    See Urethral Stenosis

Stricturoplasty
Intestines 44615

Stroboscopy
Larynx 31579

STS 86592-86593
See Syphilis Test

Stuart-Prower Factor 85260

Study, Color Vision
See Color Vision Examination

Sturmdorf Procedure 57520

Styloidectomy
Radial 25230

Styloid Process
Radial
    Excision 25230

Stypven Time
See Russell Viper Venom Time

Subacromial Bursa
Arthrocentesis .20610

Subclavian Arteries
See Artery, Subclavian

Subcutaneous Injection
See Injection, Subcutaneous

Subcutaneous Mastectomies
See Mastectomy, Subcutaneous

Subcutaneous Tissue
Excision 15831-15839

Subdiaphragmatic Abscess
See Abscess, Subdiaphragmatic

Subdural Electrode
Insertion .61531-61533
Removal 61535

Subdural Hematonia
See Hematoma, Subdural

Subdural Puncture 61105-61108

Subdural Tap 61000-61001

Sublingual Gland
Abscess
    Incision and Drainage 42310-42320
Calculi (Stone)
    Excision 42330
Cyst
    Drainage 42409
    Excision 42408
Excision 42450

Subluxation
Elbow 24640

Submandibular Gland
Calculi (Stone)
    Excision 42330-42335
Excision 42440

Submaxillary Gland
Abscess
    Incision and Drainage 42310-42320

Submucous Resection of Nasal Septum
See Nasal Septum, Submucous Resection

Subperiosteal Implant
Reconstruction
    Mandible 21245-21246
    Maxilla 21245-21246

Subphrenic Abscess
See Abscess, Subdiaphragmatic

Substance S, Reichstein's
See Deoxycortisol

Subtrochanteric Fracture
See Femur, Fracture, Subtrochanteric

Sucrose Hemolysis Test
See Red Blood Cell (RBC), Fragility, Osmotic

Suction Lipectomies
See Liposuction

Sudiferous Gland
See Sweat Glands

Sugars 84375-84379

Sugar Water Test
See Red Blood Cell (RBC), Fragility, Osmotic

Sugiura Procedure
See Esophagus, Repair, Varices

Sulfate
Chondroitin
    See Chondroitin Sulfate
DHA
    See Dehydroepiandrosterone Sulfate
Urine 84392

Sulfation Factor
See Somatomedin

Sulphates
See Sulfate

Sumatran Mite Fever
See Scrub Typhus

Superficial Musculoaponeurotic System (SMAS) Flap
Rhytidectomy .15829

Supernumerary Digit
Reconstruction 26587
Repair 26587

Supply
Chemotherapeutic Agent 96545
    See Chemotherapy
Contact Lenses 92391, 92396
Educational Materials 99071
Low Vision Aids 92392
    See Spectacle Services
Materials 99070
Ocular Prosthesis 92393
Prosthesis
    Breast 19396
Radionuclide 78990
Radionuclide Therapy 79900
Radiopharmaceutical 78990
Radiopharmaceutical Therapy 79900
Spectacles 92390
Spectacle Prosthesis 92395

Suppositories, Vaginal
See Pessary

Suppression 80400-80408

Suppression/Testing
See Evocative/Suppression Test

Suppressor T Lymphocyte Marker
See CD8

Suppurative Hidradenitides
See Hidradenitis, Suppurative

Suprahyoid
Lymphadenectomy 38700

Supraorbital Nerve
Avulsion 64732
Incision 64732
Transection 64732

Supraorbital Rim and Forehead
Reconstruction 21179-21180

Suprapubic Prostatectomies
See Prostatectomy, Suprapubic

Suprarenal
Gland
    See Adrenal Gland
Vein
    See Vein, Adrenal

Suprascapular Nerve
Injection
    Anesthetic .64418

Suprasellar Cyst
See Craniopharyngioma

Surface CD4 Receptor
See CD4

Surface Radiotherapy
See Application, Radioelement, Surface

Surgeries
Breast-Conserving
    See Breast, Excision, Lesion
Conventional
    See Celiotomy
Laser
    See Laser Surgery
Mohs
    See Mohs Micrographic Surgery
Repeat
    See Reoperation

Surgical
Avulsion
    See Avulsion
Cataract Removal
    See Cataract, Excision
Collapse Therapy; Thoracoplasty
    See Thoracoplasty
Diathermy
    See Electrocautery
Galvanism
    See Electrolysis
Incision
    See Incision

Microscopes
   See Operating Microscope
Pathology
   See Pathology, Surgical
Planing
   Nose
      Skin 30120
Pneumoperitoneum
   See Pneumoperitoneum
Removal, Eye
   See Enucleation, Eye
Revision
   See Reoperation
Services
   Post-Op Visit 99024

Surveillance
See Monitoring

Suspension
Aorta...........................33800
Kidney
   See Nephropexy
Vagina
   See Colpopexy

Suture
See Repair
Abdomen 49900
Aorta 33320-33322
Bile Duct
   Wound 47900
Bladder
   Fistulization 44660-44661, 45800-45805,
                  51880-51925
      Vesicouterine 51920-51925
      Vesicovaginal 51900
   Wound 51860-51865
Cervix 57720
Colon
   Diverticula 44604-44605
   Fistula 44650-44661
   Plication 44680
   Stoma 44620-44625
   Ulcer 44604-44605
   Wound 44604-44605
Esophagus
   Wound 43410-43415
Eyelid 67880
   Closure of 67875
   with Transposition of Tarsal Plate 67882
   Wound
      Full Thickness 67935
      Partial Thickness 67930
Facial Nerve
   Intratemporal
      Lateral to Geniculate Ganglion 69740
      Medial to Geniculate Ganglion 69745
Foot
   Tendon 28200-28210
Gastroesophageal 0008T, 43405
Great Vessel 33320-33322
Hemorrhoids 46945-46946
Hepatic Duct
   See Hepatic Duct, Repair

Intestine
   Large
      Diverticula 44605
      Ulcer 44605
      Wound 44605
Intestines
   Large
      Diverticula 44604
      Ulcer 44604
      Wound 44604
   Small
      Diverticula 44602-44603
      Fistula 44640-44661
      Plication 44680
      Ulcer 44602-44603
      Wound 44602-44603
      Stoma 44620-44625
Iris
   with Ciliary Body 66682
Kidney
   Fistula 50520-50526
   Horseshoe 50540
   Wound 50500
Leg, Lower
   Tendon 27658-27665
Leg, Upper
   Muscle 27385-27386
Liver
   Wound 47350-47361
Mesentery 44850
Nerve 64831-64876
Pancreas 48545
Pharynx
   Wound 42900
Rectum
   Fistula 45800-45825
   Prolapse 45540-45541
Removal
   Anesthesia 15850-15851
Spleen
   See Splenorrhapy
Stomach
   Fistula 43880
   Laceration 43501-43502
   Stoma 43870
   Ulcer 43501, 43840
   Wound 43840
Tendon
   Foot 28200-28210
   Knee 27380-27381
Testis
   Injury 54670
   Suspension 54620-54640
Thoracic Duct
   Abdominal Approach 38382
   Cervical Approach 38380
   Thoracic Approach 38381
Throat
   Wound 42900
Tongue
   to Lip 41510
Trachea
   Fistula
      without Plastic Repair 31820
      with Plastic Repair 31825
   Stoma
      without Plastic Repair 31820
      with Plastic Repair 31825

   Wound
      Cervical 31800
      Intrathoracic 31805
Ulcer 44604-44605
Ureter 50900
   Deligation 50940
   Fistula 50920-50930
Urethra
   Fistula 45820-45825, 53520
   Stoma 53520
   to Bladder 51840-51841
   Wound 53502-53515
Uterus
   Fistula 51920-51925
   Rupture 58520, 59350
   Suspension 58400-58410
Vagina
   Cystocele 57240, 57260
   Enterocele 57265
   Fistula
      Rectovaginal 57300-57307
      Transvesical and Vaginal Approach ..57330
      Urethrovaginal 57310-57311
      Vesicovaginal 51900, 57320-57330
   Rectocele 57250-57260
   Suspension 57280
   Wound 57200-57210
Vas Deferens 55400
Vein
   Femoral 37650
   Iliac 37660
   Vena Cava 37620
Wound 44604-44605

Swallowing
Evaluation 92526, 92610-92613,
92616-92617
Cine 74230
Treatment 92526
Video 74230

Swanson Procedure 28309

Sweat Collection
Iontophoresis 89360

Sweat Glands
Excision
   Axillary 11450-11451
   Inguinal 11462-11463
   Perianal 11470-11471
   Perineal 11470-11471
   Umbilical 11470-11471

Sweat Test 82435
See Chloride, Blood

Swenson Procedure 45120

Syme Procedure 27888

Sympathectomy
Artery
   Digital 64820
   Radial 64821
   Superficial Palmar Arch 64823
   Ulnar 64822
Cervical 64802
Cervicothoracic 64804

Tarsal Bone
See Ankle Bone

Tarsal Joint
See Foot
Arthrodesis 28730-28735, 28740
   with Advancement 28737
   with Lengthening 28737
Craterization 28122
Cyst
   Excision 28104-28107
Diaphysectomy 28122
Dislocation 28540-28545, 28555
   Percutaneous Fixation 28545-28546
Excision 28116, 28122
Fracture
   Open Treatment 28465
   without Manipulation 28450
   with Manipulation 28455-28456
Fusion 28730-28735, 28740
   with Advancement 28737
   with Lengthening 28737
Repair 28320
   Osteotomy 28304-28305
Saucerization 28122
Tumor
   Excision 28104-28107, 28171

Tarsal Strip Procedure 67917

Tarsal Tunnel Release 28035

Tarsometatarsal Joint
Arthrodesis 28730-28735, 28740
Arthrotomy 28020, 28050
Dislocation 28600-28605, 28615
   Percutaneous Fixation 28606
Exploration 28020
Fusion 28730-28735, 28740
Removal
   Foreign Body 28020
   Loose Body 28020
Synovial
   Biopsy 28050
   Excision 28070

Tarsorrhaphy 67875
Median 67880
Severing 67710
   with Transposition of Tarsal Plate 67882

Tattoo
Cornea 65600
Skin 11920-11922

TBG
See Thyroxine Binding Globulin

TBS
See Bethesda System

TB Test
Antigen Response 0010T
Skin Test 86580-86585

TCT
See Thrombin Time

Td Shots
See Tetanus Immunization; Vaccines

Team Conference
Case Management Services 99361-99373

Tear Duct
See Lacrimal Duct

Tear Gland
See Lacrimal Gland

Technique
Pericardial Window
   See Pericardiostomy
Projective
   See Projective Test

Teeth
X-Ray 70300-70320

Telangiectasia
Chromosome Analysis 88248
Injection 36468

Telangiectasia, Cerebello-Oculocutaneous
See Ataxia Telangiectasia

Telephone
Case Management Services 99361-99373
Pacemaker Analysis 93733, 93736
Transmission of ECG 93012

Teletherapy
Dose Plan 77305-77321

Temperature Gradient Studies 93740

Temporal, Petrous
Excision
   Apex 69530

Temporal Arteries
See Artery, Temporal

Temporal Bone
Electromagnetic Bone Conduction Hearing Device
   Implantation/Replacement 69710
   Removal/Repair 69711
Excision 69535
Resection 69535
Tumor
   Removal 69970
Unlisted Services and Procedures 69979

Temporomandibular Joint (TMJ)
Arthrocentesis 20605
Arthrography 70328-70332
   Injection 21116
Arthroplasty 21240-21243
Arthroscopy
   Diagnostic 29800
   Surgical 29804
Arthrotomy 21010
Cartilage
   Excision 21060
Condylectomy 21050
Coronoidectomy 21070
Dislocation
   Closed Treatment 21480-21485
   Open Treatment 21490
Injection
   Radiologic 21116

Magnetic Resonance Imaging (MRI) 70336
Meniscectomy 21060
Prostheses
   See Prosthesis, Temporomandibular Joint
Reconstruction
   See Reconstruction, Temporomandibular Joint
X-Ray with Contrast 70328-70332

Tenago Procedure 53431

Tendinosuture
See Suture, Tendon

Tendon
Achilles
   See Achilles Tendon
Arm, Upper
   Revision 24320
Finger
   Excision 26180
Forearm
   Repair 25260-25274
Graft
   Harvesting 20924
Insertion
   Biceps Tendon 24342
Lengthening
   Ankle 27685-27686
   Arm, Upper 24305
   Elbow 24305
   Finger 26476, 26478
   Forearm 25280
   Hand 26476, 26478
   Leg, Lower 27685-27686
   Leg, Upper 27393-27395
   Toe 28240
   Wrist 25280
Palm
   Excision 26170
Release
   Arm, Lower 25295
   Arm, Upper 24332
   Wrist 25295
Shortening
   Ankle 27685-27686
   Finger 26477, 26479
   Hand 26477, 26479
   Leg, Lower 27685-27686
Transfer
   Arm, Lower 25310-25312, 25316
   Arm, Upper 24301
   Elbow 24301
   Finger 26497-26498
   Hand 26480-26489
   Leg, Lower 27690-27692
   Leg, Upper 27400
   Pelvis 27098
   Thumb 26490-26492, 26510
   Wrist 25310-25312, 25316
Transplant
   Leg, Upper 27396-27397
Wrist
   Repair 25260-25274

Tendon Origin
Insertion
   Injection 20551

Tendon Pulley Reconstruction of Hand
See Hand, Reconstruction, Tendon Pulley

Tendon Sheath
Arm
　　Lower
　　　　Repair 25275
Finger
　　Incision .26055
　　Incision and Drainage 26020
　　Lesion 26160
Foot
　　Excision 28086-28088
Hand Lesion 26160
Injection 20550
Palm
　　Incision and Drainage 26020
Removal
　　Foreign Body 20520-20525
Wrist
　　Excision, Radical 25115-25116
　　Incision 25000-25001
　　Repair 25275

Tenectomy, Tendon Sheath
See Excision, Lesion, Tendon Sheath

Tennis Elbow
Repair 24350-24356

Tenodesis
Biceps Tendon
　　at Elbow 24340
　　Shoulder 23430
Finger 26471-26474
Wrist 25300-25301

Tenolysis
Ankle 27680-27681
Arm, Lower 25295
Arm, Upper 24332
Finger
　　Extensor 26445-26449
　　Flexor 26440-26442
Foot 28220-28226
Hand Extensor 26445-26449
　　Flexor 26440-26442
Leg, Lower 27680-27681
Wrist 25295

Tenomyotomy
Shoulder 23405-23406

Tenon's Capsule
Injection 67515

Tenoplasty
Anesthesia 01714

Tenorrhaphy
See Suture, Tendon

Tenosuspension
See Tenodesis

Tenosuture
See Suture, Tendon

Tenotomy
Achilles Tendon 27605-27606
Ankle 27605-27606
Arm, Lower 25290
Arm, Upper 24310
Finger 26060, 26455-26460
Foot .28230, 28234
Hand 26450, 26460
Hip
　　Iliopsoas Tendon 27005
Hip, Abductor .27006
Hip, Adductor 27000-27003
Leg, Upper 27306-27307, 27390-27392
Toe 28010-28011, 28232-28234, 28240
Wrist 25290

TENS
See Application, Neurostimulation; Physical Medicine/Therapy/Occupational Therapy

Tensilon Test 95857-95858

Tension, Ocular
See Glaucoma

Tentorium Cerebelli
Section 61440

Terman-Merrill Test 96100

Termination, Pregnancy
See Abortion

Test
Antiglobulin
　　See Coombs Test
Aphasia
　　See Aphasia Testing
Bender Visual-Motor Gestalt
　　See Bender-Gestalt Test
Binet
　　See Binet Test
Blood
　　See Blood Tests
Blood Coagulation
　　See Coagulation
Breath
　　See Breath Test
Cervical Mucus Penetration
　　See Cervical Mucus Penetration Test
Clinical Chemistry
　　See Chemistry Tests, Clinical
Complement Fixation
　　See Complement, Fixation Test
Exercise
　　See Exercise Stress Tests
Fern
　　See Smear and Stain, Wet Mount
Fetal, Nonstress
　　See Fetal Non-Stress Test
Function, Vestibular
　　See Vestibular Function Tests
Gel Diffusion
　　See Immunodiffusion
Glucose Tolerance
　　See Glucose, Tolerance Test
Hearing
　　See Audiologic Function Tests

Hemagglutination Inhibition
　　See Hemagglutination Inhibition Test
Ink Blot
　　See Inkblot Test
Intelligence
　　See Intelligence Test
Lung Function
　　See Pulmonology, Diagnostic
Neutralization
　　See Neutralization Test
Papanicolaou
　　See Pap Smears
Pregnancy
　　See Pregnancy Test
Quick
　　See Prothrombin Time
Radioimmunosorbent
　　See Gammaglobulin, Blood
Rorschach
　　See Rorschach Test
Schilling
　　See Schilling Test
Skin
　　See Skin, Tests
Stanford-Binet
　　See Psychiatric Diagnosis
Tuberculin
　　See Skin, Tests, Tuberculosis

Tester, Color Vision
See Color Vision Examination

Testes
Nuclear Medicine
　　Imaging 78760-78761
Undescended
　　See Testis, Undescended

Testicular Vein
See Spermatic Veins

Testimony, Medical 99075

Testing, Histocompatibility
See Tissue Typing

Testing, Neurophysiologic
Intraoperative 95920

Testing, Neuropsychological . . .96117

Testing, Range of Motion
See Range of Motion Test

Testis
Abscess
　　Incision and Drainage 54700
Biopsy 54500-54505
Excision
　　Laparoscopic 54690
　　Partial 54522
　　Radical 54530-54535
　　Simple 54520
Hematoma
　　Incision and Drainage 54700
Insertion
　　Prosthesis .54660
Lesion
　　Excision 54512
Needle Biopsy 54500

Repair
    Injury 54670
    Suspension 54620-54640
    Torsion 54600
Suture
    Injury 54670
    Suspension 54620-54640
Transplantation
    to Thigh 54680
Tumor
    Excision 54530-54535
Undescended
    Exploration 54550-54560
Unlisted Services and Procedures ..54699, 55899

Testosterone 84402
Response 80414
    Stimulation 80414-80415
Total 84403

Testosterone Estradiol Binding Globulin
See Globulin, Sex Hormone Binding

Test Tube Fertilization
See In Vitro Fertilization

Tetanus 86280
Antibody 86774
Immunoglobulin 90389
Vaccine 90703

Tetrachloride, Carbon
See Carbon Tetrachloride

Tetralogy of Fallot ...33692-33697, 33924

Thal-Nissen Procedure 43325

Thawing
See Frozen Blood Preparation
Previously Frozen Cells 38208

Thawing and Expansion
of Frozen Cell 88241

THBR
See Thyroid Hormone Binding Ratio

Theleplasty
See Nipples, Reconstruction

Theophylline
Assay 80198

Therapeutic
Abortion
    See Abortion, Therapeutic
Apheresis
    See Apheresis, Therapeutic
Drug Assay
    See Drug Assay
Mobilization
    See Mobilization
Photopheresis
    See Photopheresis
Radiology
    See Radiology, Therapeutic

Therapies
Cold
    See Cryotherapy
Exercise
    See Exercise Therapy
Family
    See Psychotherapy, Family
Language
    See Language Therapy
Milieu
    See Environmental Intervention
Occupational
    See Occupational Therapy
Photodynamic
    See Photochemotherapy
Photoradiation
    See Actinotherapy
Physical
    See Physical Medicine/Therapy/Occupational Therapy
Speech
    See Speech Therapy
Tocolytic
    See Tocolysis
Ultraviolet
    See Actinotherapy

Therapy
Desensitization
    See Allergen Immunotherapy
Hemodialysis
    See Hemodialysis
Hot Pack
    See Hot Pack Treatment
Radiation
    See Irradiation
Speech
    See Speech Therapy

Thermocauterization
Ectropion
    Repair 67922
Lesion
    Cornea 65450

Thermocoagulation
See Electrocautery

Thermogram
Cephalic 93760
Peripheral 93762

Thermographies
See Thermogram

Thermography, Cerebral
See Thermogram, Cephalic

Thermotherapy
Prostate 53850-53853
    Microwave 53850
    Radiofrequency 53852

Thiamine 84425

Thiersch Operation 15050
See Pinch Graft

Thiersch Procedure 46753

Thigh
Fasciotomy 27025
    See Femur; Leg, Upper

Thin Layer Chromatographies
See Chromatography, Thin-Layer

Thiocyanate 84430

Third Disease
See Rubella

Third Opinion
See Confirmatory Consultations

Thompson Procedure 27430

Thompson Test
See Smear and Stain, Routine

Thoracectomy
See Thoracoplasty

Thoracentesis 32000-32002

Thoracic
Anterior Ramus
    See Intercostal Nerve
Arteries
    See Artery, Thoracic
Cavity
    See Chest Cavity
Duct
    See Lymphatics
    Cannulation 38794
    Ligation 38380
        Abdominal Approach 38382
        Thoracic Approach 38381
    Suture
        Abdominal Approach 38382
        Cervical Approach 38380
        Thoracic Approach 38381
Empyema
    See Abscess, Thorax
Surgery
    Video-Assisted
        See Thoracoscopy
Vertebra
    See Vertebra, Thoracic
Wall
    See Chest Wall

Thoracocentesis
See Thoracentesis

Thoracoplasty 32905
with Closure Bronchopleural Fistula 32906

Thoracoscopy
Diagnostic 32601-32606
    without Biopsy 32601, 32603, 32605
    with Biopsy 32602, 32604, 32606
Surgical 32650-32665
    with Control Traumatic Hemorrhage ...32654
    with Creation Pericardial Window 32659
    with Esophagomyotomy 32665
    with Excision-Plication of Bullae 32655
    with Excision Mediastinal Cyst, Tumor and/or Mass 32662
    with Excision Pericardial Cyst, Tumor and/or Mass 32661

Thymectomy 60520-60521
Sternal Split/Transthoracic
Approach 60521-60522
Transcervical Approach 60520

Thymotaxin
See Beta-2-Microglobulin

Thymus Gland 60520
Excision 60520-60521

Thyramine
See Amphetamine

Thyrocalcitonin
See Calcitonin

Thyroglobulin 84432
Antibody 86800

Thyroglossal Duct
Cyst
   Excision 60280-60281

Thyroidectomy
Partial 60210-60225
Secondary 60260
Total 60240, 60271
   Cervical Approach 60271
   for Malignancy
     Limited Neck Dissection 60252
     Radical Neck Dissection 60254
   Removal All Thyroid Tissue 60260
   Sternal Split/Transthoracic Approach ..60270

Thyroid Gland
Cyst
   Aspiration 60001
   Excision 60200
   Incision and Drainage 60000
   Injection 60001
Excision
   for Malignancy
     Limited Neck Dissection 60252
     Radical Neck Dissection 60254
   Partial 60210-60225
   Secondary 60260
   Total 60240, 60271
     Cervical Approach 60271
     Removal All Thyroid Tissue 60260
     Sternal Split/Transthoracic Approach 60270
     Transcervical Approach 60520
Metastatic Cancer
   Nuclear Imaging 78015-78018
Needle Biopsy 60100
Nuclear Medicine
   Imaging 78010
   Imaging for Metastases 78015-78018
   Imaging with Flow 78011
   Imaging with Uptake 78006-78007
   Metastases Uptake 78020
   Uptake 78000-78003
Radionuclide Therapy
   Ablation 79030
   Hyperthyroidism 79000-79001
   Metastases 79035
   Suppression 79020

Radiopharmaceutical Therapy
   Ablation 79030
   Metastases 79035
   Suppression 79020
Tumor
   Excision 60200

Thyroid Hormone Binding Ratio 84479

Thyroid Hormone Uptake 84479

Thyroid Stimulating Hormone (TSH) 80418, 80438-80440, 84443

Thyroid Stimulating Hormone Receptor ab
See Thyrotropin Releasing Hormone (TRH)

Thyroid Stimulating Immune Globulins 84445

Thyroid Stimulator, Long Acting
See Thyrotropin Releasing Hormone (TRH)

Thyroid Suppression Test
See Nuclear Medicine, Thyroid, Uptake

Thyrolingual Cyst
See Cyst, Thyroglossal Duct

Thyrotomy 31300

Thyrotropin Receptor ab
See Thyrotropin Releasing Hormone (TRH)

Thyrotropin Releasing Hormone (TRH) 80438-80439

Thyroxine
Free 84439
Neonatal 84437
Total 84436
True 84436

Thyroxine Binding Globulin ...84442

Tibia
See Ankle
Arthroscopy Surgical 29891-29892
Craterization 27360, 27640
Cyst
   Excision 27635-27638
Diaphysectomy 27360, 27640
Excision 27360, 27640
   Epiphyseal Bar 20150
Fracture 27759
Fracture
   Arthroscopic Treatment 29855-29856
     Plafond 29892
   Closed Treatment 27824-27825
   Distal 27824-27828
   Intercondylar 27538-27540
   Malleolus 27760-27766, 27808-27814
   Open Treatment 27535-27536, 27758-27759, 27826-27828
   Plateau 29855-29856
     Closed Treatment 27530-27536
   Shaft 27752-27759
   without Manipulation 27824
   with Manipulation 27825

Incision 27607
Osteoplasty
   Lengthening 27715
Prophylactic Treatment 27745
Reconstruction 27418
   at Knee 27440-27443, 27446
Repair 27720-27725
   Epiphysis 27477-27485, 27730-27742
   Osteochondritis Dissecans
     Arthroscopy 29892
     Osteotomy 27455-27457, 27705, 27709-27712
   Pseudoarthrosis 27727
Saucerization 27360, 27640
Tumor
   Excision 27635-27638, 27645
X-Ray 73590

Tibial
Arteries
   See Artery, Tibial
Nerve
   Repair/Suture
     Posterior 64840

Tibiofibular Joint
Arthrodesis 27871
Dislocation 27830-27832
Disruption
   Open Treatment 27829
Fusion 27871

TIG
See Immune Globulins, Tetanus

Time
Bleeding
   See Bleeding Time
Prothrombin
   See Prothrombin Time
Reptilase
   See Thrombin Time

Tissue
Culture
   Chromosome Analysis 88230-88239
   Homogenization 87176
   Non-neoplastic Disorder 88230, 88237
   Skin Grafts 15100-15121, 15342-15343
   Solid Tumor 88239
   Toxin/Antitoxin 87230
   Virus 87252-87253
Enzyme Activity 82657
Examination for Ectoparasites 87220
Examination for Fungi 87220
Expander
   Breast Reconstruction with 19357
   Insertion
     Skin 11960
   Removal
     Skin 11971
   Replacement
     Skin 11970
Grafts
   Harvesting 20926
Granulation
   See Granulation Tissue
Homogenization 87176
Hybridization In Situ 88365

Mucosal
  See Mucosa
Preparation
    Drug Analysis 80103
Soft
    Abscess 20000-20005
Transfer
    Adjacent
      Eyelids 67961
      Skin 14000-14350
    Facial Muscles 15845
    Finger Flap 14350
    Toe Flap 14350
Typing
    HLA Antibodies 86812-86817
    Lymphocyte Culture 86821-86822

Tissue Factor
See Thromboplastin

TLC
See Chromatography, Thin-Layer
Screen 84375

TMJ
See Temporomandibular Joint (TMJ)
Prostheses
  See Prosthesis, Temporomandibular Joint

Tobramycin
Assay 80200

Tocolysis 59412, 99553
External Cephalic Version 59412

Tocopherol 84446

Toe
See Interphalangeal Joint, Toe;
Metatarsophalangeal Joint; Phalanx
Amputation 28810-28825
Capsulotomy 28270-28272
Fasciotomy 28008
Fracture
  See Fracture, Phalanges, Toe
Lesion
    Excision 28092
Reconstruction
    Angle Deformity 28313
    Extra Toes 28344
    Hammertoe 28285-28286
    Macrodactyly 28340-28341
    Syndactyly 28345
    Webbed Toe 28345
Repair
    Bunion 28290-28299
    Muscle 28240
    Tendon 28232-28234, 28240
    Webbed 28280
    Webbed Toe 28345
Tenotomy 28010-28011, 28232-28234
Unlisted Services and Procedures 28899

Toes
Arthrocentesis 20600
Dislocation
  See Specific Joint
Magnetic Resonance Imaging
(MRI) 73721-73723

Reconstruction
    Extra Digit 26587
Repair
    Extra Digit 26587
    Macrodactylia 26590
Reposition to Hand 26551-26556
Strapping 29550
X-Ray 73660

Toe Flap
Tissue Transfer 14350

Tolbutamide Tolerance Test 82953

Tolerance Test
Glucagon 82946
Glucose 82951-82952
    with Tolbutamide 82953
Heparin-Protamine 85530
Insulin 80434-80435
Maltose 82951-82952
Tolbutamide 82953

Tomodensitometries
See CT Scan

Tomographic Scintigraphy, Computed
See Emission Computerized Tomography

Tomographic SPECT
Myocardial Imaging 78469

Tomographies, Computed X-Ray
See CT Scan

Tomography, Computerized Axial
Abdomen
  See Abdomen, CT Scan
Head
  See Head, CT Scan

Tomography, Emission Computed
See Positron Emission Tomography
Single Photon
  See SPECT

Tompkins Metroplasty 58540
See Uterus, Reconstruction

Tongue
Abscess
    Incision and Drainage ..41000-41006, 41015
Biopsy 41100-41105
Cyst
    Incision and Drainage 41000-41006,
                       41015, 60000
Excision
    Complete 41140-41155
    Frenum 41115
    Partial 41120-41135
    with Mouth Resection 41150-41153
    with Radical Neck 41135, 41145,
                      41153-41155
Fixation 41500
Hematoma
    Incision and Drainage ..41000-41006, 41015
Incision
    Frenum 41010
Lesion
    Excision 41110-41114

Reconstruction
    Frenum 41520
Repair
  See Repair, Tongue
    Laceration 41250-41252
    Suture 41510
Suture 41510
Unlisted Services and Procedures 41599

Tonography 92120
with Provocation 92130

Tonometry, Serial 92100

Tonsil, Pharyngeal
See Adenoids

Tonsillectomy 42820-42826

Tonsils
Abscess
    Incision and Drainage 42700
Excision 42825-42826
    Lingual 42870
    Radical 42842-42845
    Tag 42860
    with Adenoids 42820-42821
Lingual
    Destruction 42870
Unlisted Services and Procedures 42999

Topiramate
Assay 80201

Torek Procedure
See Orchiopexy

Torkildsen Procedure 62180

TORP (Total Ossicular Replacement Prosthesis) 69633, 69637

Torsion Swing Test 92546

Torula
See Cryptococcus

Torus Mandibularis
Tumor Excision 21031

Total
Abdominal Hysterectomy
  See Hysterectomy, Abdominal, Total
Bilirubin Level
  See Bilirubin, Total
Catecholamines
  See Catecholamines, Urine
Cystectomy
  See Bladder, Excision, Total
Dacryoadenectomy
  See Dacryoadenectomy, Total
Elbow Replacement
  See Replacement, Elbow, Total
Esophagectomy
  See Esophagectomy, Total
Gastrectomy
  See Excision, Stomach, Total
Hemolytic Complement
  See Complement, Hemolytic, Total
Hip Arthroplasty
  See Hip, Total Replacement

Knee Arthroplasty
  See Prosthesis, Knee
Mastectomies
  See Mastectomy
Ostectomy of Patella
  See Patellectomy
Splenectomy
  See Splenectomy, Total

Touroff Operation 37615
See Ligation, Artery, Neck

Toxicology Screen 80100-80103

Toxin, Botulinum
See Chemodenervation

Toxin Assay 87230

Toxoplasma
Antibody 86777-86778

Trabeculectomies
See Trabeculoplasty

Trabeculectomy ab Externo
in Absence of Previous Surgery 66170
with Scarring Previous Surgery 66172

Trabeculoplasty
by Laser Surgery .65855

Trabeculotomy ab Externo
Eye 65850

Trachea
Aspiration 31720
  Catheter 31720-31725
Catheterization 31700
Dilation 31630-31631
Endoscopy
  via Tracheostomy 31615
Excision
  Stenosis 31780-31781
Fistula
  without Plastic Repair 31820
  with Plastic Repair 31825
Fracture
  Endoscopy 31630
Incision
  Emergency 31603-31605
  Planned 31600-31601
  with Flaps 31610
Instillation
  Contrast Material 31708
Introduction
  Needle Wire .31730
Puncture
  Aspiration and/or Injection 31612
Reconstruction
  Carina 31766
  Cervical 31750
  Fistula 31755
  Intrathoracic .31760
Repair
  Cervical 31750
  Fistula 31755
  Intrathoracic .31760
  Stoma 31613-31614

Revision
  Stoma
    Scars .31830
Scar
  Revision 31830
Stenosis
  Excision 31780-31781
  Repair 31780-31781
Stoma
  Repair
    without Plastic Repair 31820
    with Plastic Repair 31825
  Revision
    Scars .31830
Tumor
  Excision
    Cervical 31785
    Thoracic 31786
Unlisted Services and Procedures
  Bronchi 31899
Wound
  Suture
    Cervical 31800
    Intrathoracic 31805

Tracheal
Stent
  Placement 31631
Tubes
  See Endotracheal Tube

Trachelectomy 57530
Radical 57531

Tracheloplasty
See Cervicoplasty

Trachelorrhaphy 57720

Tracheo-Esophageal Fistula
See Fistula, Tracheoesophageal

Tracheobronchoscopy
through Tracheostomy 31615

Tracheoplasty
Cervical 31750
Intrathoracic 31760
Tracheopharyngeal Fistulization 31755

Tracheostoma
Revision .31613-31614

Tracheostomy
Emergency 31603-31605
Planned .31600-31601
Revision
  Scar 31830
Surgical Closure
  without Plastic Repair 31820
  with Plastic Repair 31825
Tracheobronchoscopy through 31615
with Flaps 31610

Tracheotomy
Tube Change 31502

Tracking Tests (Ocular) 92545
See Ear, Nose and Throat

Tract, Urinary
See Urinary Tract

Traction Therapy
See Physical Medicine/Therapy/Occupational
Therapy
Manual 97140
Mechanical 97012

Tractotomy
Medulla 61470
Mesencephalon 61480

Training
Activities of Daily Living 97535, 99509
Biofeedback 90901-90911
Cognitive Skills .97532
Community/Work Reintegration 97537
Home Management 97535, 99509
Orthoptic/Pleoptic 92065
Orthotics 97504
Prosthetics 97520
Self Care 97535, 99509
Sensory Integration 97533
Walking (Physical Therapy) 97116
Wheelchair Management/Propulsion 97542

TRAM Flap
Breast Reconstruction 19367-19369

Trans-Scaphoperilunar
Fracture/Dislocation
  Closed Treatment 25680
  Open Treatment 25685

Transaminase
Glutamic Oxaloacetic 84450
Glutamic Pyruvic 84460

Transcatheter
Biopsy 37200
Closure
  Percutaneous
    Heart 93580-93581
Embolization
  Percutaneous 37204
    Cranial 61624-61626
Occlusion
  Percutaneous 37204
    Cranial 61624-61626
Placement
  Intravascular Stents 0005T-0007T,
                      37205-37208
Therapy
  Embolization .75894
  Infusion 37201-37202, 75896-75898
  Perfusion
    Cranial 61624-61626
  Retrieval 75961

Transcatheter Foreign Body
Retrieval 37203

Transcortin 84449

**Transcutaneous Electric Nerve
Stimulation**
See Application, Neurostimulation

Transdermal Electrostimulation
See Application, Neurostimulation

Transection

Artery
Carotid 61610, 61612
Blood Vessel
Kidney 50100
Carotid
with Skull Base Surgery 61609
Nerve 64732-64772
Vagus 43640-43641
Pulmonary Artery 33922

Transesophageal

Doppler Echocardiography 93312-93318

Transfer

Blastocyst
See Embryo Transfer
Gamete Intrafallopian
See GIFT
Jejunum
with Microvascular Anastomosis
Free 43496
Preparation
Embryo 89255
Cryopreserved 89256
Surgical
See Transposition
Tendon
See Tendon, Transfer
Toe to Hand 26551-26556

Transferase

Aspartate Amino 84450
Glutamic Oxaloacetic 84450

Transferrin 84466

Transformation

Lymphocyte 86353

Transfusion

Blood 36430
Exchange 36450-36455
Fetal 36460
Push
Infant 36440
Blood Parts
Exchange 36511-36516
Unlisted Services and Procedures 86999
White Blood Cells 86950

Transfusion of, Blood, Autologous

See Autotransfusion

Transluminal

Angioplasty
Arterial 75962-75968
Atherectomies
See Artery, Atherectomy
Coronary Balloon Dilatation
See Percutaneous Transluminal Angioplasty

Transmyocardial Laser Revascularization 33140-33141

Transosteal Bone Plate

Reconstruction
Mandible 21244

Transpeptidase, Gamma-Glutamyl

See Gamma Glutamyl Transferase

Transplant

See Graft
Bone
See Bone Graft
Hair
See Hair, Transplant

Transplantation

See Graft
Allogenic
See Homograft
Autologous
See Autograft
Bone Marrow 38240-38242
Cartilage
Allograft
Knee 0013T
Autograft
Knee 0012T
Knee 0014T
Cornea
Autograft/Homograft
Lamellar 65710
Penetrating 65730-65755
for Aphakia 65750
Hair
Punch Graft 15775-15776
Strip 15220-15221
Heart 33945
Heart-Lung 33935
Heterologous
See Heterograft
Intestines
Allotransplantation 44135-44136
Donor Enterectomy 44132-44133
Liver 47135
Heterotopic 47136
Lung
Anesthesia 00580
Donor Pneumonectomy 32850
Double, without Cardiopulmonary
Bypass 32853
Double, with Cardiopulmonary
Bypass 32854
Single, without Cardiopulmonary
Bypass 32851
Single, with Cardiopulmonary
Bypass 32852
Muscle
See Muscle Flaps
Pancreas 48160, 48550-48556
Parathyroid 60512
Renal
Allotransplantation 50360
with Recipient Nephrectomy 50365
Autotransplantation 50380
Donor Nephrectomy 50300-50320, 50547
Recipient Nephrectomy 50340
Removal Transplanted Renal Allograft .50370
Skin
See Dermatology
Stem Cells 38240-38242
Cell Concentration 38215
Cryopreservation 38207
Harvesting 38205-38206
Plasma Depletion 38214
Platelet Depletion 38213
Red Blood Cell Depletion 38212

T-cell Depletion 38210
Thawing 38208
Tumor Cell Depletion 38211
Washing 38209
Testis
to Thigh 54680
Tissue, Harvesting
See Graft, Tissue, Harvesting

Transpleural Thoracoscopy

See Thoracoscopy

Transposition

Arteries
Carotid 0037T, 35691, 35694-35695
Subclavian 0037T, 35693-35695
Vertebral 35691-35693
Cranial Nerve 64716
Eye Muscles 67320
Great Arteries
Repair 33770-33781
Nerve 64718-64721
Ovary 58825
Peripheral Nerve
Major 64856
Vein Valve 34510

Transthoracic Echocardiography

See Echocardiography

Transthyretin

See Prealbumin

Transureteroureterostomy 50770

Transurethral Balloon Dilation

Prostatic Urethra 52510

Transurethral Fulguration

Postoperative Bleeding 52606

Transurethral Procedure

See Specific Procedure
Prostate
Incision 52450
Resection 52612-52614
Thermotherapy 53850-53853
Microwave 53850
Radiofrequency 53852

Trapezium

Arthroplasty
with Implant 25445

Travel, Unusual 99082

Treacher-Collins Syndrome

Midface Reconstruction 21150-21151

Treatment, Tocolytic

See Tocolysis

Trendelenburg Operation

See Varicose Vein, Removal, Secondary Varicosity

Trephine Procedure

Sinusotomy
Frontal 31070

Treponema Pallidum
Antibody
    Confirmation Test 86781
Antigen Detection
    Direct Fluorescence 87285

TRH
See Thyrotropin Releasing Hormone (TRH)

Triacylglycerol
See Triglycerides

Triacylglycerol Hydrolase
See Lipase

Tributyrinase
See Lipase

Trichiasis
Repair 67825
    Epilation, by Forceps 67820
    Epilation, by Other than Forceps 67825
    Incision of Lid Margin 67830
       with Free Mucous Membrane Graft .67835

Trichina
See Trichinella

Trichinella
Antibody 86784
Trichogram 96902

Trichrome Stain 88313

Tricuspid Valve
Excision 33460
Repair 33463-33465
Replacement 33465
Repositioning 33468

Tridymite
See Silica

Trigeminal Ganglia
See Gasserian Ganglion

Trigeminal Nerve
Destruction 64600-64610
Injection
    Anesthetic 64400
    Neurolytic 64600-64610

Trigeminal Tract
Stereotactic
    Create Lesion 61791

Trigger Finger Repair 26055

Trigger Point
Injection
    One or Two Muscles 20552
    Two or More Muscles 20553

Triglyceridase
See Lipase

Triglycerides 84478

Triglyceride Lipase
See Lipase

Trigonocephaly 21175

Triiodothyronine
Free 84481
Reverse 84482
Total 84480
True 84480

Triolean Hydrolase
See Lipase

Trioxopurine
See Uric Acid

Tripcellim
See Trypsin

Trisegmentectomy 47122

Trocar Biopsy
Bone Marrow 38221

Trochanteric Femur Fracture
See Femur, Fracture, Trochanteric

Trophoblastic Tumor GTT
See Hydatidiform Mole

Troponin 84484
Qualitative 84512
Quantitative 84484

Truncal Vagotomies
See Vagotomy, Truncal

Truncus Arteriosus
Repair 33786

Truncus Brachiocephalicus
See Artery, Brachiocephalic

Trunk, Brachiocephalic
See Artery, Brachiocephalic

Trypanosomiases
See Trypanosomiasis

Trypanosomiasis 86171, 86280

Trypsin
Duodenum 84485
Feces 84488-84490

Trypsin Inhibitor, Alpha 1-Antitrypsin
See Alpha-1 Antitrypsin

Trypure
See Trypsin

Tsalicylate Intoxication
See Salicylate

TSH
See Thyroid Stimulating Hormone

TSI
See Thyroid Stimulating Immunoglobulin

Tsutsugamushi Disease
See Scrub Typhus

TT
See Thrombin Time

TT-3
See Triiodothyronine, True

TT-4
See Thyroxine, True

Tubal Embryo Stage Transfer
See Embryo Transfer

Tubal Ligation 58600
Laparoscopic 58670
with Cesarean Delivery 58611

Tubal Occlusion
See Fallopian Tube
with Cesarean Delivery
    See Fallopian Tube, Occlusion; Occlusion
    Create Lesion
        See Fallopian Tube, Occlusion; Occlusion,
        Fallopian Tube

Tubal Pregnancy 59121
with Salpingectomy and/or
Oophorectomy 59120

Tuba Auditoria (Auditiva)
See Eustachian Tube

Tube, Fallopian
See Fallopian Tube

Tubectomy
See Excision, Fallopian Tube

Tubed Pedicle Flap
Formation 15570-15576

Tubercleplasty
Tibia
    Anterior 27418

Tubercle Bacilli
Culture 87116

Tuberculin Test
See Skin, Tests, Tuberculosis

Tuberculosis
Antigen Response Test 0010T
Culture 87116
Skin Test 86580-86585

Tuberculosis Vaccine (BCG) 90585-90586

Tubes
Endotracheal
    See Endotracheal Tube
Gastrostomy
    See Gastrostomy Tube

Tube Change
Tracheotomy 31502

Tube Placement
Endoscopic
    Bile Duct, Pancreatic Duct 43268
    Nasobiliary, Nasopancreatic
        for Drainage 43267
Gastrostomy Tube 43750
Nasogastric Tube 43752
Orogastric Tube 43752

Tudor 'Rabbit Ear'
See Urethra, Repair

Tuffier Vaginal Hysterectomy
See Hysterectomy, Vaginal

Tumor
See Craniopharyngioma
Abdomen
    Destruction/Excision 49200-49201
Abdominal Wall
    Excision 22900
Acetabulum
    Excision 27076
Ankle 27615-27619
Arm, Lower 25075-25077
Arm, Upper
    Excision 24075-24077
Back/Flank
    Excision 21930
    Radical Resection 21935
Bile Duct
    Destruction 43272
    Extrahepatic 47711
    Intrahepatic 47712
Bladder 52234-52240
    Excision 51530, 52355
Brain 61510
    Excision 61518, 61520-61521,
               61526-61530, 61545, 62164
Breast
    Excision 19120-19126
Bronchi
    Excision 31640
Calcaneus 28100-28103
    Excision 27647
Carpal 25130-25136
Cheekbone 21030, 21034
Chest Wall
    Excision 19260-19272
Clavicle
    Excision 23140, 23200
      with Allograft 23146
      with Autograft 23145
Coccyx 49215
Colon
    Destruction 44393, 45383
Cranial Bone
    Reconstruction 21181-21184
Destruction
    Chemosurgery 17304-17310
    Urethra 53220
Ear, Middle
    Extended 69554
    Transcanal 69550
    Transmastoid .69552
Elbow
    Excision 24075-24077
Esophagus
    Ablation 43228
Excision
    Femur .27355-27358
Facial Bone 21029-21030, 21034
Fallopian Tube
    Resection 58950, 58952-58954
Femoral .27355-27358
Femur 27065-27067
    Excision 27365

Fibroid
    See Leiomyomata
Fibula 27635-27638
    Excision 27646
Finger
    Excision 26115-26117
Foot 28043-28046
Forearm
    Radical Resection 25077
Gastrostomy
    See Lesion
Gums
    Excision 41825-41827
Hand
    Excision 26115-26117
Heart
    Excision 33120-33130
Hip 27047-27049, 27065-27067
    Excision 27075-27076
Humerus
    Excision 23150, 23220-23222, 24110
      with Allograft 23156, 24116
      with Autograft 23155, 24115
Ileum .27065-27067
Immunoassay for Antigen 86294, 86316
    CA 125 86304
    CA 15-3 86300
    CA 19-9 86301
Innominate
    Excision 27077
Intestines, Small
    Destruction 44369
Ischial
    Excision 27078-27079
Kidney
    Excision 50562, 52355
Knee
    Excision 27327-27329, 27365
Lacrimal Gland
    Excision
      Frontal Approach 68540
      with Osteotomy 68550
Larynx
    Excision 31300
      Endoscopic 31540-31541, 31578
      Incision 31300
Leg, Lower 27615-27619
Leg, Upper
    Excision 27327-27329
Localization
    Nuclear Medicine 78800-78803
Mandible .21044-21047
Maxilla 21030, 21034, 21048-21049
Maxillary Torus Palatinus 21032
Mediastinal
    Excision 39220
Mediastinum 32662
Meningioma 61512
    Excision 61519
Metacarpal 26200-26205, 26250-26255
Metatarsal 28104-28107
    Excision 28173
Neck
    Excision 21555-21556
    Radical Resection 21557
Olecranon
    Excision 24120

Olecranon Process
    with Allograft
      Excision 24126
    with Autograft
      Excision 24125
Ovary
    Resection 58950-58954
Pancreatic Duct
    Destruction 43272
Parotid Gland
    Excision 42410-42426
Pelvis 27047-27049
Pericardial
    Endoscopic 32661
    Excision 33050
Peritoneum
    Resection 58950, 58952-58954
Phalanges
    Finger 26210-26215, 26260-26262
    Toe 28108
    Excision 28175
Pituitary Gland
    Excision 61546-61548, 62165
Positron Emission Tomography (PET) 78810
Pubis 27065-27067
Radiation Therapy 77295
Radius 25120-25126, 25170
    Excision 24120
    with Allograft
      Excision 24126
    with Autograft
      Excision 24125
Rectum
    Destruction 45190, 45320, 46937-46938
    Excision 45160-45170
Resection
    Face 21015
    Scalp 21015
    with Cystourethroscopy 52355
Retroperitoneal
    Destruction/Excision 49200-49201
Sacrum 49215
Scapula
    Excision 23140, 23210
      with Allograft 23146
      with Autograft 23145
Shoulder
    Excision 23075-23077
Skull
    Excision 61500
Soft Tissue
    Elbow
      Excision 24075
    Finger
      Excision 26115
    Forearm
      Radical Resection 25077
    Hand
      Excision 26115
    Wrist
      Excision 25075
      Radical Resection 25077
Spinal Cord
    Excision 63275-63290
Stomach
    Excision 43610-43611
Talus 28100-28103
    Excision 27647

Tarsal 28104-28107
   Excision 28171
Temporal Bone
   Removal 69970
Testis
   Excision 54530-54535
Thorax
   Excision 21555-21556
   Radical Resection 21557
Thyroid
   Excision 60200
Tibia 27365-27638
   Excision 27645
Torus Mandibularis 21031
Trachea
   Excision
     Cervical 31785
     Thoracic 31786
Ulna 25120-25126, 25170
   Excision 24120
   with Allograft
     Excision 24126
   with Autograft
     Excision 24125
Ureter
   Excision 52355
Urethra 52234-52240, 53220
   Excision 52355
Uterus
   Excision 58140-58146
Vagina
   Excision 57135
Vertebra
   Additional Segment
     Excision 22116
   Cervical
     Excision 22100
   Lumbar 22102
   Thoracic
     Excision 22101
Wrist 25075-25077, 25135-25136
   Radical Resection 25077

Tunica Vaginalis
Hydrocele
   Aspiration 55000
   Excision 55040-55041
   Repair 55060

Turbinate
Excision 30130-30140
Fracture
   Therapeutic 30930
Injection 30200
Submucous Resection
   Nose Excision 30140

Turbinate Mucosa
Cauterization 30801-30802

Turcica, Sella
See Sella Turcica

Turnbuckle Jacket 29020-29025
Removal 29715

TURP
See Prostatectomy, Transurethral

Tylectomy
See Breast, Excision, Lesion

Tylenol
Urine 82003

Tympanic Membrane
Create Stoma 69433-69436
Incision 69420-69421
Reconstruction 69620
Repair 69450, 69610

Tympanic Nerve
Excision 69676

Tympanolysis 69450

Tympanometry 92567
See Audiologic Function Tests

Tympanoplasty
See Myringoplasty
Radical or Complete 69645
   with Ossicular Chain Reconstruction ..69646
without Mastoidectomy 69631
   with Ossicular Chain Reconstruction ..69632
     and Synthetic Prosthesis 69633
with Antrotomy or Mastoidotomy 69635
   with Ossicular Chain Reconstruction ..69636
     and Synthetic Prosthesis 69637
with Mastoidectomy 69641
   with Intact or Reconstructed Wall 69643
     and Ossicular Chain Reconstruction ..69644
   with Ossicular Chain Reconstruction ..69642

Tympanostomy 69433-69436

Tympanotomy
See Myringotomy

Typhoid Vaccine 90690-90693
AKD 90693
Oral 90690
Polysaccharide 90691

Typhus
Endemic
   See Murine Typhus
Mite-Borne
   See Scrub Typhus
Sao Paulo
   See Rocky Mountain Spotted Fever
Tropical
   See Scrub Typhus

Typing, Blood
See Blood Typing

Typing, HLA
See HLA Typing

Typing, Tissue
See Tissue Typing

Tyrosine 84510

Tzank Smear 87207

T Cell Leukemia Virus I, Human
See HTLV I

T Cell Leukemia Virus II, Human
See HTLV II

T Cell Leukemia Virus II Antibodies, Human
See Antibody, HTLV-II

T Cell Leukemia Virus I Antibodies, Adult
See Antibody, HTLV-I

T Lymphotropic Virus Type III Antibodies, Human
See Antibody, HIV

U

Uchida Procedure
See Tubal Ligation

UDP Galactose Pyrophosphorylase
See Galactose-1-Phosphate, Uridyl Transferase

UFR
See Uroflowmetry

Ulcer
Anal
   See Anus, Fissure
Decubitus
   See Debridement; Pressure Ulcer (Decubitus);
   Skin Graft and Flap
Pinch Graft 15050
Pressure 15920-15999
Stomach
   Excision 43610

Ulcerative, Cystitis
See Cystitis, Interstitial

Ulna
See Arm, Lower; Elbow; Humerus; Radius
Arthrodesis
   Radioulnar Joint
     with Resection 25830
Arthroplasty
   with Implant 25442
Centralization or Wrist 25335
Craterization 24147, 25150-25151
Cyst
   Excision 24125-24126, 25120-25126
Diaphysectomy 24147, 25150-25151
Excision 24147
   Abscess 24138
   Complete 25240
   Epiphyseal Bar 20150
   Partial 25145-25151, 25240
Fracture
   Closed Treatment 25530-25535
   Olecranon 24670-24675
     Open Treatment 24685
   Open Treatment 25545
   Shaft 25530-25545
     Open Treatment 25574
   Styloid
     Closed Treatment 25650
     Open Treatment 25652
     Percutaneous Fixation 25651

Lacrimal System 68899
Laparoscopy 38129, 38589, 43289, 43659,
    44238-44239, 44979, 47379, 47579, 49329,
    49659, 50549, 50949, 54699, 55559, 58578,
                            58679, 59898, 60659
Larynx 31599
Lip 40799
Liver 47379, 47399
Lungs 32999
Lymphatic System 38999
Magnetic Resonance 76498
Maxillofacial 21299
Maxillofacial Prosthetics 21089
Meckel's Diverticulum 44899
Mediastinum 39499
Mesentery Surgery 44899
Microbiology 87999
Mouth .40899, 41599
Musculoskeletal 25999, 26989
Musculoskeletal Surgery
    Abdominal Wall 22999
    Neck 21899
    Spine 22899
    Thorax 21899
Musculoskeletal System 20999
    Ankle 27899
    Arm, Upper 24999
    Elbow 24999
    Head 21499
    Knee 27599
    Leg, Lower 27899
    Leg, Upper 27599
Necropsy 88099
Nervous System Surgery 64999
Neurology/Neuromuscular Testing 95999
Nose 30999
Nuclear Medicine 78999
    Blood 78199
    Bone 78399
    Endocrine System 78099
    Genitourinary System 78799
    Heart 78499
    Hematopoietic System 78199
    Lymphatic System 78199
    Musculoskeletal System 78399
    Nervous System 78699
    Therapeutic 79999
Obstetrical Care 59898-59899
Omentum 49329, 49999
Ophthalmology 92499
Orbit 67599
Otorhinolaryngology 92700
Ovary 58679, 58999
Oviduct 58679, 58999
Palate 42299
Pancreas Surgery 48999
Pathology 89399
Pelvis 27299
Penis 55899
Peritoneum 49329, 49999
Pharynx 42999
Physical Therapy 97039, 97139, 97799
Pleura 32999
Pressure Ulcer 15999
Preventive Medicine 99429
Prostate 55899
Psychiatric 90899
Pulmonology 94799

Radiation Physics 77399
Radiation Therapy 77499
    Planning 77299
Radiology, Diagnostic 76499
Radionuclide Therapy 79999
Radiopharmaceutical Therapy 79999
Rectum 44239, 45999
Salivary Gland 42699
Scrotum 55899
Seminal Vesicle .55899
Shoulder Surgery 23929
Sinuses 31299
Skin 17999
Special Services and Reports 99199
Spine 22899
Stomach 43659, 43999
Strapping 29799
Surgical Pathology 88399
Temporal Bone 69979
Testis .54699, 55899
Throat 42999
Tongue 41599
Tonsil/Adenoid 42999
Trachea 31899
Transfusion 86999
Ultrasound 76999
Ureter 50949
Urinary System 53899
Uterus 58578-58579, 58999
Uvula 42299
Vagina 58999
Vascular 37799
Vascular Endoscopy 37501
Vascular Injection 36299
Vascular Studies .93799
Vas Deferens 55899
Wrist 25999

Unna Paste Boot 29580
Removal 29700

UPP
See Urethra Pressure Profile

Upper
Digestive System Endoscopy
    See Endoscopy, Gastrointestinal, Upper
Extremity
    See Arm, Upper; Elbow; Humerus
Gastrointestinal Bleeding
    See Gastrointestinal, Upper, Hemorrhage
Gastrointestinal Endoscopy, Biopsy
    See Biopsy
        See Biopsy, Gastrointestinal, Upper
        Endoscopy; Endoscopy, Gastrointestinal
GI Tract
    See Gastrointestinal Tract, Upper

Urachal Cyst
See Cyst, Urachal

Urea Breath Test 78267-78268, 83014

Urea Nitrogen
See Blood Urea Nitrogen
Clearance 84545
Quantitative 84520

Semiquantitative .84525
Urine 84540

Urea Nitrogen, Blood
See Blood Urea Nitrogen

Urecholine Supersensitivity Test
See Cystometrogram

Ureter
Anastomosis
    to Bladder 50780-50785
    to Colon 50810-50815
    to Intestine 50800, 50820-50825
    to Kidney 50740-50750
    to Ureter 50760-50770
Biopsy 50955-50959, 50974-50978, 52007
Catheterization .52005
Continent Diversion 50825
Creation
    Stoma 50860
Destruction
    Endoscopic 50957-50959, 50976-50978
Dilation 52341-52342, 52344-52345
    Endoscopic 50553, 50572, 50953, 50972
Endoscopy
    Biopsy 50955-50959, 50974-50978,
                                    52007, 52354
    Catheterization 50953, 50972, 52005
    Destruction 50957-50959, 50976-50978,
                                        52354
    Dilation 52341-52342, 52344-52345
    Excision
        Tumor 52355
    Exploration .52351
    Injection of Implant Material 52327
    Insertion
        Stent 50947, 52332-52334
    Lithotripsy 52353
    Manipulation of Ureteral Calculus 52330
    Radioactive Substance 50959, 50978
    Removal
        Calculus 50961, 50980, 52320-52325,
                                            52352
        Foreign Body 50961, 50980
    Resection 52355
    via Incision 50970-50980
    via Stoma 50951-50961
Exploration 50600
Incision and Drainage 50600
Injection
    Radiologic 50684, 50690
Insertion
    Catheter 50393
    Stent 50393, 50947, 52332-52334
    Tube 50688
Lesion
    Destruction .52354
Lithotripsy 52353
Lysis
    Adhesions 50715-50725
Manometric Studies
    Pressure 50686
Meatotomy 52290
Nuclear Medicine
    Reflux Study 78740
Postcaval
    See Retrocaval Ureter

Reconstruction 53445
Removal
  Prosthesis 53446-53447
Repair
  Prosthesis .53449
Replacement
  Prosthesis .53448
Suture
  Fistula 45820-45825, 53520
  to Bladder 51840-51841
  Wound 53502-53515
Tumor
  Destruction 53220
  Excision 53220
Unlisted Services and Procedures 53899
Urethrocystography 74450-74455
Urethrotomy 52270-52276
X-Ray with Contrast 74450-74455

Urethral
Diverticulum
  Marsupialization 53240
Meatus, Dorsal
  See Epispadias
Sphincter
  Biofeedback Training 90911
  Insertion
    Prosthesis .53444
  Removal
    Prosthesis 53446-53447
  Replacement
    Prosthesis .53448
Stenosis
  Dilation 52281
Stent
  Insertion 52282
  Removal
    Bladder 52310-52315
    Urethra 52310-52315
Stricture
  Dilation 52281, 53600-53621
  Injection
    Steroids 52283
Syndrome
  Cystourethroscopy 52285

Urethrectomy
Total
  Female 53210
  Male 53215

Urethrocele
See Urethra, Prolapse

Urethrocystography 74450-74455
Contrast and/or Chain 51605
Retrograde 51610
Voiding 51600

Urethrocystopexy
See Vesicourethropexy

Urethromeatoplasty 53450-53460

Urethropexy 51840-51841

Urethroplasty 46744-46746
First Stage 53400
One Stage
  Hypospadias 54322-54328

Reconstruction
  Female Urethra 53430
  Male Anterior Urethra . . . . : . . .53410
  Prostatic/Membranous Urethra
    First Stage 53420
    One Stage 53415
    Second Stage 53425
  Second Stage 53405
    Hypospadias 54308-54316
  Third Stage
    Hypospadias 54318

Urethrorrhaphy 53502-53515

Urethroscopy
See Endoscopy, Urethra

Urethrostomy 53000-53010

Urethrotomy 53000-53010
Direct Vision
  with Cystourethroscopy 52276
Internal 52601, 52647-52648
with Cystourethroscopy
  Female 52270
  Male 52275

Uric Acid
Blood 84550
Other Source .84560
Urine 84560

Uridyltransferase, Galactose-1-Phosphate
See Galactose-1-Phosphate, Uridyl Transferase

Uridylyltransferase, Galactosephosphate
See Galactose-1-Phosphate, Uridyl Transferase

Urinalysis 0041T, 81000-81099
Automated 81001, 81003
Glass Test 81020
Microalbumin 82043-82044
Microscopic .81015
Pregnancy Test 81025
Qualitative 81005
Routine 81002
Screen 81007
Semiquantitative 0041T, 81005
Unlisted Services and Procedures 81099
Volume Measurement 81050
without Microscopy 81002

Urinary Bladder
See Bladder

Urinary Catheter Irrigation
See Irrigation, Catheter

Urinary Concentration Test
See Water Load Test

Urinary Sphincter, Artificial
See Prosthesis, Urethral Sphincter

Urinary Tract
X-Ray with Contrast 74400-74425

Urine
Albumin
  See Albumin, Urine
Blood
  See Blood, Urine
Colony Count .87086
Pregnancy Test 81025
Tests 81001

Urobilinogen
Feces 84577
Urine 84578-84583

Urodynamic Tests
Bladder Capacity
  Ultrasound .51798
Cystometrogram 51725-51726
Electromyography Studies
  Needle 51785
Residual Urine
  Ultrasound .51798
Stimulus Evoked Response 51792
Urethra Pressure Profile 51772
Uroflowmetry 51736-51741
Voiding Pressure Studies
  Bladder 51795
  Intra-Abdominal 51797

Uroflowmetry 51736-51741

Urography
Antegrade 74425
Infusion 74410-74415
Intravenous 74400-74415
Retrograde 74420

Uroporphyrin 84120

Urothromboplastin
See Thromboplastin

Uterine
Adhesion
  See Adhesions, Intrauterine
Cervix
  See Cervix
Endoscopies
  See Endoscopy, Uterus
Haemorrhage
  See Hemorrhage, Uterus

Uterus
Ablation
  Endometrium 0009T, 58353
Biopsy
  Endometrium 58100
  Endoscopic 58558
Catheterization
  X-Ray 58340
Chromotubation 58350
Curettage
  Postpartum 59160
Dilation and Curettage 58120
  Postpartum 59160
Ectopic Pregnancy
  Interstitial
    Partial Resection Uterus 59136
    Total Hysterectomy 59135

UTP Hexose 1 Phosphate Uridylyltransferase

See Galactose-1-Phosphate, Uridyl Transferase

Uvula

Uvulectomy 42140

UV Light Therapy

See Actinotherapy

V

V, Cranial Nerve

See Trigeminal Nerve

V-Y Operation, Bladder, Neck

See Bladder, Repair, Neck

V-Y Plasty

See Skin, Adjacent Tissue Transfer

Vaccination

See Allergen Immunotherapy; Immunization; Vaccines

Vaccines

Vagina

Repair
  Aneurysm 36834
  Angioplasty 75978
  Graft 34520
Sampling
  Venography 75893
Sinus
  Venography 75870
Skull
  Venography 75870-75872
Spermatic
  Excision 55530-55540
  Ligation 55550
Splenic
  Splenoportography 75810
Stripping
  Saphenous 37720-37735
Subclavian
  Thrombectomy 34471-34490
Thrombectomy
  Other than Hemodialysis Graft
  or Fistula 35875-35876
Unlisted Services and Procedures 37799
Valve Transposition 34510
Varicose
  See Varicose Vein
Vena Cava
  Thrombectomy 34401-34451
  Venography 75825-75827

Velpeau Cast 29058

Vena Cava
Catheterization 36010
Reconstruction 34502
Resection with Reconstruction 37799

Vena Caval
Thrombectomy 50230

Venereal Disease Research Laboratory
See VDRL

Venesection
See Phlebotomy

Venipuncture
See Cannulation; Catheterization
Breast
  Cytology 0045T
Child/Adult
  Cutdown 36425
  Percutaneous 36410
Infant
  Cutdown 36420
  Percutaneous 36400-36406
Routine 36415

Venography
Adrenal 75840-75842
Arm 75820-75822
Epidural 75872
Hepatic Portal 75885-75887
Injection 36005
Jugular 75860
Leg 75820-75822
Liver 75889-75891
Neck 75860
Nuclear Medicine 78445, 78457-78458
Orbit 75880

Renal 75831-75833
Sagittal Sinus 75870
Vena Cava 75825-75827
Venous Sampling 75893

Venorrhaphy
See Suture, Vein

Venotomy
See Phlebotomy

Venous Access Device
Obstruction Removal 75901-75902

Venous Access Port
Insertion 36533
Obstruction Clearance 36536-36537
Removal 36535
Revision 36534

Venous Blood Pressure
See Blood Pressure, Venous

Venovenostomy
See Anastomosis, Vein

Ventilating Tube
Insertion 69433
Removal 69424

Ventilation Assist ...94656-94657, 99504
See Pulmonology, Therapeutic

Ventricular Puncture 61020-61026,
61105-61120

Ventriculocisternostomy 62180,
62200-62201

Ventriculography
Anesthesia
  Brain 00214
  Cardiac 01920
Nuclear Imaging 78635

Ventriculomyectomy 33416

Ventriculomyotomy 33416

Vermiform Appendix
See Appendix

Vermilionectomy 40500

Verruca(e)
See Warts

Verruca Plana
See Warts, Flat

Version, Cephalic
See Cephalic Version

Vertebra
See Spinal Cord; Spine; Vertebral Body; Vertebral Process
Additional Segment
  Excision 22103, 22116
Arthrodesis
  Exploration 22830
  Posterior 22590-22802
  Spinal Deformity
    Anterior Approach 22808-22812
    Posterior Approach 22800-22804

Cervical
  Excision
    for Tumor 22100, 22110
    Fracture 23675-23680
  Fracture/Dislocation
    Additional Segment
      Open Treatment 22328
    Cervical
      Open Treatment 22326
    Lumbar
      Open Treatment 22325
    Thoracic
      Open Treatment 22327
Kyphectomy 22818-22819
Lumbar
  Excision
    for Tumor 22102, 22114
Osteoplasty
  CT Scan 76013
  Fluoroscopy 76012
  Lumbar 22521-22522
  Thoracic 22520-22522
Osteotomy
  Additional Segment
    Anterior Approach 22226
    Posterior/Posterolateral Approach ..22216
  Cervical
    Anterior Approach 22220
    Posterior/Posterolateral Approach ..22210
  Lumbar
    Anterior Approach 22224
    Posterior/Posterolateral Approach ..22214
  Thoracic
    Anterior Approach 22222
    Posterior/Posterolateral Approach ..22212
Thoracic
  Excision
    for Tumor 22101, 22112

Vertebrae
Arthrodesis
  Anterior 22548-22585
  Spinal Deformity 22818-22819

Vertebral
Arteries
  See Artery, Vertebral
Body
  Biopsy 20250-20251
  Excision
    Decompression 63081-63091
    Lesion 63300-63308
    with Skull Base Surgery 61597
  Fracture/Dislocation
    Closed Treatment 22305
      without Manipulation 22310
  Kyphectomy 22818-22819
Column
  See Spine
Corpectomy 63081-63308
Fracture
  See Fracture, Vertebra
Process
  Fracture/Dislocation
    Closed Treatment
      with Manipulation, Casting and/or
      Bracing 22315

Very Low Density Lipoprotein
See Lipoprotein, Blood

Voice Button 31611

Voiding Pressure Studies
Abdominal 51797
Bladder 51795

Volatiles 84600

Volhard's Test
See Water Load Test

Volkman Contracture 25315-25316

Volume Reduction, Lung
See Lung Volume Reduction

Von Kraske Proctectomy
See Proctectomy, Partial

VP
See Voiding Pressure Studies

Vulva
Abscess
  Incision and Drainage 56405
Colposcopy 56820
  Biopsy 56821
Excision
  Complete 56625, 56633-56640
  Partial 56620, 56630-56632
  Radical 56630-56631, 56633-56640
    Complete 56633-56640
    Partial 56630-56632
  Simple
    Complete 56625
    Partial 56620
Lesion
  Destruction 56501-56515
Perineum
  Biopsy 56605-56606
  Incision and Drainage 56405
Repair
  Obstetric 59300

Vulvectomy
Complete 56625, 56633-56640
Partial 56620, 56630-56632
Radical 56630-56631, 56633-56640
  Complete
    with Bilateral Inguinofemoral
    Lymphadenectomy 56637
    with Inguinofemoral, Iliac, and Pelvic
    Lymphadenectomy 56640
    with Unilateral Inguinofemoral
    Lymphadenectomy 56634
  Partial
    with Bilateral Inguinofemoral
    Lymphadenectomy 56632
    with Unilateral Inguinofemoral
    Lymphadenectomy 56631
  Simple
    Complete 56625
    Partial 56620

VZIG
See Immune Globulins, Varicella-Zoster

V Flap Procedure
One Stage Distal Hypospadias Repair 54322

W

W-Plasty
See Skin, Adjacent Tissue Transfer

WADA Activation Test 95958
See Electroencephalography

WAIS-R 96100

Waldius Procedure 27445

Wall, Abdominal
See Abdominal Wall

Walsh Modified Radical Prostatectomy
See Prostatectomy

Warts
Flat
  Destruction 17110-17111

Washing
Sperm 58323

Wasserman Test
See Syphilis Test

Wassmund Procedure
Osteotomy
  Maxilla.........................21206

Waterston Procedure 33755

Water Load Test 89365

Water Wart
See Molluscum Contagiosum

Watson-Jones Procedure 27695-27698

Wave, Ultrasonic Shock
See Ultrasound

WBC
See White Blood Cell

Webbed
Toe
  Repair 28280

Wedge Excision
Osteotomy 21122

Wedge Resection
Ovary 58920

Well-Baby Care 99381, 99391, 99432

Wellness Behavior
See Evaluation and Management, Health Behavior

Wernicke-Posadas Disease
See Coccidioidomycosis

Westergren Test
See Sedimentation Rate, Blood Cell

Western Blot
HIV 86689
Protein 84181-84182
Tissue Analysis 88371-88372

Wheelchair Management/Propulsion
See Physical Medicine/Therapy/Occupational Therapy
Training 97542

Wheeler Knife Procedure
See Discission, Cataract

Wheeler Procedure
See Blepharoplasty, Entropion
Blepharoplasty 67924
Discission Secondary Membranous Cataract 66820

Whipple Procedure 48150

Whirlpool Therapy 97022
See Physical Medicine/Therapy/Occupational Therapy

Whitemead Operation
See Hemorrhoidectomy, Complex

White Blood Cell
Alkaline Phosphatase 85540
Antibody 86021
Count 85032, 85048, 86348
Differential 85004-85007, 85009
Histamine Release Test 86343
Phagocytosis 86344
Transfusion
  See Leukocyte, Transfusion

Whitman Astragalectomy
See Talus, Excision

Whitman Procedure 27120

Wick Catheter Technique 20950

Widal Serum Test
See Agglutinin, Febrile

Window
Oval
  See Oval Window
Round
  See Round Window

Window Technic, Pericardial
See Pericardiostomy

Windpipe
See Trachea

Winiwarter Operation
See Anastomosis, Gallbladder to Intestines

Winter Procedure 54435

Wintrobe Test
See Sedimentation Rate, Blood Cell

X

X-Ray Tomography, Computed
See CT Scan

Xa, Coagulation Factor
See Thrombokinase

Xenoantibodies
See Antibody, Heterophile

Xenograft 15400-15401

Xenografts, Skin
See Heterograft, Skin

Xenotransplantation
See Heterograft

Xerography
See Xeroradiography

Xeroradiography 76150

XI, Coagulation Factor
See Plasma Thromboplastin, Antecedent